Medical Microbiology
Volume 1

Medical Microbiology

Volume 1

edited by

C. S. F. EASMON
Wright Fleming Institute
St Mary's Hospital Medical School
London

J. JELJASZEWICZ
National Institute of Hygiene
Warsaw
Poland

ACADEMIC PRESS · 1982

A Subsidiary of Harcourt Brace Jovanovich, Publishers

London · New York · Paris · San Diego · San Francisco
São Paulo · Sydney · Tokyo · Toronto

ACADEMIC PRESS INC. (LONDON) LTD
24/28 Oval Road, London NW1 7DX

United States Edition published by
ACADEMIC PRESS INC.
111 Fifth Avenue, New York, New York 10003

British Library Cataloguing in Publication Data

Medical microbiology. — Vol. 1
1. Medical microbiology
616.01'05   QR46

ISBN 0–12–228001–6

Composed in Monophoto Times by
Latimer Trend & Company Ltd, Plymouth
Printed in Great Britain by
St Edmundsbury Press, Bury St Edmunds, Suffolk

4-1-86

Contributors

J. D. Band
Bacterial Diseases Division
Center for Infectious Diseases
Centers for Disease Control
US Department of Health and Human
  Services
Public Health Service
Atlanta
Georgia 30333

J. G. Bartlett
Department of Medicine
Johns Hopkins University School of
  Medicine
Baltimore, Maryland
and
Tufts University School of Medicine
Boston, Massachusetts

J. S. Finlayson
Bureau of Biologics
Food and Drug Administration
Bethesda
Maryland 20205

R. A. Gleckman
Department of Medicine
University of Massachusetts Medical
  School and Division of Infectious
  Disease
Saint Vincent Hospital
Worcester, Massachusetts 01604

J. Y. Homma
The Kitasato Institute
5–9–1 Shirokane
Minato–Ku
Tokyo 108

J. Jeljaszewicz
Department of Bacteriology
National Institute of Hygiene
00–791 Warsaw

H. J. Jennings
Division of Biological Sciences
National Research Council of Canada
Ottawa
Ontario

D. L. Kasper
Division of Infectious Diseases
Beth Israel Hospital and Channing
  Laboratory
Brigham and Women's Hospital
Harvard Medical School
Boston, Massachusetts

I. Kato
Department of Bacterial Infection
Institute of Medical Science
University of Tokyo
Tokyo

R. B. Kohler
Infectious Diseases Division
Wishard Memorial Hospital
Indiana University Medical Center
1001 West 10th Street
Indianapolis, Indiana 46202

O. R. Pavlovskis
Naval Medical Research Institute
Bethesda
Maryland 20014

H. Platt
Equine Research Station
PO Box 5
Snailwell Road
Newmarket
Suffolk CB8 7DW

G. Pulverer
Institute of Hygiene
University of Cologne
5000 Cologne 41

A. L. Reingold
Bacterial Diseases Division
Center for Infectious Diseases
Centers for Disease Control
US Department of Health and Human
  Services
Public Health Service
Atlanta
Georgia 30333

K. Roszkowski
Department of Radiotherapy
Postgraduate Medical Centre
00–909 Warsaw

W. Roszkowski
Department of Immunology
Institute of Tuberculosis
00–138 Warsaw

S. Szmigielski
Center for Radiobiology and
  Radioprotection
00–909 Warsaw

C. E. D. Taylor
Clinical Microbiology and Public Health
  Laboratory
Addenbrooke's Hospital
Cambridge CB2 2QW

N. S. Taylor
Department of Medicine
Johns Hopkins University School of
  Medicine
Baltimore, Maryland
and
Tufts University School of Medicine
Boston, Massachusetts

L. J. Wheat
Infectious Disease Division
Wishard Memorial Hospital
Indiana University Medical Center
1001 West 10th Street
Indianapolis, Indiana 46202

A. White
Infectious Disease Division
Wishard Memorial Hospital
Indiana University Medical Center
1001 West 10th Street
Indianapolis, Indiana 46202

B. Wretlind
Department of Bacteriology
Karolinska Hospital
S104 01 Stockholm

Preface

Medical microbiology has developed rapidly over the past decade. Immunological and biochemical techniques have been applied to the early diagnosis of infectious disease and to monitoring antimicrobial therapy. The importance of non-sporing anaerobes in causing infection has been recognized. There has been renewed interest in the beta-lactam antibiotics in which the basic penicillin and cephalosporin nucleus has been manipulated to increase both their spectrum of activity and resistance to beta lactamases. Effective antiviral chemotherapy now seems likely to become a reality. The theoretical background provided by cellular immunology is now being applied to the development of new improved vaccines. Medical microbiologists have, of course, not had things all their own way. Hospital-acquired infection, particularly in the immunocompromised patient, is an increasing problem and is often the limiting factor in the management of other diseases. Allied to this is the increase in antibiotic resistance not only in the hospital flora but in organisms such as *Neisseria gonorrhoeae* and *Haemophilus influenzae*. New infectious agents such as *Legionella pneumophila* and Lassa, Marburg and Ebola viruses have been described.

It is our aim in this open-ended series to include major review articles, not only by established authorities, but also by younger active research workers, which will reflect this diversity and be of interest to medical microbiologists and their veterinary colleagues. We plan two types of volume: the first consisting of subjects chosen for their topicality and general interest with no particular theme, and the second of a series of articles related to a common theme.

Volume 1 is of the first type. The dangers of colitis associated with particular antibiotics and the importance of *Clostridium difficile* and its toxin in this condition are discussed by Drs Bartlett and Taylor. Although its role in the pathogenesis of antibiotic-associated colitis is a recent finding, *C. difficile* is not a newly discovered organism. *Legionella pneumophila* and the bacterium causing contagious equine metritis are newly described bacterial pathogens. Their discovery, properties and the diseases they cause are discussed by Drs Reingold and Band and Platt and Taylor respectively. In contrast the problem of urinary tract infections, covered by Dr Gleckman, is one of the oldest and commonest in microbiology, but nevertheless still presents many difficulties. We have included two chapters on *Pseudomonas aeruginosa*. Drs Pavlokis and

Wretlind deal with extracellular toxins and their role in pathogenicity, Dr Homma with the exploitation of pseudomonal products as vaccine components. Four other chapters have an immunological flavour. Dr Finlayson covers the use of immunoglobulins as therapeutic agent. Drs Kohler, Wheat and White their use as diagnostic reagents. The type-specific antigens of group B streptococci, prime candidates for a vaccine, are discussed by Drs Kasper and Jennings. A rather different strategy, that of non-specific immunostimulation with propionibacteria (better known as *Corynebacterium parvum*), is covered by Dr Roszkowski and his colleagues. Finally, Dr Kato describes the use of staphylococcal alpha toxin as a biological probe for membrane studies.

We hope that this volume will be of interest to medical microbiologists. With the steady expansion of this discipline review articles are needed and there are very few review publications that deal exclusively with medical microbiology.

We should like to thank the authors for their contributions to this volume and we would appreciate any comments and suggestions for future volumes.

Janusz Jeljaszewicz   *Charles Easmon*
                                                                   August 1982

Contents

1 Antibiotic-associated colitis

JOHN G. BARTLETT and NANCY S. TAYLOR

Colitis is one of the most frequent and potentially severe adverse reactions associated with antimicrobial drug usage. A spectrum of pathological changes have been noted, the most characteristic lesion being pseudomembranous colitis. This lesion was described long before antimicrobial drugs were available and a variety of risk factors were noted at that time, but the vast majority of cases encountered currently are antibiotic associated. There has been marked progress during the past decade in our understanding of this complication. Initial studies made extensive use of endoscopy to provide extensive descriptions of pathology and the clinical features of the disease. In more recent years, *Clostridium difficile* has become the recognized pathogen in the vast majority of cases. The role of this microbe was initially detected in experiments utilizing an animal model of antibiotic-associated colitis in 1977. Clinical applications of these findings quickly followed, and by 1978 the culprit was defined, a sensitive diagnostic assay was described, and specific forms of treatment became readily available. There are few diseases in medicine in which this much progress was made over such short interval. There are also few medical conditions in which the lessons learned from animal experiments proved so directly applicable to the clinical setting. This chapter will review the topic of antibiotic-associated colitis with emphasis on these more recent developments.

I. HISTORICAL PERSPECTIVE

Studies of pseudomembranous lesions of the bowel may be divided into three periods (Table 1). The initial reports antedated the antibiotic era with the

Table 1   Observations with pseudomembranous enterocolitis during three study periods

		Antibiotic era	
	Preantibiotic era	1952–1965	1970–1980
Major risk factor	Intestinal surgery Others (see text)	Antibiotics Chloramphenicol Tetracycline	Antibiotics Ampicillin Clindamycin Cephalosporins
Anatomy			
Location of lesions	Small bowel and/or colon	Small bowel and/or colon	Primarily colon
Histology	←——————————————— Similar or identical ———————————————→		
Suspected cause	Ischaemia(?)	*S. aureus*	*C. difficile*
Diagnosis			
Anatomical	Autopsy	Clinical features (often poorly established)	Endoscopy
Agent	—	Stool Gram stain and culture	Stool toxin assay
Treatment	Supportive only	Oral vancomycin	Oral vancomycin Cholestyramine

original description by Finney (1893) who noted "pseudodiphtheritic enteritis" in a patient who had undergone a gastro-enterostomy. Numerous reports followed in which a variety of risk factors were identified, primarily intestinal surgery complicated by hypotension, but also spinal fracture, intestinal obstruction, colonic carcinoma, uraemia, heavy metal poisoning, the haemolytic-uraemic syndrome and ischaemic cardiovascular disease (Bartlett and Gorbach, 1977). Many of these associated conditions suggested ischaemia of the bowel as an aetiological factor, although this was never proven. The disease at this time was relatively infrequent, but the mortality rate was high, possibly reflecting the fact that most cases were established only at autopsy examination (Penner and Bernheim, 1939; Pettet *et al.*, 1954).

The second period of study followed shortly after the availability of antimicrobials when the terms "antimicrobial-induced pseudomembranous enterocolitis", "post-operative enterocolitis" and "staphylococcal enteritis" were often used interchangeably. *Staphylococcus aureus* was the commonly accepted pathogen on the basis of Gram stains of stool showing clusters of Gram-positive cocci and stool cultures which yielded this microbe (Altemeier *et al.*, 1963; Azar and Drapanas, 1968; Hummel *et al.*, 1964; Wakefield and Sommers, 1953; Prohaska *et al.*, 1956). The majority of stool isolates produced an enterotoxin (Surgalla and Dacti, 1955) and the majority of typable strains were phage type 80/81, 53/77 or U-18 (Hummel *et al.*, 1963; Dearing and Needham, 1960). Oral administration of either the enterotoxin or *S. aureus* isolates combined with antibiotics produced lethal enterocolitis in chinchillas (Wood *et al.*, 1956; Prohaska *et al.*, 1959; Tan *et al.*, 1959; Warren *et al.*, 1963). Many patients were treated with oral vancomycin with good results to provide further support for the etiological role of *S. aureus* (Kahn and Hall, 1966). "Staphylococcal enterocolitis" became a common diagnosis, especially in post-operative patients receiving antibiotics where reports of incidence were as high as 14% in one study (Azar and Drapanas, 1968) and 30% in another (Hummel *et al.*, 1964).

Critical analysis of the reports noted above cast doubt on the frequency of the complication and some now question the aetiological role of *S. aureus*. Investigators even at that time noted that most of the patients with this diagnosis who died of other causes had no demonstrable intestinal lesions at autopsy (Dearing *et al.*, 1960) and those who did have anatomically confirmed disease often had no evidence of staphylococci in their stool (Pettet *et al.*, 1954; Valberg and Truelove, 1961). Furthermore, *S. aureus* is found in the normal faecal flora of 15–30% of healthy adults (Finegold *et al.*, 1974; Hummel *et al.*, 1964), and colonization rates may exceed 90% in patients receiving some antibiotics (Hummel *et al.*, 1964). It is possible that the attention focussed on this organism reflected the widespread concern for staphylococci which was responsible for widespread epidemics of infections at the time. Although it is not possible to confirm or refute the conclusions of these prior studies, it does appear that even if *S. aureus* was once responsible for antibiotic-associated pseudomembranous colitis (PMC), it no longer represents an important agent of the disease.

There was a lull in reporting of antibiotic-associated PMC in the 1960s. However, this was followed by a flurry of reports in the 1970s which often emphasized the role of clindamycin in this complication. Initial work primarily concerned incidence data and anatomical descriptions made possible by the extensive use of endoscopy (Slagle and Boggs, 1976; Stroeghlein *et al.*, 1974; Scott *et al.*, 1973; Totten *et al.*, 1978; Tedesco *et al.*, 1974; LeFrock *et al.*, 1975). A striking feature in this work was that *S. aureus* was infrequently recovered (Keusch and Present, 1976) although extensive microbiological studies of the faecal flora failed to elucidate any alternative agent (Marr *et al.*, 1975; Allen *et al.*, 1977). This experience led to studies designed to demonstrate a transferable toxin in an animal model which eventually revealed the role of *C. difficile.*

II. CLINICAL AND PATHOLOGICAL OBSERVATIONS

A. Pathology

1. Pseudomembranous colitis (PMC)

The usual finding with gross inspection is multiple elevated yellowish-white plaques which vary in size from a few millimetres to 15–20 mm in diameter (Fig. 1). The intervening mucosa may appear normal or show hyperaemia and oedema. Occasionally, the pseudomembranes coalesce to involve large segments of the colonic mucosa. These may slough, leaving large, denuded areas of the mucosa. According to recent descriptions, PMC usually involves the distal colon and often involves the entire colon, but there may be rectal sparing. Small-bowel involvement appears to be infrequent.

Histological studies (Goulson and McGovern, 1965; Sumner and Tedesco, 1975) show the pseudomembrane arises from a point of superficial ulceration on an intact mucosa. There is an acute or chronic inflammatory infiltrate in the lamina propria with the submucosa showing oedema and vascular dilatation. The pseudomembrane is composed of fibrin, mucin, sloughed mucosal epithelial cells, and inflammatory cells. Price and Davies (1977) have classified the histological features of PMC into three categories which appear to be rather uniform in an individual patient. The earliest or most mild form consists of focal necrosis with polymorphonuclear cells and an eosinophilic exudate within the lamina propria. Splaying out from the necrotic focus is a collection of fibrin and polymorphonuclear cells which form the characteristic "summit lesion". The second category, representing more advanced disease, shows disrupted glands containing mucin and polymorphonuclear cells surmounted with typical pseudomembranes. Both types of lesions show areas of intervening normal mucosa and the inflammatory changes are limited to the superficial portion of the lamina propria, predominantly subepithelial in location. The third and most advanced form of the disease shows complete structural necrosis with extensive involvement of the lamina propria, which is overlaid by a thick confluent pseudomembrane.

Crypt abscesses are not a feature of PMC. There is one report showing fibrin thrombi in the mucosal capillaries, suggesting bowel ischaemia in the pathogenesis (Bogomoletz, 1976). However, this has not been a consistent finding by most observers; furthermore, the clinical presentation and other features of the pathological findings do not suggest ischaemia. There is no bacterial invasion of the bowel mucosa, and no typical bacterial morphotype is seen within the pseudomembrane.

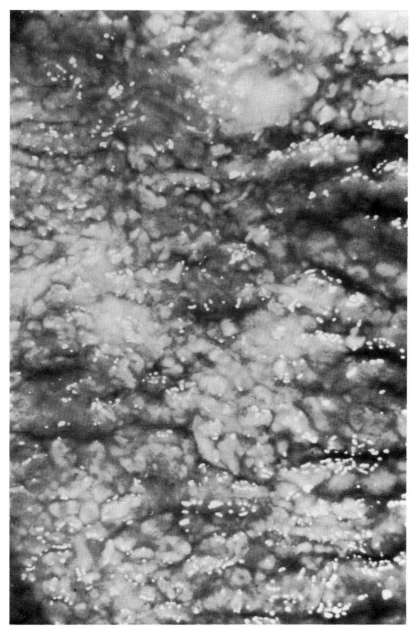

Fig. 1 Typical plaque lesions of pseudomembranous colitis.

2.   Colitis without pseudomembrane formation

Histological studies may show many of the features noted above except for the typical pseudomembrane. This often represents situations where pseudomembranes were dislodged in preparation for endoscopy or the point of attachment was missed in obtaining the biopsy (Tedesco, 1976). Another form of "non-specific colitis" is a lesion showing granularity and friability with histological changes resembling idiopathic ulcerative colitis (Pittman *et al.*, 1974; Manashil and Kern, 1973; Koltz *et al.*, 1953). In less severe forms of "colitis" there is simply hyperaemia and oedema of the intestinal mucosa on gross inspection.

B.   Signs and symptoms

1.   Antibiotic-associated diarrhoea

The single symptom which is found in nearly all patients with antibiotic-associated colitis, is diarrhoea. The onset of diarrhoea is initially noted during the course of antibiotic treatment in one-half to two-thirds of cases; the remaining patients never detect a change in bowel habits until after the implicated drug has been discontinued. The temporal limit between the time an antibiotic is discontinued and its implication as a cause of diarrhoea appears to be 4–6 weeks.

Diarrhoea is variously described on the basis of the total stool volume, percentage water content, and the frequency and character of stooling. For practical purposes, the most frequent definition used in clinical studies is: (1) there are 2–5 stools per day which are semi-solid or liquid in character; (2) this must represent a change in the patient's usual bowel pattern; (3) there should be no alternative explanation for diarrhoea; and (4) the onset of symptoms should occur either during antimicrobial administration or within 4–6 weeks after these drugs have been discontinued. Using this definition, the incidence of antibiotic-associated diarrhoea according to prospective studies is 5–10% for ampicillin and 7–26% for clindamycin (Table 2). Similar data from prospective studies are not available for most other antimicrobials. Among those with antibiotic-associated diarrhoea, the incidence of colitis varies from 5–50% depending to a large extent on the frequency of endoscopic examination.

The diarrhoea ascribed to antibiotics generally consists of relatively large volumes of loose or watery stools, sometimes with mucus but rarely with grossly evident blood. The duration of diarrhoea following discontinuation of the implicated agent is variable, but the average is 8–12 days. Some patients with severe disease have up to 30 stools per day and the course may be protracted to 4 weeks or longer. Other patients have less severe symptoms which resolve rapidly. With clindamycin, which has been the most extensively

Table 2   Incidence of antibiotic-associated diarrhoea

	Cases	No. with diarrhoea	Percentage
Clindamycin			
Swartzberg *et al.* (1976)	1000	66	6.6
Neu *et al.* (1977)	200	27	13
Tedesco *et al.* (1974)	200	42	21
Gurwith *et al.* (1977)	343	61	18
Lusk *et al.* (1977)	62	16	26
Brause *et al.* (1980)	143	10	7
Leigh *et al.* (1980)	281	33	12
Ampicillin			
Tedesco *et al.* (1975)	200	9	4.5
Gurwith *et al.* (1977)	140	9	6
Lusk *et al.* (1977)	96	4	9
Brause *et al.* (1980)	318	16	5

studied, there may be two patterns with considerable overlap. One pattern is watery stools without colitis which occurs during antimicrobial administration, resolves promptly when the drug is discontinued, and may be dose related. A possible mechanism is a direct effect of the drug to cause altered intestinal water and electrolyte transport (Giannella *et al.*, 1981). The second pattern is diarrhoea, often with colitis, which is not dose related, is more likely to start after the drug has been discontinued, and often follows a protracted course. A major mechanism for this latter form is the toxin produced by *C. difficile* to be described below.

2. Systemic symptoms

Some patients with antibiotic-associated colitis have few symptoms other than diarrhoea. However, many individuals will experience abdominal cramps, abdominal tenderness, fever, and leucocytosis (Tedesco *et al.*, 1974; Mogg *et al.*, 1979). Fever is usually low grade, but may be as high as 106°F. Peripheral leucocyte counts are variable, often range from 10 000–20 000 mm^{-3} and may be 40 000 mm^{-3} or greater. Late and serious complications include severe dehydration, electrolyte imbalance, hypotension, hypo-albuminaemia with anasarca or toxic megacolon. Extra-intestinal symptoms appear to be extremely rare with antibiotic-associated colitis except for the complications which may be ascribed to fluid, electrolyte and albumin losses. However, there is an interesting case report of polyarthritis involving the shoulders, elbows, knees and ankles in a patient with clindamycin-associated colitis (Rollins and Moeller, 1975).

3. Prognosis

The prognosis for antibiotic-associated PMC without specific therapy is highly variable, depending to a large extent on the methods used to establish the diagnosis. In the report by Tedesco *et al.* (1974) where there was extensive use of endoscopy to detect this diagnosis even among patients with trivial symptoms, all patients with antibiotic-associated PMC recovered with simply supportive care. Nevertheless, many of these individuals suffered prolonged bouts of diarrhoea which often required hispitalization for extended periods. Other studies which focus attention on more severely ill patients indicate mortality rates as high as 20% (Mogg *et al.*, 1979). Mortality at the present time even for seriously ill patients is virtually nil reflecting the recognition of a microbial pathogen and the availability of specific forms of treatment to be discussed below.

C. Diagnosis

1. Endoscopy

The diagnosis of antibiotic-associated colitis should be suspected in any patient who has otherwise unexplained diarrhoea which occurs either during or up to 4–6 weeks following antibiotic administration. The favoured method for establishing the pathological changes noted in the colon is with endoscopy to detect typical mucosal plaque-like lesions (Sumner and Tedesco, 1975). There may be copious amounts of mucus, which must be removed with caution to avoid separation of the stalk attachment. Analogous precautions are necessary in the colon preparation prior to the procedure for the same reasons. Care must also be exercised to include the entire lesion in a biopsy, since the stalk attachment is necessary for microscopic confirmation. The distal colon is involved in the majority of cases so that sigmoidoscopy is generally adequate. However, occasional patients will have pseudomembranes restricted to the right colon necessitating the use of colonoscopy (Tedesco, 1980; Burbige and Radigan, 1981). Endoscopic observations in patients with antibiotic-associated diarrhoea without pseudomembranes include a normal mucosa, erythema and oedema, and friability, ulceration or haemorrhage. These latter findings may be very suggestive of idiopathic ulcerative colitis.

2. Radiology

Radiological findings may be helpful in establishing the diagnosis of PMC (Stanley *et al.*, 1974; Tully and Feinberg, 1974). Plain films in advanced disease often show a markedly oedematous colon, distorted haustral markings and distension of the entire colon. Occasionally, there are small irregularities which represent pseudomembranous plaques in profile. Barium enema may show rounded filling defects which outline the pseudomembranous plaques. However, this examination is often non-diagnostic due to underpenetration of barium, excessive mucous secretions, confluence of the pseudomembrane or minimal involvement. Diagnostic accuracy is improved with air contrast studies, but this procedure must be performed with caution because of the potential complication of colonic perforation.

D. Antibiotics implicated

1. Antibiotic-associated diarrhoea

Nearly all antimicrobials with an antibacterial spectrum have been implicated in both diarrhoea and colitis. Exceptions are parenterally administered aminoglycosides and vancomycin which, to our knowledge, have not been associated with colitis. The most complete data for the incidence of diarrhoea and colitis based on prospective surveys are available for ampicillin and clindamycin as summarized in Table 2. The wide ranges noted in different studies presumably reflect vagaries in the definition of diarrhoea, the frequency of endoscopic examination, and epidemiological patterns. There is minimal variation in the incidence according to the route of drug administration so that parenteral usage confers the same risk noted with oral treatment. Most studies also show no good evidence for a dose relationship. Analysis of patients and their underlying diseases have failed to reveal any characteristics other than increasing age which is associated with an increased incidence of antibiotic-associated diarrhoea.

2. C. difficile-*induced diarrhoea and colitis*

A review of the antimicrobial agents implicated in 243 patients with *C. difficile*-induced diarrhoea or colitis showed the most frequent were ampicillin (82 patients), clindamycin (56), and cephalosporins (55) (Bartlett, 1981a). The cephalosporin group included virtually all compounds in this class which are currently marketed in the United States. Less frequent drugs which were implicated in 8 to 20 cases were penicillins other than ampicillin or amoxicillin, erythromycin, sulphamethoxazole-trimethoprim and sulphasalazine. It is of interest to note that there were only two cases associated with tetracycline and no cases which could be clearly ascribed to chloramphenicol or oral neomycin. This is emphasized due to the disparency noted with this series compared to the reports of PMC from the 1950s and 1960s showing chloramphenicol, tetracycline and oral neomycin to be the most frequently implicated drugs in antibiotic-associated PMC (Reiner *et al.*, 1952; Hale and Cosgriff, 1957; Altemeier *et al.*, 1963; Hummel *et al.*, 1964).

The results of our studies as well as those of others have shown that the only drugs which appear to be responsible for *C. difficile*-induced colitis are those with a spectrum of activity against bacteria. This includes some antineoplastic compounds which have antibacterial activity (Cudmore *et al.*, 1979), rifampin (Boriello *et al.*, 1980), and miconazole. Drugs with a spectrum restricted to mycobacteria, fungi or parasites do not appear to cause this complication.

III.   *CLOSTRIDIUM DIFFICILE* AND ANTIBIOTIC-ASSOCIATED COLITIS

Rapidly evolving evidence during the late 1970s showed compelling evidence that *C. difficile* is responsible for most cases of antibiotic-associated colitis. This work occurred at a time when the only implicated agent according to previous studies was *Staphylococcus aureus*. However, the role of this organism was questioned when the observations of the earlier work could not be confirmed. The most serious problem was that *S. aureus* simply could not be recovered from the stools of most patients with this complication. The original work implicating *C. difficile* was performed in an animal model of antibiotic-associated colitis. The observations were then applied to patients resulting in the definition of a new enteric pathogen.

A.   Antibiotic-associated colitis in guinea pigs and hamsters

1.   *Initial observations*

Hambre *et al.* (1943) first reported that penicillin was usually lethal to guinea pigs shortly after this drug became available. Subsequent studies indicated that guinea pigs were susceptible to challenge with a variety of other antimicrobials as well, and hamsters were found to be equally susceptible (Ambrus *et al.*, 1952; Bartlett *et al.*, 1978b; DeSomer *et al.*, 1955; Ebright *et al.*, 1981; Eyssen *et al.*, 1957; Farrar and Kent, 1965; Fekety *et al.*, 1979; Green, 1974; Kaipainen and Faine, 1951; Schneierson and Perlman, 1956; Silva, 1979; Small, 1968; Toshniwal *et al.*, 1979). Antimicrobial agents which are commonly lethal for hamsters (the most extensively studied model) include lincomycin, clindamycin, erythromycin, tetracyclines, ampicillin, penicillin, virtually all cephalosporins, metronidazole, vancomycin, and orally administered aminoglycosides.

Experiments with both hamsters and guinea pigs have shown similar observations among animals which develop the toxic consequences of antimicrobial administration. The animals become anorexic, dehydrated and hypothermic, with ruffled fur and an unsteady gait. Death usually ensues within 1–3 days after the onset of symptoms, most commonly at 3–7 days after challenge. The only consistent finding at necropsy is a hyperaemic caecum which is distended with bloody liquid contents (Fig. 2). Histological studies of

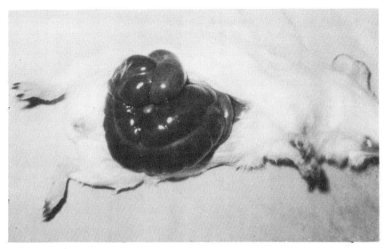

Fig. 2 Typical necropsy finding of haemorrhagic caecitis in a guinea pig which expired five days following penicillin challenge.

the caeca and ilea of moribund animals shows mucosal haemorrhage, leucocytic cell infiltration in the lamina propria, epithelial hyperplasia, and occasional ulceration with an overlying inflammatory exudate (Humphrey *et al.*, 1979b; Lusk *et al.*, 1978; Price *et al.*, 1979; Abrams *et al.*, 1980). Features which are somewhat disparent compared to the anatomy of colonic lesions in patients with PMC are: (1) the profound mucosal haemorrhage and proliferative chances noted in animals; (2) the infrequency of superficial crypt necrosis with exudation and typical pseudomembranes; and (3) the localization of the major pathology to the caecum and terminal ileum. The gross and histological changes appear to be similar for guinea pigs and hamsters with antibiotic-induced typhlitis.

2. Aetiology

The initial studies implicating *C. difficile* in antibiotic-associated colitis were performed using the hamster model of clindamycin-induced disease (Bartlett *et al.*, 1977b; Rifkin *et al.*, 1977). This work showed that clindamycin was usually lethal with all routes of administration including intramuscular, intraperitoneal, oral, direct injection in the caecum, and even topical application to the dermis. The LD_{50} with clindamycin hydrochloride was found to be approximately 50 µg (Bartlett *et al.*, 1979). These data provide testimony of the extraordinary sensitivity of the animal to antibiotic exposure. In retrospect, this may be analogous to the susceptibility of some animals to proliferation and toxin production of bacteria in the stagnant segment of the caecum as seen with *C. botulinum* (Miyazaki and Sakaguchi, 1978).

Attempts to define a pathological mechanism in this model utilized a series of experiments designed to detect a transferable agent using intracaecal inoculations (Table 3) (Bartlett *et al.*, 1977a; Bartlett, 1979). It was noted that the disease could be serially transferred using caecal contents from animals with typical disease for 5 sequential passes. The substance responsible for transferable disease could be filtered through a 0.02 μm membrane filter and this was neutralized with gas-gangrene polyvalent antitoxin. These experiments suggested a clostridial toxin leading to stool cultures for clostridia with the objective of detecting an organism which would reproduce typical disease with intracaecal inoculum of the broth culture. One organism, *C. difficile*, satisfied this criterion. Subsequent work showed cultures of caecal contents yielded *C. difficile* in each of 35 hamsters with clindamycin-induced disease, whereas stools from ten healthy hamsters prior to clindamycin challenge were uniformly negative. Other investigators have detected *C. difficile* in stools from 5 of 92 healthy hamsters which were not exposed to antimicrobials (Toshniwal *et al.*, 1979) indicating a 6% carrier rate.

3. Cytotoxicity assay

During the early course of these investigations with hamsters, an attempt was made to recover a viral agent as well as a bacterial pathogen (Chang *et al.*, 1978). Interest in the possible viral aetiology was aroused by a previous report by Green (1974) indicating that tissue specimens from guinea pigs and hamsters with penicillin-induced caecitis contained a substance which was cytopathic to WI-38 cells. The author's conclusion was that a latent virus was responsible, although no specific viral agent could be identified. On the basis of this earlier study, caecal contents from hamsters were examined in tissue culture which showed cytopathic changes using a variety of cell lines. However, evidence that a virus was responsible could not be supported because the cytopathic substance could be passed through a 0.02 μm membrane, it was resistant to RNase and DNase and could not be propagated. More importantly, the cytopathic changes were found to be neutralized by *C. sordellii* antitoxin.

The tissue culture assay was subsequently performed on 540 hamsters with clindamycin-induced caecitis and these were uniformly positive for a cytopathic toxin which was neutralized by *Clostridium sordellii* antitoxin. Sequential analysis of faecal pellets obtained from 30 hamsters at 12-hour intervals after a single challenge dose of clindamycin showed all animals had positive specimens at 36 hours, and titres of this toxin gradually increased as the disease progressed to reach a mean of $10^{-6.4}$ dilutions in caecal contents at necropsy (Bartlett *et al.*, 1979a). The tissue culture assay was also performed on animals challenged with a variety of additional antimicrobial agents. These studies showed that all animals which expired had positive tissue culture assays which mean titres ranging from $10^{-5\pm0.6}$ to $10^{-6.7\pm0.4}$ dilutions at necropsy (Bartlett *et al.*, 1978b). Thus, the same cytopathic toxin is detected in stool from virtually all hamsters with antibiotic-induced caecitis, implicating a common mechanism regardless of the agent used to induce the disease.

4. Microbial source of cytotoxin

The initial experiments to detect a transferable agent in antibiotic-induced caecitis in hamsters implicated *Clostridium difficile* was the responsible pathogen. However, the toxin in cell-free supernate of stool from afflicted animals could be neutralized with *C. sordellii* antitoxin according to several assays of biological activity including tissue cultures, colitis induction with intracaecal injection or lethality tests with intraperitoneal injection (Bartlett *et al.*, 1977b; Rifkin *et al.*, 1977). These studies suggesting differing clostridial species in the aetiology of this disease initially posed problems in interpretation. Evidence against a pathogenic role of *C. sordellii* was based on the fact that this organism was recovered in stool from diseased animals on only rare occasions (Lusk *et al.*, 1978) and the vast majority of strains fail to produce a cytotoxin *in vitro* (Bartlett *et al.*, 1978d; Allo, 1980). The apparent disparency was subsequently clarified by the observation that *Clostridium difficile* produces a cytopathic toxin *in vitro* which is neutralized by *C. sordellii* antitoxin, thus indicating antigenic cross-reactivity (Bartlett *et al.*, 1978).

5. Experiments in guinea pigs

The classic description of antibiotic-associated colitis in experimental animals was the guinea pig challenged with penicillin as originally described by Hambra *et al.* (1943). The previously noted studies in hamsters were therefore repeated in guinea pigs to detect a similar mechanism (Lowe *et al.*, 1980). This work showed 7 of 8 animals challenged with aqueous penicillin G expired at 3 to 8 days (Table 3). Necropsy examination revealed haemorrhagic caeca with a mean caecal weight of 57 g, accounting for approximately 20% of the total body weight. Caecal contents from all 7 animals showed a cytopathic toxin which was neutralized by *C. sordellii* antitoxin and cultures yielded *C. difficile*. Intracaecal injection of the isolates reproduced the anatomical lesions noted with penicillin administration.

6. Summary of experiments implicating C. difficile *in antibiotic-induced caecitis in animals*

The experiments cited above provide compelling evidence that *C. difficile* is responsible for antibiotic-associated colitis in both hamsters and guinea pigs following antimicrobial administration. It should be noted that the studies described from our group were performed in three different laboratory facilities using animals from three different suppliers in order to limit

Table 3 Studies of antibiotic-induced caecitis in hamsters and guinea-pigs

	Hamsters	Guinea-pig
Antimicrobial challenge		
Agent, dose	Clindamycin, 5 mg IP	Penicillin G, 200 000 units IM
No. tested	35	8
No. expired	35 (100%)	7 (87%)
Day of death past challenge	3–6 days	3–8 days
Necropsy for haemorrhagic caecitis	35/35	7/8[a]
Stool culture for C. difficile		
Pre-challenge	0/10	0/8
Post-challenge	35/35	7/8[a]
Concentration in stool at necropsy	$10^{6.8}-10^{8.8}$ g^{-1}	$10^{5.3}-10^{7.3}$ g^{-1a}
Sensitivity in vitro		
Clindamycin	64 µg ml^{-1}	—
Penicillin	—	0.5 µg ml^{-1}
Tissue culture assay for cytotoxin neutralized by C. sordellii *antitoxin*		
No. positive	35/35	7/8[a]
Concentration (dilutions)	$10^{-6}-10^{-7}$	$10^{-3}-10^{-5}$
Rechallenge with C. difficile *injected intracaecally*		
Whole cells	16/16	3/3
Cell-free supernatant	10/10	3/3
Cell-free supernatant plus C. sordellii antitoxin	0/10	0/3

[a] Positive results apply to the 7 animals that expired; one survived and had a negative necropsy examination, and caecal contents failed to show C. difficile or the cytotoxin.

idiosyncrasies that might be inherent in a particular animal source or environment. The evidence implicating *C. difficile* as responsible for antibiotic-induced caecitis in hamsters and guinea pigs is based on the following observations:

(a) Serial transfer was achieved for 5 passes using intracaecal injection of caecal contents from animals with antibiotic-induced caecitis and the fraction responsible for transferable pathogenicity could be passed through a 0.02 µm membrane filter.

(b) Cultures of stools from animals with antibiotic-induced caecitis have uniformly yielded *C. difficile* in high concentrations, although this organism is infrequently found in stool specimens from healthy animals.

(c) Intracaecal injections of *C. difficile* or the cell-free supernatant of these cultures produces haemorrhagic caecitis which is identical by gross and histological criteria to the lesions noted with antibiotic exposure.

(d) Tissue culture assays of stools from animals with antibiotic-induced caecitis show a cytopathic toxin which may be neutralized with *C. sordellii* antitoxin. The same antitoxin preparation also prevents transferable disease using intracaecal inoculations of stool supernatant.

(e) Broth cultures of *C. difficile* show a cytopathic toxin which may be neutralized with *C. sordellii* antitoxin with animal challenge and tissue cultures indicating antigenic cross-reactivity.

7. Related studies in other animals

Clostridium difficile has been implicated as a cause of lethal diarrhoea in newborn hares (Dabard *et al.*, 1979). Studies by Bornside *et al.* (1964) showed that the intestines of rabbits, rats, guinea pigs, and dogs with strangulation obstruction contain a toxin which is lethal to mice and is neutralized by *C. sordellii* antitoxin. This is consistent with *C. difficile*-induced disease, although *C. sordellii* may also be responsible (Allo, 1980). With these exceptions, *C. difficile* has been implicated in enteric disease in animals only with antibiotic exposure. It is of interest to note that rats, mice and rabbits are susceptible to *Clostridium difficile* toxin and expire when the cell-free supernatant or purified toxin is given systemically (Taylor *et al.*, 1981). These animals also develop typical haemorrhagic lesions of the large and small bowel when the toxin is administered into the intestinal lumen. Nevertheless, mice and rats are remarkably tolerant of antimicrobials and simply do not develop bowel complications which are so characteristic of hamsters and guinea pigs. Rabbits may develop typical intestinal lesions when given antimicrobials, but the aetiology of the disease has not been thoroughly examined. One report suggests a possible role of *C. perfringens* type E, but the data to support this conclusion is tenuous (Katz *et al.*, 1978; LaMont *et al.*, 1979). Chinchillas develop lethal colitis with exposure to tetracyclines and possibly other antibiotics; prior studies implicated *S. aureus*, although this conclusion has not been reexamined in the light of the more recent observations regarding *C. difficile* (Tan *et al.*, 1959).

B. Studies in patients

The clinical relevance of the studies in experimental animals became apparent when *C. difficile* and its cytotoxin were found in stools of patients with antibiotic-associated colitis. This has led to extensive work directed at determining carrier rates of the organism, the incidence of *C. difficile* toxin, and epidemiological studies to detect environmental sources of the microbe.

1. *Historical perspective on* Clostridium difficile

C. difficile was originally described as a component of the normal faecal flora of newborn infants by Hall and O'Toole (1935). Although these investigators recognized the toxigenic potential of their isolates, there was little subsequent attention focused on *C. difficile* because its role in clinical disease remained elusive. A review of clinical experience at Cook County Hospital by Gorbach and Thadepalli (1975) showed this microbe accounted for only one of 65 strains of *Clostridia* recovered from blood cultures and 3 of 87 strains recovered from soft-tissue infections. Smith and King (1962) reviewed the clinical observations in seven patients with infections involving *C. difficile* and noted no particularly characteristic lesion. Since all cultures yielded other microbes the authors concluded that *C. difficile* was of uncertain pathogenic significance. Hafiz subsequently reported recovering the organism from infant stool, faecal specimens from several animal species, and the normal vaginal flora in 72% of women, as well as numerous environmental sources, including soil, hay and sand (Hafiz, 1974; Hafiz and Oakley, 1976; Hafiz *et al.*, 1975). Hafiz also found *C. difficile* in urethral discharge from 42 patients with "non-specific urethritis" but not in urethral specimens from 100 controls (Hafiz *et al.*, 1975). However, the potential role of *C. difficile* in this disease has not been supported in subsequent studies (Halen *et al.*, 1977), which suggest that *C. difficile* plays no well-defined role in extra-intestinal diseases.

2. *Stool cultures for* Clostridium difficile

(a)   Culture techniques

C. difficile was originally detected in the faecal flora of newborn infants with non-selective media (Hall and O'Toole, 1934). These workers experienced extreme difficulty in recovering the organism and maintaining it in their stock collection, thus accounting for the original appellation applied: "*Bacillus difficilis*". The recent work showing the role of *C. difficile* as an enteric pathogen has led to the use of several techniques to facilitate its recovery in the faecal flora:

(1) *Paracresol-containing media.* One of the first attempts to develop a selective technique to recover *C. difficile* was reported by Hafiz (1974) in work that actually antedated information regarding the role of this microbe in antibiotic-associated colitis. Hafiz noted that *C. difficile* had the virtually unique property of producing paracresol from phenylalanine, leading to the use of 0.2% paracresol in reinforced clostridial broth cultures as a selective medium. High isolation rates of

C. difficile were noted from a variety of sources (Hafiz, 1974; Hafiz and Oakley, 1976; Hafiz *et al.*, 1976). A more recent report by W. L. George *et al.* (1979) indicated that 0.2% paracresol inhibited *C. difficile* growth and selectivity was lost with lower concentrations. However, these investigators used agar media rather than the broth as originally described.

(2) *Laked blood agar containing kanamycin, menadione and haemin.* Investigators at the General Hospital in Birmingham, England have used this relatively non-selective media and recovered *C. difficile* from 27 of 30 stools which contained the toxin (R. H. George *et al.*, 1978; Keighley *et al.*, 1978). The high recovery rate may have been facilitated by an epidemic of *C. difficile*-induced PMC at their hospital which obviously allowed ample access to fresh samples.

(3) *Heat shock.* Larson *et al.* (1978) have reported good recovery rates for *C. difficile* with heat shock at 75°C for 20 minutes or 80°C for 10 minutes to select sporulating bacteria in frozen samples prior to subculture.

(4) *Selective agar containing cycloserine and cefoxitin.* W. L. George *et al.* (1979c) developed a selective media utilizing antibiotics based on *in vitro* susceptibility tests of *C. difficile* isolates. The media which proved superior in their studies was egg yolk–fructose agar containing 500 µg of cycloserine ml^{-1} and 16 µg of cefoxitin ml^{-1}. Quantitative cultures of stock strains showed that the counts of antibiotic-incorporated media were comparable to the counts on non-selective brucella base blood agar. Using stool, *C. difficile* grew within 24–48 hours, and this was the only organism detected in 8 of 13 faecal specimens. Even when other bacteria were present, *C. difficile* was readily distinguished by unique colonial characteristics including chartreuse fluorescence with ultraviolet light, filamentous edge, low umbonate in profile, and yellow coloration of the medium. Quantitation using frozen specimens from PMC patients showed concentrations ranging from 10^3–10^7 g^{-1} (mean $10^{4.2}$ g^{-1}) with this organism accounting for an average of 0.1% of the total cultivatable flora.

(b) Comparison of culture techniques
The previously noted culture techniques were examined to compare relative merits for recovering *C. difficile* using frozen stools from 18 patients with antibiotic-associated PMC and positive toxin assays (Willey and Bartlett, 1979). Non-selective media (brucella base blood agar) was often successful, but the recovery rate was largely dependent upon diligence of the micro-biologist in picking multiple colony types for subsequent subculture and identification. Indeed, *C. difficile* was readily recognized on the primary

isolation plate in only 33% of the specimens. The use of ethanol shock prior to culture on non-selective media offered little advantage as a selective method. Optimal results were achieved with selective agar incorporating cycloserine and cefoxitin since all 18 specimens yielded strains of *C. difficile* which were readily detected. The unique colonial morphology, the distinctive odour of paracresol, and the paucity of other colony forms on the selective media obviously simplified the detection. Incubation of specimens in broth containing 0.2% paracresol or ethanol shock prior to plating on to the antibiotic-incorporated media proved to be no advantage, but simply added additional steps to the culture technique which appeared to be superfluous.

(c)   Stability of C. difficile *in stool*
The concentrations of *C. difficile* with various storage conditions have been studied using stools from hamsters with antibiotic-associated colitis (Willey and Bartlett, 1979). Fresh specimens yielded concentrations of $10^{6.9}$–$10^{7.7}$ g^{-1}, with refrigeration for 48 hours the decrease in viable counts never exceeded $10^{0.3}$ organisms g^{-1}, and freezing at $-40°C$ resulted in losses of $10^{0.6}$ to $10^{2.1}$ CFU ml^{-1}. This indicates that the storage conditions obviously affect concentrations of *C. difficile* and that fresh or refrigerated specimens would be preferable for accurate quantitation. Nevertheless, the selective media incorporating cycloserine and cefoxitin proved adequate for detecting this microbe despite freezing, often for extended periods, prior to culture. A review of our experience with this media using frozen specimens which contained the cytotoxin indicates that *C. difficile* was recovered from 139 of 144 (96%). Five of the culture positive specimens were originally obtained from an outbreak of antibiotic-associated PMC in 1973 (Tedesco *et al.*, 1974) in which the stools had been stored for 5 years in unspecified conditions prior to culture.

3.   Colonization rates
Several studies are now available regarding colonization rates of *C. difficile* for various patient populations (Table 4). Among patients with antibiotic-associated diarrhoea or colitis with positive toxin assays the yield of *C. difficile* has been uniformly high. Combining data from six investigations the overall recovery rate in specimens from 184 patients was 95%. In contrast, the recovery rate of this microbe in the stools of healthy adults is only about 2% (Larson *et al.*, 1978; Willey and Bartlett, 1979; W. L. George *et al.*, 1979a; Viscidi *et al.*, 1981). Higher rates of 15–20% are noted in adults who have recently had antibiotic exposure with no gastro-intestinal complications (Viscidi *et al.*, 1981). The organism has not been found with increased frequency among patients with a variety of diarrhoeal diseases which are ascribed to conditions other than antibiotic exposure. The largest series

Table 4   Isolation rates of *C. difficile* in stools

Patient category	Culture technique[a]	No. with *C. difficile/* No. tested	
Antibiotic-associated diarrhoea or colitis with positive toxin assay			
George, R. H. *et al.* (1978)	NSM	8/8	
Keighley *et al.* (1978)	NSM	16/17	
Larson *et al.* (1978)	HS	4/5	
Viscidi *et al.* (1981)	C&C	125/130	90–100%
Gilligan *et al.* (1981)	C&C	13/14	
Lishman *et al.* (1981)	C&C	9/10	
Antibiotic-associated diarrhoea with negative toxin assay			
Viscidi *et al.* (1981)	C&C	13/85	
Keighley *et al.* (1978)	NSM	5/28	0–15%
Borriello (1979)	HS	0/14	
Antibiotic administration without diarrhoea			
Viscidi *et al.* (1981)	C&C	12/56 (21%)	
Miscellaneous intestinal diseases unrelated to antimicrobial exposure			
Larson *et al.* (1978)	HS	0/20	
Falsen *et al.* (1980)[b]	C&C	81/2390	0–3%
Gilligan *et al.* (1981)	C&C	2/100	
Borriellio (1979)	HS	0/60	
Healthy adults			
George, W. L. *et al.* (1978)	NSM	4/137	
Larson *et al.* (1978)	HS	0/11	2–3%
Viscidi *et al.* (1981)	C&C	0/60	
Keighley (1981)	NSM	3/109	
Healthy neonates			
Hall and O'Toole (1935)	NSM	4/10	
Larson *et al.* (1978)	Heat shock	5/8	29–71%
Viscidi *et al.* (1981)	C&C	13/45	
Kim *et al.* (1981)	C&C	15/21	

[a] Indicates method for primary isolation NSM=Non-selective media, HS=heat shock, C&C=agar media containing cycloserine plus cefoxitin.
[b] See text for explanation.

examining such individuals is the report by Falsen *et al.* (1980) in which stool samples submitted to a reference laboratory in Sweden were routinely examined for a variety of enteric pathogens. Clinical information is notably sparse in this report, but an assumption is made that the majority had diarrhoea due to causes other than antibiotic exposure. The overall recovery rate of *C. difficile* in 2390 samples was 3%, approximating the recovery rate noted in healthy adults. High rates of isolation have been noted in healthy neonates who appear to have a colonization rate of approximately 30–40% (Hall and O'Toole, 1935; Kim *et al.*, 1981; Larson *et al.*, 1978; Viscidi *et al.*, 1981). The duration of this relatively high rate of carriage in newborn infants is not well defined. However, samplings obtained in various paediatric populations indicate a progressive decline with the establishment of the "normal" adult flora (Snyder, 1940; Hafiz, 1974; Viscidi *et al.*, 1981). Snyder (1940) examined the faecal flora sequentially in 22 children from the ages two weeks to one year and found *C. difficile* in 19% of 142 specimens from weaned infants compared to no isolations in 21 specimens from breast-fed infants. These data are of interest in the light of more recent work showing colostrum specimens may contain IgA which neutralizes *C. difficile* cytotoxin (Wada *et al.*, 1980). As expected, concentrations of *C. difficile* in stool show considerable variations which may reflect, in part, storage conditions prior to culture. Nevertheless, counts as high as $10^{6.7}$ to $10^{8.9}$ g^{-1} have been reported in asymptomatic patients receiving cefoxitin (Mulligan *et al.*, 1981). In our experience, the mean concentrations of *C. difficile* in frozen stool were $10^{4.6}$ g^{-1} in 13 healthy neonates, $10^{5.3}$ g^{-1} in 14 asymptomatic adults and $10^{5.6}$ g^{-1} in 76 patients with PMC (Viscidi *et al.*, 1981). Thus, available data suggest that concentrations of the putative agent do not distinguish patients who are carriers and those with disease.

4. In vitro *susceptibility*

In vitro susceptibility testing of *C. difficile* has shown some unexpected findings. The original isolate of *C. difficile* recovered in hamsters with clindamycin-induced caecitis was clindamycin resistant, suggesting superinfection as the pathophysiological mechanism (Bartlett *et al.*, 1977a). However, subsequent work with the animal model has shown that the antimicrobial used to induce the disease often proved to be quite active against the strain subsequently isolated. This was noted, for example, in guinea pigs given penicillin where the strains of *C. difficile* recovered at necropsy were sensitive to penicillin at ≤ 0.5 µg ml^{-1} (Table 3). With some drugs which cause lethal typhlitis in hamsters, the stool levels achieved are several hundredfold higher than the minimum inhibitory concentration (Ebright *et al.*, 1981). A partial explanation of this apparent contradiction is that animals challenged with antibiotics which are active against *C. difficile* do not generally develop evidence of typhlitis or positive toxin assays until the inducing agents is discontinued (Bartlett *et al.*, 1979a). This is seen with vancomycin where hamsters remain healthy when the drug is continued for up to three months, but then expire when it is discontinued (Browne, 1977).

A similar paradox appears to apply to some patients with antibiotic-associated colitis due to *C. difficile*. *In vitro* sensitivity tests of *C. difficile* from patients from a variety of sources shows the most active drugs are metronidazole, vancomycin, ampicillin and penicillin G (Burdon *et al.*, 1979; W. L. George *et al.*, 1978; Dzink and Bartlett, 1980; Fekety, 1979; Shattleworth *et al.*, 1980). Over 90% of strains are susceptible to each of these agents at concentrations of $2 \, \mu g \, ml^{-1}$ or less. Cephalosporins are considerably less active with MIC values which usually exceed $8 \, \mu g \, ml^{-1}$. Cefoxitin and moxalactam are especially inactive. Erythromycin shows a bimodal distribution, with about 90% of strains being sensitive and the rest being highly resistant. Most strains are susceptible to tetracycline, although transferable tetracycline resistance has been described (Smith *et al.*, 1981). Activity of clindamycin is variable since 50–60% are susceptible at $1 \, \mu g \, ml^{-1}$ while 10–12% are resistant at $128 \, \mu g \, ml^{-1}$. It is noteworthy that ampicillin, which is commonly responsible for this complication, is active *in vitro* against virtually all strains, including those from patients with ampicillin-associated colitis. Similarly, many patients with clindamycin-induced colitis have *C. difficile* isolates which are highly susceptible (Dzink and Bartlett, 1980). These observations suggest that sensitivity profiles of *C. difficile* isolates are not useful in determining the drugs which are likely to cause this complication.

5. *Tissue culture assay for* C. difficile *toxin*

(a) *Historical perspective*
The original description of a cytopathic toxin in antibiotic-induced caecitis in animals was reported by Green (1974), who ascribed this observation to a latent virus. More recent studies with these animals utilized stool and demonstrated that cytotoxicity was a result of a toxin which could be neutralized by *C. sordellii* antitoxin as noted above. With regard to patients, Larson *et al.* (1977) were the first to report that stools from patients with antibiotic-associated PMC contained a heat-labile cytotoxin. The authors hypothesized this to be a bacterial toxin, but no specific bacterial source was identified. Chang (1978) also observed cytopathic changes in tissue cultures of stools from similar patients, but made the important additional observation that the cytotoxin could be neutralized with gas gangrene polyvalent antitoxin. This antitoxin preparation is composed of equine serum immunoglobulins to the five species of clostridia which cause gas gangrene. Subsequent work indicated that the fraction of the polyvalent antitoxin responsible for

neutralization is *C. sordellii* antitoxin (Chang *et al.*, 1978a). These observations were initially reported in 1977 (Bartlett *et al.*, 1977a; Larson and Price, 1977); within one year the published clinical experience with this assay from three laboratories had shown that stools from 71 or 72 patients with anatomically confirmed cases of antibiotic-associated PMC contained a cytopathic toxin which was neutralized by *C. sordellii* antitoxin (Bartlett *et al.*, 1978a; Bartlett, 1979a; R. H. George *et al.*, 1978; Keighley *et al.*, 1978; Larson *et al.*, 1978).

(b)   Method for performing the tissue culture assay
Virtually all tissue culture cell types are susceptible to *C. difficile* toxin (Chang *et al.*, 1979a). These include primary human amnion, baby hamster kidney (BHK-21), HeLa, monkey kidney (LLC Mk-2), mouse fibroblast (L-929), rabbit kidney, human diploid lung fibroblasts (WI-38), baby mouse kidney, baby hamster kidney, human chorion and human brain cells. Relative sensitivity of the first seven cell types noted were compared with TCD-50 values which proved to be very similar. These data suggest that almost any cell line may be employed for clinical testing. The test may be done with tissue culture tubes obtained commercially or with the microtitre system, depending on the number of samples and resources of the laboratory. Neutralization by the antitoxin is regarded as a critical feature of the test because stools from even healthy persons may contain non-specific cytopathic substances. Antitoxin preparations which have been found to neutralize *C. difficile* toxin include gas gangrene polyvalent antitoxin (providing this includes *C. sordellii* antitoxin), *C. sordellii* antitoxin, or *C. difficile* antitoxin (Chang *et al.*, 1979a). The potency of these antitoxins varies with different sources, and the activity of *C. sordellii* antitoxin in this assay does not correlate with values reported for activity against *C. sordellii* in mouse lethality tests. Antitoxin to *C. difficile* has obvious theoretical advantages, but the current supply is meagre (Ehrich *et al.*, 1980). Toxin neutralization occurs almost immediately, so that preincubation of the toxin–antitoxin mixture is not necessary (Chang *et al.*, 1978b). Results are generally interpreted at 18–24 hours, although high titre specimens may show changes within 4 hours and occasional specimens have no demonstrable changes for 48 hours. Interpretation should not be delayed beyond 48 hours with *C. sordellii* antitoxin due to toxin–antitoxin disassociation (Chang *et al.*, 1978b). The criteria for a positive assay is the demonstration of a cytopathic toxin which is completely neutralized by the antitoxin (Fig. 3).

(c)   Toxin titres
Quantitation of the cytotoxin using serial 2-fold or 10-fold dilutions in PBS shows the usual titres for patients with PMC are 10^{-2} to 10^{-5} dilutions. The

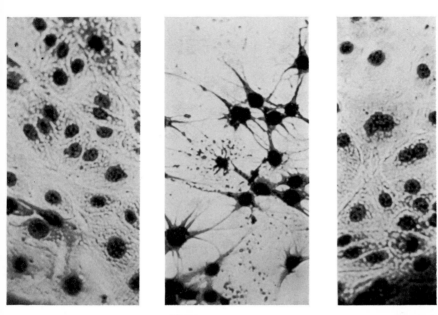

Fig. 3 Tissue culture for *Clostridium difficile* toxin using primary human amnion cells. The first panel shows a normal monolayer; the centre panel shows typical actinomorphic changes following inoculation with cell-free supernatant of stool from a patient with antibiotic-associated PMC; the right panel was inoculated with the same specimen following addition of *C. sordellii* antitoxin. Similar actinomorphic changes are noted with inocula of *C. difficile* cell-free supernatant or the purified cytopathic toxin. (Courtesy of T. W. Chang, Tufts-New England Medical Center, Boston, Massachusetts.)

highest titre recorded in our laboratory was 10^{-7} dilutions, which was the first clinical specimen examined and was from a patient with lethal PMC (Bartlett *et al.*, 1978a). Subsequent experience with this assay has shown little correlation between toxin titres and the severity of the disease. Thus, mean titres of approximately 10^{-3} dilutions were noted for patients with positive assays when categorized as PMC, antibiotic-associated diarrhoea, antibiotic recipients without diarrhoea, or healthy neonates. A similar experience has been noted by others (Larson *et al.*, 1978; Lishman *et al.*, 1981). These data suggest that the most important facet of the test is to simply demonstrate the toxin and toxin titres are of little relevance.

(d)   Methods for handling referred specimens
Most clinical laboratories lack facilities for tissue culture assays, making it necessary to submit specimens to reference laboratories, sometimes at distant locations. Sudies of specimens stored in various conditions have shown that

the cytopathic toxin is heat labile with titre decreases that correlate directly with time and temperature (Chang *et al.*, 1979a). Incubation for 5 days at −40°C showed no decrease in toxin titre, at 4°C there was a 0.5 log decrease and at room temperature there was a 1.5 log decrease. Losses at 24 hours were negligible at all temperatures examined. As a result of these observations, as well as practical considerations for patient care, it is suggested that a mailing system be used which would ensure delivery within 24 hours. Specimens which require a prolonged delay prior to processing should be maintained in frozen state.

(e)   Evidence that C. difficile *is responsible for the previously described cytotoxin*

The original observation that *C. sordellii* antitoxin neutralized the cytopathic toxin found in stool led to the premature conclusion by some that this represented "*C. sordellii* colitis" (Leigh, 1977; Editorial, 1977). Nevertheless, it was disturbing that *C. sordellii* was not isolated from the stools of these patients despite the fact that this organism is relatively easy to cultivate. Furthermore, studies of *C. sordellii* showed that only one of 16 strains produced a cytotoxin *in vitro*, and the toxin of this isolate failed to cause typical actinomorphic changes (Bartlett *et al.*, 1978d). Data implicating *C. difficile* and based on stool cultures of both experimental animals and patients was reported at approximately the same time. The disparency between these studies was subsequently clarified by the demonstration that broth cultures of *C. difficile* contained a toxin which produced actinomorphic changes in tissue cultures and was neutralized with *C. sordellii* antitoxin (Bartlett *et al.*, 1978d). Studies by Ehrich *et al.* (1980) have shown that antisera to partially purified *C. difficile* toxin will neutralize *C. sordellii* with mouse lethality testing, although activity against the homologous species was greater. Strains of *C. difficile* and *C. sordellii* have also been shown to share a common EDTA extractable antigen (Poxton and Byrne, 1981). These studies indicate that, despite marked differences in biochemical profiles used for taxonomic classification, these two clostridial species have antigentically related toxins.

The demonstration of antigenic cross-reactivity suggests the possibility that other clostridial species may also be responsible for the cytopathic toxin noted in stools from patients with PMC including *C. sordellii*. To examine this thesis a total of 109 strains of clostridia representing 23 identifiable species were tested for *in vitro* production of a cytopathic toxin (Bartlett *et al.*, 1978d). The source of these isolates was stool from experimental animals or patients with antibiotic-induced diarrhoea or colitis. *C. difficile* was the only strain which produced the typical cytopathic changes which were completely neutralized by the *C. sordellii* antitoxin. On the basis of these observations, combined with

:covery of *C. difficile* in over 95% of stool specimens which are positive in the
ssue culture assay, it is concluded that a positive tissue culture assay is
irtually diagnostic of *C. difficile* toxin.

f) Clinical experience with the tissue culture assay
  (1) *Patients with antibiotic-associated diarrhoea and colitis.* Studies from
       multiple laboratories have shown that stools from nearly all patients
       with antibiotic-associated PMC contain the previously noted toxin
       (Table 4). In our experience, this toxin has been observed in 137 of 141
       (97%) patients with antibiotic-associated PMC and approximately
       25% of patients with antibiotic-associated diarrhoea and no documen-
       ted pseudomembrane formation (Bartlett *et al.*, 1981). These results
       implicate *C. difficile* in the full spectrum of pathological changes noted
       with antibiotic-associated diarrhoea, although the incidence is ob-
       viously far greater among those with PMC.
  (2) *Healthy adults.* Approximately 3% of healthy adults harbour *C.*
       difficile, but these individuals have negative toxin assays. Some
       patients with *C. difficile*-induced diarrhoea or colitis will continue to
       excrete *C. difficile* toxin following recovery. We have observed one
       patient who continued to have positive toxin assays in stools obtained
       up to 9 months after complete resolution of symptoms (Bartlett,
       1981b). Antibiotic recipients who do not develop clinically apparent
       gastro-intestinal complications have a relatively high rate of *C. difficile*
       carriage (Viscidi *et al.*, 1981), and some of these individuals have
       positive toxin assays despite the absence of symptoms (Viscidi *et al.*,
       1981; W. L. George *et al.*, 1979b; Lishman *et al.*, 1980). The carriage of
       C. difficile without detectable toxin cannot usually be explained by the
       lack of toxigenic potential since the vast majority of strains produce the
       cytotoxin *in vitro* (Viscidi *et al.*, 1981).
  (3) *Healthy neonates.* In contrast to the experience with adults, healthy
       newborn infants often have *C. difficile* and its toxin with no apparent
       consequences (Borriello, 1979; Kim *et al.*, 1981; Larson *et al.*, 1978;
       Rietra *et al.*, 1978; Suttleworth *et al.*, 1980; Viscidi *et al.*, 1981). The
       frequency of the toxin in this population is generally 25–50% (Table
       5). Furthermore, toxin titres are generally high. Prior reports have
       implicated *C. difficile* in neonatal necrotizing enterocolitis (Cashmore
       et al., 1981), neonatal antibiotic-associated colitis (Donta *et al.*, 1981)
       and sudden infant death (Scopes *et al.*, 1980). However, the signific-
       ance of *C. difficile* toxin in stools of such patients is difficult to interpret
       due to the high rate of positive tissue culture assays among healthy
       infants. Available evidence suggests a decline in the incidence of the

Table 5 Tissue culture assays of stools for a cytopathic toxin which is
neutralized by *C. sordellii* antitoxin

Patient category	No. positive/ No. tested	
Antibiotic-associated PMC		
Larson *et al.* (1977)	9/9	
George, R. H. *et al.* (1978)	8/8	97–100%
Keighley *et al.* (1978)	16/16	
Bartlett *et al.* (1980)	137/141	
Antibiotic-associated diarrhoea without *confirmed PMC*		
Bartlett *et al.* (1980)	193/710	
Gilligan *et al.* (1981)	15/59	17–25%
Lishman *et al.* (1981)	9/52	
Gastro-intestinal diseases unrelated to *antibiotic exposure*		
Miscellaneous conditions		
Bartlett *et al.* (1980)	9/562	2%
Gilligan *et al.* (1981)	2/100	
Post-operative diarrhoea		
Keighley *et al.* (1978)	0/28	
Inflammatory bowel disease relapse[a]		
Bolton *et al.* (1980)	5/25	
Trnka and LaMont (1980)	11/59	
Meyer *et al.* (1980)	0/44	
Bartlett (unpublished data)	18/110	
Lishman *et al.* (1981)	0/34	
Healthy adults		
Bartlett *et al.* (1981)	0/60	
Lishman *et al.* (1981)	0/27	
Antibiotic exposure without diarrhoea		
Bartlett *et al.* (1980)	2/110	2–8%
Lishman *et al.* (1981)	4/53	
Healthy neonates		
Viscidi *et al.* (1981)	12/45	
Larson *et al.* (1978)	5/8	27–63%
Borriello (1979)	10/19	
Kim *et al.* (1981)	9/21	

[a] See text for details.

toxin during the first year of life (Viscidi *et al.*, 1981), so that toxin assays are more meaningful for clinical correlation for children over 2–5 years (Batts *et al.*, 1980; Viscidi and Bartlett, 1981).

(4) *Inflammatory bowel disease.* The initial studies suggesting a role for *C. difficile* in relapses of inflammatory bowel disease (IBD) were reported by LaMont and Trnka (1980) and Bolton *et al.* (1980). A subsequent series by Trnka and LaMont (1981) showed that the frequency of *C. difficile* toxin correlated with the severity of the relapse. Quite incredibly, 9 of 15 patients categorized as having severe symptoms had positive assays. However, these results were not supported according to another study (Meyers *et al.*, 1981) which showed no evidence of *C. difficile* toxin in stool specimens from 44 patients with IBD including 20 with severe symptoms. One explanation for this apparent discrepancy is that many of the patients with IBD and positive toxin assays have had recent antibiotic exposure, suggesting the superimposition of antibiotic-related gastro-intestinal complications (Bartlett, 1981b). Our own experience with IBD patients is compatible with this interpretation: positive assays were noted in stools from 15 of 57 patients with relapses of IBD who had recently received antimicrobials, compared to 3 of 53 who lacked this history of antibiotic exposure (Table 5).

(5) *PMC not associated with antibiotic exposure.* PMC was initially described long before the availability of antimicrobial agents, and a variety of risk factors other than these drugs have been described. This is now regarded as a relatively rare form of the disease. Nevertheless, our experience with 7 such patients who denied antimicrobial exposure for at least 3 months prior to the onset of symptoms indicated the uniform presence of *C. difficile* cytotoxin. (Moskovitz and Bartlett, 1981; Peiken *et al.*, 1980; Wald *et al.*, 1980.)

(g) Alternative methods for toxin detection

The tissue culture assay poses the disadvantage of requiring facilities which are not generally available in most clinical microbiology laboratories. Bacterial cultures are considered an inadequate substitute due to the expertise necessary and the time required. There also appears to be reduced specificity compared to toxin assays when comparing results in Tables 4 and 5. Counterimmunoelectrophoresis (CIE) is an alternative to tissue cultures for *C. difficile* toxin detection. Welch *et al.* (1980) used this method with *C. sordellii* antitoxin versus *C. difficile* culture filtrates and found precipitin lines with each of 17 strains. However, cross reactions were also noted with *C. sordellii* and *C. bifermentans* and no stool specimens were examined. Ryan *et al.* (1980) examined CIE using *C. difficile* antitoxin (Ehrich *et al.*, 1980) versus ten stool specimens which were positive with the tissue culture assay and 32 which were negative. The two methods appeared equally sensitive and specific. However, it now appears that the antigen detected with CIE does not represent the cytotoxin, since the immunogen used to prepare C. difficile antitoxin contained multiple proteins (Libby et al., 1981). It also seems unlikely that CIE would be as sensitive as tissue cultures for detecting a toxin which is cytopathic in concentrations of 170 pg ml $^{-1}$ or less. Another antigen detection method which has undergone more extensive clinical testing is enzyme immunoassay (EIA) (Yolken et al., 1981). The standard sandwich technique was used with C. difficile antisera prepared in goats and rabbits. Initial results with 277 specimens showed almost perfect correlation with tissue culture assays. The only exceptions were 3 "false positive" EIA assays in which there was alternative evidence for C. difficile infection. Again, it is not certain that the antigen detected with this method is the cytotoxin due to the lack of monospecific antibody.

IV. TREATMENT

The detection of a bacterial pathogen antibiotic-associated diarrhoea and colitis provides the rationale for specific forms of therapy. The greatest experience has been with two entirely different forms of treatment: anti-microbials directed against the putative agent and the use of anion exchange resins to bind C. difficile toxin.

1. Vancomycin

Orally administered vancomycin has been used extensively on the basis of several theoretical advantages. First, the original suspicion of a bacterial aetiology in antibiotic-associated colitis in animals was based on the protection afforded with vancomycin (Bartlett et al., 1977c; Browne et al., 1977). Subsequent studies with over 200 strains of C. difficile showed all were susceptible to vancomycin at concentrations of 16 µg ml $^{-1}$ or less (George et al., 1979a; Burdon et al., 1979; Fekety, 1979; Dzink and Bartlett, 1980). The drug is poorly absorbed with oral administration so that the mean stool level with 500-mg doses is approximately 3000 µg g $^{-1}$ (Tedesco et al., 1978) and with 125-mg doses is 350–500 µg g $^{-1}$ (Burdon et al., 1979; Keighley et al., 1978). Serum levels are negligible with oral treatment and so systemic toxicity is virtually nil (Bryan and White, 1978; Tedesco et al., 1978). Finally, there was considerable precedent for this type of therapy since oral vancomycin was used extensively with good results in the treatment of antibiotic-associated PMC in the 1960s when S. aureus was a suspected pathogen (Kahn and Hall, 1966).

The clinical experience reported to date with oral vancomycin in daily doses of 500 mg to 2 g have been extremely good. A controlled trial reported Keighley *et al.* (1978) using the lower dosage (125 mg four times daily) showed 8 of 9 patients had rapid clinical response with elimination of the toxin, the organism and histological evidence of PMC by the fifth treatment day. In contrast, 5 of 7 untreated control patients had persistence of symptoms, *C. difficile* and the toxin. A review of our experience with 90 patients, most of whom received 500 mg 4 times daily, showed 87 (97%) responded well (Bartlett *et al.*, 1979b). In general, there was a prompt eradication of fever within 24–48 hours, and diarrhoea resolved over 1–13 days with a mean of 4.5 days. The only major problem encountered was that 17 patients (19%) developed a relapse characterized by a recurrence of symptoms following discontinuation of vancomycin.

2. Relapses following vancomycin treatment

Relapses following vancomycin therapy were initially reported by W. L. George *et al.* (1979d) and have subsequently been noted in about 15–20% of patients (Bartlett *et al.*, 1979b). These relapses tend to follow a stereotyped pattern with a good initial response and recurrence of diarrhoea at 2–21 days following discontinuation of treatment. Analysis of stools at the time of relapse shows the presence of *C. difficile* toxin and cultures yield *C. difficile* strains which are susceptible to vancomycin. Endoscopy often shows PMC, and this may be noted in some patients with a normal intervening endoscopy examination at the completion of vancomycin treatment. Comparison of patients with and without relapses following vancomycin therapy showed no difference in terms of the total daily dose of vancomycin, or the duration of treatment. Patients with a relapse may be treated with another course of vancomycin and will almost always respond, but 20–30% of these individuals will suffer another relapse (Bartlett *et al.*, 1979b).

Two possible mechanisms for relapse are reacquisition of *C. difficile* or the failure to eradicate the putative agent. Serial collections of stools for culture show elimination of *C. difficile* in sequentially collected specimens during the course of vancomycin, thus supporting the latter mechanism (Keighley *et al.*, 1978). Such studies are, of course, subject to the potential problem of detecting small numbers of bacteria in stools and so conclusions are somewhat limited. Gnotobiotic mice which were monoassociated with *C. difficile* were used to examine the potential utility of vancomycin for eliminating the organism (Onderdonk *et al.*, 1980). In this experiment, colonization with *C. difficile* (without antibiotic exposure) resulted in faecal concentrations of 10^9 CFU g^{-1} of stool, cytotoxin levels of 10^{-6} dilutions and severe colitis. Treatment of these animals with vancomycin resulted in elimination of the cytotoxin and improvement in the histological changes in the caecal mucosa.

However, bacteriological studies showed persistence of *C. difficile* spores, and discontinuation of vancomycin resulted in the return of vegetative forms, cytotoxin levels of 10^{-6} dilutions and a recurrence of severe colitis. This experiment suggests that vancomycin may not eliminate spores from the gastro-intestinal tract, and since toxin production is associated with replication of vegetative forms, this appeared to provide an alternative explanation for at least some relapses.

3. Anion exchange resins

A potential utility of cholestyramine in antibiotic-associated colitis was initially reported by Burbige and Milligan (1975) before the role of *C. difficile* was known. These investigators noted that patients with this condition given oral cholestyramine in a dose of 4 g three times daily for 5 days had a prompt improvement in symptoms, with the only side effect being constipation. Subsequent studies have shown that this drug, like other anion exchange resins, binds the toxin produced by *C. difficile*, thus providing a plausible explanation for the favourable results noted clinically (Chang *et al.*, 1978c; Humphrey *et al.*, 1979a; Taylor and Bartlett, 1980). The clinical experience of multiple investigators has shown variable results with these resins. Keusch and Present (1976) noted that only about 50% of patients responded, multiple failures were reported by Tedesco *et al.* (1979), and Keighley (1981) observed almost universal failure with cholistipol. (Cholistipol is another anion exchange resin which appears to be somewhat superior to cholestyramine in the ability to bind *C. difficile* cytotoxin *in vitro* (Chang *et al.*, 1978c).) Nevertheless, Milligan and his associates (Kreutzer and Milligan, 1980) have reported an update of their original experience which showed excellent responses in each of 12 patients. Our interpretation of these data is that nearly uniform success has been achieved with vancomycin, the major problems being the excessive cost of the agent, its noxious taste, and the high rate of relapses. Cholestyramine appears to be less universally effective, but it is substantially less expensive, and relapses, although they do occur (Hutcheon *et al.*, 1978) appear to be less common.

4. Vancomycin combined with cholestyramine

The distinctive modes of action for these two agents suggests the combination might provide superior results. However, *in vitro* experiments have shown that cholestyramine binds vancomycin as well as *C. difficile* toxin (Taylor and Bartlett, 1980). This type of treatment was examined in the hamsters challenged with clindamycin and then treated with vancomycin or vancomycin in combination with cholestyramine. The results showed that cholestyramine reduced the mean level of biologically active vancomycin in stool from 550 to 77 $\mu g\ g^{-1}$. The addition of cholestyramine had no influence on toxin levels in stool or on mortality rates, which were independent of those which were observed with vancomycin alone (Taylor and Bartlett, 1980). This suggests that the concurrent administration of vancomycin with an anion exchange resin has the theoretical disadvantage of reducing local antimicrobial activity, although the clinical significance of this remains obscure since the levels achieved, especially with the higher recommended doses, may still be well above the inhibitory concentration.

5. Bacitracin

Bacitracin has many of the potential advantages described for vancomycin: it is poorly absorbed when administered orally, levels in the colonic lumen are high, and *in vitro* activity against *C. difficile* is good (Chang *et al.*, 1980). The reported experience with this drug is limited, but results to date appear promising. There is no evidence that bacitracin is superior to vancomycin, although the cost is somewhat less and it may be purchased in many countries where vancomycin is not available.

6. Metronidazole

Metronidazole is extremely active against *C. difficile in vitro* since nearly all strains tested to date are susceptible at 1 µg ml^{-1} or less. However, it is well absorbed when taken orally so that concentrations in the colon lumen are minimal (Arabi *et al.*, 1979). This represents a theoretical disadvantage since *C. difficile*-induced colitis is a toxin mediated disease in which there is no mucosal invasion and the organism is restricted to the intestinal lumen. There are several anecdotal case reports indicating favourable results with metronidazole (Matuchansky *et al.*, 1978; Trinh *et al.*, 1978; Bolton, 1979; Oldenburger and Miller, 1980; Pashby *et al.*, 1979). However, it is disturbing that this drug has also been implicated as the causal agent in at least 9 patients who developed antibiotic-associated colitis with positive toxin assays while receiving orally administered metronidazole (Keighley *et al.*, 1979; Keighley and Burdon, 1979; Sanginur *et al.*, 1980; Thompson *et al.*, 1981).

7. Antitoxin

Antitoxin to *C. difficile* or *C. sordellii* neutralizes *C. difficile* toxin and might be effective therapeutically. We are aware of the use of *C. sordellii* antitoxin only in experimental animals, where the results have been disappointing. Systemic administration has proven ineffective in reducing the mortality rate in hamsters challenged with clindamycin (Bartlett *et al.*, 1978c). This could be accomplished only with intralumenal injections requiring repeated laparotomy (Allo *et al.*, 1979). Even here, the results were less impressive than traditional treatment with vancomycin.

8. Manipulations of the faecal flora

C. difficile-induced diarrhoea or colitis presumably reflects the loss of colonization resistance which is presumed to be an important factor in maintaining stable microbial populations in the colon. Evidence for this assumption is based on the fact that the *C. difficile*-toxin-mediated enteric disease occurs almost exclusively in both rodents and man in the presence of antibiotic exposure. The lack of a competing flora also appears to account for the high colonization rate noted in neonates. Analogous observations apply to experimental animals where colonization with *C. difficile* is readily achieved only in neonates (Dabard *et al.*, 1979), gnotobiotes (Onderdonk *et al.*, 1980), or coonventional adult animals given antibiotics (Larson *et al.*, 1978). With regard to antibiotics, Larson *et al.* (1978) noted that fatal colitis could be induced by oral administration of one colony-forming unit of *C. difficile* following vancomycin treatment; oral challenge using large concentrations without antibiotics results in no detectable disease. Numerous colonic bacteria have also been shown to inhibit growth of *C. difficile in vitro* (Rolfe *et al.*, 1981). These observations suggest that re-establishment of the normal flora may be an important goal in treatment. This has been attempted with faecal enemas with reportedly good results in 13 of 16 patients (Bowden *et al.*, 1981).

V.   EPIDEMIOLOGICAL CONSIDERATIONS

A.   Epidemiology of antibiotic-induced colitis in animals

The susceptibility of hamsters and guinea pigs to antibiotics has been noted by multiple investigators at diverse locations for nearly four decades. However, these observations have been inconsistent since others have utilized the same antibiotics in these animals with no deleterious consequences (Fraser *et al.*, 1978). The divergent experience is presumably explained on the basis of the epidemiology of *C. difficile* as initially reported by Larson *et al.* (1980). These investigators challenged hamsters with clindamycin and then distributed the animals in a variety of locations. The mortality rate for hamsters housed in the facility where previous experiments had been conducted was 96% compared to 27% for animals placed in cages with a bacterial barrier. A similar observation was noted by Toshniwal *et al.* (1981) who also reported that cultures from 14 of 73 (19%) environmental sources yielded *C. difficile* in the "conventional room" where the incidence of this complication was extremely high. These studies suggest that it may be difficult to produce caecitis with antibiotics in animals at locations where the organism is not prevalent or easily transmitted, an observation which has important potential implications in clinical studies.

B.   Epidemiology of antibiotic-associated colitis in patients

There is compelling evidence for epidemiological patterns in antibiotic-induced colitis in patients as well as experimental animals. "Outbreaks" of this complication have been reported in hospitals in St Louis (Tedesco *et al.*, 1974), Dallas (Ramirez-Ronda, 1974), Chicago (Kabins and Spira, 1975), Birmingham, England (Mogg *et al.*, 1979) and London (Greenfield *et al.*, 1981). The experience at the General Hospital in Birmingham, England is particularly instructive (Kappas *et al.*, 1978; Mogg *et al.*, 1979; Keighley, 1980). At this hospital, 66 surgical patients acquired antibiotic-associated colitis during a 4-year period, including 27 from one ward who developed the complication during a 6-month period. The "epidemic" was eventually brought under control, presumably as a result of sterilization of ward sigmoidoscopes and vancomycin treatment of asymptomatic carriers of *C. difficile* (Keighley, 1980). These observations suggest that *C. difficile*-induced colitis may result from cross-infection as well as sporadically, and this may account for sharp differences in incidence data according to various observers.

C.   Source of *C. difficile*

Observations regarding the epidemiology of *C. difficile*-induced diarrhoea and colitis raised questions regarding the source of the microbe as an important facet of the epidemiology. As noted above, stool cultures indicate that approximately 3% of healthy adults harbour *C. difficile*, and these individuals are at presumed risk when receiving antimicrobial agents. However, temporally defined outbreaks in some hospitals suggest an environmental source of contamination. To investigate this, Mulligan *et al.* (1979, 1981) cultured environmental sites of 8 patients with *C. difficile*-induced diarrhoea. This microbe was recovered in 37 of 114 (32%) case-associated sites compared to 6 of 445 (1.3%) control sites. Similar studies reported by Fekety *et al.* (1981) showed positive cultures for *C. difficile* in 110 of 1086 (10%) environmental samplings obtained from case-associated hospital wards compared to 14 of 489 (2.5%) control sites. The primary sources for positive cultures were toilets, bed pans and floors. The organism was also isolated from the hands and stools of asymptomatic hospital personnel working in case-associated areas. Cultures of air, food and walls were uniformly negative. These observations with patient areas parallel the findings with experimental animals by the Ann Arbor group. It would appear that the disease often occurs sporadically, but the high yield of the putative agent in case-associated areas probably accounts for the high incidence sometimes reaching epidemic proportions among hospitalized patients. Optimal methods for prevention of transmission have not been adequately studied. However, a common current suggestion is for enteric isolation precautions with careful hand washing and rigorous cleansing of potentially contaminated surfaces.

VI.   *CLOSTRIDIUM DIFFICILE* TOXIN

A.   Historical perspective

In their original description, Hall and O'Toole (1935) noted that *C. difficile* isolates from the stool of healthy infants produced a toxin which was lethal to both guinea pigs and rabbits. Subsequent work by Snyder (1937) indicated this toxin was heat labile, there were marked strain variations in the amount of toxin produced, and susceptible species included the cat, dog, rat and pigeon. The challenges to experimental animals in these studies were made by intradermal or subcutaneous injections resulting in local oedema with central necrosis at 24–48 hours, followed by death at 2–9 days. Necropsy examination of these animals failed to show any demonstrable pathological changes except at the injection site. Oral administration of *C. difficile* broth cultures to guinea pigs and rats, as well as injections into the small bowel in dogs, caused no detectable systemic toxicity (Snyder, 1937). This led the author to conclude that this toxin, like that of *C. tetani*, was not absorbed through the gastro-intestinal tract.

Although the toxigenic potential of *C. difficile* was clearly established for over four decades, any role in naturally occurring disease in either animals or patients escaped detection until the studies cited above which identified its role as an enteric pathogen, primarily in the setting of antibiotic exposure. This more recent work has provided the impetus to examine the cytotoxin, presumably reflecting the fact that tissue cultures are relatively easy to perform and the belief that the same toxin which is responsible for the morphological changes in tissue cultured cells is also responsible for systemic toxicity and intestinal pathology. However, at the risk of retrospective iconoclasm, this latter assumption now appears to be erroneous. More recent studies indicate that *C. difficile* produces at least two toxins with differing biological activities.

B. Cytotoxin

1. In vivo *production*

Studies were performed using a variety of broth media to determine the optimal method to induce cytotoxin production (Bartlett *et al.*, 1978d). Aliquots of the cultures were taken at daily intervals for five days for optical density measurement and tissue culture assays using both cell sonicates and cell-free supernatants. In general, the highest titres of cytotoxin (10^{-3} to 10^{-5} dilutions) were noted with glucose-containing media using sonicates obtained at 24–48 hours, and broth supernatants obtained at 72–96 hours. Studies of *C. difficile* toxin levels during continuous cultivation showed increases of 100–1000-fold in adverse conditions such as increasing E_h (-360 to $+100$ mV), increasing temperature (37 to 45°C) and addition of subinhibitory concentrations of bactericidal antibiotics such as vancomycin and penicillin (Onderdonk *et al.*, 1979). In contrast, and of some interest in terms of the understanding of the pathophysiology of this disease, clindamycin had no effect on toxin levels. This work suggests that the cytotoxin is protoplasmic and released with autolysis. It also suggests that a direct effect of antimicrobials on the organism cannot be implicated in the pathophysiology of *C. difficile*-induced disease.

2. *Incidence of toxigenic strains*

The fact that some patients harbour *C. difficile* with negative tissue culture assays of stool suggests that some strains lack the ability to produce the cytopathic toxin. However, available evidence indicates that this applies to only a small portion of isolates. Our experience with tissue culture assays performed on cell-free supernatant after five days of incubation in chopped meat–glucose broth showed 306 of 312 strains produced cytotoxin (Bartlett, unpublished data). Toxin-producing isolates in this study included numerous strains which were recovered from the normal flora of healthy persons who had no detectable toxin on direct analysis of stool. However, isolates from stools which lack detectable cytotoxin often produce relatively small amounts of toxin; with toxin positive specimens there is a crude correlation between toxin titres in stool and *in vitro* toxin production by the stool isolate (Viscidi *et al.*, 1981). Neither the toxigenic potential of the strain nor the toxin titre of the specimen correlate with the severity of disease. Investigations by Burdon *et al.* (1978) indicated only 10 of 27 strains produced cytotoxin and Shuttleworth *et al.* (1980) noted 33 of 78 strains were non-toxigenic. However, critical analysis suggests either that the conditions for *in vitro* testing were suboptimal or that the strains may have been misidentified.

3. Characterization of cytotoxin

The cytopathic toxin has been partially purified by several groups using a variety of biochemical techniques (Taylor and Bartlett, 1979; Rolfe and Finegold, 1979; Humphrey *et al.*, 1979; Aswell *et al.*, 1979; Taylor *et al.*, 1981). All of these reports indicate a protein which is sensitive to heat (56°C, 1 hour), acid conditions (pH 3, 1 hour), alkaline conditions (pH 9, 1 hour) and trypsin (50 μg ml^{-1}, 1 hour). The isoelectric point has been measured at 5.0 (Rolfe and Finegold, 1979) and 5.4–5.6 (Aswell *et al.*, 1979). Molecular weight determinations have varied widely and include estimates of 95 000–125 000 (Humphrey *et al.*, 1979), 240 000 (Taylor and Bartlett, 1979), 530 000 (Rolfe and Finegold, 1979) and 600 000 (Aswell *et al.*, 1979). These differences presumably reflect variations in the methods and conditions used for purification. Rolfe and Finegold (1979) noted that the cytotoxin disassociated into components with molecular weights of 185 000 and 50 000 daltons. The more highly purified preparations have shown the minimum quantity required for typical cytopathic activity is 170 pg ml^{-1}.

4. Mechanism of cytotoxin

Studies with stool, broth cultures of *C. difficile* or partially purified preparations the cytotoxin show cytotoxicity to all cell lines tested, regardless of tissue cell type or animal species of origin. The rapidity and extent of changes in tissue cultured cells is related to toxin concentration, cell density and the composition of the incubation medium (Chang *et al.*, 1979a; Florin and Thelestam, 1981). Scanning electronmicroscopy with high concentrations of the cytotoxin shows ultrastructural changes reach a maximum at one hour, although conventional light microscopy indicate a latent period of at least three hours, with progression to a maximum at 24–48 hours (Chang *et al.*, 1979b). The type of morphological alteration induced varies with the cell line examined and may show actinomorphic changes or cell rounding. The toxin induces actinomorphic changes with fibroblasts which presumably result from disruption of the stress fibres formed by actin microfilaments (Thelestam and Bronnegard, 1980). This change in the morphology and cytoskeleton resembles the effect produced by fungal alkaloid cytochalasins (Miranda *et al.*, 1974). There appears to be irreversible intoxication, although there is no cell death according to vital staining with trypan blue and evidence of residual metabolic function with RNA and protein synthesis (Thelestam and Bronnegard, 1980). Metabolic effects, such as depression of membrane transport function and inhibition of protein synthesis, do not appear to be the primary cause of morphological changes, since this appears to occur only after toxin induced CPE is observed. According to Donta and Shaffer (1980), *C. difficile* toxin produces morphological changes with YI adrenal cells and HeLa cells that are identical to those noted with cholera or *E. coli* enterotoxins, but these changes are not associated with increased levels of cyclic AMP and steroidogenesis. A report by Vesely *et al.* (1981) showed that *C. difficile* cytotoxin in concentrations as low as 1.7 pg ml^{-1} stimulates guanylate cyclase activity. To our knowledge, this is the only study to demonstrate a potential mechanism of diarrhoea using standardized methods for examining enteric toxins. Critical analysis of the report indicates that this fails to explain the inflammatory reaction which is a prominent feature in most cases. There is also inadequate assurance that the purified cytotoxin did not contain Toxin A to be described below.

5. Antibody to cytotoxin

The experience of multiple investigators, including our own group (Taylor and Bartlett, 1979), indicates extreme difficulty in raising antibody which neutralizes cytopathic effects using *C. difficile* toxin preparations as immunogens in animals. This has been accomplished only by Erich *et al.* (1980). Similarly, such neutralizing antibody has not been observed in clinical specimens using convalescent sera and stools from patients with *C. difficile*-induced diarrhoea or colitis (Bartlett, 1979c). An exception is serum from a single patient reported by Lishman *et al.* (1981). Neutralizing copro-antibody would appear uncommon, owing to the prolonged carriage of the toxin noted in many patients, especially when untreated. Nevertheless, Wada *et al.* (1980) noted neutralizing activity in 5 of 60 cultured colostral cell specimens which was ascribed to IgA.

C. Toxin A

1. Detection and activity

Much of the work summarized above was conducted with the notion that the cytopathic toxin is responsible for the biological activity of *C. difficile*. However, there is now evidence that the organism also produces a second toxin which may be more important in the pathophysiology of *C. difficile*-induced enteric disease (Taylor *et al.*, 1981; Bartlett *et al.*, 1981). A clue to the presence of a second toxin resulted from the tests of biological activity using a number of assays during sequential stages in the purification of the cytotoxin from cell-free supernatant of *C. difficile*. These included the rabbit ileal loop assay, hamster caecitis assay using intracaecal injections, mouse lethality testing, and the standard tissue culture assay. The purification scheme included ultrafiltration, Sephadex G-200 chromatography, and ion exchange chromatography using DEAE Sepharose CL6B. This resulted in a 75% recovery and a 200–1500-fold purification of cytotoxin compared with starting material. All of the previously noted animal assays of biological activity were positive with the starting material and after Sephadex G-200 chromatography, but there was a major loss in animal assays following ion exchange chromatography despite good recovery of the cytotoxin. Stepwise elution with a NaCl gradient following this final stage showed two major protein peaks, designated peak I and peak II, the latter containing the cytotoxin. Repeat testing with peak I material showed that this contained another toxin which was further purified using DAVIS-PAGE. The biologically active protein, designated Toxin A, had a mouse LD_{50} of 10 ng, and 50 ng was sufficient to cause haemorrhagic caecitis with intracaecal injection into hamsters. Comparative values for the partially purified cytotoxin indicated a mouse LD_{50} of 4400 ng, and the minimum amount of protein required to produce haemorrhagic caecitis in hamsters was 125 000 ng. The greatest difference in biological activity between these two proteins was found in ligated intestinal loops in hamsters and rabbits (Fig. 4). Toxin A was consistently positive in both models, with accumulation of bloody fluid and severe haemorrhagic necrosis of the intestinal mucosa. By contrast, the cytotoxin has been negative using loop inoculations with inocula containing up to 150 μg in rabbits and 20 μg in hamsters. Peak I material did cause cytopathic changes in tissue culture, but was approximately 10 000-fold less potent compared to the partially purified cytotoxin in peak II preparations.

2. Toxin A antisera

Antisera prepared with purified Toxin A as the immunogen completely neutralized the biological activity of the homologous protein in the mouse lethality test and the ligated loop assays. This antisera failed to neutralize the cytopathic effects of purified cytotoxin in the tissue culture assay. Our attempts to prepare antisera which will neutralize cytopathic changes using purified cytotoxin have not been successful. However, antisera to partially purified cytotoxin supplied by Ehrich *et al.* (1979) neutralized the activity of Toxin A in mouse lethality testing and the cytopathic changes of the cytotoxin. This suggests that both toxins were present in their immunogen.

3. Properties of Toxin A

Toxin A and cytotoxin co-purify with Sephadex G-200 chromatography suggesting similar molecular weights which are estimated at 240 000 daltons. Stability tests show that Toxin A and the cytotoxin are both heat labile (56°C, 1 hour). Toxin A is stable with acid conditions (pH 4.0, 1 hour), alkaline conditions (pH 10, 1 hour), and trypsin (50 μg ml^{-1}, 1 hour). By contrast, cytotoxin is inactivated when exposed to these conditions. Additionally, Toxin A has proven to be considerably more stable than the cytotoxin with repeated freezing and thawing.

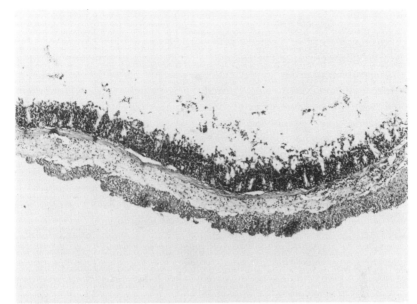

Fig. 4a

Fig. 4 Histology of hamster ligated colonic loop injected with 20 µg protein of toxin A (4a) or cytotoxin (4b). There is acute inflammation and haemorrhage with destruction of the mucosal lining and sloughing of tissue in the animal challenged with toxin A. The loop injected with the cytotoxin in comparable quantities shows preservation of the normal architecture.

Fig. 4b

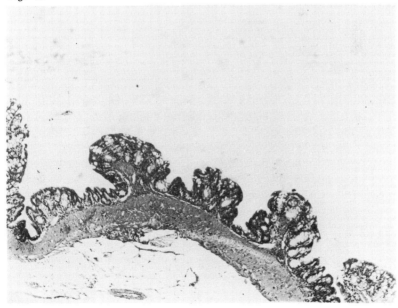

4. Interrelationship of Toxin A and cytotoxin

The results summarized above indicate that *C. difficile* produces two toxins which may be separated by ion exchange chromatography. One toxin, designated cytotoxin, is extremely potent in tissue culture assays and appears to serve as a relatively sensitive and specific marker for *C. difficile*-induced enteric disease (Table 5). The second toxin, designated Toxin A, appears to be substantially more potent in biological assays of enteric toxins using animal models. These data suggest that Toxin A may be more important in the clinical expression of *C. difficile*-induced gastro-intestinal complications. This may also account for several disturbing factors noted with clinical correlations and results of tissue culture assays such as: the lack of a correlation between disease severity and titre of cytotoxin; occasional patients with PMC, negative toxin assays and positive cultures for *C. difficile*; occasional adults with positive toxin assays and no symptoms; and the high rate of positive toxin assays in healthy neonates. Evidence that the two toxins are different is based on the previously summarized data concerning biological activities, differences in physical properties and, perhaps most importantly, antigenic differences. Nevertheless, the interrelationship of these two toxins is not clear. Small amounts of cytotoxic activity is found with purified Toxin A preparations which is not neutralized by antisera to Toxin A, and re-electrophoresis of purified Toxin A preparations shows two protein bands, including one which appears to migrate with purified cytotoxin. Thus, the two toxins resist separation even after ion exchange chromatography. This type of complexing may explain the weak cytopathic activity of Toxin A and may also explain the substantial differences in molecular weight determinations for cytotoxin reported by various observers.

SUMMARY

Clostridium difficile was originally described in 1935 and was noted to produce a potent toxin that was lethal for experimental animals at that time. However, the role of this microbe in veterinary or clinical medicine remained obscure until recent studies which show this to be an important enteric pathogen. Studies since 1977 indicate that *C. difficile* is responsible for nearly all cases of antibiotic-associated PMC and approximately 25% of antibiotic-associated diarrhoeal disease. The evidence to date suggests that *C. difficile* is rarely involved in extra-intestinal infections, and it causes enteric disease almost exclusively in the presence of antibiotic exposure. Exceptions include the possible role of *C. difficile* in occasional patients with relapses of inflammatory bowel disease, PMC which is not associated with antibiotic exposure and an enigmatic role in gastro-intestinal diseases of neonates. The close association with antibiotic exposure is unexplained, although the loss of colonization resistance remains an attractive theory in the pathophysiology. Stool cultures indicate that approximately 3% of healthy adults harbour *C. difficile* in the colonic flora, and these individuals are presumably at risk with antibiotic exposure. However, there are also epidemics of *C. difficile*-induced disease in which acquisition of the putative agent from environmental sources appears to be responsible. Specific forms of therapy include non-absorbed antimicrobial agents directed against *C. difficile* and ion exchange resins to bind the toxin.

There are two facets of the *C. difficile* story that merit emphasis. First, it illustrates the difficulty encountered in detecting new enteric pathogens with conventional stool cultures, because this was done unsuccessfully for three decades using stool from patients and experimental animals with antibiotic-associated colitis. It is instructive to note that *C. difficile* was originally detected by experiments designed to reveal a transferable toxin, and subsequent analyses were based primarily on methods to detect an antigenic marker, the cytotoxin, rather than stool bacteriology. The second major instructive lesson concerns the utility of animal experiments using the hamster model of antibiotic-induced colitis that has provided critical information that proved clinically applicable for virtually all facets of current knowledge concerning *C. difficile*-induced enteric disease. This includes the initial detection of the responsible agent, the development of a tissue culture assay for clinical detection, the use of vancomycin for therapy, the intimate association of disease with antibiotic usage, and the potential importance of epidemiological spread. Animal models also provided the initial clue to the presence of a second toxin which is of considerable interest in our understanding of pathophysiological mechanisms. It now appears that the cytotoxin serves as a sensitive and specific marker of *C. difficile*-induced disease, but the second toxin, Toxin A, may play a more important role in the clinical expression of enteric complications.

REFERENCES

Abrams, G. D., Allo, M., Rifkin, G. D., Fekety, R. and Silva, J., Jr. (1980). *Gut* **21**, 493–499.

Allen, S. A., Dunn, G. D., Page, D. L. and Wilson, F. A. (1977). *Gastroenterology* **73**, 158–163.

Allo, M. (1980). *J. Surg. Res.* **28**, 421–425.

Allo, M., Silva, J., Jr., Fekety, R., Rifkin, G. and Waskin, H. (1979). *Gastroenterology* **76**, 351–355.

Alpers, D. H. and Grimme, N. (1978). *J. Infect. Dis.* **137**, 756–763.

Altemeier, W. A., Hummel, R. P. and Hill, E. O. (1963). *Ann. Surg.* **157**, 847–857.

42   *J. G. Bartlett and N. S. Taylor*

Ambrus, C. M., Sideri, C. N., Johnson, G. C. and Harrison, E. (1952). *Antibiot. Chemother.* **2**, 521–527.
Arabi, T., Dimock, F., Burdon, D. W., Alexander-Williams, J. and Keighley, M. R. B. (1979). *J. Antimicrob. Chemother.* **5**, 531–537.
Aswell, J. E., Ehrich, M., Van Tassell, R. L., Tsai, C. C., Holdeman, L. V. and Wilkins, T. D. (1979). "Microbiology 1979", Amer. Soc. Microbiol., Washington, DC. pp. 272–275.
Azar, H. and Drapanas, T. (1968). *Amer. J. Surg.* **115**, 209.
Bartlett, J. G. (1979c). *Clin. Gastroenterol.* **8**, 783–801.
Bartlett, J. G. (1979). *Rev. Infect. Dis.* **1**, 530–539.
Bartlett, J. G. (1981a). *Johns Hopkins Med. J.* **149**, 6–9.
Bartlett, J. G. (1981b). *Gastroenterology* **80**, 863–865.
Bartlett, J. G. and Gorbach, S. L. (1977). Pseudomembranous colitis. In "Advances in Internal Medicine" (G. H. Stollerman, ed.) Yearbook Medical Publishers, Chicago. pp. 455–476.
Bartlett, J. G., Kasper, D. L., Cisneros, R. and Onderdonk, A. B. (1977a). Proceedings of the 17th Interscience Conference on Antimicrobial Agents and Chemotherapy, New York, N.Y. October, 1977. (Abstract #170).
Bartlett, J. G., Onderdonk, A. B., Cisneros, A. B. and Kasper, D. L. (1977b). *J. Infect. Dis.* **136**, 701–705.
Bartlett, J. G., Onderdonk, A. B. and Cisneros, R. L. (1977c). *Gastroenterology* **73**, 772–776.
Bartlett, J. G., Chang, T. W., Gurwith, M., Gorbach, S. L. and Onderdonk, A. B. (1978a). *New Engl. J. Med.* **298**, 531–534.
Bartlett, J. G., Chang, T. W., Moon, N. and Onderdonk, A. B. (1978b). *Amer. J. Vet. Res.* **39**, 1525–1530.
Bartlett, J. G., Chang, T. W. and Onderdonk, A. B. (1978c). *J. Infect. Dis.* **138**, 81–86.
Bartlett, J. G., Moon, N., Chang, T. W., Taylor, N. S. and Onderdonk, A. B. (1978d). *Gastroenterology* **75**, 778–782.
Bartlett, J. G., Chang, T. W., Taylor, N. S. and Onderdonk, A. B. (1979a). *Rev. Infect. Dis.* **1**, 370–378.
Bartlett, J. G., Tedesco, F. J., Shull, S. and Lowe, B. (1979b). *Gastroenterology* **78**, 431–434.
Bartlett, J. G., Taylor, N. W., Chang, T. W. and Dzink, J. A. (1981). *Amer. J. Clin. Nutr.* **33**, 2521–2526.
Batts, D. H., Martin, D., Holmes, R., Silva, J. and Fekety, F. R. (1980). *J. Ped.* **97**, 151–153.
Bogomoletz, W. V. (1976). *Gut* **17**, 483.
Bolton, R. P. (1979). *Brit. Med. J.* **2**, 1479–1480.
Bolton, R. P., Sherrief, R. J. and Read, A. E. (1980). *Lancet* **1**, 383–384.
Bornside, R. H., Floyd, E. and Cohn, I., Jr. (1964). *J. Surg. Res.* **4(95)**, 233–239.
Borriello, S. P. (1979). *Research Clin. Forums* **1**, 33–36.
Boriello, S. P., Jones, R. H. and Phillips, I. (1980). *Brit. Med. J.* **281**, 1180–1181.
Bowden, T. A., Jr., Mansberger, A. R., Jr. and Lykins, L. E. (1981). *Amer. Surg.* **47**, 178–183.
Brause, B. D., Romankiewicz, J. A., Gotz, V., Franklin, J. E., Jr. and Roberts, R. B. (1980). *Amer. J. Gastroenterol.* **73**, 244–248.
Brown, R. L. (1975). *Antibiot. Chemother.* **2**, 5.
Browne, R., Fekety, R., Jr., Silva, J., Jr., Boyd, D. I., Work, C. O. and Abrams, G. D. (1977). *Johns Hop. Med. J.* **141**, 183–192.

Bryan, C. S. and White, W. L. (1978). *Antimicrob. Ag. Chemother.* **14**, 634–635.
Burbige, E. J. and Milligan, F. D. (1975). *J. Amer. Med. Assoc.* **231**, 1157–1158.
Burbige, E. J. and Radigan, J. J. (1981). *Dis. Colon Rectum* **23**, 198–200.
Burdon, D. W., Brown, J. G., George, R. H., Abari, Y., Alexander-Williams, J. and Keighley, M. R. B. (1978). *New Engl. J. Med.* **19**, 48–49.
Burdon, D. W., Brown, J. D., Youngs, D., Arabi, Y., Shinagawa, N., Alexander-Williams, J. and Keighley, M. R. B. (1979). *J. Antimicrob. Chemother.* **5**, 307–310.
Cashore, W. J., Peter, G., Lauermann, M., Stonestreet, B. S. and Oh, W. (1981). *J. Pediatr.* **98**, 308–311.
Chang, T. W. (1978). *J. Infect. Dis.* **137**, 854.
Chang, T. W., Bartlett, J. G., Gorbach, S. L. and Onderdonk, A. B. (1978a). *Infect. Immun.* **20**, 526–529.
Chang, T. W., Gorbach, S. L. and Bartlett, J. G. (1978b). *Infect. Immun.* **22**, 418–422.
Chang, T. W., Onderdonk, A. B. and Bartlett, J. G. (1978c). *Lancet* **2**, 258–259.
Chang, T. W., Lauermann, M. and Bartlett, J. G. (1979a). *J. Infect. Dis.* **140**, 765–770.
Chang, T. W., Lin, P. S., Gorbach, S. L. and Bartlett, J. G. (1979b). *Infect. Immun.* **23**, 795–798.
Chang, T. W., Gorbach, S. L., Bartlett, J. G. and Saginur, R. (1980). *Gastroenterology* **78**, 1584–1586.
Cudmore, M. A., Silva, J., Jr. and Fekety, R. (1979). Proceedings of the 19th Interscience Conference on Antimicrobial Agents and Chemotherapy. Boston, 1979. (Abstract #379.)
Dabard, J., Dubos, F., Martinet, L. and Ducluzeau, R. (1979). *Infect. Immun.* **24**, 7–11.
Dearing, W. H., Baggenstoss, A. H. and Weed, L. A. (1960). *Gastroenterology* **38**, 441–451.
Dearing, W. H. and Needham, G. M. *J. Amer. Med. Assoc.* **174**, 1597–1602.
DeJesus, R. and Peternel, W. W. (1978). *Gastroenterology* **74**, 818–820.
DeSomer, P., Van de Voorde, H., Eyssen, H. and Van Dijck, P. (1955). *Antibiotic Chemother.* **5**, 463–469.
Donta, S. T. and Shaffer, S. J. (1980). *J. Infect. Dis.* **141**, 218–222.
Dpnta, S. T., Stuppy, M. S. and Meyers, M. G. (1981). *Amer. J. Dis. Child* **135**, 181–182.
Dzink, J. A. and Bartlett, J. G. (1980). *Antimicrob. Ag. Chemother.* **17**, 695–698.
Ebright, J. R., Fekety, R., Silva, J., Jr. and Wilson, K. (1981). *Antimicrob. Ag. Chemother.* **19**, 980–986.
Editorial (1977). *Lancet* **2**, 1113–1114.
Ehrich, M., Van Tassell, R. L., Libby, J. M. and Wilkins, T. D. (1980). *Infect. Immun.* **28**, 1041–1043.
Eyssen, H., DeSomer, P. and Van Dijck, P. (1957). *Antibiot. Chemother.* **7**, 55–63.
Falsen, E., Kaijser, B., Nehls, L., Nygren, B. and Svedhem, A. (1980). *J. Clin. Microbiol.* **12**, 297–300.
Farrar, W. E., Jr. and Kent, T. H. (1965). *Amer. J. Path.* **47**, 629.
Fekety, R. (1979). *In* "Microbiology 1979" Amer. Soc. Microbiol., Washington, D.C. pp. 276–279.
Fekety, R., Silva, J., Jr., Toshniwal, R., Allo, M., Armstrong, J., Browne, R., Ebright, J. and Rifkin, G. D. (1979). *Rev. Infect. Dis.* **1**, 386–396.
Fekety, R., Kim, K-H., Brown, D., Batts, D. H., Cuctmore, M. and Silva, J., Jr. (1981). *Amer. J. Med.* **70**, 906–908.
Finegold, S. M., Attebery, H. R. and Sutter, V. L. (1974). *Amer. J. Clin. Nutr.* **27**, 1456–1469.

Finney, J. M. T. (1893). Bull. Johns Hopkins Hosp. **4**, 53–55.

Florin, I. and Thelestam, M. (1981). *Infect. Immun.* **33**, 67–74.

Fraser, D. W., Wachsmuth, I. K., Bopp, C., Feeley, J. C. and Tsai, R. F. (1978). *Lancet* **1**, 175–177.

George, R. H., Symonds, J. M., Dimock, F., Browne, J., Arabi, D., Shinagawa, N., Keighley, M. R. B., Alexander-Williams, J. and Burdon, D. W. (1978). *Brit. Med. J.* **1**, 695.

George, W. L., Sutter, V. L. and Finegold, S. M. (1978). *Current Microbiol.* **1**, 55–58.

George, W. L., Kirby, B. D., Sutter, V. L. and Finegold, S. M. (1979a). *In* "Microbiology 1979" Amer. Soc. Microbiol., Washington, D.C. pp. 267–271.

George, W. L., Rolfe, R. D., Mulligan, M. and Finegold, S. M. (1979b). *Clin. Res.* **27**, 344A.

George, W. L., Sutter, V. L., Citron, D. and Finegold, S. M. (1979c). *J. Clin. Microbiol.* **9**, 214–219.

George, W. L., Volpicelli, N. A., Stiner, D. B., Richman, D. D., Liechty, E. J., Mok, H. Y., Rolfe, R. D. and Finegold, S. M. (1979d). *New Engl. J. Med.* **301**, 414–415.

Giannella, R. A., Serumaga, J., Walls, D. and Drake, K. W. (1981). *Gastroenterology* **80**, 907–913.

Gilligan, P. H., McCarthy, L. R. and Genta, V. M. (1981). *J. Clin. Microbiol.* **14**, 26–31.

Gorbach, S. L. and Thadepalli, H. (1975). *J. Infect. Dis.* **131**, 581–585.

Goulson, S. J. M. and McGovern, V. J. (1965). *Gut* **6**, 207–212.

Green, R. (1974). *Yale J. Biol. Med.* **3**, 166–188.

Greenfield, C., Szawathowski, M., Noone, P., Burroughs, A., Bass, N. and Pounder, R. (1981). *Lancet* **1**, 371–372.

Gurwith, M., Rabin, H. R. and Love, K. (1977). *J. Infect. Dis.* **135**, S104–S110.

Hafiz, S. L. (1974). *Clostridium difficile* and its toxins. Ph.D. Thesis, University of Leeds.

Hafiz, S. L. and Oakley, C. L. (1976). *J. Med. Microbiol.* **9**, 129–137.

Hafiz, S. L., McEntegart, M. G., Morton, R. S. and Waitkins, S. A. (1975). *Lancet* **1**, 420–421.

Hale, H. W., Jr. and Cosgriff, H. J., Jr. (1957). *Amer. J. Surg.* **94**, 710–717.

Hall, I. C. and O'Toole, E. (1935). *Amer. J. Dis. Child.* **49**, 390–402.

Halen, A., Ryden, A. C., Schwan, A. and Wallin, J. (1977). *Brit. J. Venereal Dis.* **53**, 367–371.

Hambre, D. M., Rake, G. and McKee, E. M. (1943). *Amer. J. Med. Sci.* **206**, 642–652.

Hummel, R. P., Hill, E. O. and Altemeier, W. A. (1963). *J. Surg. Res.* **3**, 289.

Hummel, R. P., Altemeier, W. A. and Hill, E. O. (1964). *Ann. Surg.* **160**, 551.

Humphrey, C. D., Condon, C. W., Cantey, J. R. (1979a). *Gastroenterology* **76**, 468–476.

Humphrey, C. D., Lushbaugh, W. B., Condon, C. W., Pittman, J. C. and Pittman, F. E. (1979b). *Gut* **20**, 6–15.

Hutcheon, D. F., Milligan, F. D., Yardley, J. H. and Hendrix, T. R. (1978). *Amer. J. Dig. Dis.* **23**, 321–326.

Kabins, A. and Spira, T. J. (1975). *Ann. Intern. Med.* **83**, 830–831.

Kahn, M. Y. and Hall, W. H. (1966). *Ann. Intern. Med.* **65**, 1–7.

Kaipainen, W. J. and Faine, S. (1951). *Nature* **5**, 463–469.

Kappas, A., Shinagawa, N., Arabi, Y., Thompson, H., Burdon, D. W., Dimock, F., George, R. H., Alexander-Williams, J. and Keighley, M. R. B. (1978). *Brit. Med. J.* **1**, 675–678.

Katz, L., LaMont, J. T., Trier, J. S., Sonnenblick, E. B., Rothman, S. W., Broitman, S. A. and Rieth, S. (1978). *Gastroenterology* **74**, 246–252.

Keighley, M. R. B. (1980). *Drugs* **20**, 49–56.

Keighley, M. R. B. (1981). Antibiotic-associated colitis. *In* "Infection in Surgery" Watts, J. McK., McDonald, P. J., O'Brien, P. E., Marshall, V. R. and Finlay-Jones, J. J. (Eds) Churchill-Livingstone, Edinburgh, pp. 129–137.

Keighley, M. R. B. and Burdon, D. W. (1979). *Lancet* **2**, 607.

Keighley, M. R. B., Burdon, D. W., Arabi, Y., Alexander-Williams, J., Thompson, H., Youngs, D., Johnson, M., Bently, S., George, R. H. and Mogg, G. A. G. (1978). *Brit. Med. J.* **2**, 1667–1669.

Keighley, M. R. B., Arabi, Y., Alexander-Williams, J., Youngs, D. and Burdon, D. W. (1979). *Lancet* **1**, 894–897.

Keusch, G. T. and Present, D. H. (1976). *J. Infect. Dis.* **133**, 578–587.

Kim, K-H., Fekety, R., Botts, D. H., Brown, D., Cudmore, M., Silva, J., Jr. and Waters, D. (1981). *J. Infect. Dis.* **143**, 42–50.

Koltz, A. P., Palmer, W. L. and Kirsner, J. B. (1953). *Gastroenterology* **25**, 44–49.

Kreutzer, E. W. and Milligan, F. D. (1978). *Johns Hopkins Med. J.* **143**, 67–72.

LaMont, J. T. and Trnka, Y. M. (1980). *Lancet* **1**, 381–383.

LaMont, J. T., Sonnenblick, E. B. and Rothman, S. (1979). *Gastroenterology* **76**, 356–361.

Larson, H. E. and Price, A. B. (1977). *Lancet* **2**, 1312–1314.

Larson, H. E., Parry, J. V., Price, A. B., Davies, J. and Tyrell, D. A. J. (1977). *Brit. Med. J.* **1**, 1246–1248.

Larson, H. E., Price, A. B., Honour, P. and Borriello, S. P. (1978). *Lancet* **1**, 1063–1066.

Larson, H. E., Price, A. B. and Boriello, S. P. (1980). *J. Infect. Dis.* **142**, 408–413.

LeFrock, J. L., Klainer, A. S., Chen, S., Gainer, R. B., Omar, M. and Anderson, W. (1975). *J. Infect. Dis.* **131**, S108–S115.

Leigh, D. A. (1977). *Antimicrob. Ag. Chemother.* **15**, 195–198.

Leigh, D. A., Simmons, K. and Williams, S. (1980). *J. Antimicrob. Chemother.* **6**, 639–645.

Libby, J. M., Sullivan, N., Van Tassell, R. L. and Wilkins, T. D. (1981). Proceedings of the 81st Annual Meeting of the American Society for Microbiology, Dallas, Texas, March, 1981. (Abstract # B44.)

Lishman, A. H., Al-Jumaili, I. J. and Record, C. O. (1981). *J. Clin. Pathol.* (in press).

Lishman, A. H., Al-Jumaili, I. J. and Record, C. O. (1981). *Gut* **22**, 34–37.

Lowe, B., Fox, L. and Bartlett, J. G. (1980). *Amer. J. Veterin. Res.* **41**, 1277–1279.

Lusk, R. H., Fekety, R., Jr., Silva, J., Jr., Bodendorfer, T., Devine, B. J., Kawanishi, H., Korff, L., Nakauchi, D., Rogers, S. and Siskin, S. B. (1977). *J. Infect. Dis.* **135**, S111–S119.

Lusk, R. H., Fekety, R., Silva, J., Browne, R. A., Ringler, D. H. and Abrams, G. D. (1978). *J. Infect. Dis.* **137**, 464–475.

Manashil, G. B. and Kern, J. A. (1973). *Amer. J. Gastroent.* **60**, 394.

Marr, J. J., Sans, M. D. and Tedesco, F. J. (1975). *Gastroenterology* **69**, 352–358.

Matuchansky, C., Aries, J. and Maire, P. (1978). *Lancet* **2**, 580–581.

Meyers, S., Mayer, L., Bottone, E., Desmond, E. and Janowitz, H. D. (1981). *Gastroenterology* **80**, 697–700.

Miranda, A. F., Godman, G. C. and Tanenbaum, S. W. (1974). *J. Cell. Biol.* **62**, 406–423.

Miyazaki, S. and Sakaguchi, G. (1978). *Japan J. Med. Sci. Biol.* **31**, 1–15.

Mogg, G. M., Keighley, M., Burdon, D., Alexander-Williams, J., Youngs, D., Johnson, M., Bentley, S. and George, R. (1979). *Brit. J. Surg.* **66**, 738.

Mosleovitz, M. and Bartlett, J. G. (1981). *Arch. Intern. Med.* **141**, 663–664.

Mulligan, M. E., George, W. L., Rolfe, R. D. and Finegold, S. M. (1981). *Amer. J. Clin. Nutr.* **33**, 2533–2538.

Mulligan, M. E., Rolfe, R. D., Finegold, S. M. and George, W. L. (1979). *Curr. Microbiol.* **3**, 173–175.

Neu, H. C., Prince, A., Neu, C. O. and Garvey, G. J. (1977). *J. Infect. Dis.* **135**, S120–S125.

Newton, W. L., Steinman, H. G. and Brandriss, M. W. (1964). *J. Bacteriol.* **88**, 537–538.

Novak, E., Lee, J. G., Seckman, C. E., Phillips, J. P. and DiSanto, A. R. (1976). *J. Amer. Med. Assoc.* **235**, 1451–1454.

Oldenburger, T. R. and Miller, M. S. (1980). *Amer. J. Gastroenterol.* **74**, 359–360.

Onderdonk, A. B., Lowe, B. R. and Bartlett, J. G. (1979). *Appl. Environ. Microbiol.* **38**, 637–641.

Onderdonk, A. B., Cisneros, R. L. and Bartlett, J. G. (1980). *Infect. Immuno.* **28**, 227.

Pashby, N. L., Bolton, R. P. and Sherriff, R. J. (1979). *Brit. Med. J.* **1**, 1605–1606.

Peikin, S. R., Galdibini, J. and Bartlett, J. G. (1980). *Gastroenterology* **79**, 948–951.

Penner, A. and Bernheim, A. (1939). *Arch. Path.* **27**, 966.

Pettet, J. D., Baggenstoss, A. H., Dearing, W. H. and Judd, E. S. (1954). *Surg. Gynecol. Obstet.* **8**, 546.

Pittman, F. E., Pittman, J. C. and Humphrey, C. D. (1974). *Arch. Intern. Med.* **134**, 368.

Poxton, I. R. and Byrne, M. D. (1981). *J. Gen. Microbiol.* **122**, 41–46.

Price, A. B. and Davies, D. R. (1977). *J. Clin. Path.* **30**, 1–12.

Price, A. B., Larson, H. E. and Crow, J. (1979). *Gut* **20**, 467–475.

Prohaska, J. V., Jacobson, M. J., Drake, C. T. and Tan, T.-L. (1959). *Surg. Gynec. Obstet.* **109**, 73–77.

Prohaska, J. V., Long, E. T. and Nelson, T. S. (1956). *Arch. Surg.* **72**, 977–983.

Ramirez-Ronda, C. H. (1974). *Ann. Intern. Med.* **81**, 860.

Reiner, L., Schlesinger, M. J. and Miller, G. M. (1952). *Arch. Path.* **54**, 39–67.

Rietra, P. J., Souterus, K. W. and Zanen, H. C. (1978). *Lancet* **2**, 189.

Rifkin, G. D., Fekety, F. R., Silva, J., Jr. and Sack, R. B. (1977). *Lancet* **2**, 1103–1106.

Rolfe, R. D. and Finegold, S. M. (1979). *Infect. Immun.* **25**, 191–201.

Rolfe, R. D., Helebian, S. and Finegold, S. M. (1981). *J. Infect. Dis.* **143**, 470–475.

Rollins, D. E. and Moeller, D. (1975). *J. Amer. Med. Assoc.* **231**, 1228.

Ryan, R. R., Kwasnik, I. and Tilton, R. C. (1980). *J. Clin. Micro.* **12**, 776–779.

Saginur, R., Hawley, C. R. and Bartlett, J. G. (1980). *J. Infect. Dis.* **141**, 772–774.

Schneierson, S. S. and Perlman, E. (1956). *Proc. Soc. Exp. Biol. Med.* **91**, 229–230.

Scopes, J. W., Smith, M. F. and Beach, R. C. (1980). *Lancet* **1**, 1144.

Scott, A. J., Nicholson, G. I. and Kerr, A. R. (1973). *Lancet* **2**, 1232–1234.

Shuttleworth, R., Taylor, M. and Jones, D. M. (1980). *J. Clin. Path.* **33**, 1002–1005.

Silva, J., Jr., (1979). Animal models of antibiotic-induced colitis. *In* "Microbiology 1979" Amer. Soc. Microbiol., Washington, D.C. pp. 258–263.

Slagle, G. W. and Boggs, H. W. (1976). *Dis. Colon Rectum* **19**, 253–255.

Small, J. D. (1968). *Lab. Animal Care* **18**, 411–420.

Smith, J. C., Markowitz, S. M. and Macrina, F. L. (1980). *Antimicrob. Ag. Chemother.* **19**, 997–1003.

Smith, L. D. S. and King, E. O. (1962). *J. Bacteriol.* **84**, 65–67.
Snyder, M. D. (1937). *J. Infect. Dis.* **60**, 223–229.
Snyder, M. L. (1940). *J. Infect. Dis.* **66**, 1–16.
Stanley, R. J., Melson, G. L. and Tedesco, F. J. (1974). *Radiology* **111**, 519–524.
Stroehlein, J. R., Sedlack, R. E., Hoffman, H. N. and Newcomer, A. D. (1974). *May. Clin. Proc.* **49**, 240–243.
Sumner, H. W. and Tedesco, F. J. (1975). *Arch. Path.* **99**, 237.
Surgalla, M. J. and Dach, G. M. (1955). *J. Amer. Med. Assoc.* **158**, 149.
Sutter, V. L. and Finegold, S. M. (1974). The effect of antimicrobial agents on human faecal flora. *In* "The Normal Microbial Flora of Man" (Skinner, F. A. and Carr, J. G., Eds) Academic Press, New York, N.Y. pp. 229–240.
Swartzberg, J. E., Maresca, R. M. and Remington, J. W. (1976). *Arch. Intern. Med.* **136**, 876–879.
Tan, T.-L., Drake, C. T., Jacobson, M. J. and Prohaska, J. V. (1959). *Surg. Gynecol. Obstet.* **108**, 415–420.
Taylor, N. S. and Bartlett, J. G. (1979). *Rev. Infect. Dis.* **1**, 379–385.
Taylor, N. S. and Bartlett, J. G. (1980). *J. Infect. Dis.* **141**, 92–97.
Taylor, N. S., Thorne, G. and Bartlett, J. G. (1981). *Infect. Immun.* (in press).
Tedesco, F. J. (1975). *Amer. J. Dig. Dis.* **20**, 295–297.
Tedesco, F. J. (1976). *Amer. J. Dig. Dis.* **21**, 26–31.
Tedesco, F. J. (1980). *Gastroenterology* **7**, 295–297.
Tedesco, F. J., Barton, R. W. and Alpers, H. D. (1974). *Ann. Intern. Med.* **81**, 429–433.
Tedesco, F. J., Markam, R., Gurwith, M., Christie, D. and Bartlett, J. G. (1978). *Lancet* **2**, 226–228.
Tedesco, F. J., Napier, J., Gamble, W., Chang, T. W. and Bartlett, J. G. (1979). *Ann. Gastroenterology* **1**, 51–54.
Thelestam, M. and Bronnegard, M. (1980). *Scand. J. Infect. Dis. Suppl.* **22**, 16–29.
Thompson, G., Clark, A. H., Hare, K. and Spilg, W. G. S. (1981). *Brit. Med. J.* **282**, 804–805.
Toshniwal, R., Fekety, R. and Silva, J., Jr. (1979). *Antimicrob. Ag. Chemother.* **16**, 167–170.
Toshniwal, R., Silva, J., Jr., Fekety, R. and Kim, K.-H. (1981). *J. Infect. Dis.* **143**, 51–54.
Totten, M. A., Gregg, J. A., Fremont-Smith, P. and Legg, M. (1978). *Amer. J. Gastro.* **69**, 311–319.
Trinh, D., Kernbaum, S. and Frottier, J. (1978). *Lancet* **1**, 338–339.
Trnka, Y. M. and LaMont, J. T. (1981). *Gastroenterology* **80**, 693–696.
Tully, T. E. and Feinberg, S. B. (1974). *Amer. J. Roent.* **121**, 291.
Valberg, L. S. and Truelove, S. C. (1961). *Amer. J. Dig. Dis.* **5**, 729–738.
Vesely, D. L., Straub, K. D., Nolan, C. M., Rolfe, R. D., Finegold, S. M. and Monson, T. P. (1981). *Infect. Immun.* **33**, 285–291.
Viscidi, R. P. and Bartlett, J. G. (1981). *Pediatrics* **67**, 381–386.
Viscidi, R., Willey, S. and Bartlett, J. G. (1981). *Gastroenterology* **81**, 5–9.
Wada, N., Nishida, N., Iwaki, S., Ohi, H., Miyawaki, T., Taniguchi, N. and Migita, S. (1980). *Infect. Immun.* **29**, 545–550.
Wakefield, R. D. and Sommers, S. C. (1953). *Ann. Surg.* **138**, 249.
Wald, A., Mendelow, H. and Bartlett, J. G. (1980). *Ann. Intern. Med.* **92**, 798–799.
Warren, S. E., Sugiyama, H. and Prohaska, J. V. (1963). *Surg. Gynec. Obstet.* **114**, 29–33.

Welch, D. F., Menge, S. K. and Matsen, J. M. (1980). *J. Clin. Microbiol.* **11**, 470–473.
Willey, S. H. and Bartlett, J. G. (1979). *J. Clin. Microbiol.* **10**, 880–884.
Wood, J. S., Jr., Bennett, I. L., Jr. and Yardley, J. H. (1956). *Johns Hop. Med. J.* **98**, 454–463.
Yolken, R. H., Whitcomb, L. S., Libby, J., Ehrich, M., Wilkins, T., Marien, G. and Bartlett, J. G. (1981). *J. Infect. Dis.* (in press).

2 Contagious equine metritis

H. PLATT and C. E. D. TAYLOR

I. INTRODUCTION

Infections of the reproductive tract of animals have been studied principally in species of economic importance such as horses, cattle, sheep and pigs. Although these domestic animals in some ways resemble human beings in their susceptibility to such infections, they often differ in respect of the microbial agents concerned and the particular sites affected. This applies especially to the venereally transmitted infections, which tend to be species-specific.

In all species studied, many infections of the endometrium are opportunistic. Retention of the products of conception, failure of the uterus to involute post-partum, or the presence of foreign bodies may all predispose to infection; in the human being, intra-uterine contraceptive devices may sometimes be responsible. In the absence of such circumstances, however, acute endometritis is rare in women during reproductive life. This may be in some way related to the fact that, unlike other mammals, which have an oestral cycle, reproductive periodicity in the female human being and other primates is expressed in a menstrual cycle during which there is shedding and renewal of the endometrium.

In horses, opportunistic endometrial infections by streptococci, *Escherichia coli*, and other commensal or environmental organisms are common. Some mares, possibly because of deficiencies in the natural defences of the genital tract, appear to be particularly susceptible to these. Metritis is also seen in several types of genital infections that are transmitted venereally. These transmissible infections usually occur in outbreaks involving the mares recently served by a particular stallion. Several such infections are recognized in horses.

(i) *Klebsiella infections.* Certain strains of *Klebsiella pneumoniae*, especially those of capsular types 1, 2 and 5 give rise to a transmissible form of metritis (Platt *et al.*, 1976). The stallion is clinically unaffected and transmission is usually the result of transient contamination of the surfaces of the penis and prepuce. Occasionally, an ascending infection of the mucosal surfaces of the urinary tract becomes established in the stallion, leading to a permanent carrier state (Crouch *et al.*, 1972).

(ii) *Pseudomonas aeruginosa.* Although this organism is sometimes present in the bacterial flora of the penis and prepuce without obvious venereal infection in the mares (Hughes *et al.*, 1967), transmission by the stallion sometimes occurs, leading to small outbreaks of *Pseudomonas* endometritis. The stallions responsible show no clinical signs of infection.

(iii) *Equine Coital Exanthema* is a herpesvirus infection (*Equine Herpesvirus 3*) characterized by papulovesicular lesions and ulceration in the external genitalia in both sexes. The disease has a low incidence in Britain, but is a well recognized condition.

(iv) *Dourine*, a disease with considerable mortality, is caused by *Trypanosoma equiperdum*. Inflammatory lesions of the external genitalia are seen in mares and stallions, to be followed by plaque-like cutaneous lesions, peripheral neuropathy and emaciation. The disease has been eradicated from Britain and Western Europe but is still found in many parts of the world.

In the spring of 1977, on stud farms in the vicinity of Newmarket, Suffolk, England there was a major outbreak of a highly contagious genital infection which was clearly distinct from any previously recognized disease. This was an event of some significance, not only on account of the serious financial and other implications for horse breeding, but also because the causal agent proved to be a hitherto unknown species of micro-organism. To distinguish this newly recognized disease, it was originally designated Contagious Equine Metritis (1977), now shortened to Contagious Equine Metritis (CEM).

Because the disease first appeared in Thoroughbred horses, the organization and procedures involved in Thoroughbred breeding in the UK will be briefly outlined.

Thoroughbred breeding is organized to provide a wide choice of sires for service to mares. This involves a considerable degree of movement and mixing of brood-mares. Artificial insemination of bloodstock is not practised, since by international agreement among studbook authorities, only foals conceived by natural service are eligible for registration. At the beginning of the year, each mare is sent to a selected stallion, resident at a particular stud, with a view to service during the official breeding season (February 15 to July 15). Mares are frequently sent for service to Ireland and France or sometimes other countries. The timing of service depends upon that of oestrus, and in mares that arrive pregnant service will not take place until one or two oestral periods after foaling. Most mares are served during March and April. They remain at stud for 2–3 months but mares from "boarding studs" or other local premises are "walked-in" for service when in oestrus, returning home immediately afterwards. It has been common practice for all mares to be checked before service for freedom from genital infections, but until 1977 examinations were principally based on bacteriological cultures of cervical swabs on blood agar medium incubated aerobically only, because the principal infections of concern were caused by aerobic bacteria. At the stud where the disease appeared the vaginal specula used in taking these swabs were immersed in cetrimide solution after use in each animal.

II. THE RECOGNITION OF CEM AND ITS CAUSAL AGENT

A. Epidemiological and clinical features of the outbreak in 1977

Contagious equine metritis first appeared in 1977, at a large, modern Thoroughbred stud where 6 stallions were resident and there were 209 visiting mares from different parts of the UK, the Republic of Ireland, France, Germany, Italy and the USA. Most of these mares were stabled at the stud, but some were "walked-in" from other local premises.

The beginning of the outbreak was somewhat insidious. Although in retrospect the first case was probably seen at the end of March (Simpson, 1977), it was in early April that several mares which had been served were found to have come back into oestrus after a shortened interoestrus interval, a phenomenon associated with uterine infection (Hughes and Loy, 1969). By mid-April, an increasing number of mares were showing varying amounts of mucopurulent uterine exudate, which in some cases was very copious, with vulval discharge coating the hind quarters and tail. There was usually some degree of vaginitis (Crowhurst, 1977). Affected mares were infertile but showed no constitutional disturbances, and the stallions appeared clinically normal. By the first week of May about 40% of newly served mares were showing signs of infection (Powell, 1978) and on 11th May the decision was taken to suspend breeding until the nature of the condition had been established and the stallions could be declared free from infection. Although in most cases clinical signs appeared a few days after service, occasionally they were seen in mares which had not been served, indicating the probability of spread in some instances by handling and examination.

By this time, cases had appeared on other studs in Newmarket. It is likely that mares "walked-in" to the affected stud had returned infected to boarding studs where cross-infection of other mares had occurred, and these in turn were probably responsible for infecting stallions on other studs in Newmarket. Altogether, 29 studs in the Newmarket area, involving 200–250 mares were affected (Powell and Whitwell, 1979). The true figure was probably higher, since in the early stages bacteriological diagnosis could not be made.

B.   Identification of the causal agent

The unusual nature of this outbreak was recognized from an early stage. The condition was highly contagious by coitus but bore no resemblance to dourine or coital exanthema, and initially a bacterial causal agent could not be cultivated. O'Driscoll *et al.* (1977) reported the isolation of *Proteus mirabilis* from the cervix of affected mares and from the urethra of implicated stallions, but this organism was considered by others as unlikely to be the causative agent.

Samples of vaginal discharge from infected mares submitted for laboratory examination were found to contain large numbers of polymorphs, ciliated and other uterine epithelial cells, and a variable number of small bacilli or coccobacilli. In the early stages, the significance of these bacteria was uncertain. The possible role of viruses, chlamydia, mycoplasmas and trichomonads had to be considered, and workers in several veterinary and medical laboratories collaborated with field investigators to explore, and eventually to exclude, these possibilities. Notwithstanding the presence of bacteria in smears of exudate, initial attempts to cultivate a significant organism were unsuccessful, except for the isolation of a *Bacteroides* sp. on serum agar under anaerobic conditions. This organism was probably a vaginal commensal, and its isolation highlighted the unsuitability of vaginal exudate as material for investigation. Henceforth attention was focussed on the bacteriology of samples from the cervix and uterus.

Samples were collected by veterinary colleagues on cotton-tipped swabs from the cervical canal and endometrium of typical cases of the disease, with careful precautions to avoid any contact with pools of vaginal exudate. The swabs were placed immediately in Stuart's Transport Medium (Stuart *et al.*, 1954) and conveyed to the Public Health Laboratory, Cambridge, within an hour and plated on a variety of media under differing atmospheric conditions. A scanty but pure growth of an unidentified Gram-negative coccobacillus was present on "chocolate" (heated blood) agar after 4 days' incubation in an atmosphere containing carbon dioxide. Cervical swab samples from other affected mares, collected during the next few days, yielded a similar organism, often in pure culture. In cervical swabs from a series of 10 mares with metritis, the unidentified organism was present in 9 cases; from 1 mare a haemolytic streptococcus was cultured (Platt *et al.*, 1977).

The pathogenic significance of the organism was confirmed by experimental transmission of infection to healthy pony mares. The organism in pure culture was introduced on swabs into the cervix of each of two pony mares which were in oestrus and had been shown by pre-infection bacteriological examination not to be carrying the organism. Two days later both showed evidence of cervicitis and vaginitis, and in one there was purulent exudate in the vagina. A swab from the cervix of one of these mares, inserted into the cervix of a third mare, also gave rise to the disease. The organism was re-isolated under appropriate cultural conditions from all three ponies. The results of these experiments fulfilled the requirements of Koch's postulates (Wilson and Miles, 1975a), and it was concluded that the unidentified organism isolated was the pathogen responsible for the outbreak (Platt *et al.*, 1977), and pending identification and classification, it was designated the contagious equine metritis organism (CEMO).

The same organism was then sought in swabs from the external genitalia of the stallions associated with the infected mares but at first considerable problems were encountered due to heavy contamination of the cultures by commensal and environmental organisms. With the aid of a selective medium containing streptomycin (a drug to which the strains first isolated were found to be highly resistant), this difficulty was overcome and it was possible to demonstrate that all 6 stallions were still carrying the organism 40 days after service of mares had been discontinued.

It may be worth considering, with the benefit of hindsight, some of the factors which played a part in the successful isolation of this organism. Such a fastidious and relatively slow-growing organism is particularly liable to be overgrown or inhibited (Swerczek, 1978b; Atherton, 1978) in the presence of large numbers of other bacteria and fungi. Initial isolation from the stallions without a selective medium would almost certainly have been impossible, while in the mares commensals were a potential source of confusion in the examination of vaginal discharges. In the uterus and cervix, however, the organism was present in profusion and often isolated in pure culture. The importance of cleanly collected samples from the site of primary multiplication of the organism is evident. Preservation of the organism in transport medium and rapid conveyance to the laboratory were also important. In the cultivation of the organism, the use of various media incubated under differing atmospheric conditions was especially necessary for growth of a fastidious organism with rather specific cultural requirements.

III. THE CHARACTERISTICS OF CEM

A. Natural History of CEM

1. The mare

CEM appears to be exclusively a genital infection and, in its acute form, it manifests itself as a purulent endometritis which is usually transmitted by coitus. In the acute stage, the endometrium is the principal site of multiplication of the causative organism and the mare is infertile. The organism can usually be cultured also from the vagina, urethral vestibule and clitoris, but the extent to which the more posterior regions of the genital tract are capable of supporting multiplication is uncertain. Clinical and pathological observations have yielded no evidence of significant salpingitis or ovarian involvement.

The mare will accept the stallion only at oestrus, so this is when infection usually occurs. At oestrus the cervix is relaxed, and the organism is likely to be introduced directly into the uterus with the ejaculate. However, the susceptibility of the uterus to infections in general tends to be greater during dioestrus than at oestrus (Rowson *et al.*, 1953), and experimentally CEM can be readily initiated outside the period of oestrus if the inoculum is introduced into the uterine lumen.

It has been suggested that CEM can be transmitted by contamination of the vulva with the causal organism, but experimental evidence (see below) suggests that ascending infection does not take place spontaneously. Coitus or the insertion of a speculum, however, might well displace organisms present on the vulva into the more anterior part of the genital tract and lead to infection of the uterus.

In typical CEM, signs of acute infection become apparent two or more days after service. In the more severe cases there is vulval discharge which is encrusted on the hind quarters and hairs of the tail. Sometimes, however, discharge may be slight or absent, and signs of infection may be seen only on vaginoscopic examination. Usually there are inflammatory changes in the folds of the cervical mucosa and exudation, varying from slight mucoid coating of the cervix to mucopurulent discharge from the cervical canal. There is often some vaginitis, and pools of mucopurulent exudate may be present in the vaginal floor. Infection is not accompanied by pyrexia or other constitutional disturbances (Simpson, 1977). The acute signs of infection usually subside within 1–2 weeks, but in untreated mares uterine infection persists for a variable period after the clinical signs have abated. Eventually infection can no longer be demonstrated in the uterus and some mares become completely free of infection. In others, however, a symptomless carrier state develops. In the Newmarket outbreak in 1977 about 20–25% of the mares thought to have been infected became carriers. Two types of carrier have been recognized:

Uterine carriers are rare and are possibly due to sequestration of infection in the depth of the endometrium, or elsewhere in the reproductive tract, because occasional mares, after a period of apparent freedom from infection, have started once again to excrete the organism from the uterus in association with mucopurulent discharge.

Clitoral carriers constitute the majority of CEM carriers, and recognition of the significance of the clitoris as a site where the organism of CEM may be harboured for long periods has important implications for the control of the disease. The clitoris of the mare contains a deep fossa, partly enclosing the glans clitoridis, and there are small inconspicuous diverticuli, the clitoral sinuses, in the frenulum clitoridis (Simpson and Eaton-Evans, 1978b). The clitoral fossa and sinuses contain smegma-like material and are lined by a glandless epidermoid mucous membrane containing lymphoid tissue. The CEM organism becomes established in the clitoral secretions during the acute exudative stage of the disease and in some mares it persists there for considerable periods. Platt *et al.* (1978a) and Simpson and Eaton-Evans (1978a) isolated the organism from the clitoral fossa after it had been eliminated from other regions of the genital tract. Subsequently, Simpson and Eaton-Evans (1978b) found that sometimes the organism was harboured in the clitoral sinuses even though it could not be isolated from the clitoral fossa. The presence of the organism in the clitoris does not elicit specific local changes or serological response. Whether there is multiplication of the organism is unknown, nor is it clear whether there is any invasion of the superficial layers of the epithelium.

The effects of the disease on fertility can be attributed to acute endometrial inflammation. The duration of the infertile state has not been defined but is probably only a few weeks. Mares which were infected in 1977 conceived readily in 1978, and up to the present there have been no published reports of any long-term effects on fertility. During the outbreak in 1977 occasional mares conceived in spite of exposure to infection but some of these had received intra-uterine antibiotic treatment after service. There is little information on the fertility of clitoral carriers because mares that are found to be carriers are not served until infection has been eliminated by treatment. However, an experimental pony mare which was a symptomless clitoral carrier 11 months after primary infection conceived after a single service and produced a normal foal (Platt and Simpson, unpublished observation). In such a case the organism might be displaced from the clitoris during coitus and re-introduced into the uterus, but endometritis would be unlikely to develop in view of the marked post-infection immunity which the uterus exhibits (Timoney *et al.*, 1979b; Fernie *et al.*, 1980; Sahu *et al.*, 1980).

2. The stallion

The organism of CEM (CEMO) appears to have no pathogenic effects in stallions, but it is clear that it is capable of surviving for a variable, sometimes considerable, period on the surface of the external genitalia.

The organism is harboured particularly in the smegma in the fossa glandis (urethral fossa), a deep fold surrounding the tip of the urethra with a diverticulum, the urethral sinus. In carrier stallions, CEMO can often be cultured also from the terminal urethra and the internal surface of the prepuce. Samples of pre-ejaculatory fluid (the secretion of Cowper's glands) may contain the organism, but this is probably due to contamination in the terminal urethra, since there is no evidence of ascending infection.

The surface of the external genitalia seems to provide a favourable environment for the survival and possibly slow multiplication of the organism.

3. Fetus and placenta

The pathogenicity of CEMO in the pregnant uterus is not clearly defined. In 1977, a few infected mares conceived, but in most of them endometrial infection was probably subsiding or had already been eliminated by the time conception occurred. Newborn foals and placentae from 10 such mares have been examined (Whitwell, 1979; Powell and Whitwell, 1979). Two of these mares had vaginal discharge from which CEMO was isolated during pregnancy, and the remaining 8 were identified as clitoral carriers. The offspring of all these mares were clinically normal, but in the placentae of the two foals whose dams had vaginal discharge, a low-grade chorionitis was present at the cervical pole of the allantochorion and there were raised focal areas in the amnion. CEMO was isolated from the chorion, allantois, and amnion in both cases. It was also found in the prepuce of one of the foals at 36, 48, 86 and 105 days after birth; it was then eliminated by treatment. In two other mares, both clitoral carriers, CEMO was also isolated from the placenta at full term but no placentitis was found. In one it was present in the chorion, allantois and amnion, and in the other as a scanty growth in the chorion alone (Whitwell, 1979 and unpublished).

It is evident that the CEM organism may sometimes invade the placenta, and the possibility of intra-uterine transmission exists but has not yet been conclusively demonstrated. Up to the present, CEMO has not been implicated as a cause of abortion, fetal infection, malformation, or retarded fetal growth. It has not been found in 200 aborted fetuses and young foals submitted for autopsy to the Equine Research Station since 1977, nor in numerous placentae from normal full-term foals unassociated with CEM outbreaks (Whitwell, 1979).

4. Infections in young horses

The CEM organism has occasionally been isolated from the external genitalia of young adult thoroughbreds which, so far as is known, have not been used for breeding. Most of these cases have been colts born in the Republic of Ireland from 1974 onwards, and two were the offspring of the same mare in successive years. In addition to the foal with preputial infection previously mentioned, two colts born in England were identified as CEM carriers when they were 4 years old. Retrospective inquiry revealed that both had been on the same infected stud during the CEM outbreak in 1977. One was born at the stud, and the other arrived there with its dam, 5 days after birth.

The mode of infection in these cases is uncertain, and more than one mechanism may be involved. Some cases possibly arise from congenital infections acquired via the placenta, or from the clitoris of the dam during birth. However during outbreaks of CEM, a more important means of infection, especially for male foals, may be through direct genital contact with straw bedding or pasture contaminated by discharge from infected mares.

5. Susceptibility of non-equine species

(a) Animals

CEMO has not yet been implicated as a cause of spontaneous disease in any species other than the horse. Experimentally, however, the disease can be reproduced in donkeys (Timoney et al., 1979a). Intravaginal inoculation of the organism produced no clinical signs of infection in rabbits, guinea pigs, or mice, but after being introduced into the uterus, CEMO could be isolated for a few days from the genital tract of rabbits and for up to 41 days from mice (Timoney et al., 1978c). Attempts to transmit the infection to heifers, ewes, and a young sow were unsuccessful (Timoney et al., 1978a).

In view of the apparent insusceptibility of cattle, it is of interest that Corbel and Brewer (1980) have found serological reactions to CEMO in a proportion of cattle sera. In the course of a study undertaken to identify potential causative agents of reproductive failure in cattle, they examined 688 sera, 596 of which had been submitted for routine tests for brucellosis and 92 from cases of abortion. Nearly all samples of serum tested contained agglutinins for the CEM organism, titres ranging from 1 in 10 to 1 in 160, with the majority between 1 in 20 and 1 in 40. Furthermore in 13.6% of the samples submitted for routine Brucella testing, presumed to come from healthy animals, and in 5.4% of the samples from animals after abortion, precipitin lines were obtained on diffusion in agar against the CEM organism. Most of the positive samples came from Scotland and South-West England. The authors suggest that the antibody activity they found represented a cross-reaction between antigens of commensal or other organisms and those of the CEM organism.

Currently available evidence indicates that CEM is a natural disease of

Equidae, but information on the susceptibility of most other genera is lacking. That the organism may have susceptible hosts other than the horse and donkey cannot be excluded.

(b) Humans

Attempts to isolate the CEM organism from the genital tract of patients attending clinics for sexually transmitted diseases have been unsuccessful (Taylor and Rosenthal; Taylor-Robinson, personal communications). This may simply reflect technical difficulties or problems in obtaining suitable specimens at the appropriate time. Because of its susceptibility to penicillin and other commonly used antibiotics, the organism would probably be eliminated in treating gonorrhoea, so it is most unlikely to be a cause of post-gonococcal urethritis. Possibly, however, there may be some patients with a condition resembling gonorrhoea, in whom the gonococcus is not found, but who respond to antibiotic treatment, and are regarded as having had a gonococcal infection. Alternatively, the organism of CEM may possibly be transmitted among humans, especially the sexually promiscuous, without causing clinical disease.

Evidence of human infection with the CEM organism, or with organisms antigenically related to it, has been sought serologically. Taylor and Rosenthal (1978a) have looked for agglutinins to the CEM organism in the sera of various population groups. In an initial study of patients attending a genito-medical clinic, including patients with venereal disease, they found agglutinins at a dilution of 1 in 20 or more in 22% of female patients and 13% of male patients. These figures compared with 7% and 4% for healthy female and male blood donors respectively and only 2% for women attending antenatal clinics. In contrast, they did not find any evidence of agglutinins at the same dilution in the sera of four veterinary surgeons who had had particularly close contact with infected horses.

Wilkinson and Rodin (1978) tested 423 sera from similar groups of patients by an indirect fluorescence antibody test. A total of 49 (11.6%) were positive at a dilution of 1 in 20 or more, comprising 35/248 (14.1%) male and 11/114 (9.7%) female patients attending a venereal disease clinic, and 3/61 (5%) of women attending antenatal clinics. The authors concluded that antibody reactive with the CEM organism is present in the sera of an appreciable number of patients attending an urban venereal disease clinic.

Taylor and Rosenthal (1978b) tested the sera of 220 men with non-gonococcal urethritis (NGU): 37% were found to have agglutinins to the CEM organism at a dilution of 1 in 20, and several had titres greater than 1 in 20 — some as high as 1 in 320. Both groups of authors point out that such serological results must be interpreted with caution. They do not necessarily mean that those concerned had been infected by the CEM organism: the agglutinins might equally well be due to cross-reaction with other, undetermined, organisms sharing common antigens with the CEM organism.

In a further study, in 223 patients with NGU, Taylor *et al.* (1979) found agglutinins in the sera of 84 (37.6%); in 12.5% of patients there was a four-fold or greater rise in titre during the course of their illness. There was no evidence that these agglutinins resulted from infection by chlamydiae or ureaplasmas. Certain patients with agglutinins seemed to respond better to therapy with antibiotics effective against the CEM bacterium *in vitro* than patients without agglutinins. The findings suggest that the CEM bacterium or a microorganism related to it may be aetiologically involved in a proportion of patients with NGU.

In contrast to these findings, Mardh *et al.* (1980) did not find serum agglutinins in 40 consecutive Swedish male patients with NGU or in 30 patients with sexually acquired reactive arthritis. They point out the difficulty in interpreting agglutination tests with the CEM organism and the need to examine serum for antibodies by another technique.

Füzi (1980) suggested that genital infections with *Haemophilus influenzae* and *Haemophilus parainfluenzae* might account for some of the serological responses to the CEM organism that have been reported in patients with NGU. Some degree of cross-reactivity between the CEM organism and *H. influenzae*, and also with *Haemophilus influenzaemurium*, was described by Taylor *et al.* (1978), although the reactions with *H. influenzae* were found only with recent isolates and not with the type strain. Füzi reported that *H. influenzae* and *H. parainfluenzae* can often be isolated from the genital tract in patients with sexually transmitted diseases and drew attention to the evidence that they may sometimes be pathogenic. In other cases, infections may be mild or asymptomatic with persistent excretion of the organisms in genital discharges or urine.

B.   Experimental transmission of CEM

1.   Mares

Several groups of investigators have reproduced CEM experimentally by introducing pure cultures of streptomycin-resistant strains of CEMO into the uterus of healthy mares (Platt *et al.*, 1978b; Timoney *et al.*, 1978b; Dawson *et al.*, 1978; Pierson *et al.*, 1978; Ricketts, 1979). The disease produced was very similar to that of field cases of CEM (Fig. 1).

The incubation period after experimental infection ranged from 1–4 days. The response varied in severity in different animals and sometimes was relatively inconspicuous. In some, the changes tended to be more exudative than inflammatory. In most instances, clinical signs of infection had subsided within two weeks, but infection of the uterus persisted for a variable period

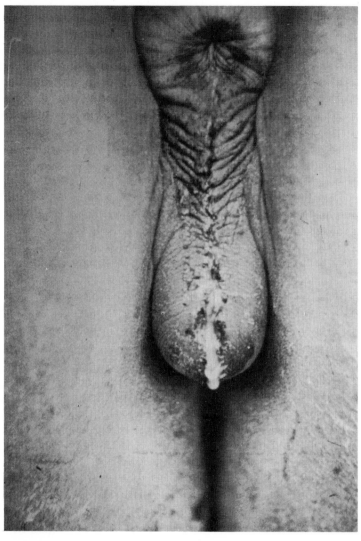

Fig. 1 Vulval discharge in a pony mare, 7 days after intra-uterine inoculation with the organism of CEM. (Courtesy of Mr D. J. Simpson.)

after clinical abatement. Usually, infection was eliminated from the uterus spontaneously within 4–6 weeks but sometimes it persisted for as long as 4 months. Even in severely affected animals, no pyrexia or other constitutional disturbances were detected except occasionally some transient neutrophilia or leucocytosis.

After disappearance of the organism from the uterus, some animals became free of infection, but in others symptomless infection persisted in the clitoris. In experiments at the Equine Research Station, Newmarket, four out of eight ponies inoculated with streptomycin-resistant strains developed clitoral infection for periods varying from 85–677 days after disappearance of the organism from the uterus. The mare infected for 677 days eventually eliminated the organism spontaneously, and at 1001 days was free from detectable infection.

In experimental infections with streptomycin-sensitive strains of CEMO (Platt and Simpson, unpublished) there were differences in response between the two deposited streptomycin-sensitive strains (NCTC 11225 and NCTC 11226). Infection with NCTC 11226 produced acute endometritis similar in character and severity to the effects of the streptomycin-resistant type strain NCTC 11184, and the organism could be isolated from the uterus until 28 days after infection. In contrast, NCTC 11225, inoculated at an approximately similar dose (3×10^8 CFU) gave rise to changes of minimum clinical severity without obvious purulent exudate and only slight cervicitis. The organism was still present in the uterus at 24 days after infection when the animal was humanely killed. Isolation of these streptomycin-sensitive strains from the mixed flora of the clitoris on unselective media presented considerable difficulty (Dr M. E. Mackintosh, personal communication). Nevertheless, it is reasonable to assume that some animals may harbour streptomycin-sensitive strains of CEMO in the clitoris after clinical recovery and that clitoral carriers of these strains may exist.

Attempts to produce the disease by deposition of streptomycin-resistant strains of the organism in the clitoris or the urethral vestibule were unsuccessful, with cultured organisms, infective exudate, or an infected clitoral swab (Platt and Simpson, unpublished). In these experiments, care was taken to avoid mechanical displacement of the inoculum into the more anterior regions of the genital tract, and the animals were not examined vaginoscopically for at least 2 weeks. During this time there were no external signs of infection, and the organism was not found in cervical swabs taken at 2–3 weeks after inoculation. There was also no serological evidence of infection. The organism deposited in the clitoris appeared not to multiply and after 7–18 days could no longer be recovered.

The organism also failed to survive for more than 3–9 days after introduction into the conjunctival sacs or nasal passages and could not be re-isolated from the mouth after oral inoculation. No evidence of local or other infection was observed in these experiments and serological conversion was not detectable. Neither transmission of infection nor serological conversion was found in a healthy mare housed in the same loose-box with infected mares (Platt and Simpson, unpublished).

2. Stallions and colts

Four pony colts were experimentally infected by introducing a streptomycin-resistant strain of the CEM organism (NCTC 11184) into the fossa glandis. None showed clinical signs of infection, but the organism survived in the external genitalia for varying periods. At autopsy performed on one pony after 3 weeks the organism was recovered from the fossa glandis, terminal urethra and prepuce. In two ponies, infection persisted at least 28 and 46 days respectively before disappearing spontaneously. The fourth animal was still infected after 28 months, and at autopsy, the organism was recovered in profusion from the fossa glandis and terminal urethra, in small numbers from the inguinal skin, but not from the prepuce. In the two ponies examined at autopsy, infection had remained localized near the site of inoculation, and although extensive histological and bacteriological examinations of the genito-urinary tract were made, no evidence of tissue invasion or ascending infection was detected (Platt et al., 1978b and unpublished observations).

One of the stallions was allowed to serve a healthy mare while still infected. The mare developed typical CEM 2 days later.

The establishment and persistence of infection on the external genital skin of the male probably depend upon several factors, but the number of organisms acquired seems to be especially important. An uninfected stallion which served a clitoral carrier mare was swabbed immediately post coitum and the organism was recovered from several sites on the surface of the penis but the following day and subsequently, it could no longer be demonstrated in the external genitalia.

C. The pathology of CEM in the mare

The pathology of CEM has been studied at autopsy of pony mares after experimental infections (Platt et al., 1978b) and in endometrial biopsies from field cases of CEM (Ricketts et al., 1978; Samuel et al., 1979).

From autopsy studies it was evident that the principal lesions were in the uterus; no significant changes were found in the fallopian tubes, fimbriae, ovaries, the urinary tract, or elsewhere in the body. In the uterus, there was widespread endometritis with local erosion of surface epithelium (Fig. 2), but the glands were unaffected. Surviving epithelium often appeared pseudostratified with "foamy" epithelial cells containing intracytoplasmic droplets of

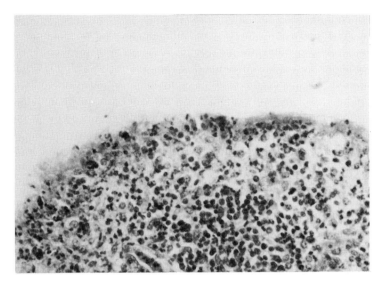

Fig. 2   Epithelial erosion and acute endometritis in the uterus of a pony mare, 4 days after intra-uterine inoculation with the organism of CEM (NCTC 11184). H & E × 425.

mucin. In the acute stage of infection, there were subepithelial vacuoles, and the endometrial stroma was oedematous and densely infiltrated by polymorphs, eosinophils, and mononuclear cells. There was emigration of polymorphs into the uterine lumen where a profuse purulent exudate was present (Fig. 3). The acute endometrial changes subsided fairly rapidly and endometrial regeneration took place from glandular and surviving luminal epithelium.

Ricketts *et al.* (1978) and Samuel *et al.* (1979) observed similar changes in endometrial biopsies. By electronmicroscopy, they found nuclear enlargement, cytoplasmic vacuolation and apical blebs in ciliated and microvillous cells of the epithelium; ciliary clumping, myelin figures, and inclusions resembling lysosomes were also seen. The plasma membranes were fragmented or detached, and there was loss of apical microvilli.

In chronic clitoral carriers, histological examination of the clitoris revealed some infiltration of macrophages and plasma cells into the epithelium, but the specificity and significance of these changes were doubtful (Platt, unpublished observations).

From these findings, it appears that the specialized epithelium of the uterus is the predilection site for CEMO, while the squamous epithelium in other regions of the genital tract appears to be resistant to the infection.

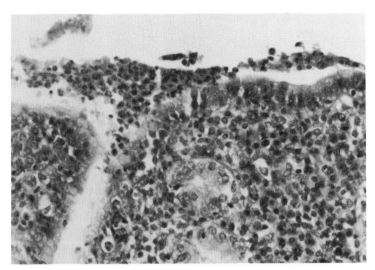

Fig. 3 Acute endometritis and purulent exudation into the uterine lumen in a pony mare 4 days after intra-uterine inoculation with the organism of CEM (NCTC 11184). H & E × 435.

D.   Immunological responses and immunity in CEM

1.   Humoral antibody

In primary infections with CEMO serum antibodies appear and can be demonstrated by several techniques. In field cases, Benson *et al.* (1978) titrated antibody by direct agglutination and antiglobulin techniques, using an antigen prepared by boiling CEMO in isotonic saline for 2 hours followed by suspension in 0.5% phenol-saline. The antibody response was also studied in two experimentally infected ponies (Dawson *et al.*, 1978) in both of which agglutinin and/or antiglobulin titres began to rise at 7 days and reached peaks between 21 and 24 days; thereafter they steadily declined. In one pony only low agglutination and antiglobulin titres were found but there was a good complement fixation (CF) titre. In the other animal there was a significant titre in all three tests. Antibody tended to persist in a significant amount for longer in CF than in agglutination and antiglobulin tests. Croxton-Smith *et al.* (1978) found that in 5 of 6 mares CF antibody was still demonstrable after 6 months. Bryans *et al.* (1979), using a CF antigen which appeared to be associated with the bacterial surface, confirmed these findings, and found that significant titres sometimes remained for as long as 244 days.

Fernie *et al.* (1979) have developed a passive haemagglutination test that includes the use of formalinized, tanned turkey erythrocytes sensitized with an extract of sonicated organisms.

Serological surveys for antibody against CEMO have been based on agglutination, antiglobulin, complement fixation, and passive haemagglutination tests. Antibody can be demonstrated in only a few recovered animals and chronic clitoral carriers: of 1140 mares which had been exposed to CEM in the previous 1–2 years, 4.7% were serologically positive in one or more of these tests (Frank, 1979b).

An enzyme-linked immunosorbent assay (ELISA), developed by Sahu *et al.* (1979b), detected antibody at higher dilutions of serum than did other techniques, and some sera which gave negative results by tube agglutination, plate agglutination or antiglobulin techniques had significant titres of antibody by the ELISA method.

2. Antibody in genital mucus

Local antibody, demonstrable in vaginal mucus 2–3 weeks after experimental infection and in field cases of the disease, may reach high titres (Platt, unpublished data; Timoney *et al.*, 1979b). This antibody has not yet been characterized immunochemically. The persistence of local antibody has not been determined, and there is insufficient evidence on which to assess its usefulness as a means of detecting carrier animals.

3. Post-infection and -vaccination immunity

After recovery from CEM, mares are relatively resistant to re-infection. When the organism is re-introduced into the uterus after several months, the clinical response is less than in primary infections and the numbers of organisms recoverable from the genital tract is reduced (Timoney *et al.*, 1979b). In mares challenged after 7–15 months, Fernie *et al.* (1980) also observed a reduced clinical response and found that re-infection of the endometrium either did not occur or was less severe than in primary infections. In the same study, four previously uninfected ponies were vaccinated with a formalinized culture of the streptomycin-resistant type strain of the organism (NCTC 11184). Although they developed good humoral antibody responses, three reacted with typical signs of CEM when challenged by intra-uterine inoculation. However, the severity of the clinical response and the degree of bacterial shedding were less in the vaccinated ponies than in unvaccinated control ponies. There was no close correlation, either in the vaccinated or the recovered ponies, between the response to challenge and the amounts of humoral antibody before re-infection. It seems likely that serum antibody plays a less important role than local antibody and cell-mediated immunity in determining resistance. Similar findings in vaccinated ponies have been reported by Sahu (1981).

In experiments with mice, and using implanted plastic chambers, Arko and Wong (1980) were able to induce some degree of immunity to CEMO by vaccination. They found that the immune response did not depend upon complement and suggested that antibody-complement-mediated bacteriolysis may be less important than cell-mediated immunity. However, the mechanism of immunity was not fully defined, and some differences were noted between CEMO and *Neisseria gonorrhoeae* as regards the state of immunity and the ability of organisms to survive in the chambers.

IV. DISTRIBUTION AND PROVENANCE OF CEM

Knowledge of the geographical distribution of CEM is still incomplete because in many countries surveys for its presence that have included appropriate bacteriological methods have not been undertaken. In Europe it has been recognized in the UK, the Republic of Ireland, France, Germany, Belgium, Italy, Yugoslavia, Denmark and Austria. It is also present in Australia, the USA and Japan (Table 1).

In the UK the disease is believed to have been introduced in 1977 with infected carrier mares, probably from the Republic of Ireland. This has not been established with certainty, since mares from several countries were present on the affected stud during the outbreak at Newmarket, but an unusual genital infection, clinically similar to CEM, was present on several Thoroughbred studs in the Republic of Ireland in 1976 (O'Driscoll *et al.*, 1977).

The outbreaks in Thoroughbreds in the USA in 1978 resulted from the importation of infected carrier stallions from France (Knowles, 1979), and in 1979 there was an outbreak in Missouri on a Trakehner stud following importation of a Trakehner stallion from West Germany (Fales *et al.*, 1979). In Australia, the disease was probably present before 1977 and is believed to have originated from Europe although details of the source of infection are lacking (Hazard *et al.*, 1979). Thoroughbred breeding in Japan has developed only recently, from horses imported over several years from the UK, the Republic of Ireland, France, the USA and other countries with established Thoroughbred populations. The source of CEM infection in Japan has not been made known.

It is likely that CEM had existed in the Republic of Ireland, France, Australia and probably some other countries for an unknown period before 1977. It seems unlikely, however, that it could have been present in the Republic of Ireland for very long because of the considerable interchange of Thoroughbred and other horses between that country and the UK. No evidence has emerged to suggest that CEM existed in the UK before 1977. Moreover, the infectivity and severity of the disease in the Newmarket

Table 1 Reported geographical distribution of CEM

Region	Breeds and types of horse						References
	Thoroughbred	Trakehner	Trotter	Half-bred	Pony	Not known	
WESTERN EUROPE							
UK	*(R)	—	—	—	—	—	Platt et al. (1977)
Eire	*(R)	—	—	—	—	—	Timoney et al. (1977)
France	*(R) (S[a])	—	*	*	*	—	Pitre et al. (1979)
Germany	—	*(S)[a]	*(R) (S)	*(S)	—	—	Blobel et al. (1978) / Blobel et al. (1979) / Mumme & Ahlswede (1979) / Sonnenschein & Klug (1979)
Belgium	—	—	*(S)	—	—	—	
Italy	*(R)	—	—	—	—	—	Codazza et al. (1980)
Yugoslavia	—	—	—	—	—	*(S)	
Denmark	—	—	*(S)	—	—	—	
Austria	—	—	*(R)	—	—	—	Anon (1981)
AMERICA							
USA	*(R) (S)	*(S)	—	—	—	—	Swerczerk (1978a,c) / Fales et al. (1979)
AUSTRALASIA							
Australia	*(R)	—	—	—	—	—	Hughes et al. (1978) / Hazard et al. (1979)
ASIA							
Japan	*(R)	—	—	—	—	—	Sugimoto et al. (1980) / Kikuchi et al. (1982)

[a] Inferred from epidemiological evidence on outbreaks in USA.
* CEM organism isolated; R=Streptomycin-resistant strain; S=Streptomycin-sensitive strain.
— No reported isolations.

outbreak suggest that the mares on the affected stud were highly susceptible and without immunological experience of the infection.

At present there is a paucity of information on the prevalence of the infection in most countries, especially in types of horses where there is no economic incentive to investigate the causes of genital infections in detail. CEM may well be present in some horse populations as an endemic infection, perhaps masquerading as other types of genital infection, of which the causal agents can be more readily demonstrated. In several European countries, the disease is present in trotters, riding horses and ponies. Both streptomycin-resistant and streptomycin-sensitive strains of CEMO have been isolated from these breeds. It may well be that CEM has existed in certain types of horse for a considerable period, and introduction of infection into the Thoroughbred breed was a relatively recent event.

V. TREATMENT AND CONTROL OF CEM

A. Treatment

Most mares with acute CEM recover spontaneously without treatment and eventually eliminate the organism from the endometrium after a variable period. Usually, however, treatment is given to curtail infection of the uterus, to avert development of the carrier state, and so reduce the risk of spread of the disease.

Treatment usually consists in uterine infusion on several occasions with solutions of chlorhexidine, or with penicillin, ampicillin or other antibiotics, in conjunction with topical treatment of the clitoris. In the acute stage, parenteral antibiotic treatment has also been used (Crowhurst *et al.*, 1979).

B. Control

In 1977, a UK working party chaired by Sir David Evans DSc, FRS was set up by the Horserace Betting Levy Board to co-ordinate research on the disease and to formulate a policy for its control. It was recognized from an early stage that effective control depended upon prompt and accurate diagnosis of the disease and the identification of carrier animals before service. A favourable circumstance was the fact that the disease in the UK was confined to Thoroughbred horses, the movements of which are closely supervised. The principal objective was to ensure that all mares going to stud, and all stallions, were free from infection. In order to achieve this, and in view of the carrier state that may exist in apparently healthy animals, the need for repeated bacteriological tests was recognized as imperative. A Code of

Practice prescribing the tests to be carried out on mares and stallions was drawn up to ensure, as far as possible, freedom from infection and to define the prevalence of the organism in the bloodstock population.

The Code of Practice for the breeding season of 1978 recommended that, from mares, swabs should be obtained from the cervix and urethra, and, from stallions, from the prepuce, urethra, and urethral fossa (fossa glandis), as well as of pre-ejaculatory fluid. In mares, the requirements were later extended when the importance of the clitoris as the principal site for carriage of the organism was recognized. Fortunately, this became known before the opening of the 1978 breeding season, when it was further advised that pregnant mares which might have been exposed to infection in 1977 should be isolated until they had foaled and been shown to be free from infection. In the event of abortion, the fetus and placenta were to be submitted to laboratory examination for the presence of CEMO. Recommendations were also made for improving the standards of hygiene on stud farms, and the practice of "walking-in" of mares for service was discouraged. To ensure that adequate facilities were widely available in the UK, about 40 laboratories were recognized, on the basis of their performance in a quality control scheme organized by the Ministry of Agriculture, Fisheries and Food, as centres where swabs could be examined for the presence of CEMO in order to comply with the Code of Practice.

The universal acceptance of these proposals reflected a recognition of the potential seriousness of the disease. In the period between 1st September 1977 and 31st July 1978, swabs were examined in the UK from 17 306 Thoroughbred mares, 1046 Thoroughbred stallions and about 2500 non-Thoroughbred horses. The CEM organism was isolated from 52 Thoroughbred mares and 2 Thoroughbred stallions during this period; it was not found in any of the non-Thoroughbred horses. Forty-nine of the infected mares were carriers and were detected before service. Three were acute cases sampled during two small outbreaks of CEM in the spring of 1978. Each outbreak resulted from the presence of an undetected carrier mare (Powell et al., 1978).

It was evident that the disease in the UK was probably confined to Thoroughbred horses and that nearly all isolations of the organism were from animals which had been on studs known to have been infected in 1977. Some others had been on studs in the Republic of Ireland or France, and in three mares the source of infection could not be identified.

Modified Codes of Practice were adopted for the 1979 and 1980 breeding seasons. There were two outbreaks in England in 1979, each arising from undetected carrier mares, and in 1980 no outbreaks were reported although several mares were identified as carriers before being served (Table 2). Some of these were mares involved in outbreaks the previous year, or which had been

Table 2 Reported CEM in Thoroughbred horses in the United Kingdom (1977–1981)

| | | | Outbreaks | Incidence of carriers (carriers/nos examined bacteriologically) | | |
	Studs	Animals	Mares	Stallions and colts	Total	
Spring 1977	29	200–250	—	—	—
Sept 1977– July 1978	2	4	49/17 303 (0.28%)	2/1046 (0.19%)	51/18 349 (0.28%)
Sept 1978– July 1979	2	20	11/13 389 (0.08%)	0/872 (0%)	11/14 261 (0.08%)
Sept 1979– July 1980	0	0	8/13 848 (0.06%)	1/887 (0.11%)	9/14 735 (0.06%)
Sept 1980– July 1981	1	23	0/13 483 (0%)	0/330 (0%)	0/14 562 (0%)

Powell *et al.* (1978); Frank (1979a); Anon (1980).

imported. In 1981 there was one outbreak, probably due to an undetected carrier mare.

Control measures similar to those adopted in the UK have been applied in the Republic of Ireland and other countries. Experience of the disease since 1977 has shown that its control depends principally upon detecting symptomless carrier animals, but until more information becomes available on the distribution of the disease in various countries, the dangers of re-importation of infection will remain.

At present, diagnosis of the disease rests upon bacteriological identification of the causal agent. However, the organism is fastidious, and unless careful attention is paid to maintaining optimum conditions for its cultivation, its presence in swabs, especially those from carrier animals, may escape detection. This is particularly so in respect of the streptomycin-sensitive strains. Isolation of these strains may pose no particular problem in acute cases of the disease, when the organisms are present in the uterus in large numbers, often in more or less pure culture, but their detection in carrier mares and stallions may present considerable problems, because the sites where the organism is harboured have an abundant local flora which may overgrow or inhibit cultures of the organism. For the isolation of streptomycin-resistant strains, streptomycin-containing media can be used, but selective media applicable to streptomycin-sensitive strains are still being developed (see p. 87).

VI. CHARACTERISTICS OF THE CAUSAL ORGANISM OF CEM

A. Microscopy

In Gram-stained smears of pus from the cervix uteri of infected mares, appearances are those of a typical Gram-negative coccobacillus with occasional short filamentous forms. Most of the organisms are free-lying, but occasionally some may be found phagocytosed in polymorphonuclear leucocytes (Fig. 4). Under appropriate conditions of cultivation (see below), the organism is a Gram-negative, non-acid-fast, non-motile coccobacillus with a mean diameter of 0.8 μm (range 0.7–1.0 μm) with occasional filaments 5–6 μm in length.

The organism has been studied morphologically by means of transmission and scanning electronmicroscopy (Taylor *et al.*, 1978; Swaney and Breese, 1980). In scanning electronmicrographs Swaney and Breese reported differences in bacterial morphology in primary cultures from cervical exudate, according to the culture medium on which the organisms had been growing. Bacteria cultivated on heated blood ("chocolate") agar containing tryptose

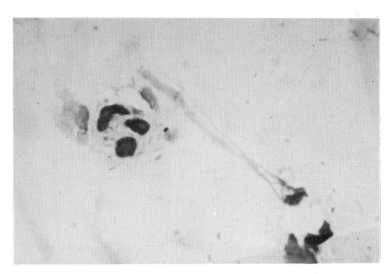

Fig. 4 CEM organisms in exudate from the cervix uteri of an infected mare. Some of the organisms have been phagocytosed by a polymorph. Gram ×1550.

were predominantly coccal in shape, whereas those taken from heated blood ("chocolate") agar containing Eugon were more rodlike. Apparently the composition of the growth medium influenced the predominant shape of the organisms during their first passage from an infected mare. It was further evident that some cells taken from both media adhered to one another. In electronmicroscopy studies (Taylor *et al.*, 1978; Swaney and Breese, 1980) neither pili nor flagellae were observed.

The proportion of coccal to bacillary forms and the length of the bacillary forms appear to depend on the culture medium and possibly the conditions of incubation and age of the culture. It is well-known that with *H. influenzae* coccal forms predominate when the organism has been growing under preferential conditions, as in cerebrospinal fluid *in vivo* in a patient with meningitis, whereas rod-shaped and filamentous forms often appear in old cultures (Wilson and Miles, 1975b) and in cultures of sputum from patients with chronic bronchitis.

In negatively stained preparations in the electron microscope, the surface of the organism bears a coarse pattern of wrinkles (Taylor *et al.*, 1978; Swaney and Breese, 1980), as in many Gram-negative bacteria (Glauert and Thornley, 1969) (Fig. 5). The surface pattern on the organism of CEM does not appear to be in any way characteristic.

Swaney and Breese (1980) have studied the ultrastructure of the organism in considerable detail. In thin sections stained with uranyl acetate, a multilayered cell membrane was evident. The outer membrane was slightly wavy, and in places small fibres appeared to be attached to it. In thin sections stained with ruthenium red, readily distinguishable outer and cytoplasmic membranes, as well as a dense intermediate layer, were evident. The stain also revealed a fringe 20 to 30 nm wide composed of threads around the outside of the organism. These threads did not obscure the outline of the outer membrane and were regarded by Swaney and Breese as capsular material. The outer and cytoplasmic membranes were triple-layered, each layer being about 7 nm in width. The dense intermediate layer was about 4 nm wide and was separated from the outer membrane by a thin, electronlucent zone, giving a bilaminar appearance.

In thin sections of organisms that had been allowed to react with ferritin-tagged antibody before being stained with uranyl acetate, ferritin particles formed a layer 15 to 20 nm from the outer membrane. This distance corresponds approximately to the width of the structure revealed by ruthenium red staining, regarded by Swaney and Breese as a capsule, and visible to a lesser extent in areas lacking ferritin but clearly demonstrated in thin sections additionally stained with ruthenium red.

After heating the organism, suspended in phosphate buffered saline, for four hours at 90–97°C, the outer membrane was indistinguishable in thin sections stained with uranyl acetate. The dense intermediate layer surrounded the cytoplasmic membrane and in some cells was separated from it. However, in sections stained by ruthenium red, outer membranes that had become detached during the process of heating were visible and appeared grossly stretched and distorted, although still surrounding the cells. Furthermore, the capsular material was not demonstrable, which would suggest that it had dissolved in the phosphate-buffered saline during heating. Cytoplasmic membranes were still surrounded by the dense intermediate layer.

Although capsules have not been observed with the light microscope in preparations of the organism mixed with Indian ink, the evidence presented by Swaney and Breese strongly suggests that under appropriate conditions the organism produces a capsular substance. Its reaction with ruthenium red suggests that it contains an acidic polysaccharide (Luft, 1971).

It is worth noting in retrospect that, although not mentioned by the authors, a structure suggesting a capsule may be seen in the electronmicrographs published earlier by Taylor *et al.* (1978) (Fig. 6). Professor R. W. Horne, who was responsible for these electronmicrographs, did in fact draw attention to this structure (personal communication), but the authors did not feel that the evidence for a capsule at that time was sufficiently strong to warrant mention of it.

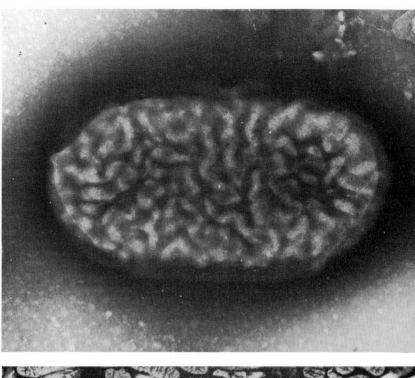

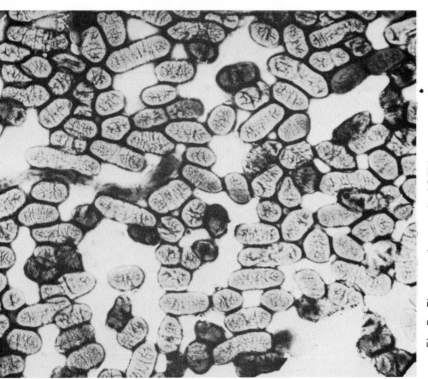

Fig. 5 Electron micrograph of CEM organisms (NCTC 11184) negatively stained with phosphotungstic acid. *Left* × 9000; *right* × 80 000. (Courtesy of Dr T. G. Wreghitt.)

B. Isolation, growth requirements and cultural characteristics

The CEM organism was first isolated and recognised as the likely cause of CEM in the Public Health Laboratory, Cambridge, UK in May 1977. Smears from swabs of cervical exudate were stained by Gram's method, and then each swab was inoculated on two plates of blood agar, one plate of heated blood ("chocolate") agar and one plate of MacConkey agar. All these cultures, except for one of the blood agar plates, were incubated at 37°C in an atmosphere of air containing 5–10% V/V carbon dioxide. One of the blood agar plates relating to each swab was incubated anaerobically in an atmosphere of hydrogen 90% and carbon dioxide 10% V/V plus a palladium catalyst. After 66 hours, small colonies about 0.5 mm diameter were observed on the heated blood ("chocolate") agar that had been incubated in an atmosphere of air containing 5–10% V/V carbon dioxide. In 9 of 10 mares examined initially, a heavy and in most cases a pure growth of the putative pathogen was obtained. It was clear from the circumstances surrounding the first isolation of the organism that it was relatively fastidious as regards nutritional requirements and atmospheric conditions. In particular, heated blood ("chocolate") agar contained one or more substances, not present in unheated blood agar, which improved growth; also an atmosphere composed of 5–10% V/V carbon dioxide in air was preferable to one composed of 10% V/V carbon dioxide in hydrogen with a palladium catalyst. Subsequently, it was reported from the UK National Collection of Type Cultures that cultures incubated at 37°C for three to four days in a McIntosh and Fildes' jar evacuated to 570 mmHg and refilled with 90% hydrogen and 10% V/V carbon dioxide, but with the palladium catalyst omitted (i.e. micro-aerophilic conditions), yielded more growth initially than either aerobic or strictly anaerobic conditions or those of an incubator containing an atmosphere of 5–10% V/V carbon dioxide in air. This report from the UK National Collection of Type Cultures has apparently caused the organism to be regarded as micro-aerophilic. Nevertheless, after several subcultures in the UK National Collection of Type Cultures, the organism was propagated in an incubator containing an atmosphere of 5–10% V/V carbon dioxide in air. It is therefore questionable whether the organism can be correctly described as micro-aerophilic, for this would imply that micro-aerophilic conditions are obligatory for growth, as they are for example with *Campylobacter jejuni*.

Swabs from the urethra, the urethral fossa and the prepuce of each of six apparently healthy stallions which had served infected mares, together with a swab that had been dipped into a freshly collected sample of pre-ejaculatory fluid, were similarly processed at the Public Health Laboratory, Cambridge. After 24 hours of incubation, the culture plates were found to be heavily overgrown with a mixed flora that included *Proteus* spp., coliform bacilli,

Staphylococcus aureus, micrococci and faecal streptococci, all presumed to be derived from the normal external genital flora of the stallions. It was quickly discovered, however, that the strains of the putative pathogen were resistant to more than 512 mg l^{-1} streptomycin. The stallions were therefore re-sampled and the swabs inoculated on heated blood ("chocolate") agar medium containing 100 mg l^{-1} streptomycin. When the plates were incubated at 37°C in an atmosphere of air containing 5–10% carbon dioxide V/V, an

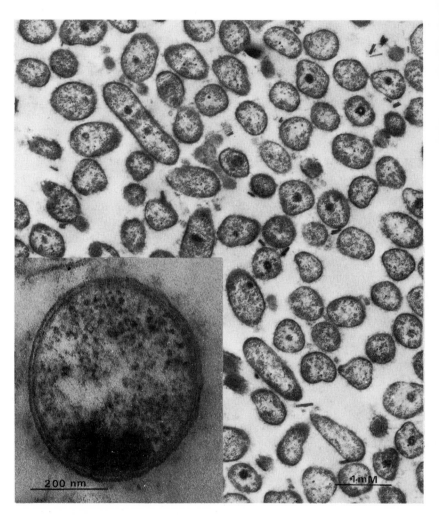

Fig. 6 Electron micrograph of ultra-thin section of CEM organisms (NCTC 11184). (Courtesy of Prof. R. W. Horne.)

organism morphologically indistinguishable from that isolated from the mares was isolated from one or more sites in each stallion. Subsequently, the strains isolated from the stallions were shown to be biochemically and otherwise similar to those isolated from the infected mares. Gram-stained smears of the swabs taken from stallions proved of little help in revealing the presence of the putative pathogen because of the many contaminating organisms.

On heated blood ("chocolate") agar incubated at 37°C in an atmosphere of air containing 5–10% carbon dioxide V/V, small opalescent glistening colonies less than 0.5 mm in diameter appear within 48 hours. On further incubation, colonies reach a maximum size of 1–2 mm in diameter in three to four days (Fig. 7). A high degree of humidity does not improve growth. On prolonged incubation, colonies retain an entire edge and the surface remains un-differentiated. When touched with a straight wire, colonies have a mainly butyrous consistency but with a slight "stickiness". According to Sahu and Dardiri (1980), colonies glided on the agar surface when pushed with a loop and gelled in water, colonies up to 5 days of age gelling faster than older colonies.

Growth has been observed over the temperature range of 30–41°C with an optimum of 37°C, but is very poor or absent at 22°C (Taylor *et al.*, 1978).

The ability of the organism to grow on various media after several subcultures was investigated in the UK National Collection of Type Cultures and the results are shown in Table 3. Of those media tested, the best for supporting growth was heated Columbia blood ("chocolate") agar (Columbia base: Ellner *et al.*, 1966), but varying degrees of growth were obtained also on unheated blood agar, serum agar, starch agar, casein agar, egg-yolk (LV) agar, and Casman's blood agar. Media not supporting growth included MacConkey agar, poly-β-hydroxy-butyrate agar, Tween agars (Tween 20, 40, 80), 3.5% W/V sodium chloride agar, and 1% W/V glycine agar. Initially, growth was not observed on nutrient agar, but in X, V and XV requirement tests, made on nutrient agar, and with prolonged incubation (14 days), a film of growth was seen, with some stimulation of growth around the X and XV discs but not around the V disc. Unlike Shreeve (1978), however, the organism was not found to be *dependent* on either X or V factors. A lack of dependence on X factor was judged by a positive result with the D-amino-laevulinic acid test (Kilian, 1976). Furthermore, Dr M. Kilian (Aarhus, Denmark) confirmed a lack of dependency on X or V factors for growth of the organism (personal communication).

The film of growth on nutrient agar after prolonged incubation could be explained by the presence of a very small amount of X factor, either as a contaminant in the medium, or as a result of transfer in the inoculum from medium containing X factor.

Table 3 Characteristics of the CEM organism and description of the type strain: NCTC 11184

GROWTH ON (OR AT)

Columbia 'chocolate' blood agar	+ (preferred)
Columbia unheated blood agar	+
'Chocolate' blood agar	+
Unheated blood agar	±
Columbia serum agar	±
Nutrient agar, 14 d	±
Nutrient agar, 14 d, plus X factor	± (some stimulation)
Nutrient agar, 14 d, plus V factor	± (no stimulation)
Nutrient agar, 14 d, plus XV factors	± (some stimulation)
Starch agar	±
Casein agar	±
[a]Egg-Yolk (LV) agar	±
[a]Tween 20, 40, 80 agars	−
MacConkey agar	−
Poly-β-hydroxybutyrate agar	−
[a]3.5% NaCl agar	−
[a]1% glycine agar	−
'Chocolate' blood agar, aerobic incubation	±
'Chocolate' blood agar, anaerobic incubation	±
[a]'Chocolate' blood agar, microaerophilic incubation	+
[a]'Chocolate' blood agar, 5% CO_2 in air incubation	+
[a]'Chocolate' blood agar, aerobic, added moisture	±
22°C	±
30°C	+
37°C	+ (optimum)
41°C	+

MISCELLANEOUS CHARACTERISTICS

Motility (22°C, 30°C, 37°C)	−
Haemolysis, horse blood agar	−
[a]D-aminolaevulinic acid test	+
Slide agglutinations with:	
(a) Brucella abortus, unabsorbed antiserum	−
(b) Brucella abortus, absorbed antiserum	−
(c) Brucella melitensis, absorbed antiserum	−
(d) Brucella ovis antiserum	−
(e) 1 in 500 acriflavine	+
Tube agglutinations with NTC 11184 antiserum (see Table 4)	
Slide agglutinations with NCTC 11184 antiserum (see Table 5)	
Susceptibility to antimicrobial agents (see Table 6)	

BIOCHEMICAL CHARACTERISTICS

[a]Cytochrome oxidase production	+
[a]Catalase production	+
Starch hydrolysis	—
Casein hydrolysis	—
[a]Urease production	—
Lecithinase production	No growth
Aesculin hydrolysis	No growth
Gelatinase production (tube test)	—
Gelatinase production (plate test, heavy inoculum)	—
Hydrogen sulphide production, lead acetate strips over:	
(a) chocolate blood agar slopes	—
(b) peptone water, nutrient broth	No growth
Indole production:	
(a) oxalic acid strip over chocolate blood agar slope	—
[b](b) in peptone water, Kovac's reagent	—
(c) in 5% serum peptone water, Ehrlich's reagent	—
[b]Nitrate reduction	—
Nitrite reduction (5% serum added to nitrite broth)	—
Nitrate reduction (Cook's, 1950)	—
Citrate utilization (Koser's)	—
Serum liquefaction (Loeffler's)	—
Arginine desimidase (Thornley, 1960)	—
Arginine dihydrolase (Moller, 1955)	—
Lysine decarboxylase (Moller, 1955)	—
Ornithine decarboxylase (Moller, 1955)	—
[a]Methyl red and Voges-Proskauer	No growth
[a]Gluconate oxidation	No growth
[a]Malonate utilization	No growth
[a]Phenylalanine deamination	No growth
Deoxyribonuclease production (heavy inoculum)	—
β-galactosidase production	—
Phosphatase	+
Acid from:	
glucose (Neisseria media)	—
maltose (Neisseria media)	—
sucrose (Neisseria media)	—
glucose, aerobic (Hugh and Leifson, 1953, medium)	—
glucose, anaerobic (Hugh and Leifson, 1953, medium)	—
glucose (serum water medium)	—
glucose (peptone water medium)	No growth
glucose (ammonium salt medium)	No growth
glucose (phenol red broth base, 5% Fildes' extract)	—

[a] See text. (Taylor, et al., 1978.)
[b] Test repeated with 5% horse serum added to media.
Other tests, as in Cowan (1974).

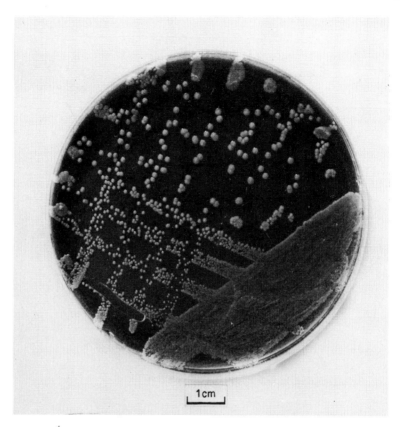

Fig. 7 6-day culture of the CEM organism on heated blood (Eugon) agar. (Courtesy of Mr J. G. Atherton.)

Swaney and Sahu (1978) compared the growth of the coccobacillus on heated blood ("chocolate") agar prepared from tryptose blood agar base (Difco Laboratories) and Eugonbroth (Baltimore Biological Laboratory). To prepare Eugon agar, they added Noble agar (Difco) to a final concentration of 1.5% to Eugonbroth. Both media were autoclaved, cooled at 50°C, supplemented with 10% oxalated horse blood, heated to 75°C for 10 minutes, and cooled again to 50°C; 200 mg l^{-1} streptomycin was then added. Before use, petri dishes containing the media were incubated in air overnight at 37°C to detect contamination.

Colonies of the coccobacillus were visible under ×15 magnification on heated blood ("chocolate") Eugon agar after 24 hours of incubation in a humid atmosphere containing 5% carbon dioxide and 95% air. None was visible on heated blood ("chocolate") tryptose agar.

After 48 hours of incubation, colonies on heated blood ("chocolate") Eugon agar were 1 mm in diameter; after 72 hours they were 1.5 mm. Colonies on similar medium containing tryptose were less than 1 mm after 72 hours of incubation. Similar numbers of colonies grew on both media from the same inoculum. The size of colonies on either agar was related to their density: the fewer the numbers, the larger the colonies. Although there was some variation in colonial size and morphology, the characteristics of the different colonial types were not always maintained on subculture (Sahu, 1980; Mackintosh, personal communication). On prolonged incubation variation in colonial morphology tends to increase (Sahu, 1980).

Colonies on heated blood ("chocolate") tryptose agar were visible under $\times 15$ magnification in 24 hours when 0.2 g sodium sulphite and 0.3 g L-cystine were added per litre. Both chemicals are constituents of Eugonbroth.

The coccobacillus multiplied in the absence of blood on Eugon agar containing 25 mg l^{-1} recrystallized haemin. This characteristic parallels the haem requirement of some members of the *Haemophilus* genus.

Since the organism was first described (Taylor *et al.*, 1978), streptomycin-sensitive strains of the organism have been isolated. Two streptomycin-sensitive strains have been deposited in the UK National Collection of Type Cultures: (1) NCTC 11225 (Equine Research Station 5304) submitted by Dr M. E. Mackintosh in 1978 and obtained by her from Kentucky, USA (Swerczek, 1978a,c); (2) NCTC 11226 (Equine Research Station 5192) submitted by Dr M. E. Mackintosh in 1978 and obtained by her from Ghent, Belgium.

When examined in the National Collection of Type Cultures, both these strains showed minor variations when compared with the type strain NCTC 11184. NCTC 11225 failed to grow on nutrient agar with X and V factors discs added, grew slightly on TSI agar, and failed to grow on casein agar. NCTC 11226 produced very small colonies, failed to grow on nutrient agar with X and V factors and failed to grow on 2% sodium chloride agar or casein agar. Both strains were similar to NCTC 11184 in being catalase-, oxidase- and phosphatase-positive, asaccharolytic, and in being negative or failing to grow in the other tests performed. Both were agglutinated by antiserum to NCTC 11184.

According to Dr M. E. Mackintosh (personal communication), NCTC 11225 appears to be less fastidious than other strains. It is less demanding of carbon dioxide, cystine and sulphite and will grow aerobically, although not to single colonies. On Eugon agar, containing 5% heated horse blood, the culture appears brownish-green and the green colour may extend into the agar. This effect is more pronounced under aerobic conditions of incubation. Cultures of other strains of CEMO are brownish-pink and have no effect on the agar. All strains of CEMO grow to some extent in Eugon broth, usually in the depth of the culture, without any addition of blood or serum even if incubated aerobically. Strain NCTC 11225 grows to a greater density than other strains and gives a more uniform turbidity in broth. Dr M. E. Mackintosh noted the "greening effect" on receipt of the culture, but other strains subcultured in her laboratory for over 2 years have not shown this effect, nor has she adapted any other strains to grow better in broth culture.

A comprehensive account of the bacteriological techniques applicable to the isolation of the CEM organism from mares and stallions is given by Mackintosh (1981), who recommends for primary isolation the use of a glucose-free medium containing L-cystine (300 mg l^{-1}) or L-cysteine hydrochloride (100 mg l^{-1}), sodium sulphite (200 mg l^{-1}) and 2–5% heated horse or sheep blood. The use of Eugon agar for primary isolation is contraindicated.

C. Survival at various temperatures

The CEM organism, suspended in isotonic saline, was killed by heating for 1 hour at 56°C. On the surface of nutrient agar which does not support growth, the bacterium could not be recovered after 48 hours in an atmosphere of air at 20°C or 37°C, but remained viable for up to 6 days at 4°C. When stored on swabs without transport medium, it survived 4 days at 4°C, 2 days at 20°C, but only 1 day at 30°C or 37°C (Rosenthal, unpublished observations). Sahu et al. (1979a), using a strain of the CEMO which originated in the Republic of Ireland, reported that the numbers of bacteria in phials of infective exudate decreased 15-fold within 1 day at 22°C but only 2-fold at 4°C.

At temperatures less than 37°C, the use of transport medium extended the survival time of the organism. In Stuart's Transport Medium, the organism survived on swabs at least 21 days at 4°C, 5 days at 20°C, and 2 days at 30°C. At 37°C, the use of transport medium did not influence the survival time, and the organism could not be grown after 1 day (Rosenthal, unpublished observations).

Sahu et al. (1979a) compared the efficacy of various transport media and found that survival at −70°C, 4°C or 22°C was longer in Amies Modified Transport (AMT) medium with charcoal (Amies, 1967), than AMT medium without charcoal, or in Stuart's Transport Medium. They recommended that samples on cotton-tipped swabs should be immersed in AMT medium containing charcoal and stored frozen on dry ice during transport to the laboratory.

D. Effect of pH on survival

According to Sahu and Dardiri (1980), the CEM organism is extremely susceptible to acid pH up to 4.5. Growth was not observed after the bacteria had been incubated at pH 3, 3.5 and 4 for 5 minutes. At pH 4.5 a 6.5 $\log_{10}$ inactivation was found. The bacteria were not inactivated, however, at pH 6 and 7.

E.   Biochemical properties

The CEM organism proved to be relatively unreactive in some forty tests done in the UK National Collection of Type Cultures (Table 3). Only those for catalase, cytochrome oxidase and phosphatase were positive. In particular, the organism was asaccharolytic in all the media tested.

Tests performed by Dr R. W. A. Feltham (personal communication) for cellular enzymes by means of an APIZYM strip revealed the presence of acid and alkaline phosphatases, leucine aminopeptidase, phosphoamidase and esterase.

F.   DNA base composition

The DNA base composition as estimated in the UK National Collection of Type Cultures from the melting temperature was 36.1% GC. (The value of approximately 39% GC originally given in personal communications, and quoted by Platt *et al.* (1977) and Shreeve (1978) was derived from an initial, crude DNA extract.)

G.   Antigenic properties

The type strain of the organism NCTC 11184 was not agglutinated in slide tests by antisera to *Brucella abortus* (absorbed and unabsorbed antisera), to *Brucella melitensis* (absorbed antiserum), or to *Brucella ovis*, but was agglutinated by 1 in 500 acriflavine (Taylor *et al.*, 1978).

An antiserum against the type strain NCTC 11184 was prepared by intramuscular and intravenous inoculation of a rabbit. The results of testing this antiserum in tube agglutination tests against suspensions of various organisms are shown in Table 4 and by slide agglutination in Table 5. Although in tube tests all the cross-reactions were weak, slightly more agglutination was obtained with a strain of *Haemophilus influenzae* than with strains of *Pasteurella multocida* and *Brucella abortus* which in turn gave stronger reactions than the other organisms tested. In the slide tests, a few cross-reactions were observed, but the greatest was only at a 1 in 2 dilution of the antiserum with *H. influenzaemurium*, *Neisseria elongata glycolytica* and *Pasteurella pneumotropica*. Smith and Young (1978) reported cross-reactions between CEMO and *Moraxella liquifaciens* and *Mima polymorpha (Acinetobacter calcoaceticus)*.

Table 4 The CEM organism: tube agglutinations with NCTC 11184 (Cambridge 61717/77) and other antisera

Antiserum	Antigen	Reciprocal dilutions of antiserum										
		10	20	40	80	160	320	640	1280	2560	5120	Control
Cambridge 61717/77	61717/17	++	++	++	++	++	++	++	+	−	−	−
Cambridge 61717/77	B. abortus, NCTC 8226	+	±	−	−	−	−	−	−	−	−	−
Cambridge 61717/77	P. multocida, recent isolate	+	±	−	−	−	−	−	−	−	−	−
Cambridge 61717/77	H. influenzae, recent isolate	++	+	±	−	−	−	−	−	−	−	−
Cambridge 61717/77	Y. pseudotuberculosis, stock strain	+	−	−	−	−	−	−	−	−	−	−
Cambridge 61717/77	Y. enterocolitica, PHLS Quality Control strain	+	−	−	−	−	−	−	−	−	−	−
Legionnaires' Disease, convalescent serum	Cambridge 61717/77	−	−	−	−	−	−	−	−	−	−	−
[a]B. abortus	61717/77	±	−	−	−	−	−	−	−	−	−	−
[a]B. pertussis	61717/77	±	−	−	−	−	−	−	−	−	−	−

[a] Supplied by Standards Laboratory for Serological Reagents, Central Public Health Laboratory, Colindale, London.

Table 5 Slide agglutination of various bacteria by antiserum to the CEM organism (NCTC 11184; Cambridge 61717/77)

Antigen	Antiserum dilution		
	Undil.	1 in 2	1 in 4
Actinobacillus suis, NCTC 10843	−	NT	NT
Actinobacillus sp., NCTC 10803	+	−	NT
Haemophilus influenzae, NCTC 4560	−	NT	NT
H. influenzaemurium, NCTC 11135	+	+	−
H. parainfluenzae, NCTC 4101	−	NT	NT
H. paraphrohaemolyticus, NCTC 10670	−	NT	NT
H. paraphrophilus, NCTC 10556	−	NT	NT
H. suis, NCTC 4557	−	NT	NT
Legionnaires Disease Organism	−	NT	NT
Moraxella anatipestifer, NCTC 11014	−	NT	NT
M. atlantae, NCTC 11091	−	NT	NT
M. osloensis, NCTC 10465	+	−	NT
M. phenylpyruvica, NCTC 10526	−	NT	NT
Neisseria elongata ss. *glycolytica,* NCTC 11050	+	+	−
Pasteurella haemolytica, NCTC 10609	−	NT	NT
P. pneumotropica, NCTC 8141	+	+	−
P. ureae, NCTC 10219	−	NT	NT
Yersinia enterocolitica, NCTC 10460	−	NT	NT

Strains of further species tested were found to be rough or autoagglutinable: *Actinobacillus seminus, Haemophilus aphrophilus, H. canis, H. haemolyticus, H. parahaemolyticus, H. pleuropneumoniae, H. segnis, Moraxella nonliquefaciens, M. urethralis, Pasteurella multocida, Yersinia rodentium.*
NT not tested.

H. Susceptibility to antimicrobial agents

There are particular problems in performing disc diffusion tests with the CEM organism because of its relatively slow rate of growth. Taylor *et al.* (1978), however, found that interpretation based on the presence or absence of an obvious zone of inhibition correlates reasonably well with results of MIC tests (Table 6). As indicated by MIC tests, the streptomycin-resistant type strain of the organism was found to be highly resistant to streptomycin only, although some degree of resistance was found to lincomycin, clindamycin, sulphamethoxazole and trimethoprim. In disc tests the organism appeared resistant to metronidazole and, to a large extent, to cotrimoxazole. Chlorhexidine, however, was remarkably effective in dilutions up to 1 in 125 000 W/V. It is of interest that although the strain was resistant to streptomycin, it was sensitive to the other aminocyclitol agents tested: neomycin, kanamycin, gentamicin, tobramycin, and amikacin.

Table 6   The CEM organism: antimicrobial susceptibility of NCTC 11184 (Cambridge 61717/77)

Antimicrobial agent	Suscept. by diff. test	Minimum inhibitory concentration (mg l^{-1})		
		Strain 61717/ 77	*S. aureus* NCTC 6571	*E. coli* NCTC 10418
Penicillin	S	<0.25	0.06	32
Ampicillin	S	0.5	0.125	4
Cephaloridine	S	NT	<0.06	2
Carbenicillin	S	NT	NT	NT
Tetracycline	S	1	0.5	2
Erythromycin	S	<0.06	0.25	NT
Clindamycin	R	16	0.25	NT
Lincomycin	R	32	<0.05	NT
Gentamicin	S	0.25	0.5	0.5
Kanamycin	S	1	2	2
Neomycin	S	1	1	2
Streptomycin	R	>512	4	4
Amikacin	S	NT	NT	NT
Tobramycin	S	NT	NT	NT
Chloramphenicol	S	NT	NT	NT
Nalidixic acid	S	4	NT	2
Nitrofurantoin	S	1	16	4
Polymyxin B	S	0.25	NT	0.125
Fusidic acid	S	NT	NT	NT
Sulphamethoxazole	R	32	16	8
Trimethoprim	R	4	0.5	0.25
Cotrimoxazole	I	NT	NT	NT
Metronidazole	R	NT	NT	NT

NT not tested   S susceptible   R resistant   I   intermediate.

Rommel *et al.* (1978) reported on the *in vitro* susceptibility of an Irish strain of the organism to 37 antimicrobial agents, tested by a disc diffusion method with two different media. Their results were similar to those of Taylor *et al.* (1978), but they also found that the strain was susceptible to cephalothin, oleandomycin, bacitracin, ColyMycin (colistin), and oxolinic acid. In their hands it was completely resistant to methicillin and other similar semi-synthetic penicillins, as well as to streptomycin, lincomycin, and clindamycin.

Dabernat *et al.* (1980) tested the *in vitro* susceptibility of 17 strains of the organism by disc diffusion and agar dilution methods and obtained results similar to those of Taylor *et al.* (1978), concluding that ampicillin, gentamicin and tetracycline were the most active antibiotics against the CEM organism.

Strains susceptible to streptomycin were inhibited by $1 \, \mathrm{mg \, l^{-1}}$ of this antibiotic.

Rosenthal (unpublished observations) has explored the possibility of using trimethoprim as a selective agent for the cultivation of the CEM organism in the presence of contaminant bacteria. At concentrations up to $2.5 \, \mathrm{mg \, l^{-1}}$, growth of the CEM organism was not inhibited but there was suppression of *Proteus*, coliform bacilli, *Staph. aureus*, micrococci and faecal streptococci. At $5 \, \mathrm{mg \, ml^{-1}}$ however trimethoprim inhibited growth of the CEM organism.

I. Taxonomic position

So far it has proved impossible to identify the CEM organism as belonging to any recognized species. Even allocation to a recognized genus is difficult.

The first-stage diagnostic table of Cowan (1974) suggests four possible genera: *Acinetobacter*, *Moraxella*, *Brucella* and *Bordetella*, but the second-stage table for these genera gives apparent close fits with only *Moraxella nonliquefaciens*, *M. osloensis*, *M. urethralis*, *M. phenylpyruvica* and *Brucella suis*. These five species are excluded by several characters each (Table 7). Similarly, Skerman's key in the 8th Edition of *Bergey's Manual* (Skerman, 1974) suggests *Brucella*, *Bordetella* and *Moraxella*, but again species identification is not possible.

The serological investigations have also failed to give definite indications of any taxonomic relationship but the DNA base composition of 36.1% GC for NCTC 11184 has proved very useful in excluding certain genera:

Brucella: 56–58% GC reported for *B. abortus* and *B. melitensis* (Hoyer and McCullough, 1968).

Bordetella: 61–68% GC (Pittman, 1974).

Kingella: 47–55% GC (Snell and Lapage, 1976). This is a relatively new genus, proposed by Henriksen and Bøvre (1976) for catalase-negative, oxidase-positive, weakly saccharolytic organisms previously contained in the genus *Moraxella*.

Eikenella: 56% GC (Snell and Lapage, 1976).

Cardiobacterium: 59–60% GC (Snell and Lapage, 1976).

Branhamella: 42–47% GC (Snell and Lapage, 1976).

Although the DNA base composition is close to that of *Moraxella sensu stricto* (40–46% GC, Lautrop, 1974), inclusion of the new organism here would necessitate a widening of the criteria for admission to the genus; moreover, strain NCTC 11184 does not resemble the typical plump cells of *Moraxella* spp. and it is negative in several tests developed to assist identification in this genus. *Moraxella* is therefore also excluded.

Other genera containing organisms of varying degrees of fastidiousness in

Table 7 Differentiation of CEM organism from some apparently similar species of *Moraxella* and from *Brucella suis*

	CEM organism	M. nonlique-faciens	M. osloensis	M. phenyl-pyruvica	M. urethralis	Brucella suis
Width of cells (µm)	<1	>1	>1	>1	<1	<1
Growth						
improved by serum	–	–	–	+	–	NT
stimulated by bile	–	–	–	+	–	–
on poly-β-hydroxybutyrate	–	–	+	–	–	NT
on 4 per cent NaCl	–*	+	–	+	+	NT
on Tween agars	–	+	+	+	+	NT
anaerobically	+	+	d	+	+	–
Nitrate reduction	–	+	–	+	–	+
Nitrite reduction	–	–	–	–	+	NT
Citrate utilization	–	–	–	–	+	–
Urease production	–	–	–	d	–	+
Percentage GC of DNA[a]	36.1	43.2–43.7	43.5	42–43.5	46	NT

NT not tested   +   85–100% strains are positive   d 16–84% strains are positive.
–   0–15% strains are positive   * Assumed, since no growth occurred on 3.5% NaCl.
[a] Bøvre and Henriksen (1967); Bøvre *et al.* (1969); Snell *et al.* (1972); Snell and Lapage (1976); Taylor *et al.* (1978a).

ieir growth requirements, and which cannot be excluded on the basis of
)NA base composition, are _Francisella, Actinobacillus, Pasteurella_ and
Iaemophilus.

Francisella (33–36% GC, Normore, 1973) is a relatively poorly studied
enus which, however, is strictly aerobic; the NCTC deposited (vaccine) strain
oxidase-negative. Existing species of _Actinobacillus_ (40–42% GC, Bohacek
nd Mraz, 1967) reduce nitrates, produce acid from carbohydrates, and
roduce β-galactosidase, hydrogen sulphide and urease. _Pasteurella_ (36–43%
iC, Smith, 1974) species also reduce nitrates and produce acid from
irbohydrates. _Francisella, Actinobacillus_ and _Pasteurella_ therefore may be
ɔnsidered unsuitable genera.

According to Zinnemann and Biberstein (1974), for inclusion in the genus
Iaemophilus (37–44% GC, Kilian, 1976), an organism should be a strict
arasite requiring growth factors present in blood, especially X and/or V
ictors. Although X-dependency has been claimed for this organism (Shreeve,
978) and some stimulation of growth by X factor was observed by Taylor _et_
_l._ (1978), the D-aminolaevulinic acid test was positive, thereby indicating lack
f X dependency. Nevertheless, the genus _Haemophilus_ at present contains at
ast one species, _H. aphrophilus,_ which was originally described as X-
ependent (Khairat, 1940) but which appears to have lost such a requirement
Kilian, 1976). In this respect, it may be of some significance that the strongest
f the antigenic cross-reactions of the antiserum to strain NCTC 11184 in the
ibe agglutination tests was with _H. influenzae._

Rather than create a new genus, containing only one species and defined on
ssentially negative test results, Taylor _et al._ (1978) preferred to regard the
iusative organism of CEM as a new species of the genus _Haemophilus._ They
ierefore proposed the name _Haemophilus equigenitalis_ (e.qui.ge.ni.ta'lis:
.gen.n. _equi_ of a horse; L. adj. _genitalis_ genital) sp. n. for this organism. Their
train Cambridge 61717/77 is the type strain and has been deposited in the
'K National Collection of Type Cultures under the number NCTC 11184.
wo other streptomycin-resistant strains were subsequently deposited:
ICTC 11197 and NCTC 11198. In addition, the two streptomycin-sensitive
rains previously mentioned have been deposited by Dr M. E. Mackintosh of
ie Equine Research Station, Newmarket, in the National Collection of Type
ultures and designated NCTC 11225 and NCTC 11226 respectively.

In 1978, the proposal made by Taylor _et al._ (1978), that the causative
rganism of CEM as described by them should be included in the genus
Iaemophilus and be known as _Haemophilus equigenitalis_ was considered by
ie _Haemophilus_ subcommittee of the International Committee on Systematic
acteriology at a meeting held in Munich that year under the chairmanship of
rofessor Zinnemann. The subcommittee, however, would not accept the
rganism into the genus _Haemophilus,_ mainly because it is not X-dependent as

determined by the D-aminolaevulinic acid test and also because it does no reduce nitrate to nitrite. Furthermore, the committee held the view (Zinnemann, personal communication) that it is preferable to have a one species genus, or to create a provisional genus for at present unclassifiab species, than to open a defined genus to species that have no suitable home

The causative organism of contagious equine metritis therefore remains, a do many other organisms, the subject of unresolved taxonomic debate.

VII. GENERAL OBSERVATIONS

The appearance of an apparently new disease caused by a hithert undescribed bacterium is unusual for the second half of the twentieth century That two such diseases, legionnaires' disease and contagious equine metriti should have appeared within a few months of one another is even mor remarkable.

Circumstances leading to the recognition of new pathogens are diverse, bu often it is outbreaks of disease with unusual clinical or epidemiologic features that excite attention. When CEM first appeared, the clinical feature alone were not distinctive, but the severity of the metritis, its high degree c infectivity, and the absence of the known equine venereal pathogens indicate an unusual infection. However, the fact that the first outbreak was on a larg Thoroughbred stud farm was important in focussing attention upon it. Th numbers of animals at risk allowed the transmissibility of the infection to b ascertained, and the important financial implications were a stimulus to a fu investigation of the disease. It is quite possible that, in other circumstance the disease might have attracted less attention, since CEM is not attended b mortality, the infertility it causes is temporary, and the condition is amenab to treatment with antimicrobial agents.

CEM appears to be a new disease in the UK and the origins of the infectio are a matter of special interest to veterinarians and microbiologists. At preser there is but limited information on its geographical distribution in othe countries, but it may be endemic in horses other than Thoroughbreds in som parts of the world. It is significant that CEM was first recognized i Thoroughbreds, which, on account of their value, are subject to closer diseas control than other breeds of horse, but spread of the disease to this breed probably recent.

So far, only horses and donkeys have been shown to be susceptible, but th possibility that a reservoir of infection may exist in some other species ougl not to be overlooked. The potential survival of the organism in the inanimat environment also needs to be further explored.

Many apparently "new" pathogens may only be newly recognized, but from time to time novel or unusual types of bacteria derived by genetic change of precursor organisms undoubtedly arise. Given favourable circumstances, these will survive and ultimately, with appropriate adaption, may become parasites of a conveniently available host species. The genetic changes required may result from mutation or possibly transfer of genetic material by plasmids, transposons, phages, or other mediators from other organisms. In the present state of knowledge of CEM, it would be premature to conclude that the causal organism has recently evolved. Its characteristics, nevertheless, are sufficiently unusual to debar it from any of the genera to which recognized pathogens belong, so that at present its generic and ancestral relationships can be only a matter for speculation. In GC content and its lack of saccharolytic reactivity the organism of CEM conforms closely to the characters of *Pseudomonas cruciviae*, a soil organism isolated by Gray and Thornton (1928) in the USA (Hill, 1966). Although similarity in GC content does not necessarily imply a common ancestry, it does indicate organisms among which taxonomic affinities may eventually be established.

The recognition of CEM and legionnaires' disease has highlighted some of the problems encountered in detecting fastidious bacterial pathogens. The role of hitherto unrecognized types of bacteria in causing certain types of disease may have been neglected in recent years, partly through preoccupation with viruses and other organisms and partly through unjustified reliance on the conventional methods of bacterial culture. Successful propagation of fastidious organisms in culture depends upon a knowledge of their characteristics and growth requirements. New or unfamiliar organisms may escape detection, either through failure to grow, or because they have been overgrown by less culturally exacting organisms in the sample. In CEM, the chances of detecting the causal organism in the clitoris of symptomless carrier mares would have been low without the prior knowledge of its cultural requirements gained from study of the acute metritic form of the disease. Such a problem is relevant to sites other than the genital tract; it applies especially to mucosal surfaces having a mixed and often prolific bacterial flora. Newman *et al.* (1979), for example, have commented upon the infrequency with which fastidious organisms of the genus *Capnocytophaga* are isolated from clinical specimens, although these organisms are probably among the normal flora of the oral cavity.

The carrier state in CEM is especially interesting in that the organism can survive for long periods on the surfaces of the external genitalia. The smegma in these situations seems to provide a protective environment and may even support slow multiplication of the organism. In relation to the host, these sites are in effect extracorporeal, and the ability of the organism to survive in them confers obvious advantages to a bacterium which seems to propagate profusely only in the endometrium and to be readily susceptible to inactivation in an inanimate environment.

Symptomless carriers are a feature of many infectious diseases in which the causal organisms survive on mucous membranes, especially of the naso pharynx and bowel (Mims, 1976). In symptomless carriers of gonorrhoea, the gonococcus survives in the urethra, especially in the female. Carriage of venereally transmissible organisms exclusively in the smegma and the moist epidermoid invaginations of the external genitalia, as in CEM, is not recognized in human beings. In cattle, however, the prepuce of the bull can harbour *Campylobacter foetus* for long periods without clinical signs or local inflammatory changes, and such bulls are a source of coital infection for any cows that they serve.

In general, the resident bacterial flora of the skin does not readily accept newcomers, and intruding organisms tend to be eliminated after a short period of time. Experimentally, introducing the CEM organism into the clitoris failed to establish a persistent infection. However, the conditions of such an experiment do not reproduce the situation pertaining in the natural disease, where the clitoris is exposed to persistent and heavy contamination with infective discharge. Infections in the urethral fossa of the stallion were established more readily, although the duration of persistence varied greatly presumably depending on the degree of ecological competition with the local bacterial flora.

VIII. THE FUTURE

In the five years that have elapsed since CEM was first recognized, much has been learned about the causal organism and the natural history of the disease. There are two aspects, however, which call for closer study. One concerns the organism itself: a study of the degree of genetic homology of the organism's DNA with that of other Gram-negative bacteria might help to resolve some of the existing taxonomic problems and also perhaps throw some light upon the organism's ancestral relationships. The second question concerns the manner in which the CEM organism produces its effects in the endometrium. The pathogenesis of epithelial damage has not so far received much attention. Possibly, adherence of the organism to epithelial cell surfaces takes place as in some other Gram-negative infections of mucous membranes, but, unlike the gonococcus, pili have not as yet been observed in electronmicroscopy studies of the CEM organism. It is possible that the capsular material of the CEM organism may aid adherence to mucous surfaces as well as play a part in protecting the organism from host defence mechanisms.

In the case of infection by *Neisseria gonorrhoeae*, Veale *et al.* (1979) have demonstrated the ability of this organism to survive and multiply in human phagocytes. Novotny *et al.* (1977) have suggested that initially there is intracellular multiplication in macrophages and that aggregates of organisms and the macrophage debris constitute an infectious unit which attaches to the epithelium. The possibility exists that the CEM organism also multiplies intracellularly at some stage in the infective process. In acute CEM, however, organisms are often present extracellularly in the exudate; some appear to have been phagocytosed by polymorphonuclear leucocytes but these are usually in a minority. Similar observations have been made on chamber implant cultures by Arko and Wong (1980) who have suggested that the capsular material, described by Swaney and Breese (1980) may have antiphagocytic properties. If this is so, it may be only dead or damaged organisms which are phagocytosed. The interactions of the organism with phagocytes and uterine epithelial cells are likely to be an interesting area for future inquiry.

New diseases not only offer challenges to established ideas but may also provide signposts to new pathways of investigation of older and more familiar problems. It will therefore not be surprising if some of the questions posed by contagious equine metritis are found to have wider relevance in microbiology and the study of infection.

REFERENCES

Amies, C. R. (1967). *Can. J. publ. Hlth* **58**, 296–300.
Anon. (1980). *Vet. Rec.* **107**, 376–9. Circular no. 414 p. 18, Internat. Office of Epizootics.
Arko, R. J. and Wong, K. H. (1980). *Amer. J. Vet. Res.* **41**, 989–993.
Atherton, J. G. (1978). *Vet. Rec.* **103**, 432.
Benson, J. A., Dawson, F. L. M., Durrant, D. S., Edwards, P. T. and Powell, D. G. (1978). *Vet. Rec.* **102**, 277–280.
Blobel, H., Kitzrow, D. and Blobel, K. (1978). *Tierärztl. Umsch.* **33**, 523–524.
Blobel, H., Brückler, J., Kitzrow, D. and Blobel, K. (1979). *Compar. Immunol. Microbiol. Infect. Dis.* **2**, 551–554.
Bohacek, J. and Mraz, O. (1967). *Zentbl. Bakt. ParasitKde. Abt. 1.* orig. **202**, 468–478.
Bøvre, K. and Henriksen, S. D. (1967). *Int. J. Syst. Bact.* **17**, 343–360.
Bøvre, K., Fiandt, M. and Szybalski, W. (1969). *Canad. J. Microbiol.* **15**, 335–338.
Bryans, J. T., Darlington, R. W., Smith, B. and Brooks, R. R. (1979). *J. Equine Med. Surg.* **3**, 467–472.
Codazza, D., Giongo, P., Proverbio, E. and Lusian, F. (1980). *Clin. Vet.* **103**, 563–565.
Cook, G. T. (1950). *J. Clin. Path.* **3**, 359–362.
Corbel, M. J. and Brewer, R. A. (1980). *Vet. Rec.* **106**, 35.
Cowan, S. T. (1974). *In* Cowan and Steele's "Manual for the Identification of Medical Bacteria", 2nd edn Cambridge University Press, Cambridge.
Crouch, J. F. R., Atherton, J. G. and Platt, H. (1972). *Vet. Rec.* **90**, 21–24.

Crowhurst, R. C. (1977). *Vet. Rec.* **100**, 476.

Crowhurst, R. C., Simpson, D. J., Greenwood, R. E. S. and Ellis, D. R. (1979). *In* "Proc. Int. Symp. on Equine Venereal Diseases". Animal Health Trust pp. 40–42.

Croxton-Smith, P., Benson, J. A., Dawson, F. L. M. and Powell, D. G. (1978). *Vet. Rec.* **103**, 275–278.

Dabernat, H. J., Delmas, C. F., Tainturier, D. J. and Lareng, M. B. (1980). *Antimicrob. Ag. Chemother.* **18**, 841–843.

Dawson, F. L. M., Benson, J. A. and Croxton-Smith, P. (1978). *Equine Vet. J.* **10**, 145–147.

Ellner, P. D., Stoessel, C. J., Drakeford, E. and Vesi, F. (1966). *Amer. J. Clin. Path.* **45**, 502–504.

Fales, W. H., Blackburn, B. O., Youngquist, R. S., Braun, W. F., Schlater, L. K. and Morehouse, L. G. (1979). 22nd Annual Proc. Amer. Assn Veterinary Laboratory Diagnosticians. pp. 187–198.

Fernie, D. S., Cayzer, I. and Chalmers, S. R. (1979). *Vet. Rec.* **104**, 260–262.

Fernie, D. S., Batty, I., Walker, P. D., Platt, H., Mackintosh, M. E. and Simpson, D. J. (1980). *Res. Vet. Sci.* **28**, 362–367.

Frank, C. J. (1979). *In* "Proc. Int. Symp. on Equine Venereal Diseases", Animal Health Trust, pp. 46–48.

Füzi, M. (1980). *Lancet* **2**, 476.

Glauert, A. M. and Thornley, M. J. (1969). *A. Rev. Microbiol.* **23**, 159–198.

Gray, P. H. H. and Thornton, H. G. (1928). *Zentbl. Bakt. ParasitKde. Abt II.* **73**, 74–96.

Hazard, G. H., Hughes, K. L. and Penson, P. J. (1979). *J. Reprod. Fert. Supp.* **27**, 337–342.

Henriksen, S. D. and Bøvre, K. (1976). *Int. J. Syst. Bacteriol.* **26**, 447–450.

Hill, L. R. (1966). *J. Gen. Microbiol.* **44**, 419–437.

Hoyer, B. H. and McCullough, N. B. (1968). *J. Bact.* **95**, 444–448.

Hugh, R. and Leifson, E. (1953). *J. Bacteriol.* **66**, 24–26.

Hughes, J. P., Asbury, A. C., Loy, R. G. and Burd, H. E. (1967). *Cornell Vet.* **57**, 53–69.

Hughes, J. P. and Loy, R. G. (1969). Proc. 15th Ann. Convent. Amer. Assn of Equine Practitioners. 289–292.

Hughes, K. L., Bryden, J. D. and Macdonald, F. (1978). *Aust. Vet. J.* **54**, 101.

Khairat, O. (1940). *J. Path. Bact.* **50**, 497–505.

Kikachi, N., Tsunoda, N., Kawakami, Y., Murase, N. and Kawata, K. (1982). *Jpn J. Vet. Sci.* **44**, 107–114.

Kilian, M. (1976). *J. Gen. Microbiol.* **93**, 9–62.

Knowles, R. C. (1979). Proc. 24th Ann. Convent. Amer. Assn of Equine Practitioners. 287–290.

Lautrop, H. (1974). *In* "Bergey's Manual of Determinative Bacteriology" (R. E. Buchanan and N. E. Gibbons, co-ed.). 8th edn pp. 433–436. Williams and Wilkins, Baltimore.

Luft, J. H. (1971). *Anat. Rec.* **171**, 347–368.

Mackintosh, M. E. (1981). *Vet. Rec.* **108**, 52–55.

Mardh, P. A., Holst, E., Taylor-Robinson, D., Taylor, C. E. D. and Rosenthal, R. O. (1980). *Lancet* **2**, 310–311.

Mims, C. A. (1976). *In* "The Pathogenesis of Infectious Disease". pp. 188–189. Academic Press, London and New York.

Moller, V. (1955). *Acta. Path. Microbiol. Scand.* **36**, 158–172.

Mumme, J. and Ahlswede, L. (1979). *Dt. tierärztl. Wschr.* **86**, 257–259.

Newman, M. G., Sutter, V. L., Pickett, M. J., Blachman, U., Greenwood, J. R., Grinenko, V. and Citron, D. (1979). *J. Clin. Microbiol.* **10**, 557–562.

Normore, W. M. (1973). *In* "Handbook of Microbiology" (A. I. Laskin and H. A. Lechevailer, ed.). Vol. II, p. 585, CRS Press, Cleveland.

Novotny, P., Short, J. A., Hughes, M., Miler, J. J., Syrett, C., Turner, W. H., Harris, J. R. W. and MacLennan, I. P. B. (1977). *J. Med. Microbiol.* **10**, 347–365.

O'Driscoll, J. G., Troy, P. T., Geoghegan, F. J. (1977). *Vet. Rec.* **101**, 359–360.

Pierson, R. E., Sahu, S. P., Dardiri, A. H. and Wilder, F. W. (1978). *JAVMA* **173**, 402–404.

Pitre, J., Legendre, M. F. and Voisin, G. (1979). *Pratique Vét. Equine* **11**, 11–26.

Pittman, M. (1974). *In* "Bergey's Manual of Determinative Bacteriology" (R. E. Buchanan and N. E. Gibbons, co-ed.). 8th edn pp. 282–283. Williams and Wilkins, Baltimore.

Platt, H., Atherton, J. G. and Ørskov, I. (1976). *J. Hyg. Camb.* **77**, 401–408.

Platt, H., Atherton, J. G., Simpson, D. J., Taylor, C. E. D., Rosenthal, R. O., Brown, D. F. J. and Wreghitt, T. G. (1977). *Vet. Rec.* **101**, 20.

Platt, H., Atherton, J. G., Dawson, F. L. M. and Durrant, D. S. (1978a). *Vet. Rec.* **102**, 19.

Platt, H., Atherton, J. G. and Simpson, D. J. (1978b). *Equine Vet. J.* **10**, 153–159.

Powell, D. G. (1978). *Equine Vet. J.* **10**, 1–4.

Powell, D. G., David, J. S. E. and Frank, C. J. (1978). *Vet. Rec.* **103**, 399–402.

Powell, D. G. and Whitwell, K. E. (1979). *J. Reprod. Fert. Suppl.* **27**, 331–335.

Ricketts, S. W., Rossdale, P. D. and Samuel, C. A. (1978). *Equine Vet. J.* **10**, 160–166.

Ricketts, S. W. (1979). *In* "Proc. Int. Symp. on Equine Venereal Diseases". Animal Health Trust. pp. 27–36.

Rommel, F., Dardiri, A. H. and Sahu, S. P. (1978). *In* "Proc. 82nd Annual Meeting U.S. Animal Health Assn". pp. 237–247.

Rowson, L. E. A., Lamming, G. E. and Fry, R. M. (1953). *Vet. Rec.* **65**, 335–340.

Sahu, S. P. (1980). *Vet. Rec.* **107**, 432.

Sahu, S. P. (1981). *Amer. J. Vet. Res.* **42**, 45–48.

Sahu, S. P. and Dardiri, A. H. (1980). *Amer. J. Vet. Res.* **41**, 1379–1382.

Sahu, S. P., Dardiri, A. H., Rommel, F. A. and Pierson, R. E. (1979a). *Amer. J. Vet. Res.* **40**, 1040–1042.

Sahu, S. P., Hamdy, F. M. and Dardiri, A. H. (1979b). *In* "Proc. 83rd Ann. Meeting U.S. Animal Health Assn". pp. 243–252.

Sahu, S. P., Pierson, R. E. and Dardiri, A. H. (1980). *Amer. J. Vet. Res.* **41**, 5–9.

Samuel, C. A., Ricketts, S. W., Rossdale, P. D., Steven, D. H. and Thurley, K. W. (1979). *J. Reprod. Fert. Suppl.* **27**, 287–292.

Shreeve, J. E. (1978). *Vet. Rec.* **102**, 20.

Simpson, D. J. (1977). Proc. Special Scientific Meeting on Contagious Equine Metritis. 1977. pp. 1–7. Cambridge Nov. 19. 1977. Brit. Equine Vet. Ass. (Privately circulated).

Simpson, D. J. and Eaton-Evans, W. E. (1978a). *Vet. Rec.* **102**, 19–20.

Simpson, D. J. and Eaton-Evans, W. E. (1978b). *Vet. Rec.* **102**, 488.

Skerman, V. B. D. (1974). *In* "Bergey's Manual of Determinative Bacteriology" (R. E. Buchanan and N. E. Gibbons, co-ed.). 8th edn pp. 1098–1146. Williams and Wilkins, Baltimore.

Smith, J. E. (1974). *In* "Bergey's Manual of Determinative Bacteriology" (R. E. Buchanan and N. E. Gibbons, co-ed.). 8th edn pp. 370–373. Williams and Wilkins, Baltimore.

Smith, J. E. and Young, C. R. 1978. *Lancet* 1, 1266.

Snell, J. J. S., Hill, L. R. and Lapage, S. P. (1972). *J. Clin. Path.* 25, 959–965.

Snell, J. J. S. and Lapage, S. P. (1976). *Int. J. Syst. Bacteriol.* 26, 451–458.

Sonnenschein, B. and Klug, E. (1979). *Dt. tierärztl. Wschr.* 86, 268–270.

Stuart, R. D., Toshach, S. R. and Patsula, T. M. (1954). *Can. J. Publ. Hlth* 45, 73–83.

Sugimoto, C., Isayama, Y., Kashiwazaki, M., Fujikura, T. and Mitani, K. (1980). *Natn Inst. Anim. Hlth Q. (Jpn)* 20, 118–119.

Swaney, L. M. and Breese, S. S., Jr. (1980). *Amer. J. Vet. Res.* 41, 127–132.

Swaney, L. M. and Sahu, S. P. (1978). *Vet. Rec.* 102, 43.

Swerczek, T. W. (1978a). *Vet. Rec.* 102, 512–513.

Swerczek, T. W. (1978b). *Vet. Rec.* 103, 125.

Swerczek, T. W. (1978c). *JAVMA* 173, 405–407.

Taylor, C. E. D. and Rosenthal, R. O. (1978a). *Lancet* 1, 1038.

Taylor, C. E. D. and Rosenthal, R. O. (1978b). *Lancet* 2, 1092–1093.

Taylor, C. E. D., Rosenthal, R. O., Brown, D. F. J., Lapage, S. P., Hill, L. R. and Legros, R. M. (1978). *Equine Vet. J.* 10, 136–144.

Taylor, C. E. D., Rosenthal, R. O. and Taylor-Robinson, D. (1979). *Lancet* 1, 700–701.

Thornley, M. J. (1960). *J. Appl. Bact.* 23, 37–52.

Timoney, P. J., Ward, J. and Kelly, P. (1977). *Vet. Rec.* 101, 103.

Timoney, P. J., O'Reilly, P. J., McArdle, J. and Ward, J. (1978a). *Vet. Rec.* 102, 152.

Timoney, P. J., McArdle, J. F., O'Reilly, P. J. and Ward, J. (1978b). *Equine Vet. J.* 10, 148–152.

Timoney, P. J., Geraghty, V. P., Dillon, P. B. and McArdle, J. F. (1978c). *Vet. Rec.* 103, 563–564.

Timoney, P. J., McArdle, J. F., O'Reilly, P. J., Ward, J. and Harrington, A. M. (1979a). *Vet. Rec.* 104, 84.

Timoney, P. J., O'Reilly, P. J. McArdle, J. F., Ward. J. and Harrington, A. M. (1979b). *Vet. Rec.* 104, 264.

Veale, D. R., Goldner, M., Penn, C. W., Ward, J. and Smith, H. (1979). *J. Gen. Microbiol.* 113, 383–393.

Whitwell, K. E. (1979). *In* Proc. Int. Symp. Equine Venereal Diseases. Animal Health Trust. p. 37.

Wilkinson, A. E. and Rodin, P. (1978). *Lancet* 2, 1093.

Wilson, G. S. and Miles, A. A. (1975a). *In* "Principles of Bacteriology, Virology and Immunity" pp. 1273–1275. Edward Arnold, London.

Wilson, G. S. and Miles, A. A. (1975b). *In* "Principles of Bacteriology, Virology and Immunity" pp. 1018–1019. Edward Arnold, London.

Zinnemann, K. and Biberstein, E. L. (1974). *In* "Bergey's Manual of Determinative Bacteriology" (R. E. Buchanan and N. E. Gibbons, co-ed.). 8th edn pp. 364–368. Williams and Wilkins, Baltimore.

3 *Pseudomonas aeruginosa* toxins

OLGERTS R. PAVLOVSKIS
and BENGT WRETLIND

I. INTRODUCTION

During the last 30 years Gram-negative organisms have become the commonest cause of serious infections in hospitalized patients (Adler *et al.*, 1970; McGowan *et al.*, 1975). Infections caused by *Pseudomonas aeruginosa* have been particularly severe because a limited number of antibacterial agents are clinically effective in treatment and the patients who are most frequently involved are those whose defence mechanisms are seriously impaired. Normally commensal for humans, *P. aeruginosa* has been detected with increasing frequency in patients with serious disorders such as neoplastic diseases, cystic fibrosis, burns, severe injuries, or in patients who have received immunosuppressive therapy (Baltch and Griffin, 1977; Curtin *et al.*, 1961; Fishman and Armstrong, 1972; Flick and Cluff, 1977; Forkner *et al.*, 1958).

The pathological sequelae of these infections are not yet thoroughly understood. The pathogenicity of most Gram-negative bacteria has been attributed to endotoxin (LPS), but there is evidence that the endotoxin of *P. aeruginosa* is less toxic than that elaborated by other Gram-negative organisms. Moreover, *P. aeruginosa* does produce a number of toxic extracellular products, including exotoxin A, proteases, phospholipase, haemolysin, endotoxin, slime (Heckley, 1970; Liu, 1966b, 1974, 1979; Young and Armstrong, 1972). This chapter will review the more recent work in this field.

Because microbial products traditionally classified as toxins have been recognized as proteins, the term *toxin* will be restricted to proteins which possess properties harmful to the host (Bonventre, 1970; Bonventre *et al.*, 1967) (Table 1). The characteristics and biological activities of *P. aeruginosa* endotoxin and the common antigen (OEP) described by Homma and others

Table 1 Extracellular proteins from *P. aeruginosa*

Protein	MW $\times 10^{-3}$	pI	LD$_{50}$ (mice) (μg)	Mode of action	Proposed role in pathogenicity
Exotoxin A	54–71.5	5.0–5.1	0.06	Ribosylation of ribosomal protein EF-2	Inhibition of protein synthesis
Exoenzyme S	ND[a]	ND	ND	Ribosylation of ribosomal proteins	Possibly inhibition of protein synthesis
Elastase	25–33–39.5	5.7–6.6	60–400	Neutral metallo-proteinase	Tissue damage, degradation of coagulation and complement factors
Alkaline protease	48	4.1–5.0	100–300	Metalloproteinase	Probably same as for elastase
Phospholipase C[b]	ND	5.75–5.9	ND	Membrane damaging	Cytolytic, haemolytic, possibly destruction of lung surfactant
Leucocidin	27	5.0–5.2	1	Membrane damaging	Cytolytic, possibly induction of leucopenia

[a] ND: No data.
[b] Synonyms: lecithinase, heat-labile haemolysin.

will not be discussed in any detail (Homma, 1968; Homma and Abe, 1972; Sasaki et al., 1975; Tanato et al., 1978, 1979).

II. EXOTOXIN A

A. General remarks

Liu and associates first demonstrated that extracellular products produced by the organism might contribute to the pathogenesis of the infection (Liu et al., 1961). Detailed studies in this area were made possible by the isolation of a lethal, heat-labile exotoxin (Liu, 1966b). Injection of this exotoxin into dogs resulted in the haemodynamic and biochemical changes associated with shock and death (Atik et al., 1968). These changes included acidosis, elevated levels of circulating catecholamines, an increased arterial–venous difference in oxygen saturation, circulatory collapse, and leucopenia. These observations were similar to those made in Pseudomonas infections. This work resulted in great stimulation of interest in the Pseudomonas toxin and its role in pathogenesis.

B. Production, purification and characterization of exotoxin A

P. aeruginosa exotoxin A (toxin, lethal toxin), which is produced by over 90% of P. aeruginosa clinical isolates (Bjorn et al., 1977; Pollack et al., 1977; Sanai et al., 1980), has been purified and characterized in several laboratories (Callahan, 1974, 1976; Iglewski and Sadoff, 1979; Leppla, 1976; Liu, 1973; Lory and Collier, 1980; Vasil et al., 1976, 1977). In vitro it is secreted as a single peptide chain (Lory and Collier, 1980; Vasil et al., 1977) containing four disulphide bridges and no free sulphydryl groups. The molecular weight has been estimated to be between 54 000 and 71 500 daltons (Callahan, 1974; Chung and Collier, 1977; Leppla, 1976; Lory and Collier, 1980; Vasil et al., 1977) and pI 5.0–5.1 (Callahan, 1976; Leppla, 1976). As far as it is known, exotoxin A does not contain any unusual amino acids (Chung and Collier, 1977; Leppla, 1976) or components that would distinguish it from other non-toxic proteins.

Since nucleic acid derivatives found in laboratory media inhibit in vitro production of exotoxin A (Liu, 1973), trypticase soy broth dialysate (TSBD) plus glycerol and monosodium glutamate or modifications of this system have been used in most laboratories for exotoxin A production. In vitro exotoxin A production requires vigorous aeration, and its yields are decreased by high iron contents (50 μg ml^{-1}) (Bjorn et al., 1979b). Recently a defined medium containing three amino acids (arginine, aspartic, alanine), a carbon source, glycerol, and basal and trace salts have been used in our laboratory for exotoxin A production (DeBell, 1979; DeBell and Martin, 1979). Increasing amounts of exotoxin A were produced in cultures according to the following sequence: succinate $\geq$ citrate $>$ acetate $>$ glucose $>$ pyruvate. With 13 mM citrate, the amount of exotoxin A measured by enzyme activity and mouse lethality was approximately 90% of that produced in TSBD. A comparison of several strains of *P. aeruginosa* demonstrated that growth and exotoxin A production were essentially the same in the chemically defined medium as in TSBD. However, some strains of *Pseudomonas* do not produce good yields of exotoxin A when grown in chemically defined medium (Iglewski, personal communication). It should be noted that extracellular protease production was consistently lower in this medium. Since one of the problems encountered in large scale exotoxin A production is the proteolytic activity of the proteases produced by the organisms during growth, the chemically defined medium appears to be very well suited for exotoxin A production. Previously, in order to reduce the proteolytic activity either protease inhibitors such as nitrilotri-acetate have been added to the growth medium (Callahan, 1976) or protease-deficient mutants such as the prototype strain PA 103 have been used (Atik *et al.*, 1968; Liu, 1979). A recent report, however, indicates that two of the proteases produced by *Pseudomonas*, alkaline protease and elastase, do not have any effect on exotoxin A enzymatic activity *in vitro*. Jagger *et al.* (1980) found no reduction in either biological or enzyme activity after treatment of exotoxin A with *Pseudomonas* proteases. Another bacterial protease, thermo-lysin, rapidly inactivated exotoxin A. The discrepancy between these results and the results of Sanai *et al.* (1980), who produced non-toxic fragments of exotoxin A following treatment with *Pseudomonas* elastase, is difficult to explain. It is possible that one group studied the native exotoxin, whereas the other group used a slightly denatured exotoxin with an altered configuration, thus rendering it sensitive to degradation by proteases.

The various procedures used for exotoxin A purification have been summarized by Iglewski and Sadoff (1979). Recently purification procedures using preparative polyacrylamide gel electrophoresis or affinity chromatog-raphy have been described (Callahan, 1976; Taylor and Pollack, 1978).

C.   Biological activity of exotoxin A

Exotoxin A is toxic to cells in culture (Middlebrook and Dorland, 1977; Pavlovskis, 1972; Pavlovskis and Gordon, 1972; Pavlovskis *et al.*, 1975) and to many animal species (Atik *et al.*, 1968; Liu, 1966b; Liu *et al.*, 1973; Pavlovskis and Shackelford, 1974; Pavlovskis *et al.*, 1975; Young and Pollack, 1979), including rhesus monkeys (Pavlovskis *et al.*, 1974a). On a weight basis and the total amount in culture fluids, exotoxin A is by far the most toxic *P.*

aeruginosa product tested to date. Its average mean lethal dose (LD_{50}) for a mouse is approximately 0.06 μg (Callahan, 1976), whereas the LD_{50} for LPS is about 450 μg (Dyke and Berg, 1973) and for elastase 100 μg (Pavlovskis and Wretlind, 1979). Death usually occurs between 40 to 50 hours after an intravenous (IV) injection of exotoxin A ($2 LD_{50}$). With doses higher than $10–15 LD_{50}$ survival time remains relatively constant—about eight hours (Pavlovskis *et al.*, 1975). Other animals tested (guinea pigs, rabbits, dogs) were as sensitive to exotoxin A as mice on body weight basis. A single intravenous injection ($2 LD_{50}$) of purified exotoxin A into mice elicited necrosis, cellular swelling, and fatty change in the liver within 4–8 hours and near total hepatocellular necrosis at 48 hours (Pavlovskis *et al.*, 1976). Frequently oedematous and haemorrhagic lungs and tubular necrosis and haemorrhages in kidneys have also been observed in exotoxin-A-treated mice and dogs (Liu, 1974). Hepatic necrosis is accompanied by a parallel rise in serum levels of aspartate and alanine aminotransferases (SGOT and SGPT) and alkaline phosphatase (Pavlovskis *et al.*, 1976). Following the IV injection of exotoxin A ($2 LD_{50}$) a rapid and significant decrease of protein synthesis occurs in mouse tissues (Pavlovskis and Shackelford, 1974). During the 2–4 hour interval following toxin administration there was greater than 50% inhibition in the liver and by 16–18 hours protein synthesis was reduced to less than 20% of that of the controls (untreated mice). In kidneys, spleen, and pancreas a 50% decrease in protein synthesis was noted 18 hours post-injection. As the animals approached death, protein synthesis decreases in every tissue examined. When mice were injected with doses of exotoxin A resulting in 75% mortality, a decrease in both IgM and IgG antibodies against sheep red blood cells could be demonstrated by the Jerne plaque assay in the surviving mice (Pavlovskis *et al.*, 1980).

The first indication of the mode of action of exotoxin A was provided by Pavlovskis and associates, who demonstrated that exotoxin A inhibits amino acid uptake in cultured cells and inhibits protein synthesis in exotoxin-treated mice (Pavlovskis and Gordon, 1972; Pavlovskis and Shackelford, 1974). Later Iglewski and Kabat (1975) showed that exotoxin A inhibits protein synthesis in a manner identical to diphtheria toxin fragment A. The inhibition requires nicotinamide adenine dinucleotide (NAD) and results in a block at an elongation step of polypeptide assembly. Exotoxin A catalyses the transfer of the adenosine-5'-diphosphate-ribosyl (ADP-ribose) moiety of NAD on to elongation factor 2 (EF-2) resulting in the inactivation of EF-2 (Iglewski and Kabat, 1975; Iglewski *et al.*, 1977b):

$$NAD^+ + EF\text{-}2 \xrightleftharpoons{\text{exotoxin A}} ADP\text{-ribose-}EF\text{-}2 + nicotinamide + H^+.$$

Iglewski and associates have also demonstrated that the reaction is reversible and that the reverse reaction is favoured by low pH (Iglewski *et al.*, 1977b).

The transfer of the ADP-ribose moiety is to the same site on EF-2 in the case of both exotoxin A and diphtheria toxin, thus the reaction catalysed by one toxin can be reversed by the other (Chung and Collier, 1977; Iglewski et al., 1977b). In the case of the diphtheria toxin the ADP-ribose is attached to EF-2 via an unusual amino acid – diphthamide (Brown and Bodley, 1979; Van Ness et al., 1978). Diphthamide appears to be a derivative of histidine and is found in all EF-2 molecules examined (Brown and Bodley, 1978). It is not yet known whether this also occurs in the case of exotoxin A.

The two toxins, exotoxin A and diphtheria toxin, are distinct serologically (Iglewski and Kabat, 1975; Leppla, 1976) and exhibit different cellular specificites (Middlebrook and Dorland, 1977; Pappenheimer and Gill, 1973; Pavlovskis et al., 1975; Pavlovskis and Gordon, 1972). Studies with cells in culture using both biochemical and electron microscopy methods suggest that even though both exotoxin A and diphtherial toxins are internalized via receptor mediated endocytosis, different receptors are probably involved (Dorland et al., 1979; FitzGerald et al., 1980; Leppla et al., 1981; Middlebrook et al., 1980; Vasil and Iglewski, 1978). Furthermore, experiments with non-toxic diphtherial protein (CRM 197), which cross-reacts serologically with diphtheria toxin, showed that while CRM 197 could effectively compete with diphtheria toxin and block its toxic action, the protein had no effect on the activity of exotoxin A (Vasil and Iglewski, 1978). Recently, a mutant strain of PAO-1 has been isolated which produces a protein immunologically in-distinguishable from native exotoxin A, but is nontoxic for cultured Chinese hamster ovary cells (Cryz et al., 1980). The protein (CRM) also has no ADP-ribosylating activity. Cross-reactivity studies with CRM and diphtheria toxin or CRM 197 have not been reported.

In vitro, exotoxin A is released as a proenzyme in an enzymatically inactive form. Enzymatic activity may be effected by reduction of the disulphide bonds in the presence of urea (Leppla et al., 1978a; Lory and Collier, 1980; Vasil and Iglewski, 1976) or mild proteolysis of the exotoxin A molecule by Pseudomonas proteases in culture medium (Chung and Collier, 1977; Vasil et al., 1977). Fragments (M_r, 26 000) which inhibit enzymatic activity have been isolated from culture fluids and some preparations of purified exotoxin A after storage (Chung and Collier, 1977; Vasil et al., 1977). As the enzymatic activity of exotoxin A increases, its toxicity to cells in culture and mice decreases (Vasil et al., 1977). It appears that the lethal activity of exotoxin A depends upon the intact molecule, whereas the enzymatic activity requires structural rearrangement.

Recently, Lory and Collier (1980) were able to produce and isolate enzymatically active fragments by cleaving full or partially reduced exotoxin A molecules by proteolytic or chemical methods. Incubation of reduced toxin with chymotrypsin in the presence of oxidized NAD yielded an enzymatically active peptide (M_r, 26 000). Treatment of toxin with CNBr or 2-nitro-5-thiocyanobenzoate yielded enzymatic fragments of M_r 50 000 and 30 000 respectively. Enzymatically active non-cytotoxic fragments (M_r, 48 000) have also been isolated *in vitro* by treating exotoxin A with *P. aeruginosa* elastase followed by sodium dodecyl sulphate (SDS) polyacrylamide gel electrophoresis (Sanai *et al.*, 1980).

The lack of toxicity of the enzymatically active fragments implies that the remaining part of the exotoxin A molecule serves a function analogous to that of fragment B of diphtheria toxin. Thus exotoxin A resembles the structure–activity relationship of other bacterial toxins. That is, the molecule consists of an enzymatically active effector moiety (M_r, 26 000) and a moiety responsible for binding the toxin to the receptors on the cell surface. A receptor-binding fragment comparable to that of fragment B of diphtheria toxin has not yet been generated and isolated from purified exotoxin A, but such a fragment has been demonstrated in culture fluids (Vasil *et al.*, 1977). Thus isolation of a binding fragment may be only a technical problem in finding the appropriate conditions for the isolation and purification (Lory and Collier, 1980; Vasil *et al.*, 1977). It should be noted that although there are catalytic similarities between the enzymatic fragments of exotoxin A and diphtheria toxin (M_r, 21 145), there is no immunological cross-reactivity and they possess different pH and thermal stabilities (Lory and Collier, 1980).

To summarize, the evidence indicates that in native exotoxin A the enzymatic moiety is "buried" or distorted and that alterations in structure permit the enzymatic site to become exposed or to assume an active configuration. It is not known whether reduction or proteolytic processing of the toxin or both occur *in vivo* during the course of exotoxin A action. Although reduction of the molecule may possibly take place within the reducing environment in the cell, proteolytic processing may not only occur within the cell but also could take place prior to or after attachment to the cell receptor.

D. The pathogenic role of exotoxin A

Although the biological activity of purified exotoxin A in cells is well documented in culture and in animals, the pathogenic role of exotoxin A in human disease is not clear. Several lines of evidence, however, strongly suggest that exotoxin A contributes to the pathogenicity of the organism. It has been shown that exotoxin A, the most toxic product of the organism, is produced *in vivo* in experimental animal infections (Pavlovskis *et al.*, 1977; Saelinger *et al.*, 1977; Stieritz and Holder, 1978), as well as in human patients in sufficient amounts to elicit antibody production (Cross *et al.*, 1981; Pollack *et al.*, 1976; Pollack and Young, 1979). Mice infected with toxigenic *P. aeruginosa* strains have significantly reduced active EF-2 levels in the liver, whereas EF-2 levels were normal in infected mice pretreated with antitoxin (Pavlovskis *et al.*, 1978; Snell *et al.*, 1978) or mice infected with nontoxigenic strains (Pavlovskis *et al.*, 1978). Microscopic examinations of liver tissues from infected mice frequently revealed hepatocellular necrosis (Pavlovskis *et al.*, 1977; Wretlind and Kronevi, 1978) similar to that seen in mice injected with purified exotoxin A (Pavlovskis *et al.*, 1976). No analogous lesions were seen in mice pretreated with antitoxin. Ohman *et al.* (1980a), using nontoxigenic *Pseudomonas* mutants, has shown that exotoxin A production enhances the severity of experimental corneal infections in mice. Work in our laboratory (Pavlovskis *et al.*, 1977 and unpublished data) has produced similar results. The LD_{50} in the experimental burned mouse infection model described by Stieritz and Holder (1975) was significantly higher for nontoxigenic mutants than their corresponding toxigenic parent strains (Table 2).

Table 2   Virulence of exotoxin-A-producing *P. aeruginosa* strains and their toxin-deficient mutants[a] in mouse burn infections

Strain	Toxin	Log_{10} $LD_{50} \pm SD$[b]
PA 103	+	4.4 ± 0.9
PA 103-29	−	5.5 ± 0.4
PAO1	+	4.1 ± 0.1
PAO1-T1	−	5.8 ± 1.0

[a] PA 103-29 Isolated and characterized: Ohman *et al.* (1980c); PAO1-T1: Ohman *et al.* (1980a).
[b] $P < 0.02$.

The most convincing data regarding the pathogenic role of exotoxin A comes from immunization studies. Work in several laboratories (Liu and Hsieh, 1973; Pavlovskis *et al.*, 1977; Snell *et al.*, 1978) has demonstrated that passive immunization of mice with monospecific antitoxin resulted in significant increase in survival of mice infected with toxigenic strains as compared to control mice which received anti-bovine serum albumin (BSA) sera. Antitoxin had no protective effect on mice challenged with nontoxigenic strains of *P. aeruginosa*.

Similar results have also been obtained by actively immunizing mice with formalin inactivated highly purified (LPS-free) exotoxin A (f-toxoid) (Pavlovskis *et al.*, 1981). Three or four immunizations with the toxoid (10 µg per dose), prepared according to the procedure of Abe *et al.* (1978), and adjuvant resulted in high levels of antibody, an increase in LD_{50} (Table 3) and a significant increase in their survival rate (50–85%) (Table 4, Fig. 1) of infected

Table 3 Mean lethal doses for immunized[a] mice infected with *P. aeruginosa*

Infecting strain	Mean lethal dose ($\log_{10}$)	
	Control group[b]	Immunized group
PA 103	4.75[c]	5.55
	4.73[c]	5.93
PA 220	0.23[c]	2.03
	1.76[c]	3.36

[a] Mice immunized with f-toxoid.
[b] Control mice immunized with formalinized BSA.
[c] $P<0.01$; two-tailed Student "t" test.

Table 4 Survival of immunized[a] mice infected with *P. aeruginosa*

Infecting strain	Toxin produced	Mortality[b]		P
		Controls[c]	f-TXD	
PA 103	+	12/15	3/14	<0.01
		14/15	1/7	<0.01
PA 103-29[d]	−	15/15	15/15	>0.05
PA 220	+	14/15	3/9	<0.01
		13/15	7/15	<0.01

[a] Mice immunized with f-toxoid (F-TXD).
[b] Number of dead mice/number total mice.
[c] Control mice immunized with formalinized BSA.
[d] PA 103-29 isolated and characterized: Ohman *et al.* (1980c).

mice compared with infected controls ($<20\%$) immunized with formalinized BSA plus adjuvant. No significant differences in survival between toxoid immunized mice and their respective controls were seen when infected with nontoxigenic strains (Table 4), indicating that the protection afforded by f-toxoid is exotoxin A specific. Immunization with a glutaraldehyde-inactivated exotoxin A (g-toxoid) (Leppla *et al.*, 1978b) significantly increased the survival *time* of the toxoid immunized mice, but the survival *rate* was increased only to about 30% above the controls (Fig. 2) (Pavlovskis *et al.*, 1981). The protection of immunized mice could be improved when combined with gentamicin treatment (Figs 1 and 2) (Pavlovskis *et al.*, 1981). Virtually 100% survival was

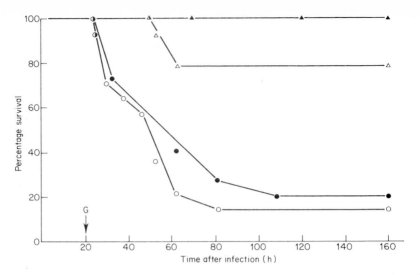

Fig. 1 Survival of burned, infected mice immunized with f-toxoid (▲, △) and controls immunized with formalinized bovine serum albumin (●, ○). Mice treated with gentamicin (●, ▲); not treated with gentamicin (○, △). G = gentamicin injection. From Pavlovskis *et al.* (1981), reprinted by permission of the American Society for Microbiology.

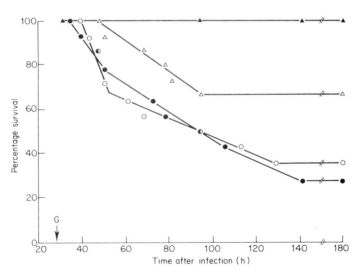

Fig. 2 Survival of burned infected mice immunized with glutaraldehyde-inactivated exotoxin A (▲, △) and controls immunized with glutaraldehyde treated bovine serum albumin (●, ○). Mice treated with gentamicin (●, ▲); not treated with gentamicin (○, △). G=gentamicin injection. From Pavlovskis *et al.* (1981), reprinted by permission of the American Society for Microbiology.

obtained when immunized mice (f- or g-toxoid) were given a single dose of gentamicin 18–20 hours post-infection. At this time gentamicin had no protective effect on the survival of control mice. Thus it appears that during the early phase of infection the immunized host effectively neutralizes the toxic effects of exotoxin A. If at approximately 20 hours post-infection the organisms are eliminated and *in vivo* exotoxin A production ceases, the host survives. In the control-BSA immunized mice, however, exotoxin A was able to continuously exert its toxicity, and by 20 hours irreversible damage had occurred and the host, regardless of the presence or absence of the organisms, died.

Cryz *et al.* (1981) have studied various toxoiding procedures of exotoxin A in detail and have produced several suitable toxoids which elicit high antitoxin levels and protect mice. They have found that formalin induces structural alterations in a region of exotoxin A molecule which is essential for cytotoxicity but distinct from a site required for enzyme activity and thus enzymatic activity was not affected. In contrast, the addition of lysine to the formalin–toxin mixtures completely destroyed enzymatic activity within 48 hours. Upon storage the formalin-derived toxoids underwent partial toxic reversion, whereas the formalin–lysine toxoid did not.

Although exotoxin has been demonstrated in the tissues of animals infected with *Pseudomonas*, circulating exotoxin A in serum has not been unequivocally demonstrated in human patients. However, as pointed out earlier, in human patients, antibody to exotoxin A has been shown to rise with *Pseudomonas* bacteremia (Pollack *et al.*, 1976) and survival has been correlated with high antitoxin titres (Cross *et al.*, 1980; Pollack and Young, 1979). Cross *et al.* (1980) showed that patients who survived bacteraemia had six times the level of antitoxin as those who died from the bacteraemia. All patients with nonbacteraemic *Pseudomonas* infections had antitoxin, and there were no deaths attributable to *P. aeruginosa*. Cross *et al.* (1980) further demonstrated that death from *P. aeruginosa* bacteraemia was significantly associated with exotoxin A production by infecting strains. Of 11 infected patients who did not produce antibodies either to exotoxin A or LPS, seven of eight died when the infecting strain produced exotoxin A. In contrast, none of three died when the infecting strain was nontoxigenic ($P < 0.001$).

The data presented indicates that exotoxin A both *in vitro* and *in vivo* acts in a highly specific manner and is extremely toxic. Observations from experimental animal infections and indirect evidence obtained from human patients strongly suggests that exotoxin A is an important virulence factor and that it contributes significantly to the pathogenic sequence of *P. aeruginosa* infections.

III. PROTEASES

One characteristic of *P. aeruginosa* is its ability to liquefy gelatin or digest casein. This property has been known to microbiologists for more than 80 years. However, the first indication that protease may contribute to the pathogenicity of the bacteria came in 1958, when Fisher and Allen described a cornea-destroying *Pseudomonas* proteolytic enzyme. Morihara (1957) was first to characterize a *Pseudomonas* protease from a strain of *P. myxogenes*, later identified as *P. aeruginosa*. The observations by Liu (1969a) that *Pseudomonas* proteases caused haemorrhagic and necrotic skin lesions were further indications that these enzymes might act as virulence factors. Most strains of *P. aeruginosa* produce several proteases including those with elastolytic activity (Morihara, 1964; Kreger and Griffin, 1974; Wretlind and Wadstrom, 1977). Two of these enzymes, elastase and alkaline protease, have been characterized and studied by several investigators.

A. Elastase

Morihara *et al.* (1965) purified and characterized a protease with elastase activity. Several investigators have confirmed Morihara's results (Balke and Sharmann, 1974; Jensen *et al.*, 1980a; Kreger and Gray, 1978; Kreger and Griffin, 1974; Scharmann and Balke, 1974; Wretlind and Wadstrom, 1977). The elastase (synonyms; protease II, protease fraction II, protease 1) can be separated from other proteases by ion exchange chromatography or isoelectric focussing and purified by ammonium sulphate precipitation or gel chromatography. More recently, affinity chromatography methods have been described (Morihara and Tsuzuki, 1975; Nishino and Powers, 1980). A completely synthetic medium for elastase production has been developed (Jensen *et al.*, 1980c). The medium contained glucose, glutamate, phenyl-alanine, valine and salts. Zinc and iron were essential for elastase production. Alkaline protease was not produced in this medium. The enzyme is a neutral, chelator-sensitive proteinase containing zinc (0.9 moles per molecule). It is active against casein, haemoglobin, elastin, fibrin and other proteins, but inactive or only weakly active against collagen. Elastase has a specificity for hydrophobic or bulky amino acids at the amino side of the splitting point (Morihara, 1974; Nishino and Powers, 1980). The molecular weight has been reported as 33 000–39 000. Sephadex chromatography gives significantly lower estimates (23 000), probably because of the interaction between the enzyme and the gel matrix resulting in retardation of the enzyme in its passage through the column. Its isoelectric point has been reported as lying between 5.7 and 6.6 (Morihara *et al.*, 1965; Kreger and Griffin, 1974; Balke and Scharmann, 1974; Wretlind and Wadstrom, 1977). The variation may be the result of autodigestion during purification.

Elastase is inhibited by chelating agents (EDTA, o-phenantroline), heavy metal ions, plasma alpha$_2$-macroglobulin, and phosphoramidon (Holder and Haidaris, 1979; Morihara and Tsuzuki, 1978).

Elastase is produced as a cell-associated inactive proenzyme early in the growth cycle and accumulates in the periplasmic space. It is converted to active enzyme *in vivo* by limited proteolysis either by alkaline protease produced by the organism or the elastase itself (Jensen *et al.*, 1980b). Yields of elastase and other exoproteins were decreased with increasing concentrations of iron in the growth medium (Bjorn *et al.*, 1979b).

B. Alkaline protease

Alkaline protease (Morihara, 1963) (synonyms: protease III, protease 2, *P. aeruginosa* proteinase) is produced by most *P. aeruginosa* strains. *In vitro* production, however, is repressed by free amino acids (Cryz and Iglewski, 1980; Morihara, 1964; Wretlind and Wadstrom, 1977). Alkaline protease was not produced in the defined medium described by Jensen *et al.* (1980c) in spite of good yields of elastase. This further emphasizes the differences in the regulation of the production of these enzymes. The molecular weight of alkaline protease is 48 400 (Inoue *et al.*, 1963; Morihara and Tsuzuki, 1977) and its isoelectric point 4.1–5.0. Alkaline protease contains 1–2 atoms of calcium per molecule. Cobalt ions have been shown to promote hydrolysis (Morihara and Tsuzuki, 1964, 1974).

C. Other proteases

Another protease (neutral protease, protease fraction I, protease I) with an isoelectric point of 8.5 and an optimum pH of 6.5 has been identified in culture fluids (Kreger and Griffin, 1974; Morihara, 1964; Wretlind and Wadstrom, 1977), however, since the enzyme is produced in small amounts, it has not yet been purified. In contrast to elastase and alkaline protease this enzyme is not inhibited by EDTA.

Several investigators have described *Pseudomonas* enzymes with collagenase activity (Schoellmann and Fisher, 1966) or collagenolytic activities of *Pseudomonas* elastase (Carrick and Berk, 1975; Jensen *et al.*, 1980a), but others have been unable to detect collagenolytic activities among *P. aeruginosa* strains (Kreger and Griffin, 1974; Morihara and Tsuzuki, 1977; Wretlind and Wadstrom, 1977). This may be due to differences in the assay methods used by the various groups. It should be noted that although few reports indicate that *Pseudomonas* proteases may possess a weak collagenolytic activity, a collagenase similar to the enzyme produced by *Clostridium histolyticum* has not been demonstrated.

D. Biological properties of proteases

The reported LD_{50} values for elastase have shown a variation 60–400 µg per mouse) depending on the preparation and the route of administration (Kawaharajo et al., 1975b; Meinke et al., 1970; Wretlind and Wadstrom, 1977). The enzyme is most toxic when administered by intrapleural or intrapulmonary routes (LD_{50} < 100 µg); it is not lethal when injected subcutaneously. On a weight basis, P. aeruginosa exotoxin A is approximately 1000 times more lethal. Elastase is inhibited by the serum protease inhibitor alpha$_2$-macroglobulin, which may explain its low toxicity (Holder and Haidaris, 1979). Injections of purified elastase into animals usually leads to haemorrhage of internal organs. In vitro treatment of rabbit alveolar macrophages with elastase leads to agglutination and vacuolization (Leake et al., 1978). However, in vitro elastase treatment does not damage the cytoplasmic membranes of HeLa cells or human diploid embryonic lung fibroblasts (Wretlind and Wadstrom, 1977). The observed changes are similar to those produced by trypsin.

Intrapulmonary and intrapleural injections of purified proteases caused extensive lung damage, with haemorrhages and necrosis of alveolar septal cells similar to that reported in cases of Pseudomonas pneumonia (Gray and Kreger, 1979; Meinke et al., 1970; Kawaharajo et al., 1975b; Shimizu et al., 1974). Thus, the results indicate that in vivo protease production may be important in eliciting lung damage. Elastase and alkaline protease cause dermonecrosis after injection of less than 10 µg of purified enzyme, suggesting a role in wound and skin infection (Kawaharajo et al., 1975a; Wretlind and Wadstrom, 1977).

Kreger and Griffin (1974) have demonstrated three cornea-damaging proteases in culture supernates of strains capable of causing kerititis. Less than 1 µg of these enzymes caused extensive colliquative necrosis of rabbit corneas after intracorneal injections. The necrosis progressed to descemetocele formation and corneal perforation. Light and electron microscopy examination of cornea showed degradation of the proteoglycan, but not of collagen fibrils (Brown et al., 1974; Kawaharajo et al., 1974; Kessler et al., 1977b; Kreger and Gray, 1978). Several plasma proteins have been shown to be substrates for Pseudomonas proteases. Fibrin and fibrinogen as well as other coagulation factors are degraded in vitro by the proteases, and this probably explains the haemorrhages observed after the injection of purified enzymes into animals (Scharmann and Kraft, 1974a). Elastase also inactivates in vitro several complement factors (C1, C3, C5, C8, and C9) (Schultz and Miller, 1974). Inactivation of human alpha$_1$-proteinase inhibitor has also been reported (Morihara et al., 1979). If this does occur in vivo, the loss of the protease inhibitor could permit leucocyte serine proteases to cause tissue damage.

E. The role of proteases in infections

P. aeruginosa infections of the eye are not common, but when they do occur they often result in loss of vision of the infected eye. Since the corneal proteoglycan is a sensitive substrate for *Pseudomonas* proteases, it has been suggested that these enzymes are the main cause of tissue damage. Experimental infections show a loss of proteoglycan ground substance with dispersal of undamaged collagen fibrils (Gray and Kreger, 1975). Similar observations have been made after intracorneal administration of proteases (Kessler *et al.*, 1977b; Kreger and Gray, 1978). Protease-producing strains have been shown to cause experimental keratitis in mice, whereas protease negative strains are avirulent (Kawaharajo and Homma, 1978). Both passive and active immunization against elastase, alkaline protease, and endotoxin-protein (OEP) protected against experimental eye infections in mice (Hirao and Homma, 1978). Recently, Ohman *et al.* (1980b) studied the role of elastase in corneal infection in mice using a mutant that produced an altered elastase due to mutation in the structural gene of the enzyme. The elastase mutant (PA01-E64) was as virulent as the wild type strain (PA01). The mutant, however, did produce alkaline protease which also has cornea-damaging activity. It should be pointed out that other *Pseudomonas* products such as exotoxin A (Iglewski *et al.*, 1977a) and heat-stable haemolysin (Johnson and Allen, 1978) may also contribute to corneal damage. It has also been suggested that host-derived proteases and collagenase may contribute to the pathogenesis of *Pseudomonas* keratitis (Kessler *et al.*, 1977a; Van Horn *et al.*, 1978).

Pseudomonas pneumonia is characterized by intra-alveolar haemorrhage, necrosis of alveolar septal cells, and infiltration of mononuclear cells suggestive of protease-induced damage (Gray and Kreger, 1979; Nordstoga, 1968; Shimizu *et al.*, 1974; Tillotson and Lerner, 1968). Sera from human patients with *Pseudomonas* pneumonia (Homma *et al.*, 1975) and cystic fibrosis (Klinger *et al.*, 1978) contained antibodies against elastase and alkaline protease. Klinger *et al.* (1978) was able to demonstrate an inverse correlation between antibody titres and the clinical severity of the disease. A vaccine containing toxoids of elastase, alkaline protease and OEP protected mink against haemorrhagic pneumonia (Aoi *et al.*, 1979; Homma *et al.*, 1978).

A role for *Pseudomonas* proteases in burn infection was suggested by Carney *et al.* (1973). Kawaharajo and Homma (1977), using an experimental protease–elastase and OEP toxoid vaccine, were able to protect mice against experimental burn infection. Snell *et al.* (1978) and Holder and Haidaris (1979) reported that injections (10 µg) of elastase, alkaline-protease or *Bacillus thermoproteolyticus* protease (thermolysin) together with protease deficient *Pseudomonas* strain (PA 103) in burned mice caused a 1000-fold reduction in LD_{50}. This effect was specific for strains of *P. aeruginosa* since the LD_{50} of other pathogenic bacteria was unaffected by the injection of proteases. The protease inhibitor alpha$_2$-macroglobulin gave a significant protection against protease positive strains (Holder, 1981).

The *in vivo* role of a product of an organism can best be studied by using mutants lacking the ability to produce that particular product. This approach has been used to define the virulence factors of salmonellas and *Staphylococcus aureus* in experimental animal infections (Forsgren, 1972; Lindberg *et al.*, 1974). Pavlovskis and Wretlind (1979) studied the role of elastase in mouse burn infections using two protease-deficient mutants of a protease-positive clinical strain, PAKS-1. Both mutants were defective in the formation of extracellular proteases and several non-toxic exo-enzymes, but produced exotoxin A. In the burned mouse model (Stieritz and Holder, 1975) the LD$_{50}$ of the mutants were one log$_{10}$ higher than that of the wild-type strain (Table 5) (Pavlovskis and Wretlind, 1979). The addition of 5–45 µg purified elastase to the infecting inoculum of elastase-deficient mutants reduced survival time and the number of surviving mice. Passive immunization with rabbit anti-elastase serum gave significant protection against the elastase-producing wild-type strain but not against the elastase-deficient mutants. Anti-elastase serum also prolonged survival time of mice infected with an elastase-deficient mutant and purified elastase. Quantitative blood cultures in mice infected with 1 LD$_{100}$ of protease-producing PAKS-1 or its protease-deficient mutants showed that the mice infected with protease-deficient strains had lower viable bacterial counts than mice infected with PAKS-1. However, when burned mice were infected with a mixture of PAKS-1 and one of the mutants at a 1:1 ratio, the number of protease-deficient organisms in the blood was considerably higher than in infections with the mutants alone.

The role of elastase in experimental burn infections was further studied in

Table 5 Virulence of elastase-producing *P. aeruginosa* strains and their elastase-deficient mutants[a] in mouse burn infections

Strains	Elastase	Log$_{10}$ LD$_{50}$[b]
PAKS-1	+	3.8
PAKS-10	(+)[c]	4.8
PAKS-17	−	4.9
PAO1	+	4.1
PAO1-E64	−	5.1

[a] PAKS-10 and PAKS-17 characterized: Pavlovskis and Wretlind (1979); PAO1-E64: Ohman *et al.* (1980b).
[b] $P<0.02$.
[c] Weakly elastase positive.

our laboratory (unpublished data) by using a mutant that produced an altered elastase. Ohman and associates (Ohman et al., 1980b) isolated a mutant that produced a temperature-sensitive elastase, probably because of a mutation in the structural gene for elastase. The LD_{50} for this mutant was one log_{10} higher than for the parent strain (Table 5). These data are in good agreement with the results from the study by Pavlovskis and Wretlind (1979) described above.

The data presented indicate that proteases, and elastase in particular, may contribute to the pathogenicity of the organism. The mechanism by which proteases exert their toxic action during an infection is not clear. Because of their high LD_{50} it is unlikely that proteases alone are responsible for the lethal effect of P. aeruginosa. The results of Pavlovskis and Wretlind (1979) suggest that elastase may be important in overcoming the host's initial defence mechanisms. This may be either as the result of proteolytic action which provides additional nutrients for the invading bacteria as suggested by Cicmanek and Holder (1979) or by the destruction of the anatomical barriers preventing the spread of the organisms. The suggestion that protease is important in overcoming the host's defences is also indirectly supported by the work of Wretlind and Kronevi (1978), who infected cyclophosphamide-treated mice with protease-positive or -negative mutants. In contrast to the work of Pavlovskis and Wretlind (1979) they found no differences in LD_{50} between the strains, nor did they find any differences in LD_{50} when protease-positive and -negative strains were injected with mucin in normal mice. Both models, however, were designed to overcome the host's initial defence mechanisms, thus negating any advantage a protease-producing strain might have. The cyclophosphamide treatment reduced the leucocyte count from approximately $8000\,mm^{-3}$ for normal mice to less than $500\,mm^{-3}$ for cyclophosphamide-treated mice (Pavlovskis and Wretlind, 1979). In the second model, the mucin protected the organisms and increased the sensitivity of the host to the invading organisms. Once the infection is established, however, proteases may contribute to local tissue damage. B. H. Iglewski, for example, found elastase in tissue homogenates from Pseudomonas-infected mice (personal communication). The role of proteases in established septicaemia is probably only marginal. In the case of Pseudomonas eye infections proteases are capable of degrading corneal proteoglycan ground substance and are responsible for the resulting structural alterations. Proteases are considered to be the cause of the rapid invasion and corneal dissolution. It has been similarly shown that proteases produced by P. aeruginosa cause dissolution of pulmonary tissue in rabbits. Both passive and active immunization of experimental animals as well as treatment with protease inhibitor alpha$_2$-macroglobulin offers a certain degree of protection against P. aeruginosa infections. Thus the data indicate that Pseudomonas proteases contribute to the pathogenic mechanism of the organism.

IV. MEMBRANE-ACTIVE TOXINS

A. Haemolysins

Most *P. aeruginosa* strains produce two haemolytic substances. One is heat-labile and is probably phospholipase C with lecithinase activity (Esselamann *et al.*, 1961; Liu, 1966a; Wretlind *et al.*, 1973) (see below); the other is a heat-stable glycolipid composed of rhamnose and β-hydroxydecanoic acid (Hisatsuka *et al.*, 1971; Jarvis and Johnson, 1949; Sierra, 1960). The phosphiolipase and the glycolipid are usually produced together in an environment low in phosphate and high in carbohydrate content (Liu, 1964). Recently a purified haemolysin preparation containing two haemolytic glycolipids has been reported (Johnson and Boese-Marrazzo, 1980). The haemolytic glycolipid is a detergent capable of solubilizing phospholipids (Hisatsuka *et al.*, 1971; Kurioka and Liu, 1967a). Its effect on cell membranes is also detergent-like (Thelestam and Mollby, 1979). Methods for production and purification of the haemolytic glycolipid have been described (Berk, 1964; Johnson and Boese-Marrazzo, 1980). It appears that the glycolipid, at least *in vitro*, may enhance the activity of the phospholipase (Kurioka and Liu, 1967a, 1967b).

The glycolipid is relatively non-toxic. Given intraperitoneally, its LD_{50} is approximately 5 mg for mice (Jarvis and Johnson, 1949) and its haemolytic activity is inhibited by serum albumin (Berk, 1964). Thus, a significant role for the glycolipid in *Pseudomonas* infections is unlikely. Johnson and Allen (1978) have presented evidence suggesting that glycolipid could contribute to tissue damage in *Pseudomonas* keratitis due to enzyme release from leucocytes. Al-Dujaili (1976) reported that *P. aeruginosa* strains isolated from the respiratory tract of patients were more strongly haemolytic than strains isolated from other sources, suggesting a role for the glycolipid in lung infections.

Although evidence indicated that the heat-labile haemolysin is phospholipase (synonyms: lecithinase, heat-labile haemolysin, haemolysin A) no direct proof of their identity had been established (Liu, 1974). Recently a heat-labile haemolysin (fraction A) was purified by isoelectric focussing and sucrose density-gradient which apparently is identical to phospholipase C (Watanabe *et al.*, 1978). This protein was shown to hydrolyse lecithin to produce phosphorylcholine (phospholipase C activity) and did not require any cofactors for its haemolytic activity. The haemolytic and phospholipase activities could not be separated indicating that the haemolytic protein is a phospholipase. Berka *et al.* (in preparation) have effectively purified *Pseudomonas* phospholipase C from low phosphate culture supernatants by adsorption with lecithin affinity gel and Sephadex G-75 gel filtration, resulting in approximately 940-fold purification. The K_m value for the enzyme was established to be 167 μM, and V_{max} to be $-2\,\mathrm{nmol\,min^{-1}}$. The isoelectric point was near 5.9, in good agreement with the value of 5.75 measured by Watanabe (1978) (Berka and Vasil, personal communication). When Berke *et al.* analysed the phospholipase by SDS-PAGE, they found that areas corresponding to enzyme activity stained diffusely with Coomassie Blue and fuschin-bisulphite suggesting that phospholipase C was either a large glycoprotein or was associated with a heterogeneous carbohydrate, possibly LPS.

The *in vitro* production of phospholipase appears to be regulated by end-product repression (Johnson and Allen, 1978). Enzyme secretion required a carbon source and ammonium, potassium or calcium ions (Stinson and Hayden, 1979) and it was repressed by inorganic but not organic phosphates (Liu, 1974; Stinson and Hayden, 1979). The calcium requirement could be substituted by magnesium or strontium ions. Gray *et al.* (in preparation) have suggested that since phospholipase C and alkaline phosphatase co-purify on the lecithin affinity column, a functional relationship to liberate inorganic phosphate from phospholipids may exist between the two enzymes. They have also found that alkaline phosphatase and phospholipase C are co-ordinately depressed by inorganic phosphate starvation.

Although phospholipase C possesses a number of toxic properties, the discussion concerning its role in pathogenesis has remained largely speculative. When phospholipase C preparations, free of protease activity, were injected into the skin of rabbits or guinea pigs, they produced, between 24–48 hours, necrosis of an area with a central abscess surrounded by a zone of erythema (Liu, 1966a). Intraperitoneal injections of the enzyme resulted in hepatic necrosis. The haemorrhagic lesions frequently observed in internal organs following protease administration have not been observed with phospholipase. However, attempts to demonstrate *in vivo* production of phospholipase in experimental animals have not been successful (Liu, 1966b), nor could phospholipase be produced *in vitro* when rabbit serum was used as source of nutrients (Liu, 1964).

The alveolar surfaces of lungs are covered with surfactants, made up mostly of lipids. Reynolds and Fick (1979) have suggested that phospholipase has the potential to destroy lung surfactants and lung tissue, thus possibly causing bronchiectasis and atelectasis. It is conceivable that the surfactants which contain phospholipids induce production of phospholipase. *P. aeruginosa* strains which produced *in vitro* significant amounts of lecithinase (phospholipase C) ($34.5 \pm 6.7\,\mu\mathrm{g\,ml^{-1}}$) when administered intranasally (via aerosol) to mice were able to multiply in the lung and were not cleared as rapidly as strains which were not excellent lecithinase producers ($8.86 \pm 1.2\,\mu\mathrm{g\,ml^{-1}}$) (Southern *et al.*, 1970). Berka and Vasil (in preparation) found that urinary tract isolates consistently produced highest amounts of phospholipase C as compared to other clinical isolates. Lung and sputum isolates also produced high levels, but greater variability existed among strains. Blood and wound isolates produced significantly lower amounts. The data suggest that alterations of pulmonary surfactants may be one factor enabling the organism to invade and colonize the lung. Baltch *et al.* (1979) reported that blood culture isolates produced greater quantities of phospholipase C and proteases than non-bacteraemic isolates. However, they were unable to show any correlation between the *in vitro* quantity of phospholipase and the prognosis of these patients. Their study suggested a local rather than systemic importance of phospholipase C in the pathogenesis.

Phospholipase C probably is not an important factor contributing to the lethality of *Pseudomonas* infections. Experimental and clinical observations suggest that phospholipase-producing strains may have an added advantage in invading the host's tissues and thus facilitate blood stream invasion. There is no statistical correlation between death or survival of experimental animals or patients and the phospholipase produced by the invading organisms.

B. Leucocidin

Scharmann (1976a, 1976b, 1976c, 1976d; Scharmann *et al.*, 1976) has characterized a cytotoxic protein active against leucocytes. This toxin designated leucocidin appears to be distinct from other *P. aeruginosa* toxins. Leucocidin does not react with anti-exotoxin A serum, and the amino acid composition of the two toxins is also different (Lutz, 1979). The toxin was produced as a cell-bound inactive precursor and released upon cell lysis and activated by proteases. Good yields of leucocidin were obtained through autolysis of washed bacterial suspensions at 37°C for 56 hours. Only 4 of 110 strains tested produced detectable amounts of the protein (Scharmann, 1976c).

Leucocidin was purified from cell autolysate by ammonium sulphate precipitation and gel chromatography. It had a molecular weight of 27 000 daltons and isoelectric point of 5.0–5.2. The purified toxin was sensitive to pronase, but resistant to several other proteases such as *Pseudomonas* elastase, trypsin, pancreatic elastase, papain, subtilisin (Scharmann, 1976c). The leucocidin exhibited the same properties as many other cytolytic toxins from bacteria. It damaged granulocytes from various animal species and human lymphocytes. Leucocidin was also cytopathogenic for different tissue culture cells, but did not cause lysis of erythrocytes or isolated leucocyte granules. After exposure to leucocidin, granulocytes became round and motility was lost. Protoplasmic extrusions appeared on the cell membrane. The final stage showed an enlarged, rounded vesicle with apparently intact plasma membrane. The cytotoxic action was studied on bovine granulocytes by following release of various intracellular markers (Scharmann, 1976a). Low-molecular markers (K^+, $^{86}Rb^+$, glucose) were lost from the granulocytes within 1–2 minutes after addition of leucocidin. The release of high molecular markers (^{51}Cr bound to proteins) occurred only after swelling of the cells. Studies with [^{125}I]-labelled toxin indicated two binding sites, one at the surface of the plasma membrane, and one that became accessible to the toxin in the course of the cytotoxic action. In the presence of Ca^{2+} the velocity of the toxin fixation was increased. The leucocidin receptor was probably an integral protein of the plasma membrane (Scharmann, 1976b). The leucocidin is relatively toxic, its LD_{50} being about 1 µg per mouse (Scharmann, 1976d). Scharmann's findings have been confirmed in a more recent paper by Lutz (1979), who also demonstrated fatty liver necrosis in mice dying after injection of leucocidin. The toxin also caused cardiovascular failure in mice and rats (Frimmer et al., 1976; Hegner et al., 1976) and loss of potassium from perfused rat livers or isolated hepatocytes (Frimmer and Scharmann, 1975).

The role of leucocidin in Pseudomonas infections is not known. Scharmann (1976a) has suggested that the neutropenia found in Pseudomonas sepsis is caused by the action of this toxin. However, Sensakovic and Bartell (1974) reported that a toxic slime fraction caused leucopenia in mice, and the relative contribution of these factors and of exotoxin A to leucopenia remains to be determined. Finally, the low incidence of leucocidin producing strains argue against any significant importance of leucocidin in Pseudomonas infections.

V. ENTEROTOXIN AND VASCULAR PERMEABILITY FACTOR

Part of the problem of studying the infectious aetiological agents of gastro-enteritis is the difficulty in identifying the pathogens among a large number of indigenous organisms. Thus, even though P. aeruginosa has been implicated in diarrhoeal conditions since the turn of the century (Williams, 1894) and a number of "diarrhoeas of unknown origin" have been attributed to the organism (Dold, 1918; Jellard and Churcher, 1967; Ensign and Hunter, 1946; South, 1971), its role in gastro-enteritis has not been clearly established. In 1971 the production of an enterotoxin by P. aeruginosa was demonstrated by its capacity to cause fluid accumulation in rabbit ileal loops following the injection of live organisms (Kubota and Liu, 1971). The amount of fluid accumulated was less than observed with Vibrio cholerae. Recently the isolation of enterotoxic P. aeruginosa strains which give positive ileal loop tests in piglets and rabbits have been reported by several laboratories (Baljer and Barrett, 1979; Shriniwas et al., 1979). We have also examined in our laboratory the ability of several Pseudomonas strains provided by Dr S. C. Sanyal (Banaras Hindu University) to induce fluid accumulation in rabbit ileal loops. We found, as did Kubota and Liu (1971), that the amount of fluid was considerably less than with *V. cholerae*. For *V. cholerae* the ratio of volume:length (approximately 8.0 cm) was between 1.0 and 1.2, whereas for the *Pseudomonas* strains it was between 0.25 and 0.47 (Merrell and Pavlovskis, unpublished data). Apparently the ability to induce fluid accumulation is very labile for *Pseudomonas* since it has already been lost in two out of four strains tested.

The enterotoxin has not been purified, but it is heat-sensitive and could be destroyed by the action of trypsin (Kubota and Liu, 1971). It appears to be distinct from any of the other toxic materials produced by *Pseudomonas* such as exotoxin A, haemolysin, or phospholipase. Okada *et al.* (1976) demonstrated a positive rabbit ileal loop test, when one-milligram quantities of purified *Pseudomonas* elastase or alkaline protease were injected into the loops. It seems unlikely, however, that proteases could be produced in such large quantities in the intestines during a natural infection.

Production of a vascular permeability factor (PF) by *P. aeruginosa* similar to the PF associated with *V. cholerae* enterotoxin has been reported (Kusama, 1974; Kusama and Huss, 1972; Shriniwas *et al.*, 1979). This factor was also destroyed by heating or treatment with trypsin and required a heat-stable cofactor for its activity. Strains producing PF tended to be more virulent in experimental mouse burn infections. The identity between PF and the enterotoxin described by Kubota and Liu (1971) has not been established. However, Shriniwas *et al.* (1979) have reported that enterotoxin-positive strains were always positive for PF suggesting that these two factors may be identical.

Because the *P. aeruginosa* enterotoxin has not yet been purified and characterized in any detail and its nature has not been established, it may be advisable to avoid the term *enterotoxin* and refer to it as a "rabbit ileal loop factor".

VI. SLIME GLYCOLIPOPROTEIN

In recent years the role of slime in *Pseudomonas* infections has been studied. The function of slime in the pathogenesis of the organisms was first reported by Liu *et al.* (1961). Bartell *et al.* (1970) isolated and purified by relatively gentle procedures a toxic slime antigen (glycolipoprotein, GLP) which caused leucopenia and death after injection into mice.

Endotoxin-free GLP (MW > 100 000) was purified from the extracellular slime layer by extraction with saline, ethanol precipitation, ion exchange chromatography, and ultracentrifugation (Bartell *et al.*, 1970). Chemical analysis showed that GLP contained hexoses, hexosamines, uronic acid, lipid and protein. Four fatty acids which were components of GLP were not present in LPS preparations from the same strains. The LPS contained one fatty acid not found in GLP (Sensakovic and Bartell, 1974). Antigenic differences between LPS and slime were demonstrated by immunodiffusion and indirect haemagglutination inhibition (Sensakovic and Bartell, 1974). Analysis of antigenic relatedness between GLPs from different strains by indirect haemagglutination inhibition demonstrated an antigenic diversity (Dimitracopoulos and Bartell, 1980). Homologous GLP showed the strongest inhibition while heterologous GLP was only slightly active. There was no correlation with the immunotype (Fisher et al., 1969) of the strains. GLP also possessed receptor-like activity for certain phages (Bartell et al., 1971) and the carbohydrate moiety appeared to be a substrate for phage depolymerase (Sensakovic and Bartell, 1975). Pseudomonas strains lysogenic for or resistant to phage 8 did not produce the depolymerase substrate and their GLPs differed quantitatively in neutral sugar, amino sugar, and protein content from the wild type GLP (Dimitracopoulos and Bartell, 1979). The GLP is distinctly different from the extracellular exopolysaccharide produced by "mucoid" strains of P. aeruginosa isolated predominantly from cystic fibrosis patients (Doggett et al., 1964; Doggett and Harrison, 1972; Hoiby, 1977; Reynolds et al., 1975). The exopolysaccharide is an alginic-acid like polysaccharide consisting mostly of D-mannuronic and L-glucoronic acids (Carlson and Matthews, 1966; Evans and Linker, 1973).

Injections of GLP into mice induced leucopenia and proved lethal. The LD_{50} of the GLP for mice was 30 μg per g (IP) of body weight, whereas the LD_{50} for LPS from the same strain was 60–90 μg per g body weight (Sensakovic and Bartell, 1974). In vitro GLP inhibited phagocytosis and exerted a mitogenic effect on human blood lymphocytes (Papamichail et al., 1980; Sensakovic and Bartell, 1980).

When GLP was treated with phenol to remove the protein, the remaining fragment still possessed all the biological activities of GLP. After acetic acid treatment which removed all of the lipid and most of the protein, the remaining carbohydrate was not toxic but retained its antigenic specificity and its ability to inhibit phagocytosis. Fragments released after treatment with phage 2-depolymerase lacked all biological activities of GLP. These results indicate that the toxic activities (leucopenia, lethality) are associated with the lipid moiety and are not due to contaminants such as exotoxin A as previously suggested (Liu, 1974). The antigenic specificity and antiphagocytic activity appears to reside in the carbohydrate portions (Sensakovic and Bartell, 1975).

Leucocytes obtained from mice injected with GLP agglutinated with rabbit anti-GLP serum indicating an in vivo association between GLP and leucocytes. This observation was also supported by fluorescein-labelled antibody studies. In vivo studies suggested that purified GLP when injected into mice enters the blood stream and becomes associated mainly with neutrophils and that the neutrophil–GLP complex is deposited in the liver leading to leucopenia (Lynn et al., 1977). It appears that GLP is an important toxic product of the organisms.

Active and passive immunization of mice against GLP protected from leucopenia and death after challenge with live organisms. Although there was some degree of cross-protection between strains, each antiserum protected most effectively against the homologous strain (Sensakovic and Bartell, 1974, 1977). LPS failed to absorb the protective antibodies from slime antiserum. The data suggest a pathogenic role for GLP.

VII. EXOENZYME S

Recently, a second extracellular protein (exoenzyme S) with ADP ribosyltransferase activity produced by some strains of P. aeruginosa has been isolated and purified about 30-fold (Bjorn et al., 1979a; Iglewski et al., 1978). The medium used for exoenzyme S production is similar to that previously developed for exotoxin A production (Thompson et al., 1980). In addition, exoenzyme S production required the presence of chelating agents such as nitrilotriacetate or EDTA, whereas exotoxin A production does not (Iglewski and Sadoff, 1979). However, EDTA inhibits the growth of the organism thus resulting in a lower overall yield. Attempts to produce exoenzyme S by growing the organism in chemically defined medium (DeBell, 1979) have not been successful (Iglewski, personal communication).

Exoenzyme S differs from exotoxin A in that it is heat-stable and does not ADP-ribosylate EF-2, but, rather, modifies one or more different proteins present in eucaryotic cell extracts. Also whereas urea and dithiothreitol treatment enhances enzymatic activity of exotoxin A, it destroys the activity of exoenzyme S. Serologically the two proteins do not cross-react. The enzymatic activities of exotoxin A and exoenzyme S cannot be neutralized by anti-S or antitoxin A respectively. The evidence suggests that exotoxin A and exoenzyme S are structurally different. It appears that in culture supernatants, exoenzyme S aggregates or associates with other proteins or lipoproteins (DeBell, personal communication; Thompson et al., 1980). Sokol and associates (personal communication) detected in vitro exoenzyme S production in 38% of 124 clinical P. aeruginosa isolates from patients with bacteraemia or burn infections. Thus production of exoenzyme S by clinical isolates of P. aeruginosa is not a rare event. The majority of strains which produce exoenzyme S also produce exotoxin A, however, 11% of strains produced only exoenzyme S.

No studies have been reported regarding the toxicity or the role of exoenzyme S in *P. aeruginosa* infections. Indirect evidence, however, does suggest that exoenzyme S may contribute to the pathogenicity of the organism. The enzyme is produced *in vivo* and in experimental infections (Bjorn *et al.*, 1979a). Skin extracts and sera from burned mice infected with a lethal dose of a non-toxigenic, exoenzyme-S-producing strain contained exoenzyme activity. Although this strain produces elastase, because of the organism's extreme lethality ($LD_{50} = 1.1 \times 10^2$) for burned mice, it is unlikely that elastase is completely responsible for its virulence. In human patients infections with exoenzyme S positive, exotoxin-A-negative strains frequently result in death (Cross *et al.*, 1980; Iglewski, personal communication). In one study, of the seven strains identified as producing exoenzyme S, five were from patients who died (Thompson *et al.*, 1980).

The role, if any, of exoenzyme S in clinical infections is not known. Data regarding the toxicity of exoenzyme *in vitro* and *in vivo* systems, its production by clinical isolates, and the protective effects of specific antibodies are still required to evaluate its relative importance and its role in the pathogenesis of the organism.

VIII. CONCLUSION

A vast amount of information on the production, isolation and characterization of *Pseudomonas* enzymes and toxins has been accumulated during recent years, but there are still important gaps in our knowledge. Although several of these toxins have been shown to contribute to the pathogenicity of the organism and their mode of action is known, little is known of the interaction of these toxins with tissues and the sequence of the pathological events.

After release from the bacterial cell, the toxin may be transported by the blood stream throughout the body and cause systemic symptoms or it may diffuse in the surrounding area and damage primarily the local tissues. Both events probably occur. Since the toxins produced by *P. aeruginosa* are considerably less powerful than those of the classical toxin-mediated diseases such as botulism or tetanus, the local effects are probably the more important ones. In a recent review, Costerton (1979) presented evidence that in nature and, very likely, in the infected host, *Pseudomonas* usually does not exist as free-floating organisms but, rather, is attached to surfaces as microcolonies enclosed in a fibrous polysaccharide matrix. If this indeed is the case, the micro-organisms would have a very efficient mechanism by which to discharge their deleterious toxins. A "free-floating" bacterium is much more susceptible to the host's defences, and the enzymes and toxins are diluted and more easily neutralized or destroyed before reaching their targets. In contrast, toxins produced by organisms growing in a dense microcolony remain sufficiently concentrated to penetrate and damage the surrounding tissue. In such a system the toxins need not be highly toxic to be effective. Furthermore, organisms growing in microcolonies are less susceptible to antibodies and antibiotics.

Because of the diversity of the *P. aeruginosa* toxins, the observed pathology in most cases cannot be attributed to a particular toxin. It appears that two of the extracellular toxins, elastase and exotoxin A, contribute significantly to the pathogenicity of the organism, whereas the role of others (phospholipase C, slime glycolipoprotein, leucocidin, exoenzyme S and the rabbit ileal loop factor) is not as clear. The proteases apparently enhance the ability of the bacteria to establish the infection, either by providing additional nutrients or by destroying anatomical barriers or by both. During the later stages of the infection the effect of exotoxin A predominates. Exotoxin A is secreted from the onset of the infection, causing a continued and irreversible damage. In experimental infections the primary organ to be affected is the liver, but in man only rarely is *Pseudomonas* infection associated with hepatic malfunction (Cross *et al.*, 1980). None the less, because the toxic action of exotoxin A — inhibition of protein synthesis — is a general biochemical function and because *in vitro* exotoxin A does not exhibit any specificity for a particular cell line, there is no reason to believe that its toxic action should be confined to only one tissue. During an infection the host is exposed to a continuous release of small amounts of exotoxin A, which may have additive biochemical and pharmacological effects on the surrounding tissues. It is therefore very probable that other organs and tissues are affected as well and that their eventual impairment contributes to the illness and death of the host. An important facet of the exotoxin A effect may be its interference with leucocyte function, as suggested by *in vitro* data showing that toxin is lethal for human macrophages derived from peripheral blood monocytes (Pollack and Anderson, 1978; Yamada *et al.*, 1977).

Experimental data show that elastase and exotoxin A elicit high levels of antibodies both in experimental animals and in patients. These results suggest that these proteins should be considered for use in a prophylactic *Pseudomonas* vaccine. Despite advances in chemotherapy and supportive treatment, *Pseudomonas* infections still constitute a major unresolved clinical problem. Several attempts to produce a vaccine from whole cells by empirical methods or from endotoxin have been made, but most of these preparations have been either too toxic or too ill-defined for use in humans. Moreover some of these antigens have the disadvantage of varying in type specificity. On the other hand, elastase and exotoxin A can be obtained in chemically pure form and do not vary with the strain type. Their biological activity can be inactivated without destroying immunogenicity. Both passive and active immunization with elastase and exotoxin A antisera or antigens protect animals against *P. aeruginosa* infections. The results with animals have been very encouraging, but the usefulness of these toxoids in a human vaccine remains to be determined. The proof, of course, will rest in the prevention of the disease.

ACKNOWLEDGEMENTS

We thank Dr Emilio Weiss for his suggestions and comments. The work was supported in part by the US Naval Research and Development Command, Research Work Unit No. M0095.PN002.5052 and the Research Institute of the Swedish National Defence.

REFERENCES

Abe, C., Shionoya, H., Hirao, Y., Okada, K. and Homma, J. Y. (1975). *Japan. J. Exptl Med.* **45**, 355–359.
Abe, C., Tanamoto, K. and Homma, J. Y. (1977). *Japan. J. Exptl Med.* **47**, 393–402.
Abe, C., Takeshi, K. and Homma, J. Y. (1978). *Japan. J. Exptl Med.* **48**, 183–186.
Adler, J. L., Burke, J. P. and Finland, M. (1970). *Arch. Intern. Med.* **127**, 460–465.
Al-Dujaili, A. H. (1976). *J. Hyg.* **77**, 211–220.
Aoi, Y., Noda, H., Yanagawa, R., Homma, J. Y., Abe, C., Morihara, K., Goda, A., Takeuchi, S. and Ishihara, T. (1979). *Japan. J. Exptl Med.* **49**, 199–207.
Atik, M. P., Liu, P. V., Hanson, B. A., Amini, S. and Rosenberg, C. F. (1968). *J. Amer. Med. Assoc.* **205**, 134–140.
Baljer, G. and Barrett, J. T. (1979). *Zbl. Vet. Med.* B **26**, 740–747.
Balke, E. and Scharmann, W. (1974). *Z. Physiol. Chem.* **355**, 958–968.
Baltch, A. L. and Griffin, P. E. (1977). *Amer. J. Med. Sci.* **274**, 119–129.
Baltch, A. L., Griffin, P. E. and Hammer, M. (1979). *J. Lab. Clin. Med.* **93**, 600–606.
Bartell, P. F., Orr, T. E. and Chudio, B. (1970). *Infect. Immun.* **2**, 543–548.
Bartell, P. F., Orr, T. E., Reese, J. F. and Imaeda, T. (1971). *J. Virol.* **8**, 311–317.
Berk, R. S. (1964). *J. Bacteriol.* **88**, 559–565.
Bjorn, M. J., Vasil, M. L., Sadoff, J. C. and Iglewski, B. H. (1977). *Infect. Immun.* **16**, 362–366.
Bjorn, M. J., Pavlovskis, O. R., Thompson, M. R. and Iglewski, B. H. (1979a). *Infect. Immun.* **24**, 837–842.
Bjorn, M. J., Sokol, P. A. and Iglewski, B. H. (1979b). *J. Bacteriol.* **138**, 193–200.
Bonventre, P. F. (1970). *In* "Microbial Toxins" (S. J. Ajl, S. Kadis and T. C. Montie, ed.) Vol. I, p. 31. Academic Press, New York and London.
Bonventre, P. F., Lincoln, R. E. and Lamana, C. (1967). *Bacteriol. Rev.* **31**, 95–109.
Brown, B. A. and Bodley, J. W. (1979). *FEBS Letters* **103**, 253–255.
Brown, S. I., Bloomfield, S. E. and Tam, W. I. (1974). *Invest. Ophthalmol. Visual Sci.* **13**, 174–180.
Callahan, L. T., III. (1974). *Infect. Immun.* **9**, 113–118.

Callahan, L. T., III. (1976). *Infect. Immun.* **14**, 55–61.
Carlson, D. M. and Matthews, L. W. (1966). *Biochemistry* **5**, 2817–2822.
Carney, S. A., Dyster, R. E. and Jones, R. J. (1973). *Brit. J. Dermatol.* **88**, 539–545.
Carrick, L., Jr. and Berk, R. S. (1975). *Biochim. Biophys. Acta* **391**, 422–434.
Chung, D. W. and Collier, R. J. (1977). *Infect. Immun.* **16**, 832–841.
Cicmanec, J. F. and Holder, I. A. (1979). *Infect. Immun.* **25**, 477–483.
Costerton, J. W. (1979). *In* "*Pseudomonas aeruginosa* the organism, diseases it causes, and their treatment" (L. D. Sabath, ed.) pp. 15–24. Huber Publishers, Bern.
Cross, A. S., Sadoff, J. C., Iglewski, B. H. and Sokol, P. A. (1980). *J. Infect. Dis.* **142**, 538–545.
Cryz, S. J. and Iglewski, B. H. (1980). *J. Clin. Microbiol.* **12**, 131–133.
Cryz, S. J., Jr., Friedman, R. L. and Iglewski, B. H. (1980). *Proc. Natl Acad. Sci. (USA)* (December).
Cryz, S. J., Jr., Friedman, R. L., Pavlovskis, O. R. and Iglewski, B. H. (1981). *Infect. Immun.* (in Press).
Curtin, J. A., Petersdorf, R. G. and Bennett, J. L. (1961). *Ann. Intern. Med.* **54**, 1077–1107.
DeBell, R. M. (1979). *Infect. Immun.* **24**, 132–138.
DeBell, R. M. and Martin, K. E. (1979). *Abstr. Annu. Meet. Amer. Soc. Microbiol.*, p. 51.
Dimitracopoulos, G. and Bartell, P. F. (1979). *Infect. Immun.* **23**, 87–93.
Dimitracopoulos, G. and Bartell, P. F. (1980). *Infect. Immun.* **30**, 402–408.
Doggett, R. G. and Harrison, G. M. (1972). *Infect. Immun.* **6**, 628–635.
Doggett, R. G., Harrison, G. M. and Wallis, E. S. (1964). *J. Bacteriol.* **87**, 427–431.
Dold, H. (1918). *Arch. Shiffs u. Tropenhyg.* **22**, 365–371.
Dorland, R. B., Middlebrook, J. L. and Leppla, S. H. (1979). *J. Biol. Chem.* **254**, 11337–11342.
Dyke, J. W. and Berk, R. S. (1973). *Z. Allg. Mikrobiol.* **13**, 307–313.
Ensign, P. R. and Hunter, C. A. (1946). *J. Pediat.* **29**, 620–628.
Esselmann, M. T. and Liu, P. V. (1961). *J. Bacteriol.* **81**, 939–945.
Evans, L. R. and Linker, A. (1973). *J. Bacteriol.* **116**, 915–924.
Fisher, E., Jr. and Allen, J. H. (1958). *Amer. J. Ophthalmol.* **46**, 249–255.
Fisher, M. W., Devlin, H. B. and Gnabasik, F. J. (1969). *J. Bacteriol.* **98**, 835–836.
Fishman, L. S. and Armstrong, D. (1972). *Cancer* **30**, 764–773.
FitzGerald, D., Morris, R. E. and Saelinger, C. B. (1980). *Cell* **21**, 867–873.
Flick, M. R. and Cluff, L. E. (1976). *Amer. J. Med.* **60**, 501–508.
Forkner, C. E., Jr., Frei, E., III, Edgecomb, J. H. and Utz, J. P. (1958). *Amer. J. Med.* **25**, 877–889.
Forsgren, A. (1972). *Acta Pathol. Microbiol. Scand. Sect. B* **80**, 564–570.
Frimmer, M. and Scharmann, W. (1975). *Naunyn-Schmiedeberg's Arch. Pharmacol.* **288**, 123–132.
Frimmer, M., Neuhof, H., Scharmann, W. and Schischke, B. (1976). *Naunyn-Schmiedeberg's Arch. Pharmacol.* **294**, 85–89.
Gray, L. D. and Kreger, A. S. (1975). *Infect. Immun.* **12**, 419–432.
Gray, L. D. and Kreger, A. S. (1979). *Infect. Immun.* **23**, 150–159.
Heckly, R. J. (1970). *In* "Microbial Toxins" (T. C. Montie, S. Kadis and S. J. Ajl, ed.) Vol. III, pp. 473–491. Academic Press, New York and London.
Hegner, D., Petter, A., Kroker, R., Anwer, M. S., Scharmann, W. and Breuninger, V. (1976). *Naunyn-Schmiedeberg's Arch. Pharmacol.* **293**, 49–55.
Hirao, Y. and Homma, J. Y. (1973). *Japan. J. Exptl Med.* **48**, 41–51.

Hisatsuka, K., Nakahara, T., Sanao, N. and Yamada, K. (1971). *Agr. Biol. Chem.* **35**, 686–692.

Hoiby, N. (1977). *Acta Pathol. Microbiol. Scand. Sect. C (Suppl.)* **262**, 1–96.

Holder, I. A. (1981). *Rev. Infect. Diseases* (in press).

Holder, I. A. and Haidaris, C. G. (1979). *Can. J. Microbiol.* **25**, 593–599.

Homma, J. Y. (1968). *Z. Allg. Mikrobiol.* **8**, 227–248.

Homma, J. Y. and Abe, C. (1972). *Japan. J. Exptl Med.* **42**, 23–34.

Homma, J. Y., Tomiyama, T., Sano, H., Hirao, Y. and Saku, K. (1975). *Japan. J. Exptl Med.* **45**, 361–365.

Homma, J. Y., Abe, C., Tanamoto, K., Hirao, Y., Morihara, K., Tsuzuki, H., Yanagawa, R., Honda, E., Aoi, Y., Fujimoto, Y., Goryo, M., Imazeki, N., Goda, A., Takeuchi, S. and Ishihara, T. (1978). *Japan J. Exptl Med.* **48**, 111–133.

Iglewski, B. H. and Kabat, D. (1975). *Proc. Natl Acad. Sci. (USA)* **72**, 2284–2288.

Iglewski, B. H. and Sadoff, J. C. (1979). *In* "Methods in Enzymology" (L. Grossman and K. Moldave, ed.) Vol. 60, pp. 780–793. Academic Press, New York and London.

Iglewski, B. H., Burns, R. P. and Gipson, I. K. (1977a). *Invest. Ophthalmol. Visual Sci.* **16**, 73–76.

Iglewski, B. H., Liu, P. V. and Kabat, D. (1977b). *Infect. Immun.* **15**, 138–144.

Iglewski, B. H., Sadoff, J. C., Bjorn, M. J. and Maxwell, E. S. (1978). *Proc. Natl Acad. Sci. (USA)* **75**, 3211–3215.

Inoue, H., Nakagawa, T. and Morihara, K. (1963). *Biochim. Biophys. Acta* **73**, 125–131.

Jagger, K., Nickol, M. M. and Saelinger, C. B. (1980). *Infect. Immun.* **28**, 746–752.

Jarvis, F. G. and Johnson, M. J. (1949). *J. Amer. Chem. Soc.* **71**, 4124–4126.

Jellard, C. H. and Churcher, G. M. (1967). *J. Hyg.* **65**, 219–228.

Jensen, S. E., Phillipe, L., Teng Tseng, J., Stemke, G. W. and Campbell, J. N. (1980a). *Can. J. Microbiol.* **26**, 77–86.

Jensen, S. E., Fecycz, I. T., Stemke, G. W. and Campbell, J. N. (1980b). *Can. J. Microbiol.* **26**, 87–93.

Jensen, S. E., Fecycz, I. T. and Campbell, J. N. (1980c). *J. Bacteriol.* **144**, 844–847.

Johnson, M. K. and Allen, J. H. (1978). *Invest. Ophthalmol. Visual Sci.* **17**, 480–483.

Johnson, M. K. and Boese-Marrazzo, D. (1980). *Infect. Immun.* **29**, 1028–1033.

Kawaharajo, K. and Homma, J. Y. (1975). *Japan J. Exptl Med.* **45**, 515–524.

Kawaharajo, K. and Homma, J. Y. (1977). *Japan J. Exptl Med.* **47**, 495–500.

Kawaharajo, K., Abe, C., Homma, J. Y., Kawano, M., Gotoh, E., Tanaka, N. and Morihara, K. (1974). *Japan J. Exptl Med.* **44**, 435–442.

Kawaharajo, K., Homma, J. Y., Aoyama, Y., Okada, K. and Morihara, K. (1975a). *Japan. J. Exptl Med.* **45**, 79–88.

Kawaharajo, K., Homma, J. Y., Aoyama, Y. and Morihara, K. (1975b). *Japan. J. Exptl Med.* **45**, 89–100.

Kessler, E., Mondino, B. J. and Brown, S. I. (1977a). *Invest. Ophthalmol. Visual Sci.* **16**, 116–125.

Kessler, E., Kennah, H. E. and Brown, S. I. (1977b). *Invest. Ophthalmol. Visual Sci.* **16**, 488–497.

Klinger, J. D., Strauss, D. C., Hilton, C. B. and Bass, J. A. (1978). *J. Infect. Diseases* **138**, 49–58.

Kreger, A. S. and Gray, L. D. (1978). *Infect. Immun.* **19**, 630–648.

Kreger, A. S. and Griffin, O. K. (1974). *Infect. Immun.* **9**, 828–834.

Kubota, Y. and Liu, P. V. (1971). *J. Infect. Dis.* **123**, 97–98.

Kurioka, S. and Liu, P. V. (1967a). *J. Bacteriol.* **93**, 670–674.

Kurioka, S. and Liu, P. V. (1967b). *Appl. Microbiol.* **15**, 551–555.
Kusama, H. (1974). *Infect. Immun.* **10**, 1185–1188.
Kusama, H. and Huss, R. H. (1972). *Infect. Immun.* **5**, 363–369.
Leake, E. S., Wright, M. J. and Kreger, A. S. (1978). *Exptl Mol. Pathol.* **29**, 241–252.
Leppla, S. H. (1976). *Infect. Immun.* **14**, 1077–1086.
Leppla, S. H., Martin, O. C. and Muehl, L. A. (1978a). *Biochem. Biophys. Res. Commun.* **81**, 532–538.
Leppla, S. H., Martin, O. C. and Pavlovskis, O. R. (1978b). *Abstr. Annu. Meet. Amer. Soc. Microbiol.* p. 29.
Leppla, S. H., Dorland, R. B., Middlebrook, J. L. and White, J. D. (1981). *Rev. Infect. Diseases* (in Press).
Lindberg, A. A., Rosenberg, I. T., Ljunggren, A., Garegg, P. J., Svensson, S. and Wallin, N.-H. (1974). *Infect. Immun.* **10**, 541–545.
Liu, P. V. (1964). *J. Bacteriol.* **88**, 1421–1427.
Liu, P. V. (1966a). *J. Infect. Dis.* **116**, 112–116.
Liu, P. V. (1966b). *J. Infect. Dis.* **116**, 481–489.
Liu, P. V. (1973). *J. Infect. Dis.* **128**, 506–513.
Liu, P. V. (1974). *J. Infect. Dis.* **130** (Suppl.), S94–S99.
Liu, P. V. (1979). *In* "*Pseudomonas aeruginosa.* Clinical Manifestations of Infection and Current Therapy" (R. G. Doggett, ed.), pp. 63–88. Academic Press, New York and London.
Liu, P. V. and Hsieh, H. (1973). *J. Infect. Dis.* **128**, 520–526.
Liu, P. V., Abe, Y. and Bates, L. J. (1961). *J. Infect. Dis.* **108**, 218–228.
Liu, P. V., Yoshii, S. and Hsieh, H. (1973). *J. Infect. Dis.* **128**, 514–519.
Lory, S. and Collier, R. J. (1980). *Infect. Immun.* **28**, 494–501.
Lutz, F. (1979). *Toxicon* **17**, 467–475.
Lynn, M., Sensakovic, J. W. and Bartell, P. F. (1977). *Infect. Immun.* **15**, 109–114.
McGowan, J. E., Jr., Barnes, M. W. and Finland, M. (1975). *J. Infect. Dis.* **132**, 316–335.
Meinke, G., Barum, J., Rosenberg, B. and Berk, R. (1970). *Infect. Immun.* **2**, 583–589.
Michaels, G. B. and Eagon, R. G. (1966). *Proc. Soc. Exptl Biol. Med.* **122**, 866–868.
Middlebrook, J. L. and Dorland, R. B. (1977). *Can. J. Microbiol.* **23**, 183–189.
Middlebrook, J. L., Dorland, R. B., Leppla, S. H. and White, J. D. (1980). *In* "Natural Toxins" (D. Eaker and T. Wadström, ed.), pp. 463–470. Pergamon Press, Oxford.
Morihara, K. (1957). *Bull. Agr. Chem. Soc. Japan* **21**, 11–17.
Morihara, K. (1963). *Biochim. Biophys. Acta* **73**, 113–124.
Morihara, K. (1964). *J. Bacteriol.* **88**, 745–757.
Morihara, K. (1974). *Adv. Enzymol.* **41**, 179–243.
Morihara, K. and Tsuzuki, H. (1964). *Biochim. Biophys. Acta* **92**, 351–360.
Morihara, K. and Tsuzuki, H. (1974). *Agr. Biol. Chem.* **38**, 621–626.
Morihara, K. and Tsuzuki, H. (1975). *Agr. Biol. Chem.* **39**, 1123–1128.
Morihara, K. and Tsuzuki, H. (1977). *Infect. Immun.* **15**, 679–685.
Morihara, K. and Tsuzuki, H. (1978). *Japan. J. Exptl Med.* **48**, 81–84.
Morihara, K., Tsuzuki, H., Oka, T., Inoue, H. and Ebata, M. (1965). *J. Biol. Chem.* **240**, 3295–3304.
Nordstoga, K. (1968). *Acta Vet. Scand.* **9**, 33–40.
Nishino, N. and Powers, J. C. (1980). *J. Biol. Chem.* **225**, 3482–3486.
Ohman, D. E., Burns, R. P. and Iglewski, B. H. (1980a). *J. Infect. Dis.* **142**, 547–555.
Ohman, D. E., Cryz, S. J. and Iglewski, B. H. (1980b). *J. Bacteriol.* **142**, 836–842.
Ohman, D. E., Sadoff, J. C. and Iglewski, B. H. (1980c). *Infect. Immun.* **28**, 899–908.

Okada, K., Kawaharajo, K., Homma, J. Y., Aoyama, Y., Kubota, Y. (1976). *Japan. J. Exptl Med.* **46**, 245–256.
Papamichail, M., Dimitracopoulos, G., Tsokos, G., Papavassiliou, J. (1980). *J. Infect. Dis.* **141**, 686–688.
Pappenheimer, A. M., Jr and Gill, D. M. (1973). *Science* **182**, 353–358.
Pavlovskis, O. R. (1972). *J. Infect. Dis.* **126**, 48–53.
Pavlovskis, O. R. and Gordon, F. B. (1972). *J. Infect. Dis.* **125**, 631–636.
Pavlovskis, O. R. and Shackelford, A. H. (1974). *Infect. Immun.* **9**, 540–546.
Pavlovskis, O. R. and Wretlind, B. (1979). *Infect. Immun.* **24**, 181–187.
Pavlovskis, O. R., Callahan, L. T., III and Meyer, R. D. (1974). *J. Infect. Dis.* **130** (Suppl.), S100–S102.
Pavlovskis, O. R., Callahan, L. T., III and Pollack, M. (1975). *In* "Microbiology 1975" (D. Schlessinger, ed.), pp. 252–256. American Society for Microbiology, Washington, D.C.
Pavlovskis, O. R., Voelker, F. A. and Shackelford, A. H. (1976). *J. Infect. Dis.* **133**, 253–259.
Pavlovskis, O. R., Pollack, M., Callahan, L. T., III and Iglewski, B. H. (1977). *Infect. Immun.* **18**, 596–602.
Pavlovskis, O. R., Iglewski, B. H. and Pollack, M. (1978). *Infect. Immun.* **19**, 29–33.
Pavlovskis, O. R., Wretlind, B. and Hale, M. L. (1980). *In* "Natural Toxins" (D. Eaker and T. Wadström, ed.), pp. 425–429. Pergamon Press, Oxford.
Pavlovskis, O. R., Edman, D. C., Leppla, S. H., Wretlind, B., Lewis, L. R. and Martin, K. E. (1981). *Infect. Immun.* **32**, 681–689.
Pollack, M. and Anderson, S. E. (1978). *Infect. Immun.* **19**, 1092–1096.
Pollack, M. and Young, L. S. (1979). *J. Clin. Invest.* **63**, 276–286.
Pollack, M., Callahan, L. T., III and Taylor, N. S. (1976). *Infect. Immun.* **14**, 942–947.
Pollack, M., Taylor, N. S. and Callahan, L. T., III. (1977). *Infect. Immun.* **15**, 776–780.
Reynolds, H. Y., Levine, A. S., Wood, R. E., Zierdt, C. H., Dale, D. C. and Pennington, J. E. (1975). *Ann. Intern. Med.* **82**, 819–831.
Reynolds, H. Y. and Fick, R. B. (1979). *In* "*Pseudomonas aeruginosa* the organism, diseases it causes, and their treatment" (L. D. Sabath, ed.), p. 79. Hans Huber Publishers, Bern.
Saelinger, C. B., Snell, K. and Holder, I. A. (1977). *J. Infect. Dis.* **136**, 555–561.
Sanai, Y., Takeshi, K., Homma, J. Y. and Kamata, H. (1978). *Japan. J. Exptl Med.* **48**, 553–556.
Sanai, Y., Morihara, K., Tsuzuki, H., Homma, J. Y. and Kato, I. (1980). *FEBS Letters* **120**, 131–134.
Sasaki, M., Ito, M. and Homma, J. Y. (1975). *Japan. J. Exptl Med.* **45**, 335–343.
Scharmann, W. (1976a). *Infect. Immun.* **13**, 836–843.
Scharmann, W. (1976b). *Infect. Immun.* **13**, 1046–1053.
Scharmann, W. (1976c). *J. Gen. Microbiol.* **93**, 283–291.
Scharmann, W. (1976d). *J. Gen. Microbiol.* **93**, 292–302.
Scharmann, W. and Kraft, W. (1974). *Blut* **28**, 90–99.
Scharmann, W. and Balke, E. (1974). *Z. Physiol. Chem.* **355**, 443–450.
Scharmann, W., Jacob, F. and Porstendörfer, J. (1976). *J. Gen. Microbiol.* **93**, 303–308.
Schoellmann, G. and Fisher, E., Jr (1966). *Biochim. Biophys. Acta* **122**, 557–559.
Schultz, D. R. and Miller, K. D. (1974). *Infect. Immun.* **10**, 128–135.
Sensakovic, J. W. and Bartell, P. F. (1974). *J. Infect. Dis.* **129**, 101–109.
Sensakovic, J. W. and Bartell, P. F. (1975). *Infect. Immun.* **12**, 808–812.
Sensakovic, J. W. and Bartell, P. F. (1977). *Infect. Immun.* **18**, 304–309.

Shimizu, T., Homma, J. Y., Aoyama, T., Onodera, T. and Noda, H. (1974). *Infect. Immun.* **10**, 16–20.
Shriniwas, Usha Menon and Bhujwala, R. A. (1979). *Indian J. Med. Res.* **70**, 380–383.
Sierra, G. (1960). *Anton. v. Leeuwenhoek J. Microbiol. Serol.* **26**, 189–192.
Snell, K., Holder, I. A., Leppla, S. H. and Saelinger, C. B. (1978). *Infect. Immun.* **19**, 839–845.
South, M. A. (1971). *J. Pediat.* **79**, 1–11.
Southern, P. M., Jr, Mays, B. B., Pierce, A. K. and Sandford, J. P. (1970). *J. Lab. Clin.* **76**, 548–559.
Stieritz, D. D. and Holder, I. A. (1975). *J. Infect. Dis.* **131**, 688–691.
Stieritz, D. D. and Holder, I. A. (1978). *J. Med. Microbiol.* **11**, 101–109.
Stinson, M. W. and Hayden, C. (1979). *Infect. Immun.* **25**, 558–564.
Tanamoto, K., Abe, C., Homma, J. Y., Kuretani, K., Hoshi, A. and Kijima, Y. (1978). *J. Biochem.* **83**, 711–718.
Tanamoto, K., Abe, C., Homma, J. Y. and Kojima, Y. (1979). *Eur. J. Biochem.* **97**, 623–629.
Taylor, N. S. and Pollack, M. (1978). *Infect. Immun.* **19**, 66–70.
Teplitz, C. and Davis, D. (1963). *U.S. Army Surg. Res. Unit Res.* MEDDH-228.
Thelestam, M. and Molby, R. (1979). *Biochim. Biophys. Acta* **557**, 156–169.
Thompson, R. M., Bjorn, M. J., Sokol, P. A., Lile, J. D. and Iglewski, B. H. (1980). *In* "Novel ADP-Ribosylations of Regulatory Enzymes and Proteins" (M. E. Smulson and T. Sugimura, ed.), pp. 425–433. Elsevier Publishers/ North Holland, Amsterdam.
Tillotson, J. R. and Lerner, A. M. (1968). *Ann. Intern. Med.* **68**, 295–307.
Van Horn, D. L., Davis, S. D., Hyndiuk, R. A. and Alpren, T. V. P. (1978). *Invest. Ophthalmol. Visual Sci.* **17**, 1076–1086.
Van Ness, B. G., Howard, J. B. and Bodley, J. W. (1978). *J. Biol. Chem.* **253**, 8687–8690.
Vasil, M. L. and Iglewski, B. H. (1978). *J. Gen. Microbiol.* **108**, 333–337.
Vasil, M. L., Liu, P. V. and Iglewski, B. H. (1976). *Infect. Immun.* **13**, 1467–1472.
Vasil, M. L., Kabat, D. and Iglewski, B. H. (1977). *Infect. Immun.* **16**, 353–361.
Watanabe, M., Murata, R. and Homma, J. Y. (1978). *Japan. J. Exptl Med.* **48**, 449–453.
Williams, E. P. and Cameron, K. (1894). *J. Pathol. Bacteriol.* **3**, 344–351.
Wretlind, B. and Kronevi, T. (1978). *J. Med. Microbiol.* **11**, 145–154.
Wretlind, B. and Wadström, T. (1977). *J. Gen. Microbiol.* **103**, 319–327.
Wretlind, B., Heden, L., Sjöberg, L. and Wadström, T. (1973). *J. Med. Microbiol.* **6**, 91–100.
Yamada, K. K., Sadoff, J. C. and Lowell, G. H. (1977) *Abstr. Annu. Meet. Amer. Soc. Microbiol.*, p. 33.
Young, L. S. and Armstrong, D. (1972). *CRC Crit. Rev. Clin. Lab. Sci.* **3**, 291–339.
Young, L. S. and Pollack, M. (1979). *In* "*Pseudomonas aeruginosa* the organism, the diseases it causes, and their treatment" (L. D. Sabath, ed.), pp. 122–123. Hans Huber Publishers, Bern.

4 Immune globulins with special reference to their role in bacterial and viral infections

J. S. FINLAYSON

I. INTRODUCTION

A. Scope and nomenclature

The immune globulins discussed in this review comprise a series of purified preparations isolated from human plasma and used for prophylactic or therapeutic purposes. As indicated below, the major protein and active ingredient in these preparations is immunoglobulin G (IgG). Indeed, in some countries, the therapeutic products themselves are designated "immuno-globulin". In the present work, however, care has been taken to distinguish between immunoglobulins *per se* (i.e., the molecular entities) and immuno-globulin *preparations*.

Use of the term immune globulins to denote commercial preparations intended for administration in the clinic is consistent with the official nomenclature employed in the United States (Code of Federal Regulations, 1980a). Although this emphasis on American products and usage pervades the review and reflects the author's experience, immune globulins used elsewhere (especially those administered intravenously) are discussed when appropriate.

To distinguish the immune globulins, which have undergone considerable purification (see Section IIB), from materials that are rich in antibodies but have not been fractionated, the latter products are referred to as immune plasmas. Excluded from most parts of this review are immunoglobulin preparations of animal origin — the antitoxins, immune sera, and similar therapeutic products. Moreover, no mention is made of antibody-containing products, regardless of origin, that are used for clinical conditions other than viral or bacterial infections. The latter category embraces antivenins and immunosuppressive agents such as antilymphocytic globulins and $Rh_0(D)$ Immune Globulin (Human). Finally, the entire focus of the review is on exogenous immune globulins intended for administration, *not* on the role an infected host's endogenous immunoglobulins may play in the course of that infection.

B. Background literature

Immune globulins have been dealt with in several recent reviews. Two of these provide overall views of the subject (Finlayson, 1979b; Stiehm, 1979). Two others resulted from deliberations of U.S. Food and Drug Administration advisory panels. The final report of one panel (Panel on Review of Viral Vaccines and Rickettsial Vaccines; S. Krugman, chairman) has been published (Goyan, 1980). The other (that of the Panel on Review of Bacterial Vaccines and Toxoids with Standards of Potency) is still in draft form, but a summary has been published by the panel chairman (Stollerman, 1978). Still other reviews have treated specific aspects of immune globulins (e.g., Aronson and Finlayson, 1980) or specific immune globulin *products* (e.g., Seeff and Hoofnagle, 1979; Ring and Duswald, 1980). In addition, recent workshops were devoted to the characteristics and uses of immune globulins prepared for intravenous administration (Alving and Finlayson, 1980; Nydegger, 1981). The reader may find these helpful for bridging gaps between the present work and the original reports.

II.   PREPARATION AND PROPERTIES

A.   Source and route of administration

Most human immune globulins used for prophylaxis of infectious disease are isolated from venous plasma and administered intramuscularly. The exceptions, however, deserve consideration. The first such preparations were isolated from placental extracts by ammonium sulphate precipitation (McKhann and Chu, 1933). They proved to be effective in the prevention or modification of measles (McKhann et al., 1935). Subsequently, other procedures were developed for obtaining immune globulin from placentas (Taylor et al., 1956). Human placentas are still used as a source for immunoglobulins (Guencheva and Manolova, 1979) and other proteins (Makula and Plan, 1979) in some parts of the world, though they are no longer fractionated for this purpose in the United States.

Because antibodies circulate freely in the bloodstream, it seemed reasonable that purified antibodies be administered intravenously. The severe reactions to human immune globulins given by this route (Cohn, 1948; Janeway, 1970), however, relegated these products to intramuscular use and indicated the need for additional work if intravenous dosage was to be considered seriously. This work was pursued on several fronts, and a number of immune globulins for intravenous use are now available (Alving and Finlayson, 1980). Some of these have been in clinical use for more than twenty years (e.g., Koch, 1963); others are still experimental. Because of the special considerations surrounding the manufacture and use of intravenous immune globulins, they are discussed in a separate section (Section VII). The present section and those immediately following it are devoted to immune globulins intended for intramuscular administration.

B.   Fractionation procedures

Large-scale isolation of immunoglobulins for clinical use became possible with the development of the cold-alcohol methods for plasma fractionation (Cohn, 1948). Although numerous modifications have been reported and subtle differences exist among the procedures utilized by individual manufacturers, most immune globulins for intramuscular administration are isolated by some variant of Cohn method 6 (Cohn et al., 1946) followed by Oncley method 9 (Oncley et al., 1949). A precipitate obtained by the former (usually fraction II + III; see Fig. 1) becomes the starting material for the latter. Fraction II, then, is the product that undergoes any pharmaceutical "finishing" steps (e.g., drying, dilution, pH adjustment, filtration) necessary to yield the final immune globulin. As in all of the Cohn procedures, separations are based on differences in solubility. The conditions for precipitation (or dissolution) of a particular protein are achieved by adjusting ethanol concentration, pH, ionic strength, temperature, and protein concentration; precipitates are generally harvested by centrifugation.

Of necessity, some alterations in the original fractionation scheme have been made to prepare additional products, e.g. Antihaemophilic Factor, from the plasma (Fig. 1). Other modifications have been introduced to streamline the process, to eliminate or combine individual steps, or to improve purity or yield. However, the reader concerned only with the use of immune globulins should avoid the trap of considering these changes mere biotechnical tinkering. For example, fraction III is rich in a variety of plasma proenzymes (Oncley et al., 1949), but differences of only a few tenths of a pH unit during the precipitation of this fraction can allow these proteins to remain in solution and, ultimately, to appear in fraction II (Painter and Minta, 1969). Their presence — either in zymogenic or activated form — in the final product can markedly affect its biochemical properties (Painter and Minta, 1969; Young et

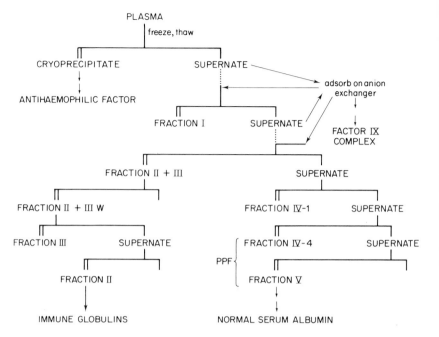

Fig. 1 Typical isolation of immune globulins from plasma. The steps summarized are based on those described by Cohn *et al.* (1946) and Oncley *et al.*
(1949). Double vertical lines indicate precipitates; dotted lines, steps at which
alternative pathways can be used. Reproduced from Finlayson (1979a) with
permission.

al., 1978; Tankersley *et al.*, 1980) and pharmacological properties (Alving *et
al.*, 1980) and thereby alter its clinical performance.

C.   Characteristics

The initial report by Oncley *et al.* (1949) indicated that 96–98% of the protein
in fraction II had the electrophoretic mobility of γ-globulin. Immunological
analyses of commercial immune globulins, conducted twenty or thirty years
later, gave values similar to these for the content of IgG; by contrast, IgA and
IgM comprised ≤1% and ≤2% of the total protein, respectively (Heiner and
Evans, 1967; Finlayson, 1979b). The recovery of either IgG (Vogelaar *et al.*,
1974) or antibody activity (Painter *et al.*, 1968) is ~60% of that in the starting
plasma. Thus if the immune globulin is prepared at a protein concentration of
165 g l^{-1} (see below), the net increase in antibody concentration is approximately 20-fold (Enders, 1944; Painter *et al.*, 1968).

   In principle immune globulins could be manufactured, distributed, and stored in a variety of forms, e.g. as dry powders for reconstitution immediately before use or as solutions prepared with any number of protein concentrations (ultimately limited by the solubility of IgG and the tolerable dosage volume) and intended for storage in the liquid or frozen state. Some of these options have been exercised. Historically, in the United States, the "broad-spectrum" immune globulin (Immune Serum Globulin) has had a protein concentration of 150–180 g l^{-1}; the specific immune globulins, of 100–180 g l^{-1}. In all cases the recommended storage temperature is 2–8°C, the solvent is 0.3 M glycine, the pH is adjusted to 6.4–7.2, and the mercurial preservative sodium ethylmercurithiosalicylate (thimerosal) is added at a concentration of 0.1 g l^{-1}.

As attention has been focused on the immune globulins, additional characteristics—not all of which are desirable—have been revealed. Early investigations showed the presence of IgG dimer (Deutsch et al., 1956), a non-native component which is found in virtually all immune globulins prepared by cold-alcohol fractionation. The amount of dimer varies with the age and manufacturing history of a particular lot, but the usual range is 10–20% of the total protein (Young et al., 1978). Higher oligomers and polymer(s) can also occur, though not necessarily at levels detectable by the usual analytical techniques.

In contrast to oligomer formation is the tendency for certain immunoglobulin preparations to undergo proteolysis during storage, even when the solutions are refrigerated. This phenomenon was first reported by Skvaril (1960a,b) and has been confirmed by many investigators (summarized by Finlayson, 1979b). Plasmin is the enzyme primarily responsible for the fragmentation (Skvaril, 1960a; Connell and Painter, 1966; Alving et al., 1980), although other enzymes may play a significant role (Alving et al., 1980; Tankersley et al., 1980). Kallikrein, as well as prekallikrein activator, has been identified in some lots of immune globulin (Alving et al., 1980). Although kallikrein does not directly attack IgG, it is a weak activator of plasminogen, hence it can enhance fragmentation when plasminogen is present and the storage period is long (Tankersley et al., 1980).

Hydrolysis of IgG by plasmin results in the formation of Fc and Fab fragments (Connell and Painter, 1966). Because Fab fragments are rapidly cleared from the body (Spiegelberg, 1970), proteolytic degradation can seriously diminish the efficacy of immune globulin (Adam and Skvaril, 1965; Painter et al., 1966; Kneapler and Cohen, 1977). Laboratory measurements of antibody activity, however, may fail to anticipate this decrease (Skvaril, 1960a; Painter et al., 1966; Brachott et al., 1972).

Little is known about the efficacy of aggregated forms of IgG, but these have been associated with adverse reactions to immune globulins (Richerson and Seebohm, 1966; Henney and Ellis, 1968; Turner et al., 1971; Kleinmann and Weksler, 1973; Bruhl, 1977). This association was reported twenty years ago in the case of intravenous immunoglobulin administration, a setting in which the reactions tend to be more frequent and more severe (Barandun *et al.*, 1962). The authors of the original report ascribed these reactions to the anticomplementary activity of IgG aggregates (Barandun *et al.*, 1962), and their conclusion has received wide acceptance despite conflicting evidence (summarized by Aronson and Finlayson, 1980).

Other investigators have surmised that multiple aetiologies are involved in the side-effects of immune globulins (Ellis and Henney, 1969; Soothill, 1971; Alving *et al.*, 1980). The data of Alving *et al.* (1980), for example, indicated that prekallikrein activator and/or kallikrein are potential mediators of vasoactive reactions. Barandun *et al.* (1980), by contrast, consider vasoactive substances to be of no causal importance in side-reactions unless high doses of immune globulin are infused rapidly. However, Cassidy *et al.* (1980) found (retrospectively) that an immunoglobulin preparation which had been withdrawn from clinical use because of the high incidence of adverse reactions was rich in prekallikrein activator.

To this controversy may be added a list of still other "contaminants" of immune globulins. Cohen and Hudson (1971) reported the presence of blood group substances, especially in placental preparations (cf. Guencheva and Manolova, 1979). Appreciable levels of blood group antibodies have also been detected, including anti-D (Lang and Veldhuis, 1973; Glassy *et al.*, 1978), as well as anti-A and anti-B (Lang and Veldhuis, 1973; Gordon *et al.*, 1980). These components appear to represent potential, rather than proven, hazards to recipients. IgA, however, which is present in all immune globulins (see above) unless specific procedures are used to remove it (Björling, 1979) can cause anaphylactic reactions in patients who lack this protein (Fudenberg, 1970; Buckley, 1980).

Thus, as in the preceding section, it becomes clear that such pedestrian issues as the chemical composition, purity, stability, and quality control of immune globulins are not far removed from clinical considerations. In the following section these issues are implicit in a brief discussion of characteristics that might be exhibited by an ultimately useful immunoglobulin preparation.

D.   "Ideal" characteristics

Proposing lists of ideal characteristics for immune globulins is not a new pastime; Table 1 includes three lists that spanned the previous decade. Although any ideal may depend on the intended use of a preparation, the similarity of these lists suggests that some features may be desirable in any immunoglobulin destined for clinical use. For example, the quest for safety

Table 1 Proposed ideal characteristics of immune globulins

Johnson (1970)	Barandun et al. (1975)[a]	Aronson and Finlayson (1980)[a]
No aggregation[b]	No aggregates	No aggregates
No fragmentation[b]	No anticomplementary activity	No fragments
Administrable either i.m. or i.v.	Normal complement-fixing activity[c]	No prekallikrein activator
No IgA	Same antibody spectrum as plasma IgG	No kallikrein
No hepatitis risk	Normal half-life	No coagulants
	Tolerance by agammaglobulinaemics	No other proteases
	Reasonable price	

[a] Proposed ideal characteristics of immune globulins for intravenous use.
[b] Either initially or during storage.
[c] In the presence of the corresponding antigen.

appears to demand freedom from aggregated (polymeric) forms of IgG; that for stability *in vitro* and a reasonable half-life *in vivo*, freedom from fragments* or enzymes that would catalyse fragmentation. In this respect "freedom" is a relative term that implies a measurement threshold (Finlayson, 1972). If possible, the latter should be lower than the threshold for an adverse response in the most sensitive recipient.

Certain other proposed characteristics (Table 1) are strongly linked to the target population. Thus the absence of IgA may be vital if the immune globulin is given to an immunodeficient individual who is specifically devoid of IgA, but may be irrelevant if it is administered to a truly agammaglobulinaemic patient. Similarly, "tolerance by agammaglobulinaemics" and "same antibody spectrum as plasma IgG" are major criteria for immunoglobulin preparations used in maintenance therapy, whereas they would be unnecessary for those which are intended to supply specific antibodies to otherwise normal patients.

It is noteworthy that only one of the lists includes freedom from the risk of hepatitis transmission (Table 1). Perhaps this is such an important characteristic that it goes without saying, or perhaps its absence merely indicates complacency. Immune globulins prepared by the Cohn-Oncley fractionation procedure (see Section IIB) have had a remarkable, albeit not perfect (Tabor and Gerety, 1979a), record of safety in this respect. The reason for this is uncertain. However, it is clear that the safety of any immune globulin manufactured by a different method must ultimately be established by an appropriate clinical trial.

III. CURRENT USES

In keeping with the emphasis of the entire chapter, this section and the next three sections are subdivided according to the infections against which particular immune globulins are used. Naturally, this organization has introduced some redundancy, especially in the case of Immune Serum Globulin, which has several indications, and of preparations that required discussion in more than one section. For the sake of consistency within each section, viral infections are considered first.

The present section is devoted to current *appropriate* uses of immune globulin, i.e., those for which prophylaxis or therapy has been shown to be efficacious or for which it can reasonably be considered effective. When controversies exist, these have been pointed out.

* If the specific therapeutic goal were renal clearance of a low molecular weight toxin (cf. Smith *et al.*, 1976) or rapid tissue penetration, a preparation consisting largely or exclusively of fragments might be useful.

A.   Maintenance of immunodeficient patients

Although routine replacement therapy in agammaglobulinaemia or hy-
pogammaglobulinaemia usually provides little information about the effectiveness of immune globulin against specific infections, this type of regimen is,
in a sense, the severest test of immunoprophylaxis. That is, unless other
prophylaxis (e.g., antibiotics) is given, the immune globulin alone must
protect the immunodeficient or immunosuppressed patient against any
infectious disease agent that the environment may harbour. That it can, in
part, meet this challenge is evidenced by the fact that agammaglobulinaemic
children receiving regular and adequate injections of Immune Serum Globulin
can enjoy relative freedom from a variety of common viral infections
(Janeway, 1970). Immune deficiency states that require such a regimen include
X-linked agammaglobulinaemia, X-linked immunodeficiency with elevated
IgM levels, common variable agammaglobulinaemia, severe combined immunodeficiency, and a syndrome characterized by near-normal serum immunoglobulin levels but impairment of antibody-forming capacity (Buckley, 1980).

The recommended maintenance dose of IgG is ~ 100 mg kg^{-1} body mass
(equivalent to 0.66 ml kg^{-1} when the protein concentration is 165 g l^{-1}) given
every 3 or 4 weeks. This dose, which was found empirically, is designed to
maintain the circulating IgG level at or above 2 g l^{-1} (Janeway and Rosen,
1966). For this reason, a loading dose of ≥ 200 mg kg^{-1} is given at the
beginning of therapy. Because the rate of IgG catabolism varies among
individuals (Waldmann and Strober, 1969), some patients may require more
frequent administration.

This dosage level has been widely used (e.g., Bruton, 1952; Nolte *et al.*,
1979) and recommended (Committee on Infectious Diseases, 1977; Stiehm,
1979), though it may not be optimal (Buckley, 1980). In a collection of cases
studied in the U.K., statistically significant additional protection was
provided by a weekly dose of 50 mg kg^{-1} (i.e., 200 mg kg^{-1} every 4 weeks),
compared with dosage at half this level (Healy, 1971), but the difference was
not considered great enough to justify the routine use of the larger quantity
(Hill and Mollison, 1971). More recently, Nolte *et al.* (1979) reported that
immunodeficient patients who received monthly doses of 150 mg kg^{-1}
developed substantially fewer acute infections than those given 100 mg kg^{-1}.
It is noteworthy that the higher dose in the latter study was given *intravenously*
and resulted in a mean elevation of the plasma IgG level nearly three times
that achieved by the lower (intramuscular) dose. Reaching this concentration
of circulating IgG by intramuscular injection would have required considerably more frequent administration or painfully large volumes of immune
globulin. The potential advantage of intravenous immunoglobulin infusion
for maintenance of immunodeficient patients is obvious. Accordingly,
intravenous products are discussed in a separate section (Section VIIC).

Regardless of the route of administration or the charge of IgG delivered, the success of immunoprophylaxis (or immunotherapy) must depend on the concentration of specific antibodies. For the routine management of immunodeficiency, a situation in which the objective is to provide an adequate level of *any* antibody needed to combat infection, the problem of quality control of the immune globulin becomes acute. Because it is impossible to test for all antibodies that might be needed, some compromise strategy is required. In the U.S., this strategy includes the requirement that each lot of Immune Serum Globulin represent at least 1000 donors, that the processing method be shown capable of concentrating tenfold (from the source material) at least two different antibodies, and that the final product meet or exceed defined levels of specified bacterial and viral antibodies (Code of Federal Regulations, 1980b).

B. Measles

The role of Immune Serum Globulin in the prophylaxis of measles is dependent on—and, in effect, reciprocal to—that of measles virus vaccine. Typically, this is the situation that obtains whenever products with proven efficacy for active and passive immunization against a single infectious agent coexist. That is, prevention and/or modification of measles was the earliest use of human immunoglobulin preparations (McKhann *et al.*, 1935), and their effectiveness for this purpose has been clearly demonstrated (Ordmann *et al.*, 1944; Stokes *et al.*, 1944). On the other hand, live measles vaccine became available for distribution in the U.S. in 1963, and within two years there began a dramatic decrease in the incidence of measles and its sequelae (Goyan, 1980). Thus the target population for passive measles prophylaxis has been reduced to exposed persons in the following categories: (1) immunodeficient patients, (2) immunosuppressed or otherwise immunocompromised patients, (3) normal children under the age of 15 months, and (4) older children or adults who are susceptible because they have not been actively immunized, either by vaccination or by contracting measles.

As alluded to previously, immunodeficient patients who receive routine injections of immune globulin will be protected against measles (Janeway, 1970). The value of passive immunization for immunosuppressed patients is illustrated by a recent report involving children who were hospitalized for acute lymphocytic leukaemia or non-Hodgkin's lymphoma and came into contact with patients suffering from measles. A group of 113 such children received a single dose (50 mg kg^{-1} body mass) of IgG intravenously; two of them developed mild cases of measles, whereas 111 showed no symptoms of the disease (Kornhuber, 1980). Under similar circumstances, the recommended intramuscular dose of Immune Serum Globulin is 0.5 ml kg^{-1} (maximum dose, 15 ml), i.e., 82.5 mg kg^{-1} (Committee on Infectious

Diseases, 1977). If the antibody concentrations of the two products were equivalent, these regimens would be expected to yield similar levels of circulating antibody (Smith *et al.*, 1972; Morell *et al.*, 1980).

The intramuscular dose recommended for a normal, susceptible individual exposed to measles is 0.25 ml kg^{-1} body mass and should be administered less than six days after the time of exposure (Public Health Service Advisory Committee on Immunization Practices, 1978). Use of Immune Serum Globulin under these conditions appears particularly important for children under one year of age: this is the group for which the risk of complications is highest. Although a much lower dose was once considered useful for "modifying" measles and thereby allowing natural, active immunity to develop, this practice is no longer recommended. Therefore, approximately three months after receiving the dose indicated above (which is no longer designated a "preventing" dose, in view of the complexity of differentiating between modification and true prevention), the child should be given measles vaccine. By this time, i.e., after four half-lives, the level of measles antibody is usually so low that it does not interfere with active immunization. Vaccination with live measles vaccine is not maximally effective unless the recipient is at least 15 months old, hence vaccination should be delayed (more than three months, if necessary) until the child reaches this age.

The same procedure and dosage apply in the case of susceptible, older children and adults. The size of this group, however, will be greatly diminished by an effective programme for active immunization. In the face of an aggressive vaccination programme, use of immune globulin for this category of recipients could virtually disappear. None the less, until "herd" immunity is complete, Immune Serum Globulin will maintain an important place in measles prophylaxis for the other categories.

C.   Hepatitis A

In the prophylaxis of hepatitis A, as in that of measles, Immune Serum Globulin has repeatedly manifested efficacy. Its effectiveness in controlling hepatitis A epidemics, which was proved more than 35 years ago (Stokes and Neefe, 1945), continues to be demonstrable (Hall *et al.*, 1977). Similarly, the ability of passive immunization to prevent infection in persons transported to areas in which hepatitis A is common was demonstrated during World War II (Gellis *et al.*, 1945b), and has since been observed in studies of both civilian travellers (Pollock and Reid, 1969; Hill and John, 1979) and military travellers (Weiland *et al.*, 1979). In fact, the latter study indicated that immune globulin can prevent even subclinical infection, despite the prevalence of hepatitis A in the local population (Weiland *et al.*, 1979).

Throughout these investigations a variety of dosage levels have been employed. At present the recommended dose is 0.02 ml kg $^{-1}$ body mass (i.e., 3.3 mg kg $^{-1}$), administered within two weeks of a household or institutional contact (Public Health Service Advisory Committee on Immunization Practices, 1977c). The same dose is used for short-term travellers to regions where hepatitis A is common; a dose of 0.05 ml kg $^{-1}$, repeated every four to six months, is recommended for persons who plan to spend more than three months in such regions. Like most of the dose levels used in field trials, these were established before laboratory tests for anti-hepatitis A virus (anti-HAV) were developed (WHO Expert Committee on Viral Hepatitis, 1977). Thus, despite studies directed toward determining the antibody concentration necessary to prevent infection (Krugman, 1976), the minimum effective dose is still unknown.

Reagents for measuring anti-HAV are now commercially available. Although, in principle, this should permit determination of the minimum effective dose, it will probably be some time before such a dosage is established. Because the currently used doses are effective (Ashley, 1955) and the current schedules for repeated immunization when re-exposure is likely can be supported (Pollock and Reid, 1969; Hill and John, 1979; Weiland et al., 1979), it appears prudent to maintain the present recommendations. If, however, the low (WHO Expert Committee on Viral Hepatitis, 1977; Frösner et al., 1979; Weiland et al., 1979) and apparently decreasing (Frösner et al., 1978, 1979) incidence of anti-HAV in the populations of developed countries were reflected by the concentration of anti-HAV in the plasma collected and, hence, in the immune globulin prepared in these countries, it is possible that the potency of the product could decrease.

For this reason, a study was undertaken to assess the situation in the U.S. Remarkably, anti-HAV titres of Immune Serum Globulin were found to have *increased* during the past 15 years (Smallwood et al., 1980, 1981). The reason for this increase is unknown, but the finding indicates that the recommendations summarized above are adequate. Thus if the concomitant use of laboratory analyses and clinical investigations allows the effective dose of anti-HAV to be established, it is likely that it will fall within or below the range that is currently employed (Smallwood et al., 1981).

D. Hepatitis B

In contrast to passive immunoprophylaxis of hepatitis A, for which both the role and effectiveness of Immune Serum Globulin are well established (Section IIIC), that of hepatitis B continues to evoke controversy (Hollinger, 1979; Krugman, 1979; Maynard, 1979; Mosley, 1979a; Favero et al., 1980). The indications that have been suggested range from narrow and cautious (Barker et al., 1978) to relatively broad (Seeff and Hoofnagle, 1979; Scheiermann and

Kuwert, 1980); the appropriate product for use in passive immunization has been discussed (Francis and Maynard, 1980; Favero *et al.*, 1980); there have been numerous calls for "re-evaluation" (e.g., Prince, 1978; Francis and Maynard, 1980); and even the mechanism of immunization has been questioned (Hoofnagle *et al.*, 1979; Mosley, 1979b). The latter item has prompted a comment entitled "How Does Hepatitis Immune Globulin Work?" (News Item, 1980). Indeed, after six years the conclusion that the results "will need fortification by long-term monitoring and continued study" (Alter *et al.*, 1975) has assumed the status of prophecy.

The current recommendations for Hepatitis B Immune Globulin use in the U.S. are limited to post-exposure prophylaxis following (1) parenteral exposure (e.g., by needle-stick), (2) oral ingestion, or (3) mucous membrane contact (e.g., by splash) involving hepatitis B surface antigen (HBsAg) positive material. In such cases, it is recommended that one dose (0.06 ml kg^{-1} body mass) be administered as soon after exposure as possible—preferably within seven days—and that an equal dose be given 28–30 days after the exposure. (The same indications and dosage schedule are suggested for Immune Serum Globulin, but *only* if Hepatitis B Immune Globulin is unavailable.)

Support for these recommendations accrued from a randomized study of 419 exposed persons (98% of whom worked in some aspect of health care) who received either Hepatitis B Immune Globulin or a lot of Immune Serum Globulin which contained no detectable antibody (anti-HBs) to hepatitis B (Seeff *et al.*, 1978). The superiority of the former appeared clear inasmuch as the incidence of either clinical hepatitis or seroconversion in its recipients was only one-fourth of that seen in the control group. Moreover, this result appeared to substantiate those obtained from an earlier study in which a direct intramuscular injection of hepatitis B virus was followed by injection of immune globulin with high or low antibody titre (Krugman *et al.*, 1971; Krugman and Giles, 1973). Later in the same year, however, Grady *et al.* (1978) reported the results of an equally large, randomized trial in which exposed medical personnel received immune globulin with a low, intermediate, or high concentration of anti-HBs. In this study the high-titre globulin gave complete protection, as assessed four months after exposure, but by nine months the differences between the groups had disappeared. The authors concluded that Hepatitis B Immune Globulin (i.e., the high-titre material) had delayed the onset but had not diminished the incidence or severity of clinical disease. Unfortunately, during storage this product underwent fragmentation (see Section IIC), a phenomenon that significantly decreases the anti-HBs titre (Grady *et al.*, 1978; Smallwood *et al.*, 1981).

Subsequently, Hoofnagle *et al.* (1979) re-analysed the study reported by Seeff *et al.* (1978). Whereas the previously observed fourfold difference in the incidence of clinical hepatitis B was confirmed, the greater incidence of *subclinical* infection in recipients of Hepatitis B Immune Globulin eliminated any difference in total infection between the two groups. Thus, contrary to the previous conclusion, it appeared that the effect of Hepatitis B Immune Globulin was not to prevent infection but rather, according to the authors (Hoofnagle *et al.*, 1979), to permit the development of passive–activity immunity.

Regardless of the mechanism by which protection is achieved, Hepatitis B Immune Globulin can be considered effective for the indications outlined above.* Much less certain is the efficacy and, because of its lower cost than the high-titre product, the proper role of Immune Serum Globulin in the prophylaxis of hepatitis B. Hoofnagle *et al.* (1979) found that the Immune Serum Globulin used as a control in their study was not only devoid of anti-HBs but also contained HBsAg; they concluded that it had induced active immunity in some recipients. This product, however, had been prepared from plasma collected before testing for HBsAg was mandatory. Although a similar lot of Immune Serum Globulin has been described (Tabor and Gerety, 1979a), this combination of characteristics — anti-HBs negative and HBsAg positive — is now extremely unlikely (Hoofnagle *et al.*, 1975b; Tabor and Gerety, 1979a; Gerety *et al.*, 1980; Hoofnagle and Waggoner, 1980). As acknowledged by Hoofnagle *et al.* (1979), with the introduction of routine testing of blood and plasma donors, the immunogenicity of Immune Serum Globulin has probably disappeared. Therefore, any recommendations for its use must be based solely on its ability to confer passive immunity.

A recent study has indicated that all lots of Immune Serum Globulin now being produced in the U.S. contain measurable anti-HBs (Gerety *et al.*, 1980). The level, however, is usually less than 1% of that in Hepatitis B Immune Globulin and is probably closer to 0.1%. These data, alone, do not argue for or against the use of Immune Serum Globulin for hepatitis B prophylaxis. Nevertheless, if such a use — either before or after exposure to infectious material — is supported by the results of future trials, it will be necessary to explain why a product nearly 1000 times as potent can still show prophylactic failures.

A number of investigations have been conducted to learn whether immune globulin is indicated for prophylaxis of other potential recipients. These

---

* Soon after the paper by Hoofnagle *et al.* (1979) was published, the results of a study of immunoglobulin prophylaxis after accidental exposure were reported from England and Wales (Medical Research Council and Public Health Laboratory Service, 1980). Although the anti-HBs titres of the preparations used were lower than that of the American Hepatitis B Immune Globulin, the incidence of hepatitis was similar to that found by Seeff *et al.* (1978). However, because there was no control group, the protective efficacy could not be assessed.

include patients and staff members of renal dialysis units (Prince *et al.*, 1978), spouses of patients with acute hepatitis B (Redeker *et al.*, 1975), and infants of hepatitis B positive mothers (Dosik and Jhaveri, 1978; Beasley and Stevens, 1978). Because these represent possible rather than established indications, the experiments are discussed in Section VIA4.

1. Impact of active immunization

The recent demonstration of efficacy for a hepatitis B vaccine (Szmuness *et al.*, 1980) holds major implications for the future uses of Hepatitis B Immune Globulin. That is, the vaccine exhibited a high degree of effectiveness (78% to 92%, depending on the criterion used) in protecting male homosexuals, a high-risk population in which re-exposure is likely. This result is consistent with earlier observations of protection afforded by pre-existing (i.e., presumably actively acquired) anti-HBs (Grady *et al.*, 1978; Seeff *et al.*, 1978; cf. Krugman and Giles, 1970). It suggests that, within either institutionally or geographically endemic settings, active immunization may be the prophylaxis of choice. Favourable results of vaccine trials would probably render moot the question of immune globulin efficacy in these situations.

The results obtained by Szmuness *et al.* (1980) also imply that the vaccine may be effective for post-exposure prophylaxis. If this proves to be so, the vaccine could supplant—or, at least, be used in consort with—Hepatitis B Immune Globulin for some of its present indications (Dienstag, 1980). In such a case, the role of Hepatitis B Immune Globulin would become analogous to that of Immune Serum Globulin in measles prophylaxis (Section IIIB).

E. Rabies

A major problem in defining the role of Rabies Immune Globulin in prophylaxis is the improbability of a controlled trial. Its efficacy is largely an assumption, albeit an eminently reasonable one, and current usage has evolved through a series of interconnected steps. An important early step was the demonstration that the combination of passive and active immunization was more beneficial for victims of head and facial bites by a rabid animal than was active immunization alone. This was shown by a study in which persons bitten by a rabid wolf were given heterologous Antirabies Serum* plus vaccine or only the vaccine. The combined treatment produced a much higher survival rate (86% or 100%, depending on the number of injections of Antirabies Serum) of persons bitten about the head than did the vaccine itself (40%).

---

* Antirabies Serum is not whole serum, but is rather a globulin fraction. Initially it was obtained by ammonium sulphate fractionation; later, it was prepared (primarily from equine serum) by this process plus pepsin digestion.

There were no deaths among victims bitten on the limbs and trunk, regardless of which regimen was employed (Baltazard and Bahmanyar, 1955).

Use of this type of combined prophylaxis has continued. Bahmanyar *et al.* (1976) described the treatment of 45 persons severely bitten by rabid dogs or wolves. All were given rabies vaccine of the human diploid cell type; 44 also received Antirabies Serum prepared from mule blood. Similarly, Selimov *et al.* (1978) reported results obtained with 31 victims of rabid wolves. Two different types of rabies vaccine were used (neither was the human diploid cell strain). All 31 patients received vaccine, and 28 were also injected with Antirabies Serum obtained from horse serum. There were no deaths in either study, indicating (by comparison with historical controls) that the total regimen is effective.

Despite this effectiveness, the incidence of serum sickness following administration of heterologous Antirabies Serum (Karliner and Belaval, 1965) provided a strong impetus to the development of a human immunoglobulin preparation (Cabasso, 1974). The recommended dose, 20 international units (IU) per kg body mass, was determined by studies with human volunteers. In these studies, a series of inoculations with rabies vaccine of the duck embryo type was preceded by a varied dose of Rabies Immune Globulin (Human) (Cabasso *et al.*, 1971; Hattwick *et al.*, 1974). Whereas doses of 10 IU kg^{-1} yielded unsatisfactorily low concentrations of circulating antibody, 40 IU kg^{-1} interfered with the active immunization. The intermediate doses apparently provided protective levels of antibody throughout the prophylactic period. Several subsequent investigations have indicated that a 20 IU kg^{-1} dose of Rabies Immune Globulin does not suppress active immunization with the human diploid cell strain vaccine (Hafkin *et al.*, 1978; Kuwert *et al.*, 1978; Nicholson and Turner, 1978).

The current recommendation is that up to half of the dose be infiltrated around the wound(s) and the remainder be injected intramuscularly. If the antibody concentration of Rabies Immune Globulin is 150 IU ml^{-1}, this amounts to a total dose of 2 ml for a 15-kg child or 10 ml for a 75-kg adult (Cabasso, 1974). This recommendation has been followed in actual clinical situations (e.g. Dempster *et al.*, 1979; Plotkin and Witkor, 1979) involving post-exposure prophylaxis with either duck embryo or human diploid cell vaccine. However, despite the favourable clinical results, it is impossible to establish the precise prophylactic contribution of passive immunization. The accumulated evidence none the less indicates that (1) the human immunoglobulin preparation is to be preferred, (2) it should be available along with vaccine, and (3) it should continue to be used with the latter at the recommended dosage.

F. Varicella

The initial studies of immunization against varicella (chickenpox) were carried out with convalescent serum, but the experimental design permitted no conclusions regarding efficacy (see review by Zaia *et al.*, 1980). More recently the analogous material, Zoster Immune Plasma, was shown to be effective (Geiser *et al.*, 1975; Balfour *et al.*, 1977), and it continues to be used in some cases today (Avenard *et al.*, 1979; Dickson and Heath, 1979). Most of the reports, however, deal with Zoster Immune Globulin, an immune globulin prepared from the plasma of persons who have recently recovered from herpes zoster (shingles). The controlled study by Brunell *et al.* (1969) showed that this product prevented varicella in normal children when it was given within 72 hours of household exposure. These authors suggested that prophylaxis with Zoster Immune Globulin might benefit several high-risk groups: children who have malignant diseases and/or are receiving immunosuppressive therapy, neonates, and susceptible adults.

Numerous subsequent investigations, mostly uncontrolled, indicated that Zoster Immune Globulin could modify varicella in immunocompromised children (Gershon *et al.*, 1974; Judelsohn *et al.*, 1974; Kay and Maycock, 1974). Because varicella is a serious — indeed, life-threatening — infection for such children, prevention or modification of clinical disease is an important step, regardless of whether seroconversion occurs. As in the case of normal children exposed to varicella, the results obtained with these patients were affected by the interval between exposure and administration of the immune globulin. When this interval exceeded three days, the attack rate rose sharply (Winsnes, 1978). The titre of the Zoster Immune Globulin may also have influenced the clinical outcome (Winsnes, 1978), a result consistent with the finding that this product was more effective than Zoster Immune Plasma (Avenard *et al.*, 1979) or Immune Serum Globulin (Brunell *et al.*, 1969).

Reports from field surveys of Zoster Immune Globulin use in children with leukaemia (Lane *et al.*, 1980) and other malignant diseases continue to emphasize its effectiveness, notwithstanding warnings that its efficacy may be overestimated (Evans *et al.*, 1980). There appears to be virtual unanimity, however, regarding the difficulty of obtaining sufficient convalescent plasma to maintain supplies of the product (Winsnes, 1978; Avenard *et al.*, 1979; Schiff, 1979).

For this reason, Zaia *et al.* (1978) screened plasma from normal blood donors and selected the individual units of plasma with the highest titres of anti-varicella-zoster for fractionation. The immune globulin obtained was named Varicella-Zoster Immune Globulin to distinguish it from the product isolated from convalescent plasma. The two types of immunoglobulin preparations showed the same antibody concentrations by several different tests (Zaia *et al.*, 1978). However, because of the possibility of qualitative differences in the antibodies present, they were compared in a randomized clinical trial. Susceptible, immunocompromised children were given either Varicella-Zoster Immune Globulin or Zoster Immune Globulin within 96 hours of exposure. There were no differences in attack rate, severity of cases that did erupt, or incidence of pneumonia, nor were there any cases of encephalitis or deaths (Zaia *et al.*, 1980).

On the basis of these observations, Varicella-Zoster Immune Globulin is recommended for susceptible, immunocompromised children (i.e. those with primary immunodeficiency or malignant disease, or undergoing immunosuppressive therapy) exposed to varicella. The dose, like that of the other immune globulins, varies with body mass; it should be given within 96 hours of exposure. In addition, Varicella-Zoster Immune Globulin is recommended for neonates whose mothers develop varicella within 120 hours before delivery or within 48 hours after delivery. The value of passive immunization under these circumstances was demonstrated by Winsnes (1978). The neonates given Zoster Immune Globulin had either mild varicella or none at all, whereas neonatal varicella is usually severe and often fatal (Stiehm and Kobayashi, 1980; Zaia *et al.*, 1980).

Because of problems such as re-exposure, inability to recognize all instances of exposure to varicella (and, hence, to administer immune globulin in all appropriate cases) or simply prophylactic failure, other modalities for prophylaxis and treatment are being explored (Gershon, 1980). These include a vaccine, transfer factor, interferon, adenine arabinoside, and acyclo-guanosine. At present it is impossible to assess the effect any of these, if successful, might exert on the use of passive immunization, especially since the agent chosen might be used in combination with immune globulin (Winsnes *et al.*, 1978).

G. Tetanus

Tetanus Immune Globulin is the only commercial immune globulin intended for use against a bacterial toxin, but it shares several dilemmas with those directed toward viral antigens. Its role and use are modulated by those of tetanus toxoid, which is probably the most efficacious of all bacterial vaccines and toxoids (Stollerman, 1978). Its efficacy for either prophylaxis or treatment has not been demonstrated unambiguously, a dilemma which it shares with the equine product, Tetanus Antitoxin. Moreover, because of the low incidence of tetanus in developed countries and the inappropriateness of placebo usage, the studies needed for such a demonstration are unlikely to be performed (Habermann, 1978).

Even the results of earlier attempts at prophylaxis with the antitoxin were clouded by difficulties of experimental design, the simultaneous introduction of improvements in hygiene and supportive care, and the occurrence of adverse reactions to heterologous protein. None the less, the weight of experience suggests that passive immunization is useful. Encouraged by the apparently complete success of a 1500-unit dose of equine antitoxin for preventing tetanus *in horses*, McComb and Dwyer (1963) attempted to determine the dose of Tetanus Immune Globulin that would provide a protective level of circulating antibody in humans. The dose chosen, 250 units, resulted in a plasma level of at least 0.01 unit ml^{-1} 28 days after administration* (McComb and Dwyer, 1963). It was endorsed by other workers (Rubbo, 1966) although subsequent measurements showed that tetanus could occur in patients with plasma antibody concentrations greater than 0.01 unit ml^{-1} (Grosbuis *et al.*, 1975). Perhaps more importantly, this dose did not interfere with the active immunization achieved by simultaneous administration of toxoid (McComb and Dwyer, 1963; Levine *et al.*, 1966; Rubbo, 1966). Levine *et al.* (1966), in fact, concluded that it was not far from the optimum for continuous protection during active–passive immunization.

If Tetanus Immune Globulin is of value in prophylaxis, when should it be employed? The various recommendations (e.g. Rubbo, 1966; Habermann, 1978) appear to be similar. Those currently used in the U.S. (Public Health Service Advisory Committee on Immunization Practices, 1977b) call for administration of 250 units intramuscularly, provided the following conditions are met: (1) the patient's tetanus immunization status is incomplete or uncertain and (2) the patient has sustained a wound other than a clean, minor one. This recommendation assumes a wound of average severity and an immunocompetent patient. The dose may require adjustment if the patient appears to be at higher risk, e.g. has a contaminated or more severe wound, or one which was not treated within 24 hours of the injury. It has been suggested that burn victims with incomplete immunization may require a higher dose (Lowbury *et al.*, 1978). In general, the 250-unit dose is also recommended for children who meet the criteria given above; however, for small children the

---

* In view of the extrapolative nature of the dose determination, it seems important to confirm its relationship to and consistency with the data available. McComb and Dwyer (1963) evidently considered 390–910 kg to be the range of body mass for horses, hence a 1500 unit dose provided 1.65–3.85 units kg^{-1}. For a 70 kg human, a 250 unit dose is near the upper extreme of this range, viz., 3.57 units kg^{-1}. If such a person had a plasma volume of 3000 ml and the maximum quantity of intravascular antibody corresponded to 40% of the injected dose (Smith *et al.*, 1972), a circulating level of 0.033 unit ml^{-1} would be achieved. If 28 days is considered to be 1.33 half-lives for IgG (see Waldmann and Strober, 1969), the level after this interval should be 0.013 unit ml^{-1}. Even if the maxumum plasma concentration corresponded to only 30% of the injected dose (Smith *et al.*, 1972; Morell *et al.*, 1980), the projected level 28 days later would be 0.01 unit ml^{-1}.

dose is sometimes adjusted to 4 units kg^{-1}. In the case of inadequate active immunization, the series of toxoid injections should, of course, be completed.

Although the treatment of clinical tetanus with Tetanus Immune Globulin has been practised for many years (Nation *et al.*, 1963) and continues to be used (Gertzen *et al.*, 1979) and recommended (Committee on Infectious Diseases, 1977), its efficacy is at least as difficult to evaluate as that of prophylaxis. Blake *et al.* (1976) summarized the conflicting, earlier results obtained by treatment with Tetanus Antitoxin as well as those accumulated from seven years of experience with the human and equine immunoglobulin preparations. This experience revealed no difference in effectiveness between the two products, but both showed case–fatality ratios of greater than 60%. Significantly, treatment with 500 units, or even less, of Tetanus Immune Globulin resulted in no poorer survival than did treatment with doses exceeding 8000 units. When the 500-unit dose was compared with a 10 000-unit dose of Tetanus Antitoxin in a controlled, randomized trial involving treatment of tetanus neonatorum, no significant differences were observed; case–fatality ratios were 42% and 43%, respectively (McCracken *et al.*, 1971). Nevertheless, for treatment with Tetanus Immune Globulin, the recommended dose is still 3000–6000 units (Committee on Infectious Diseases, 1977), i.e. the amount chosen arbitrarily 20 years ago (Nation *et al.*, 1963).

Some recent experiments suggest that the timing of administration may be as important as the dose in determining the outcome of therapy. These made use of intrathecal injection, a procedure which is enjoying a renaissance of interest after a period of dormancy. Because of its experimental nature, intrathecal administration for the treatment of tetanus is discussed in Section VIA2. If it proves to be successful, this approach may not only benefit victims of the disease but also provide, at least for some clinical situations, the long-awaited proof of efficacy.

In seeking the appropriate role for Tetanus Immune Globulin, it is essential to recognize the dominant position of tetanus toxoid. For example, the primary attack on tetanus neonatorum should begin with the active immunization of potential mothers, along with improvement of delivery, hygiene, and public health practices. When this progression has been followed, statistics have reflected a shift in the age distribution of tetanus from a "developing country pattern" to a "developed country pattern" (Fig. 2): in developing countries tetanus is primarily a disease of neonates and young children (Habermann, 1978), but in developed countries it tends to afflict the older age groups (Solmonova and Vizev, 1973; Habermann, 1978; Gertzen *et al.*, 1979). Whether the latter distribution simply reflects prior immunization practices or, as indicated by the work of Kishimoto *et al.* (1980), an age-related decline in the synthesis of anti-tetanus antibodies is uncertain. If ageing results in

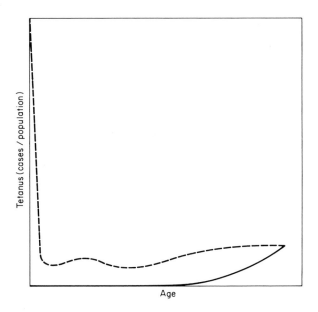

Fig. 2 Age distribution of tetanus in developing and developed countries. Schematic diagram redrawn from Habermann (1978). Broken line indicates developing country pattern; solid line, developed country pattern.

decreased immune responsiveness to tetanus toxoid, the older population may remain potential candidates for Tetanus Immune Globulin, regardless of the development of the country or the aggressiveness of its active immunization programme.

H. Summary

The current, appropriate uses of immune globulins discussed in this section are summarized in Table 2. Of necessity, the material was condensed for tabulation, hence no attempt was made to include the variations, qualifying statements, and supporting references. Accordingly, Table 2 should be regarded only as a guide to be used in conjunction with the text.

Table 2 Current appropriate uses of immune globulins[a]

Product	Indications	Dose
Immune Serum Globulin	Immunodeficiency (maintenance)	0.66 ml kg^{-1} every 3–4 weeks
Immune Serum Globulin	Measles prophylaxis	0.25 ml kg^{-1}
Immune Serum Globulin	Hepatitis A prophylaxis	0.02 ml kg^{-1} (0.05 ml kg^{-1} every 4–6 months for travel in endemic areas)
Hepatitis B Immune Globulin	Hepatitis B post-exposure prophylaxis (needle-stick, ingestion, mucous membrane exposure)	0.06 ml kg^{-1}
Rabies Immune Globulin	Rabies post-exposure prophylaxis	20 IU kg^{-1}
Varicella-Zoster Immune Globulin / Zoster Immune Globulin	Varicella (chickenpox) prophylaxis (immunosuppressed children <96 h after exposure; neonates if mother develops varicella between 120 h before and 48 h after birth)	[b]
Tetanus Immune Globulin	Tetanus prophylaxis if immunization incomplete and wound not clean, minor	250 units
Tetanus Immune Globulin	Tetanus treatment	500 units? 3000–6000 units? (see text)

[a] Immune globulins of human origin. The doses are those recommended in the U.S. Immune Serum Globulin is prepared at a protein concentration of 165 ± 15 g l^{-1}.

[b] The dose will depend on the potency of the product as manufactured in different countries. In the U.S., Varicella-Zoster Immune Globulin is vialed on the basis of unitage, and the dosage recommended is one vial per 10 kg body mass.

IV. INAPPROPRIATE USES

Stiehm (1980) has pointed out that, historically, immune globulin prophylaxis and therapy were used for a broad variety of illnesses and, with time, inappropriate uses were weeded out. Despite his counsel to the contrary, it appears that the same process is being recapitulated. Ring and Duswald (1980) recently reported that intravenous immune globulins are being promoted for more than 100 possible indications, ranging from angina through diarrhoea to zoster.

The scope of the present section is not adequate to staunch such a haemorrhage of applications, nor is it intended to discourage the quest for and validation of additional uses. Some of the latter are discussed in Section VI. The intent is rather to review certain uses of immune globulins which have been contravened by experimental results or are no longer considered good medical practice, or for which supportive data are clearly lacking.

It goes without saying that accurate diagnosis underlies the appropriate use of any drug. In the case of deficiency diseases for which replacement therapy is anticipated, this is particularly critical. More than a decade ago Fudenberg (1970) noted that much immune globulin was wasted because children were misdiagnosed as hypogammaglobulinaemic. For this section, however, it has been assumed that the diseases have been identified correctly and that the central question is the suitability of the immune globulin.

A. Immune Serum Globulin

In spite of its well-documented effectiveness in the prophylaxis of measles (Section IIIB), Immune Serum Globulin is not recommended for use in the control of measles epidemics. Moreover, although low doses can modify the clinical course of measles, the deliberate administration of a "modifying" dose is no longer recommended (Public Health Service Advisory Committee on Immunization Practices, 1978). As indicated previously (Section IIIB), the appropriate dose is $0.25\,\text{ml kg}^{-1}$ body mass, followed after at least three months by active immunization.

The clinical symptoms of rubella can be suppressed with Immune Serum Globulin (Brody *et al.*, 1965; Schiff, 1969), but it is not recommended for routine prophylaxis of rubella, even during the first trimester of pregnancy. The potential use of passive immunization against rubella is considered again in Sections VA and VIB4.

Similarly, there is no current role for passive immunization in the prophylaxis of diphtheria or poliomyelitis. Immune Serum Globulin provided some short-lived protection against poliomyelitis (Hammon *et al.*, 1953), but it proved to be an inefficient agent for prophylaxis (Stiehm, 1979) and has been discredited (Goyan, 1980). Measurement of the levels of antibodies against diphtheria and poliomyelitis in Immune Serum Globulin has been continued simply to monitor manufacturing consistency (Code of Federal Regulations, 1980b).

When Immune Serum Globulin has proved to be of value, it has been for prophylaxis rather than treatment of established infections. In fact, it is not indicated for persons whose exposure to measles occurred six or more days before presentation or for those exposed to hepatitis A more than two weeks previously.

B. Hepatitis B

The ability of Hepatitis B Immune Globulin to influence the course of clinical disease was tested in a multicentre study of fulminant hepatitis B (Acute Hepatic Failure Study Group, 1977). The immune globulin or an albumin placebo was administered (intravenously) in randomized fashion to patients at stages II, III and IV of the disease. At each stage, case–fatality ratios in the treated and placebo groups were virtually identical, thus indicating complete failure of immunotherapy with Hepatitis B Immune Globulin.

At the other extreme of the hepatitis spectrum is the person who has circulating anti-HBs and becomes exposed to hepatitis B. Such a person is already protected (Alter *et al.*, 1975; Grady *et al.*, 1978; Seeff *et al.*, 1978), hence administration of Hepatitis B Immune Globulin would be inappropriate.

C. Varicella

Although Zoster Immune Globulin was shown to prevent varicella in normal, susceptible children (Brunell *et al.*, 1969), Varicella-Zoster Immune Globulin is not indicated for this population, owing to the benign nature of the disease. Nor is it recommended for immunocompromised children with a history of varicella, unless the degree of immunosuppression is so severe as to preclude protective levels of antibodies (e.g. in bone marrow transplant recipients).

D. Mumps

The possibility of prophylaxis or treatment of mumps with exogenous antibodies has received considerable attention, but most investigators have used serum from convalescent patients rather than purified immunoglobulin (Goyan, 1980). The few studies conducted with immune globulin indicate, at best, minimal effectiveness. Reed *et al.* (1967) found that administration of Mumps Immune Globulin to seronegative recipients did not change the incidence of mumps from that of the untreated seronegative control group during an epidemic. In a sense, this result was confirmed by the recent work of Copelovici *et al.* (1979), who observed that Mumps Immune Globulin lowered the incidence of mumps, but only when the total frequency was already low.

Gellis *et al.* (1945a) reported that immune globulin prepared from the plasma of mumps-convalescent donors could influence the course of a mumps infection (i.e. lower the incidence of orchitis) if administered within 24 hours of the onset of parotitis. Immune Serum Globulin made from the plasma of control donors had no such effect. Copelovici *et al.* (1979) obtained similar results, albeit the decrease in the incidence of orchitis was very small. Reed *et al.* (1967), however, could demonstrate no change in either the incidence or severity of orchitis.

On the basis of their results, Copelovici *et al.* (1979) recommended that Mumps Immune Globulin be used only for high-risk patients. American assessment of the product has been even less favourable: it is not recommended for post-exposure prophylaxis of mumps (Committee on Infectious Diseases, 1977; Public Health Service Advisory Committee on Immunization Practices, 1977a), and its ability to diminish complications of the disease is considered unproven (Committee on Infectious Diseases, 1977; Goyan, 1980). In view of the availability of vaccines which can confer effective (Immunization Division, Bureau of State Services, 1978) and long-lasting (Weibel *et al.*, 1980) protection, the benefit–risk ratio for Mumps Immune Globulin appears unsatisfactory. Moreover, there is no evidence that Immune Serum Globulin is effective for either the prophylaxis (Public Health Service Advisory Committee on Immunization Practices, 1977a; Copelovici *et al.*, 1979) or treatment (Gellis *et al.*, 1945a; Copelovici *et al.*, 1979) of mumps (cf. Section IVA).

E. Pertussis

Pertussis Immune Globulin has been used in numerous uncontrolled investigations and a few controlled clinical trials. The latter have unequivocally demonstrated that in pertussis it fails to decrease the attack rate (Morris and McDonald, 1957), course (Place *et al.*, 1949; Hatz and Burkhardt, 1950; Balagtas *et al.*, 1971), or severity (Place *et al.*, 1949; Morris and McDonald, 1957; Balagtas *et al.*, 1971).

There appear to be at least two plausible explanations for the difference between these observations and the favourable results reported from some early trials with pertussis-convalescent serum (see Balagtas *et al.*, 1971 and references therein). One is the possibility that IgA or IgM, both of which are minor components of the fractionated immune globulins (see Section IIC), is the protective principle (Stollerman, 1978); the other is simply the uncontrolled nature of the serum studies. In either case, immune globulins have no current role in the prophylaxis or treatment of pertussis, and Pertussis Immune Globulin has no clinical *raison d'être*.

V. POSSIBLE LIMITED USES

A. Immune Serum Globulin

As the most abundant and versatile of the immune globulins for intramuscular administration, Immune Serum Globulin is probably also the immune globulin most likely to be misused. Once its use is extended beyond those listed in Section III(A,B,C), the evidence for effectiveness becomes small, and the potential for misuse grows larger. It is therefore important to recognize that the present section deals with applications for which neither controlled clinical trials nor laboratory measurements offer high likelihood of prophylactic success. Rather, these applications represent uses of Immune Serum Globulin that are justified only when relatively narrow conditions are met and when a more appropriate avenue of prophylaxis is not open.

As indicated previously (Section IIID), the appropriate agent for postexposure prophylaxis of hepatitis B following needle-stick, oral ingestion, or mucous membrane splash with HBsAg-positive material is considered to be Hepatitis B Immune Globulin. In the event that this product is unavailable and is unlikely to be available within a reasonable period of time (say, seven days) after the exposure, Immune Serum Globulin may be given. In evaluating the potential benefits of this procedure, two observations are pertinent. First, all lots of Immune Serum Globulin (at least those manufactured in the U.S.), though not routinely monitored for anti-HBs, do contain measurable levels of the antibody (Gerety *et al.*, 1980). Second, in one study, there was no difference in the degree of long-term protection conferred by equal volumes of Hepatitis B Immune Globulin and Immune Serum Globulin administered after direct exposure (Grady *et al.*, 1978). Neither of these findings provides any indication of prophylactic efficacy or the level of circulating exogenous antibody required for a protective effect. Together, however, they may offer some basis for deciding whether or not to administer Immune Serum Globulin when no alternative procedure for hepatitis B prophylaxis is available. If the decision is affirmative, the recommended dose is 0.06 ml kg^{-1} body mass, given as soon after the exposure as possible (preferably within seven days) and followed by an equal dose 25–30 days later.

The appropriate route of attack on rubella, like that against measles, is preexposure active immunization. The effectiveness of this approach is indicated by the apparent decline in the number of cases of clinical rubella or congenital rubella syndrome that have been reported since rubella virus vaccine was introduced (Goyan, 1980). Thus the role of passive immunization against rubella infection is essentially nil (Section IVA). The issue arises only when an unimmunized woman is exposed to rubella in early pregnancy. Active immunization with live virus vaccine during pregnancy is contra-indicated (Committee on Infectious Diseases, 1977; Hayden *et al.*, 1980), and in any case post-exposure vaccination may not prevent illness. Therefore, the procedure recommended in the event of confirmed exposure and susceptibility is termination of the pregnancy.

When a woman who meets these criteria will not consider a therapeutic abortion, it becomes necessary to weigh passive prophylaxis and its value, if any, for preventing fetal damage. Immune Serum Globulin is not routinely tested for antibodies against rubella. Furthermore, it can suppress the clinical disease without preventing infection (Brody *et al.*, 1965). In view of the great uncertainty surrounding its use in this situation (Goyan, 1980), Immune Serum Globulin cannot be recommended with confidence. None the less, it does contain a measurable quantity of anti-rubella (Brody *et al.*, 1965; Schiff, 1969), so administration of a large dose (20 ml) may offer some protection.

The indications for Varicella-Zoster Immune Globulin (susceptible, immunocompromised children exposed to varicella; infants of mothers who develop varicella near the time of delivery), as well as its effectiveness, were discussed in Section IIIF. The screening of plasma from normal donors to obtain starting material for manufacture appears to presage a continuous supply of the product (Zaia *et al.*, 1978). On the other hand, the exclusive use of convalescent plasma to prepare Zoster Immune Globulin may result in periodic depletion (see Section IIIF). If neither of the high-titre immune globulins is available, the use of Immune Serum Globulin should be considered. Large doses of Immune Serum Globulin ($0.6–1.2$ ml kg^{-1}) may modify varicella if given promptly after exposure (Ross, 1962; Brunell *et al.*, 1969; Gershon *et al.*, 1978). Moreover, Gershon *et al.* (1978) have reported that lots of Immune Serum Globulin suitable for passive immunization against varicella can be identified by determining the indirect immunofluorescence antibody titre of the final product.

B.   Smallpox

Vaccinia Immune Globulin, used in conjunction with smallpox vaccine, was found to make a significant contribution to the prophylaxis of smallpox (Kempe *et al.*, 1956; Kempe *et al.*, 1961). Similarly, it was shown to decrease the incidence of certain complications that followed vaccination (Nanning, 1962), and it may also have been effective in the treatment of such complications (Kempe, 1960; Kempe *et al.*, 1961; Sussman and Grossman,

1965). However, it is now a product without a disease, because global eradication of smallpox has been achieved (Breman and Arita, 1980). Only six laboratories in the world currently maintain stocks of variola virus, and only the investigators in these laboratories remain candidates for smallpox vaccination (Breman and Arita, 1980). Thus, despite the general feeling that Vaccinia Immune Globulin is useful for prevention or attenuation of the complications of vaccination (Espmark, 1979; Kempe, 1979; Neff, 1979; Netter, 1979; Wehrle, 1979), it is unlikely that it will ever be produced again on a commercial scale. This conclusion is based on (1) the extreme improbability that smallpox will recur (Meiklejohn, 1978; Breman and Arita, 1980), (2) the probability that titres of anti-vaccinia in plasma donors will decrease, (3) the fact that stimulation of such donors is no longer warranted, and (4) the recognition that the present target population is vanishingly small. One may speculate that Vaccinia Immune Globulin, if it is made at all, will be prepared from small pools of plasma obtained from persons immunized in the course of their work. Its use, then, would be restricted to such individuals at the time of primary vaccination unless an emergency demanded vaccination on a larger scale.

VI.   POSSIBLE FUTURE USES AND PRODUCTS

This section is devoted to three major, but overlapping areas that seem certain to influence the future role(s) played by immune globulins. The first of these, future uses, has been further divided to explore, sequentially, potential routes for product delivery, additional indications for current products, and future general applications for products that may or may not exist at present. Care has been taken to avoid designating these uses as "new": some represent rediscoveries of procedures that were considered, or actually employed, in the past. Among the possible routes for immunoglobulin administration, intravenous infusion commands widespread attention (see Section IIA) and has consequently been considered separately (Section VII). Here, too, some overlapping may occur; for example, a future immune globulin (Section VIB) specific for a particular antigen could be developed for intravenous use. Finally, some discussion has been directed to future preparation of immune globulins, not simply through improved fractionation procedures (Sandberg, 1978; Condie, 1980) but rather by entirely new technology—hybridoma production.

A. Possible future uses

1. *Slow subcutaneous infusion*

Berger *et al.* (1980) have recently reported the use of small, battery-operated infusion pumps to infuse Immune Serum Globulin subcutaneously at a rate of 1–2 ml hour^{-1}. Three patients with common variable immunodeficiency were treated; all were able to tolerate this regimen and thereby avoid the problems encountered with previous therapy. As a result, patient compliance improved, higher levels of circulating IgG were achieved, and infections were better controlled. Although the number of patients was small, the diversity of complications encountered during their previous treatment is sufficient to illustrate the potential value of this procedure. These complications included pain after intramuscular injection; difficult venous access, passive sensitization to allergens, and exacerbation of congestive heart failure during intravenous plasma administration; and anaphylactoid reaction to intravenous immune globulin. It is impossible, as yet, to estimate the proportion of patients for whom slow subcutaneous infusion of immune globulin will be required. None the less, it offers a valuable option for those who must receive large volumes of product, and it necessitates no modification of the product itself.

2. *Intrathecal Tetanus Immune Globulin*

Intrathecal administration of antibodies for the treatment of tetanus is not a new concept or practice (see Editorial, 1980 and references therein). Interest in the procedure has fluctuated, but it appears to be accelerating (Hughes-Davies, 1979; Editorial, 1980). More importantly, within the last few years several controlled trials of intrathecal administration have been reported. Not all of these have yielded encouraging results. In one study of tetanus neonatorum, each infant with a clinical diagnosis of tetanus was given 40 000 units of equine antitoxin, divided between the intravenous and intramuscular routes. Thirty infants received only this dosage; 30 others received, in addition, 150 units of Tetanus Immune Globulin intrathecally. No difference in mortality or severity of disease was observed (Sedaghatian, 1979). Vakil *et al.* (1979) treated patients with clinical tetanus by administering 10 000 units of equine antitoxin intravenously and penicillin intradermally; every other patient also received 250 units of Tetanus Immune Globulin intrathecally (intracisternally). After a total of 120 patients had been studied, the trial was stopped because no difference in case–fatality ratios had emerged, though the authors concluded that higher intrathecal doses should be tried.

By contrast, when Singh *et al.* (1980) used equine antitoxin intrathecally as well as intramuscularly, the results were favourable. Infants with tetanus neonatorum received 10 000 units of the antitoxin intramuscularly and supportive medication (antibiotics and sedatives). In addition, those in the experimental group were given the antitoxin intrathecally; it was administered by lumbar puncture along with an anti-inflammatory steroid (dexamethasone). The experimental group had a significantly lower case–fatality ratio than the controls, and this difference persisted when the groups were stratified according to the severity of the symptoms. More strikingly, mortality was not affected by the size of the intrathecal dose (50 or 100 units), but it varied directly with the delay in giving that dose. Intrathecal administration ≥ 24 hours after the onset of convulsions appeared to offer no benefit. Gupta *et al.* (1980) compared the effect of 250 units of intrathecal Tetanus Immune Globulin with that of 1000 units of the product given intramuscularly. Patients with symptoms of early tetanus were allocated alternately to the two regimens. Those who received the intrathecal dose showed better clinical progress and a much lower case–fatality ratio (2%) than the controls (21%), despite the fact that these same investigators found no beneficial effect of intrathecal Tetanus Immune Globulin for patients with severe spasms (Gupta *et al.*, 1980). These two studies appear to substantiate the conclusions drawn by Kryzhanovsky (1973): that during the incubation period and early stages of tetanus intrathecal administration of antitoxin is more effective than intramuscular, intravenous, or intracarotid injections, whereas at later stages antitoxin is ineffective by any route. Moreover, they suggest that there may be a role for intrathecal Tetanus Immune Globulin, at least in the treatment of mild grade tetanus.

3. Neutralization of hepatitis B virus in vitro

Although all plasma used in the manufacture of Antihaemophilic Factor (Human) and Factor IX Complex (Human) must be tested and shown to be negative for HBsAg, these products can still transmit hepatitis B (Hoofnagle *et al.*, 1975a; Gerety *et al.*, 1979). Attempts to remove the virus by a variety of methods have been unsuccessful, a result which led Tabor *et al.* (1980a) to undertake neutralization of the virus *in vitro*. Factor IX Complex was deliberately contaminated with an inoculum of hepatitis B virus, and part of the contaminated product was incubated with Hepatitis B Immune Globulin. The materials were then given intravenously to susceptible chimpanzees. Ten weeks later, the chimpanzee given contaminated Factor IX Complex developed hepatitis B, whereas the two animals that received material treated with the immune globulin showed neither clinical signs nor serological evidence of the disease during a year of observation.

Numerous factors must be considered before application of this procedure to products for human use. The minimum effective ratio of Hepatitis B Immune Globulin to coagulant is unknown. The safety of administering immune complexes is uncertain (although the animals showed no adverse reactions). Because persons with circulating anti-HBs are protected (see Section IVB), pretreatment of the coagulant administered to them would confer no benefit but could result in overuse of the immune globulin. Haemophiliacs receiving a coagulant preparation for the first time, however, are at particularly high risk for hepatitis. The vulnerability of these patients suggests that the neutralization approach deserves further exploration.

4. Hepatitis B revisited

Hepatitis B Immune Globulin, which is recommended for prophylaxis in certain situations (Section IIID) but not for the treatment of established disease (Section IVB), has been tested under still other conditions. One proposed use was for prophylaxis of the spouses of patients with acute hepatitis B. In the study conducted by Redeker et al. (1975), such spouses were observed for a period of 150 days after injection. Hepatitis B Immune Globulin appeared to be significantly more effective than Immune Serum Globulin in preventing either symptomatic or subclinical hepatitis B. Although this is not a current indication for immune globulin (Table 2), Mosley (1979b) has suggested that the administration of the high-titre product would be justified if nonpromiscuity made subsequent sexual re-exposure unlikely.

A second potential indication was prophylaxis of patients and staff members of renal dialysis units. In a randomized, multicentre trial Hepatitis B Immune Globulin was more effective in preventing infection and antigenaemia than was either Immune Serum Globulin or an immune globulin of intermediate anti-HBs titre. This result, however, persisted for only eight months after the first injection; four months later the difference was no longer significant (Prince et al., 1978). Because the experimental design involved one injection at the time of randomization and another four months later, these findings indicate that even the high-titre product was protective for only four months or less. Such observations are in accord with others obtained by studying renal dialysis patients (Kleinknecht et al., 1977) and hospital staff members (Iwarson et al., 1977). In the latter group, Hepatitis B Immune Globulin appeared to prevent clinical hepatitis B when the doses were administered three months apart (Iwarson et al., 1977). Among dialysis patients, it prevented infection, provided the interval between injections was not greater than two months (Kleinknecht et al., 1977). Under these circumstances and in view of the continuing opportunity for re-exposure, passive immunization does not appear to be an efficient method of prophylaxis. By contrast, both the patients and the staff of dialysis units, like haemophiliacs receiving their first coagulant products (Section VIA3; cf. Hoofnagle et al., 1975a), are potential candidates for hepatitis B vaccine.

Infants born to mothers who are HBsAg positive or contract acute hepatitis

B during the third trimester of pregnancy are at risk of becoming chronic HBsAg carriers, a condition associated with the development of cirrhosis or hepatoma in adult life (Beasley and Stevens, 1978). Consequently, there have been numerous attempts to interrupt this so-called vertical transmission of hepatitis B by using immune globulin. Anecdotal reports indicate both success (Dosik and Jhaveri, 1978; Iwarson *et al.*, 1979) and failure (Boxall *et al.*, 1980) of Hepatitis B Immune Globulin in preventing transmission. Immune Serum Globulin also failed to prevent infection, although the doses administered in the small study reported may have provided too little anti-HBs or delivered it too late (Tong *et al.*, 1979). The controlled studies that have been completed are encouraging and indicate that Hepatitis B Immune Globulin may indeed be an effective prophylactic agent for these infants (Beasley and Stevens, 1978; Reesink *et al.*, 1979). A trial which is underway in Taiwan (Beasley *et al.* 1981) should provide important answers. It is already apparent, however, that if this prophylactic approach is to be successful, the administration must begin very soon after birth (Beasley and Stevens, 1978; Reesink *et al.*, 1979; Tabor and Gerety, 1979c). Moreover, if it proves to be effective, its greatest value will be for areas in which hepatitis B is endemic—i.e. countries that can least afford it (de Cock, 1980). Thus, in this instance, the future role of an immune globulin in combatting infection may depend on both clinical and economic developments.

5. *Varicella/Zoster*
In the prophylaxis of varicella, the target population for Varicella-Zoster Immune Globulin is limited to neonates and susceptible, immunocompromised children (Sections IIIF and IVC). It is not, at present, recommended for administration to adults, although Preblud *et al.* (1979) have noted that susceptible adults constitute a high-risk group.

There is no established role for exogenous antibodies in the treatment of zoster infections. Nevertheless, a series of eight case reports by Dickson and Heath (1979) included some striking, favourable responses after the administration of Zoster Immune Plasma. This observation contrasts markedly with the failure of Zoster Immune Plasma to affect the severity of cutaneous disseminated zoster in immunosuppressed patients (Groth *et al.*, 1978). The optimal treatment for these patients is uncertain. A variety of therapeutic approaches are being investigated (Section IIIF), although Gallagher and Merigan (1979) have obtained good clinical results simply by stopping or reducing the immunosuppressive therapy. Winsnes *et al.* (1978) also observed little beneficial effect of Zoster Immune Globulin in patients with malignancy; however, they have suggested that it may be useful as an adjunct to treatment with transfer factor.

5. Nosocomial infections

The use of immune globulins for the prophylaxis or treatment of hospital-based infections, though not a new concept (Bennett and Brachman, 1979), may accelerate in the future. Part of this acceleration could stem from the widespread use of immunosuppressive regimens, e.g. in malignancy and transplant patients, but the availability of improved products would also have a stimulatory effect. In some cases the improvement may consist in rendering the product suitable for intravenous infusion, thereby permitting the rapid attainment of high levels of circulating antibody. In others, development may require a new product directed against a particular class of antigens. In still others, the only innovation necessary may be the proper selection of a currently available immune globulin for prophylaxis of a highly contagious infection. This usage obviously overlaps with many described elsewhere in the chapter, a fact indicative of its potential importance.

B. Possible future products

Most of the products, extant or proposed, discussed in the following sections are purified immune globulins. Some, however, are unfractionated materials, such as immune plasma (cf. Section IA). Accordingly, they are not grouped by product *per se*, but rather according to the infections or infectious agents against which they might be used.

1. Cytomegalovirus

Cytomegalovirus infections can be a major complication and cause of death in renal transplant (Condie, 1980; Zaia *et al.*, 1980) and bone marrow transplant (Ochs *et al.*, 1980b; Zaia *et al.*, 1980) patients. The possibility of administering large volumes of immune globulin intravenously for the treatment of life-threatening infections in renal transplant recipients (Condie *et al.*, 1979) has raised the hope that passive immunization, unlike other modalities (Condie, 1980), could prevent severe cytomegalovirus infection in high-risk populations (Zaia *et al.*, 1980). Cytomegalovirus Immune Globulin has been prepared from selected plasmas obtained from normal blood donors (Zaia *et al.*, 1979). This product, as well as Cytomegalovirus Immune Plasma, is currently being tested for its ability to prevent severe cytomegalovirus infections in bone marrow transplant recipients (Zaia *et al.*, 1980). The apparent success of Cytomegalovirus Immune Plasma in the treatment of cytomegalovirus pneumonitis in a renal transplant patient (Dijkmans *et al.*, 1979) suggests that passive immunization could assume a significant role in the management of these cases.

2. Haemorrhagic fevers

In view of the severity of most cases of haemorrhagic fever and the attendant high mortality, it is not surprising that a variety of therapeutic measures have been explored. At present, however, no specific preventive or therapeutic agents are available (Johnson, 1979; Maiztegui *et al.*, 1979), and much of the treatment is supportive. Therefore, the report of a controlled trial in which immune plasma provided effective treatment of Argentine haemorrhagic fever (Maiztegui *et al.*, 1979) suggests that this approach may be useful as other haemorrhagic fevers are encountered (Johnson *et al.*, 1977). This suggestion is strengthened by the recovery of an investigator who was inoculated with Ebola virus in a laboratory accident and was subsequently given convalescent serum (Emond *et al.*, 1977).

Although high-titre immune plasma or serum could be fractionated to obtain the corresponding immune globulin, it is probably premature to undertake such a preparation until more is known of these diseases and their control. The favourable results described above, however, indicate that the haemorrhagic fever immune plasmas themselves will be useful both for managing patients with these diseases and for protecting laboratory workers who are exposed during the course of their investigations.

3. Hepatitis non-A, non-B

At present, non-A, non-B hepatitis accounts for the vast majority of post transfusion hepatitis as well as a substantial portion of sporadic hepatitis case (Tabor and Gerety, 1979b). Although both transmissibility (Tabor and Gerety, 1979b and references therein) and the existence of a carrier state (Tabor *et al.*, 1980b) have been demonstrated, it is still uncertain whether non-A, non-B hepatitis is a single disease, transmitted by a single type of virus None the less, there have been reports that both the incidence of post transfusion non-A, non-B hepatitis (Knodell *et al.*, 1976; Seeff *et al.*, 1977) and the progression of the disease from an acute to a chronic stage (Knodell *et al.*, 1977) were reduced by the administration of immune globulin. Effectiveness has been claimed for both Immune Serum Globulin and Hepatitis B Immune Globulin. In one trial, however, the incidence of post-transfusion non-A, non-B hepatitis among patients who received either product differed from that of the placebo group only when the transfused blood contained anti-HBs (Conrad *et al.*, 1977). In another, Immune Serum Globulin lowered the incidence of *icteric* hepatitis but did not affect the total incidence of the disease (Seeff *et al.*, 1977).

The significance of these observations will remain uncertain until more is known of the disease(s) and the virus(es) responsible for it. Similarly, the use of immune globulin for prophylaxis of non-A, non-B hepatitis cannot be recommended until methods exist for identifying and quantitating the protective antibodies in the product. Still, the results appear encouraging. The eventual availability of suitable test methods for monitoring protective antibody should permit the preparation of a "Hepatitis non-A, non-B Immune Globulin" or, at least, the selection of lots (e.g. of Immune Serum Globulin) that could confidently be expected to show good clinical performance.

4. Rubella

Vaccination against rubella and its apparent success in reducing the frequency of congenital rubella syndrome (Goyan, 1980) was discussed in Section VA. However, even in countries with assiduous programmes for active immunization, part of the population — including women of childbearing age — has remained susceptible to rubella (Clarke et al., 1980). Thus a truly effective Rubella Immune Globulin, i.e. one which could prevent fetal damage when administered to a susceptible woman after exposure to rubella during early pregnancy, could play a small but significant role in prophylaxis. The problem, of course, would be to demonstrate effectiveness, especially in view of the ability of immune globulin to suppress clinical disease without preventing infection (Brody et al., 1965). The fact that immune globulin with a sufficiently high anti-rubella titre can prevent seroconversion in exposed volunteers (Schiff, 1969; Urquhart et al., 1978) suggests that an efficacious Rubella Immune Globulin could be developed. Key issues in such development would be identification of the level of circulating antibody needed for protection and the collection of data needed to evaluate effectiveness in actual clinical use. Whether effort is better spent in these areas or in strengthening active immunization programmes is a matter for future debate.

5. Botulism

The products currently available for use in botulism are equine antitoxins. Those directed toward botulinum toxin type E appear to be effective (Dolman and Iida, 1963), whereas those toward types A and B are more difficult to evaluate (Oberst et al., 1968; Sudre et al., 1975). The potential for adverse reactions to the equine products (Black and Gunn, 1980) has led Lewis and Metzger (1978) to prepare Botulism Immune Plasma of human origin and to undertake the production of Botulism Immune Globulin (Metzger and Lewis, 1979). The efficacy of these products will be no easier to demonstrate than that of their equine counterparts, but the need for specific therapy in addition to supportive treatment for botulism is a strong basis for pursuing their development. This is particularly true if infant botulism, as well as adult botulism, can be treated successfully with exogenous immunoglobulin (Arnon et al., 1977).

Despite their disadvantages, the equine antitoxins can be administered intravenously, thus assuring rapid attainment of the maximum possible concentration of antibodies in the circulation. In view of the desirability of speed in neutralizing botulinum toxins, a Botulism Immune Globulin suitable for intravenous administration should be a more valuable therapeutic agent than one confined to intramuscular use.

6. Diphtheria

Diphtheria, like measles and rubella, has been largely controlled through the use of active immunization; moreover, the effectiveness of the equine product, Diphtheria Antitoxin, for either prophylaxis or treatment has not been precisely established and is now probably marginal (Stollerman, 1978). Against this background, the potential role for a Diphtheria Immune Globulin appears small. Nevertheless, diphtheria still occurs, even in countries with established programmes for active immunization. Thus, if a suitable target population (e.g., unimmunized, susceptible persons; individuals, immunized or not, who have contracted diphtheria) could be identified, such a product would probably be useful. Diphtheria Immune Globulin preparations have been produced (Sgouris et al., 1969; Hartman, 1979), but they have not been tested clinically. Such testing could prove to be difficult. It would involve not only manufacture of the product and identification of a suitable study population, but also accumulation of a sufficient number of patients to provide a meaningful evaluation. The likelihood of such a study may therefore depend on the prevalence of the disease itself. If efficacy could be demonstrated, however, an intravenous diphtheria Immune Globulin might prove to be an ideal preparation for the rapid neutralization of unbound toxin (Hardegree and Cox, 1980).

7. Pseudomonas

Pseudomonas aeruginosa is a stubborn and challenging organism that can infect and colonize patients suffering from a variety of primary diseases (Doggett, 1979). Cancer patients, especially those with leukaemia or myeloma, patients with chronic diseases, such as cystic fibrosis, immunocompromised individuals, and patients treated in intensive care units have been victims of this infection. Burn patients have been considered to be at particularly high risk, although Pseudomonas infection in this group has now decreased in the U.S. (Alexander, 1979).

As one might expect, a vast array of therapeutic measures, including both active and passive immunization, have been employed (Doggett, 1979). The apparent effectiveness of the regimen, however, often varied inversely with the quality of the experimental design (Pollack, 1980). The use of exogenous immunoglobulin to protect burn patients has been diligently explored and has yielded moderate success (Jones et al., 1980 and references therein). The recent report by Jones *et al.* (1980) is especially encouraging. In this series burn victims who received *Pseudomonas* Immune Globulin, polyvalent *Pseudomonas* vaccine, or both agents showed significantly lower case–fatality ratios than did controls who received neither, despite the fact that *Pseudomonas aeruginosa* colonized at least 90% of the burns in *all* groups at some point during the hospital stay. There were no deaths of children given *Pseudomonas* Immune Globulin alone (case–fatality ratio for control children, 21%), whereas the corresponding case–fatality ratio for adults was 10% (that for control adults, 36%) and did not differ significantly from those of the other treated groups.

Although both the vaccine and the immune globulin effectively combated *Pseudomonas* in burn patients (cf. Jones *et al.*, 1979 and Jones *et al.*, 1980), use of the latter appears to offer clear advantages for immunosuppressed persons who are unable to respond normally to active immunization (Ziegler and Braude, 1980). The degree of protection achieved in this manner, however, is dependent on the vaccine used to elicit antibodies in the plasma donors (Jones *et al.*, 1980). Apparently consistent with this dependence are the observations by Pollack and Young (1979) that recovery from *Pseudomonas* septicaemia correlated with the levels of endogenous antibodies to both exotoxin A and lipopolysaccharide (endotoxin), and that the protective effects of the two types of antibodies were independent and additive. It is therefore noteworthy that Ziegler *et al.* (1981) obtained good therapeutic results with unfractionated human antiserum directed against the common core region of bacterial lipopolysaccharide (J-5 antiserum). Treatment with this antiserum produced a substantial reduction in the case–fatality ratio of patients with Gram-negative bacteraemia (major organisms, *Escherichia coli* and *Pseudomonas aeruginosa*), even among patients with septic shock. Moreover, preliminary results indicate that prophylactic administration of the antiserum to neutropenic patients with haematological malignancies decreased febrile morbidity and may have decreased Gram-negative bacteraemia as well.

The clinical successes reported suggest that either *Pseudomonas* Immune Globulin or an appropriate human antiserum that cross-reacts with *Pseudomonas* toxin(s) could have broad clinical application against *Pseudomonas* invasion. Both the safety (Ziegler and Braude, 1980) and the effectiveness of the antiserum imply that intravenous administration is the route of choice.

8. Other bacterial infections

In an editorial published more than ten years ago, Schless and Harell (1968) expressed the hope that large scale, controlled clinical trials would clarify the role of immune globulins in the treatment of systemic bacterial infections in patients without antibody deficiency. This hope was based, in part, on the therapeutic activity shown by human immunoglobulin preparations in experiments that involved mice challenged with bacteria such as *Pseudomonas aeruginosa, Escherichia coli*, and various species of *Streptococcus*. Although an objective evaluation of the ensuing clinical trials is difficult (Barandun *et al.*, 1975) and the problems inherent in conducting a medically and statistically valid study have been forcefully stated (Pirofsky, 1979), there is still reason for guarded optimism. In fact, the time for initiating such studies has probably never been more appropriate, nor the need for effective immunotherapeutic agents greater.

Potential beneficiaries of such therapy resemble those noted in Sections VIB1 and VIB7; they comprise immunosuppressed patients, those with established or impending bacteraemia, children with acute leukaemia, Hodgkin's disease, sickle cell disease, or asplenia, and children in settings with a known high incidence of bacterial infection. Organisms frequently encountered include, in addition to *Pseudomonas aeruginosa* and *Escherichia coli* (Ziegler and Braude, 1980), *Streptococcus pneumoniae* and *Haemophilus influenzae* (Siber, 1980), *Klebsiella* and *Enterobacter* (Ziegler and Braude, 1980), and other streptococci and meningococci. Antibiotics, though obviously useful, have not been completely effective; neither, in some cases, has active immunization. For example, the antibody response to pneumococcal vaccine was found to be depressed in patients treated for Hodgkin's disease, thus rendering questionable the ability of active immunization to protect them against post-splenectomy infection (Siber *et al.*, 1978). Similarly, Baker *et al.* (1980) concluded that immunization of mothers with pneumococcal vaccine is not likely to prevent neonatal infection with Group B type III streptococci, despite the antigenic similarity of the micro-organisms.

In such situations, passive immunization deserves serious consideration, especially in view of the success achieved by Ziegler and Braude (1980) in treating (and, possibly, in preventing) bacteraemia with J-5 antiserum (Section VIB7). The obstacles to such an approach, however, are multiple. One must choose the correct spectrum of bacterial polysaccharides for immunizing the donors. These must elicit antibodies not only with the desired specificities but also in sufficiently high concentration. Moreover, if the active antibodies are IgM rather than IgG (Schless and Harell, 1968; Ziegler and Braude, 1980), they will not be harvested in immune globulins prepared by the conventional procedures (Sections IIB and IIC). On the other hand, laboratory studies of Immune Serum Globulin have shown the presence of both binding and bactericidal antibodies against Gram-negative bacteria and Group B type III streptococci (Sadoff *et al.*, 1980) and protective activity against the latter (Vogel *et al.*, 1980). If that activity is high enough, clinical studies may be warranted, as Vogel *et al.* (1980) have suggested. In an extensive epidemiological trial reported in the Russian literature, prophylactic administration of Immune Serum Globulin to young children resulted in significant protection against meningococcal infection, albeit the effect was short-lived (Favorova *et al.*, 1975).

C. Hybridomas

A discussion of the future of immunotherapy would be incomplete without some mention of the potential contribution of hybridoma technology. The discovery that mouse myeloma cells could be fused with lymphocytes from the spleens of mice that had been immunized with a specific antigen to yield hybridomas (literally, hybrid-myelomas) capable of secreting monoclonal antibodies (Köhler and Milstein, 1975) has been summarized by Milstein (1980). The resulting opportunity to prepare a broad (in principle, limitless) range of specific antibodies in large quantity and high concentration has already been exploited for the production of immunological reagents. The obvious hope is that, if hybridomas of entirely human origin can be developed, the monoclonal antibodies secreted can be used for prophylaxis and treatment of human patients. In such a case, antibodies could virtually be made "to order", depending on the needs presented by the clinical situation (Merchant, 1980). Human hybridomas are now available (Olsson and Kaplan, 1980), and the rapidity of progress indicates that this hope is not misplaced. The ability of hybridomas to produce monoclonal antibodies against pathogenic bacteria (Polin, 1980) and viruses (Koprowski and Witkor, 1980) has already been demonstrated.

VII.   IMMUNE GLOBULINS FOR INTRAVENOUS USE

A.   Possibilities and problems

The rationale for considering intravenous immune globulins in a separate section was stated in Section IIA. In essence, the goal in the development of such preparations is an efficacious product that can be administered by the intravenous route without evoking adverse reactions (Section IIC). The motivation is the potentially rich clinical reward this development could yield.

The advantages of intravenous administration are many. The volume of immune globulin that can be given is larger than that possible by the intramuscular route. This is particularly important when the muscle mass available for injection is small (e.g., in paediatric or cachectic patients) or damaged (e.g., in burn patients), when intramuscular injection could result in uncontrolled bleeding (e.g. in patients with the Wiskott–Aldrich syndrome or other thrombocytopenic condition), or when the dose required is large or must be repeated at frequent intervals (e.g., in immunodeficiency). The diminished discomfort, compared with that of intramuscular injections, should lead to improved patient acceptance and consequent adherence to the therapeutic or prophylactic regimen. Finally, the rapid attainment of high levels of circulating antibody should improve the chances for clinical success when the objective is rapid neutralization of antigen (e.g. a bacterial toxin).

The reactions to intravenous infusions of immune globulins also span a considerable range, but certain symptoms have been observed so frequently that they are considered stereotypes (Barandun et al., 1962). These include chills, fever, nausea, vomiting, chest constriction and/or dyspnoea, flushing, tachycardia, back pain, and (in severe reactions) hypotension, though not all symptoms occur in every episode (Coon et al., 1961; Barandun et al., 1962; Janeway, 1970; Gislason et al., 1978; inter alia). The severity of the response is often related directly to the rate of administration, and it may abate when the infusion is slowed. Moreover, after an adverse reaction subsides, it is often possible to perform a second infusion without untoward effect. The implications of this rate-relatedness and refractory period are discussed elsewhere (Aronson and Finlayson, 1980).

B.   Preparations

There has been little disagreement with the potential advantages of intravenous immunoglobulin administration listed in the preceding section or with the ultimate goal of product development. The controversies involve the means by which these should be realized. In part, the differences of opinion stem from the lack of agreement regarding product characteristics to be sought (Table 1) and the choice of laboratory tests to predict product safety. As noted previously (Section IIC), the tests proposed have included measurements of enzymes in the contact activation (kallikrein–kinin) system (Alving et al., 1980), determination of anticomplementary activity on the assumption that the adverse reactions are mediated through the complement system (Barandun et al., 1962, 1980), and measurement of complement consumption in the belief that the reactions are not complement-mediated but rather that the consumption assays detect aggregated IgG which may elicit untoward reactions by inducing prostaglandin release (Rosen, 1970; Passwell et al., 1980). Similarly, it is not the range of side-effects that has evoked diversity, but the changes in the product or manufacturing process undertaken to eliminate them. Barandun et al. (1962) initially employed ultracentrifugation to remove aggregates, but this technique is impractical for manufacturing purposes. The following discussion is therefore confined to methods used on a production scale.

Table 3 comprises a list of immunoglobulin preparations available for intravenous use. In spite of its length, the products and processes can be

Table 3 Immunoglobulin preparations administered intravenously

Type of modification	Major agent used	Reference
Enzymic	Pepsin	Schultze and Schwick (1962)
Enzymic	Plasmin	Sgouris (1967)
pH 4	HCl[a]	Barandun et al. (1962)
Alkylation, acylation	β-Propiolactone	Stephan (1975)
Disulphide cleavage	Sulphite + tetrathionite	Masuho et al. (1977)
Disulphide cleavage	DTT,[b] iodoacetamide	Mozen et al. (1980)
None	Ethanol	Welch et al. (1980)
None	Ethanol, DEAE-Sephadex	Björling (1979)
None	Ethanol, salt, PEG	Eibl (1980)
None	DEAE-Sephadex	Hoppe et al. (1973)
None	SiO_2, QAE-Sephadex	Condie (1980)

[a] Some producers (e.g. Walsh, 1974) also add a small amount of pepsin.
[b] Abbreviations: DEAE, diethylaminoethyl; DTT, dithiothreitol; PEG, polyethylene glycol; QAE, diethyl(2-hydroxypropyl)aminoethyl.

grouped into five major categories. The first category includes immune globulins treated with proteolytic enzymes. The "standard" pepsin treatment results in relatively complete digestion, hence the product consists largely of $F(ab)_2$ fragments (Schultze and Schwick, 1962). Later enzymic treatments with pepsin (Barandun et al., 1962; Walsh, 1974) or plasmin (Sgouris, 1967) were gentler and resulted in little detectable fragmentation, if any.

The pH 4 treatment (Table 3) was developed after Barandun et al. (1962) discovered that a control tube of immunoglobulin incubated *without* pepsin was depleted of anticomplementary activity. This treatment, which was exploited to produce a product for clinical use, has recently been refined to yield a new pH-4-treated immune globulin with a still lower content of aggregated IgG (Barundun et al., 1980). The conditions chosen for treatment with β-propiolactone evidently represent a compromise between those required for eliminating anticomplementary activity and those that would damage the immunoglobulin. Although chemical modification of an immunoglobulin always carries the potential risk of creating new antigenic determinants (Wadsworth, 1976), users of the β-propiolactone-treated product evidently have not detected enhanced immunogenicity (Stephan, 1975; Kornhuber, 1980). The final examples of chemical modification of IgG are those involving selective cleavage of disulphide bridges (Table 3). In both cases an average of four bonds per molecule are broken; however, in the process developed in Japan the cleavage is oxidative (Masuho et al., 1977), but in that developed in the U.S. it is reductive (Mozen et al., 1980).

Perhaps the most intriguing approach to the production of immune globulins for intravenous use—especially in view of the early clinical experiences (Section IIA)—is the exploration of immunoglobulin preparations that have undergone no intentional modification (Table 3). The simplest of these is conventional immune globulin prepared for intramuscular use by precipitation with cold ethanol and diluted with saline before intravenous infusion (Welch et al., 1980). A somewhat more purified preparation (Björling, 1979) has been administered in similar fashion, although to minimize adverse reactions the patients are premedicated with hydrocortisone (Gislason et al., 1978). In general, the producers of these unmodified immunoglobulins have attempted to use the gentlest procedures compatible with purification. Confidence in the success of this strategy is reflected by the designation of one such product as "native IgG" (Condie, 1980).

C. Clinical experience

The clinical studies of intravenously administered immune globulins range from multicentre controlled trials to frankly anecdotal case reports. Analogous variety appears in the frequency with which these products are used. For example, usage is widespread in Germany, conservative in the U.K., extensive and exponentially increasing in Japan, and largely experimental in the U.S. Against this diverse background, objective observations are difficult; none the less, a few generalizations seem clearly substantiable. The first is that the product modifications, even if successful, may not yield a product that is free of side-effects (Magilavy et al., 1978; Eibl, 1980; Ochs, 1980). Although this situation is a natural consequence of failure to understand the mechanism of the adverse reactions, their apparently multiple aetiologies, and the lack of agreement on appropriate laboratory tests for predicting them, the empirical approach that it demands can produce encouraging results. Ochs et al. (1980a) have recently shown that simply changing the solvent (specifically, from 0.3 M glycine to 10% maltose) could dramatically lower the incidence of untoward effects.

Secondly, the need for objective evaluation criteria and stringent experimental design is obvious. Data such as the number of days absent from work or school, days with fever, and days on which antibiotics are required appear to be useful (Barandun et al., 1980). The crossover design can provide a reliable basis for comparing either the efficacy (Nolte et al., 1979) or the side-effects (Ochs et al., 1980a) of different immunoglobulin preparations. Indeed, if the patient population is heterogeneous, this may be the only technique for making a valid comparison.

Several workers, using a variety of study designs, have evaluated intravenous immune globulin for the maintenance of immunodeficient patients. In each case the preparation under investigation was judged effective (Magilavy et al., 1978; Nolte et al., 1979; Barandun et al., 1980; Eibl, 1980;

Ochs, 1980). Some conditions (e.g. bronchiectasis and upper respiratory infections) were difficult to moderate (Magilavy et al., 1978; Barandun, 1979; Ochs, 1979; Eibl, 1980; Ochs, 1980), in agreement with earlier experiences with immunodeficient patients (Barandun et al., 1975). These limitations notwithstanding, it appears certain that when efficacy data have been obtained for a particular product, it is appropriate to use that product for the maintenance of patients who are unable to produce sufficient amounts of IgG antibodies.

D. Clinical future

Certain applications of intravenous immune globulin are direct extrapolations of its use for maintenance of patients with congenital immunodeficiencies. These include routine administration in cases of immunodeficiency subsequent to malignancies, other diseases, or immunosuppressive therapy, as well as episodic administration when a patient with acquired immunodeficiency is exposed to contagious disease. In the latter situation it is uncertain whether a "broad-spectrum" immunoglobulin preparation, i.e. the intravenous equivalent of Immune Serum Globulin, will suffice (cf. Janeway, 1970 and Kornhuber, 1980) or if specific intravenous immune globulins should be sought. In either case if the exposure is to a single, identifiable agent, an objective evaluation of efficacy should be possible.

Other conditions in which successful prophylaxis and therapy, respectively, have been reported are post-operative infection (Duswald et al., 1980) and zoster (Mondorf and Duswald, 1980; cf. Pirofsky, 1979). Although the latter study was uncontrolled, its results indicate that further exploration is warranted, especially in view of the conflicting reports from previous investigations (Section VIA5).

A more theoretical, but equally deserving area for further study is the use of intravenous immune globulin in toxin-mediated disease (Hardegree and Cox, 1980). Tetanus Immune Globulin prepared for intramuscular use has been administered to tetanus patients by the intravenous route (Stollerman, 1978; Welch et al., 1980). In a controlled, randomized trial, intravenous infusion of a high-titre preparation was compared with that of a "standard" immune globulin and an albumin control. The authors found no evidence of efficacy, possibly because of the generalized state of tetanus (all patients required tracheotomy) at the time therapy was initiated (Vic Dupont et al., 1975).*

---

* Statistical analyses carried out by the present author indicated a significantly lower case–fatality ratio for patients of Vic Dupont et al. (1975) who received the high dose compared with the control group ($P < 0.05$); when patients younger than 24 and older than 75 years were excluded, this difference still approached significance ($0.07 < P < 0.08$).

The value of intravenous immune globulins in the therapy of severe bacterial infections (see Sections VIA6 and VIB8) is even more difficult to assess. The difficulties inherent in such an evaluation have been outlined (Pirofsky, 1979) and, as yet, no firm clinical data are available (Barandun, 1979; Kornhuber, 1979; Luiken, 1979; Ochs, 1979; Pirofsky, 1979). Nevertheless, it is in the area of bacterial infections that some of the greatest advances may occur. The direction of these advances cannot be predicted (Hosea *et al.*, 1981), but the striking results obtained with hyperimmune serum (Ziegler and Braude, 1980) were described previously (Sections VIB7 and 8). A major indication for immune globulins might prove to be prophylaxis against bacterial infection, whereas in the treatment of infection they might serve primarily as adjuncts to antibiotice therapy (Barandun, 1979). It is clear that definitive answers can only be obtained by controlled clinical trials and that these will be expensive and prolonged, albeit eminently worth while.

VIII. CONCLUSIONS

Immune globulins prepared from human plasma and administered intramuscularly are currently used for the maintenance of immunodeficient patients and for prophylaxis of measles and hepatitis A, though the minimum protective dose against hepatitis A has not yet been established. These indications are supported by clinical trials as well as practical experience. Among the specific immune globulins for intramuscular use, Varicella-Zoster Immune Globulin has been found effective for the post-exposure prophylaxis of susceptible, immunodeficient children and is also recommended for neonates whose mothers develop varicella near the time of delivery. Hepatitis B Immune Globulin is recommended for susceptible persons who are exposed to HBsAg-positive material by needle-stick, mucous membrane exposure, or ingestion; other indications are controversial, and use in neonates of HBsAg-positive mothers is still under study. Rabies Immune Globulin and Tetanus Immune Globulin are probably effective for post-exposure prophylaxis, but efficacy is difficult to prove because they are used in consort with rabies vaccine and tetanus toxoid, respectively. Very recent reports have indicated that intrathecal administration of Tetanus Immune Globulin or equine tetanus antitoxin may be effective in the treatment of early tetanus, provided the therapy is initiated soon enough.

There appears to be little clinical value for Mumps Immune Globulin and absolutely none for Pertussis Immune Globulin. Vaccinia Immune Globulin is an effective product left without a disease, and except for laboratory workers investigating variola or closely related viruses, a target population now that smallpox has been eradicated.

It remains to be seen whether or not immune globulins specific for non-A, non-B hepatitis, cytomegalovirus, botulinum toxins, *Pseudomonas*, or other bacteria can be proven effective. The susceptibility of immunosuppressed patients to cytomegalovirus and bacterial infections, however, suggests this as an extraordinarily fertile area for development.

A wide variety of immune globulins have been developed for intravenous use. The only indication for which objective evidence of the effectiveness of such products is available is the maintenance of immunodeficient patients. Possible future developments of these products include improved tests to predict adverse reactions, improved (e.g. safer) products, intravenous immune globulins directed against specific antigens or classes of antigens, and clinical trials to establish appropriate additional indications. Recapitulation of the route travelled in the development of intramuscular immune globulin (i.e. initial use for a plethora of indications with subsequent weeding out of the inappropriate ones) is to be avoided.

It is clear that any future progress, regardless of the direction, must be made by advances on three fronts: laboratory testing, manufacturing, and clinical investigation. Properly co-ordinated, they can define and, thereafter, continue to refine the role of immune globulins in prophylaxis and therapy of infectious disease.

REFERENCES

Acute Hepatic Failure Study Group (1977). *Ann. Intern. Med.* **86**, 272–277.

Adam, E. and Skvaril, F. (1965). *Arch. Ges. Virusforsch.* **16**, 220–221.

Alexander, J. W. (1979). *J. Trauma Suppl.* **19**, 887–889.

Alter, H. J., Barker, L. F. and Holland, P. V. (1975). *N. Engl. J. Med.* **293**, 1093–1094.

Alving, B. M. and Finlayson, J. S. (ed.) (1980). "Immunoglobulins: Characteristics and Uses of Intravenous Preparations". DHHS Publication No. (FDA)-80-9005, U.S. Government Printing Office, Washington.

Alving, B. M., Tankersley, D. L., Mason, B. L., Rossi, F., Aronson, D. L. and Finlayson, J. S. (1980). *J. Lab. Clin. Med.* **96**, 334–346.

Arnon, S. S., Midura, T. F., Clay, S. A., Wood, R. M. and Chin, J. (1977). *J.A.M.A.* **237**, 1946–1951.

Aronson, D. L. and Finlayson, J. S. (1980). *Sem. Thromb. Hemostas.* **6**, 121–139.

Ashley, A. (1955). *N. Engl. J. Med.* **252**, 88–91.

Avenard, G., Gaiffe, M. and Herzog, F. (1979). *Nouv. Presse Med.* **8**, 673–675.

Bahmanyar, M., Fayaz, A., Nour-Salehi, S., Mohammadi, M. and Koprowski, H. (1976). *J.A.M.A.* **236**, 2751–2754.

Baker, C., Kasper, D. L., Edwards, M. S. and Schiffman, G. (1980). *N. Engl. J. Med.* **303**, 173–178.

Balagtas, R. C., Nelson, K. E., Levin, S. and Gotoff, S. P. (1971). *J. Pediatr.* **79**, 203–208.

Balfour, H. H., Jr, Groth, K. E., McCullough, J., Kalis, J. M., Marker, S. C., Nesbit, M. E., Simmons, R. L. and Najarian, J. S. (1977). *Amer. J. Dis. Child* **131**, 693–696.

Baltazard, M. and Bahmanyar, M. (1955). *Bull. Wld Hlth Org.* **13**, 747–772.

Barandun, S. (1979). *Vox Sang.* **37**, 117–119.

Barandun, S., Kistler, P., Jeunet, F. and Isliker, H. (1962). *Vox Sang.* **7**, 157–174.
Barandun, S., Skvaril, F. and Morell, A. (1975). *Monogr. Allergy* **9**, 39–60.
Barandun, S., Morell, A. and Skvaril, F. (1980). *In* "Immunoglobulins: Characteristics and Uses of Intravenous Preparations" (B. M. Alving and J. S. Finlayson, ed.) pp. 31–35, DHHS Publication No. (FDA)-80-9005, U.S. Government Printing Office, Washington.
Barker, L. F., Gerety, R. J. and Tabor, E. (1978). *Adv. Intern. Med.* **23**, 327–351.
Beasley, R. P. and Stevens, C. E. (1978). *In* "Viral Hepatitis" (G. N. Vyas, S. N. Cohen and R. Schmid, ed.) pp. 333–345, Franklin Institute Press, Philadelphia.
Beasley, R. P., Hwang, L.-Y., Lin, C.-C., Stevens, C. E., Wang, K.-Y., Sun, T.-S., Hsieh, F.-J. and Szmuness, W. (1981). *Lancet* **2**, 388–393.
Bennett, J. V. and Brachman, P. S. (ed.) (1979). "Hospital Infections". Little, Brown, Boston.
Berger, M., Cupps, T. R. and Fauci, A. S. (1980). *Ann. Intern. Med.* **93**, 55–56.
Björling, H. (1979). *In* "Plasma Proteins" (B. Blombäck and L. Å. Hanson, ed.) pp. 30–37. John Wiley, Chichester.
Black, R. E. and Gunn, R. A. (1980). *Amer. J. Med.* **69**, 567–570.
Blake, P. A., Feldman, R. A., Buchanan, T. M., Brooks, G. F. and Bennett, J. V. (1976). *J.A.M.A.* **235**, 42–44.
Boxall, E., Flewett, T. H., Derso, A. and Tarlow, M. J. (1980). *Lancet* **1**, 419–420.
Brachott, D., Mosley, J. W., Lifschitz, I., Kendrick, M. A. and Sgouris, J. T. (1972). *Transfusion* **12**, 389–393.
Breman, J. G. and Arita, I. (1980). *N. Engl. J. Med.* **303**, 1263–1273.
Brody, J. A., Sever, J. L. and Schiff, G. M. (1965). *N. Engl. J. Med.* **272**, 127–129.
Bruhl, H. H. (1977). *Minnesota Med.* **60**, 673–676, 684.
Brunell, P. A., Ross, A., Miller, L. H. and Kuo, B. (1969). *N. Engl. J. Med.* **280**, 1191–1194.
Bruton, O. C. (1952). *Pediatrics* **9**, 722–728.
Buckley, R. H. (1980). *In* "Immunoglobulins: Characteristics and Uses of Intravenous Preparations" (B. M. Alving and J. S. Finlayson, ed.) pp. 3–8, DHHS Publication No. (FDA)-80-9005, U.S. Government Printing Office, Washington.
Cabasso, V. J. (1974). *J. Biol. Stand.* **2**, 43–50.
Cabasso, V. J., Loofbourow, J. C., Roby, R. E. and Anuskiewicz, W. (1971). *Bull. Wld Hlth Org.* **45**, 303–315.
Cassidy, J. T., Stein, L. D., Reynolds, R. T. and Magilavy, D. B. (1980). *In* "Immunoglobulins: Characteristics and Uses of Intravenous Preparations" (B. M. Alving and J. S. Finlayson, ed.) pp. 161–166, DHHS Publication No. (FDA)-80-9005, U.S. Government Printing Office, Washington.
Clarke, M., Stitt, J., Seagroatt, V., Schild, G. C., Pollock, T. M., Finlay, S. E. and Barbara, J. A. J. (1980). *Lancet* **1**, 537–538.
Code of Federal Regulations (1980a). Title 21, Chapter I, Part 610, Subpart F, pp. 48–53, U.S. Government Printing Office, Washington.
Code of Federal Regulations (1980b). Title 21, Chapter I, Part 640, Subpart J, pp. 134–136, U.S. Government Printing Office, Washington.
Cohen, P. and Hudson, H. H. (1971). *Vox Sang.* **21**, 311–318.
Cohn, E. J. (1948). *In* "Advances in Military Medicine" (E. C. Andrus, D. W. Bronk, G. A. Carden, Jr, C. S. Keefer, J. S. Lockwood, J. T. Wearn and M. C. Winternitz, ed.) Vol. I, pp. 364–443. Little, Brown, Boston.
Cohn, E. J., Strong, L. E., Hughes, W. L., Jr, Mulford, D. J., Ashworth, J. N., Melin, M. and Taylor, H. L. (1946). *J. Amer. Chem. Soc.* **68**, 459–475.

Committee on Infectious Diseases (1977). "Red Book". American Academy of Pediatrics, Evanston, Illinois.

Condie, R. M. (1980). *In* "Immunoglobulins: Characteristics and Uses of Intravenous Preparations" (B. M. Alving and J. S. Finlayson, ed.) pp. 179–193, DHHS Publication No. (FDA)-80-9005, U.S. Government Printing Office, Washington.

Condie, R. M., Hall, B. L., Howard, R. J., Fryd, D., Simmons, R. L. and Najarian, J. S. (1979). *Transplantation Proc.* **11**, 66–68.

Connell, G. E. and Painter, R. H. (1966). *Can. J. Biochem.* **44**, 371–379.

Conrad, M. E., Knodell, R. G., Bradley, E. L., Jr, Flannery, E. P. and Ginsberg, A. L. (1977). *Transfusion* **17**, 579–585.

Coon, W. W., Iob, V., Wolfman, E. F., Jr, Hodgson, P. E. and McMath, M. (1961). *Amer. J. Surg.* **102**, 548–553.

Copelovici, Y., Strulovici, D., Cristea, A., Tudor, V. and Armasu, V. (1979). *Virologie* **30**, 171–177.

de Cock, K. M. (1980). *Lancet* **1**, 827.

Dempster, G., Stead, S., Zbitnew, A., Rhodes, A. J. and Zalan, E. (1979). *Can. Med. Assoc. J.* **120**, 1069–1074.

Deutsch, H. F., Morton, J. I. and Kratochvil, C. H. (1956). *J. Biol. Chem.* **222**, 39–51.

Dickson, D. N. and Heath, M. (1979). *S. Afr. Med. J.* **56**, 491–494.

Dienstag, J. L. (1980). *N. Engl. J. Med.* **303**, 874–876.

Dijkmans, B. A. C., Versteeg, J., Kauffmann, R. H., van den Broek, P. J., Eernisse, J. G., van Zanten, J. J., Bakker, W., Kalff, M. W. and van Hooff, J. P. (1979). *Lancet* **1**, 820–821.

Doggett, R. G. (ed.) (1979). "*Pseudomonas aeruginosa*. Clinical Manifestations and Current Therapy". Academic Press, New York and London.

Dolman, C. E. and Iida, H. (1963). *Can. J. Public Hlth* **54**, 293–308.

Dosik, H. and Jhaveri, R. (1978). *N. Engl. J. Med.* **298**, 602–603.

Duswald, K. H., Müller, K., Seifert, J. and Ring, J. (1980). *Münch. Med. Wochenschr.* **122**, 832–836.

Editorial (1980). *Lancet* **2**, 464.

Eibl, M. (1980). *In* "Immunoglobulins: Characteristics and Uses of Intravenous Preparations" (B. M. Alving and J. S. Finlayson, ed.) pp. 23–30. DHHS Publication No. (FDA)-80-9005, U.S. Government Printing Office, Washington.

Ellis, E. F. and Henney, C. S. (1969). *J. Allergy* **43**, 45–54.

Emond, R. T. D., Evans, B., Bowen, E. T. W. and Lloyd, G. (1977). *Br. Med. J.* **2**, 541–544.

Enders, J. F. (1944). *J. Clin. Invest.* **23**, 510–530.

Espmark, J. A. (1979). *Vox Sang.* **36**, 121–122.

Evans, E. B., Pollock, T. M., Cradock-Watson, J. E. and Ridehalgh, M. K. S. (1980). *Lancet* **1**, 354–356.

Favero, M. S., Maynard, J. E. and Leger, R. T. (1980). *Crit. Care Quart.* **3**, 43–55.

Favorova, L. A., Sokova, I. N., Chernyshova, T. F., Khrometskaya, T. M., Teleshevskaya, E. A., Vinnichek, N. D., Troshina, L. D., Ershova, G. A., Obukhova, T. M., Stepanova, G. S., Kamensky, V. A., Yatsenko, V. G., Yurov, V. E. and Dolmatov, V. V. (1975). *Zh. Mikrobiol. Epidemiol. Immunobiol.* **6**, 15–18.

Finlayson, J. S. (1972). *Ann. N.Y. Acad. Sci.* **202**, 149–154.

Finlayson, J. S. (1979a). *Sem. Thromb. Hemostas.* **6**, 1–11.

Finlayson, J. S. (1979b). *Sem. Thromb. Hemostas.* **6**, 44–74.

Francis, D. P. and Maynard, J. E. (1980). *Lancet* **1**, 1086.

Frösner, G., Willers, H., Müller, R., Schenzle, D., Deinhardt, F. and Höpken, W. (1978). *Infection* **6**, 259–260.

Frösner, G. G., Papaevangelou, G., Butler, R., Iwarson, S., Lindholm, A., Couroucé-Pauty, A., Haas, H. and Deinhardt, F. (1979). *Amer. J. Epidemiol.* **110**, 63–69.

Fudenberg, H. H. (1970). *In* "Immunoglobulins. Biologic Aspects and Clinical Uses" (E. Merler, ed.), pp. 211–220, National Academy of Sciences, Washington.

Gallagher, J. G. and Merigan, T. C. (1979). *Ann. Intern. Med.* **91**, 842–846.

Geiser, C., Bishop, Y., Myers, M., Jaffe, N. and Yankee, R. (1975). *Cancer* **35**, 1027–1030.

Gellis, S. S., McGuiness, A. C. and Peters, M. (1945a). *Amer. J. Med. Sci.* **210**, 661–664.

Gellis, S. S., Stokes, J., Jr, Brother, G. M., Hall, W. M., Gilmore, H. R., Beyer, E. and Morrissey, R. A. (1945b). *J.A.M.A.* **128**, 1062–1063.

Gerety, R. J., Tabor, E., Eyster, M. E. and Drucker, J. A. (1979). *Thromb. Haemostas.* **42**, 265.

Gerety, R. J., Smallwood, L. A. and Tabor, E. (1980). *N. Engl. J. Med.* **303**, 529.

Gershon, A. A. (1980). *Rev. Infect. Dis.* **2**, 393–407.

Gershon, A. A., Steinberg, S. and Brunell, P. A. (1974). *N. Engl. J. Med.* **290**, 243–245.

Gershon, A. A., Piomelli, S., Karpatkin, M., Smithwick, E. and Steinberg, S. (1978). *J. Clin. Microbiol.* **8**, 733–735.

Gertzen, J., Huster, R. M. and Hamory, B. H. (1979). *Missouri Med.* **76**, 525–526, 530.

Gislason, D., Hanson, L. A., Kjellman, H., Ljunggren, C. and Malmberg, R. (1978). *Vox Sang.* **34**, 143–148.

Glassy, E. F., Myhre, B. A., Nakasako, Y. and Putman, L. (1978). *Transfusion* **18**, 125–126.

Gordon, J. M., Cohen, P. and Finlayson, J. S. (1980). *Transfusion* **20**, 90–92.

Goyan, J. E. (1980). *Fed. Register* **45**, 25652–25758.

Grady, G. F., Lee, V. A., Prince, A. M., Gitnick, G. L., Fawaz, K. A., Vyas, G. N., Levitt, M. D., Senior, J. R., Galambos, J. T., Bynum, T. E., Singleton, J. W., Clowdus, B. F., Akdamar, K., Aach, R. D., Winkelman, E. I., Schiff, G. M. and Hersh, T. (1978). *J. Infect. Dis.* **138**, 625–638.

Grosbuis, S., Desormeau, J. P., Girard, O. and Goulon, M. (1975). *In* "Proceedings of the Fourth International Conference on Tetanus", pp. 383–394. Fondation Mérieux, Lyon.

Groth, K. E., McCullough, J., Marker, S. C., Howard, R. J., Simmons, R. L., Najarian, J. S. and Balfour, H. H., Jr (1978). *J.A.M.A.* **239**, 1877–1879.

Guencheva, G. and Manolova, L. (1979). *Dev. Biol. Stand.* **44**, 63–67.

Gupta, P. S., Kapoor, R., Goyal, S., Batra, V. K. and Jain, B. K. (1980). *Lancet* **2**, 439–440.

Habermann, E. (1978). *In* "Handbook of Clinical Neurology" (P. J. Vinken and G. W. Bruyn, ed.) Vol. 33, Infections of the Nervous System, pp. 491–547. North-Holland, Amsterdam.

Hafkin, B., Alls, M. E. and Baer, G. M. (1978). *Dev. Biol. Stand.* **40**, 121–127.

Hall, W. T., Madden, D. L., Mundon, F. K., Brandt, D. E. L. and Clarke, N. A. (1977). *Amer. J. Epidemiol.* **106**, 75–77.

Hammon, W. M., Coriell, L. L., Wehrle, P. F. and Stokes, J. (1953). *J.A.M.A.* **151**, 1272–1285.

Hardegree, M. C. and Cox, C. B. (1980). *In* "Immunoglobulins: Characteristics and Uses of Intravenous Preparations" (B. M. Alving and J. S. Finlayson, ed.) pp. 127–132, DHHS Publication No. (FDA)-80-9005, U.S. Government Printing Office, Washington.

Hartman, L. J. (1979). *Pathology* **11**, 385–387.

Hattwick, M. A., Rubin, R. H., Music, S., Sikes, R. K., Smith, J. S. and Gregg, M. B. (1974). *J.A.M.A.* **227**, 407–410.

Hatz, F. and Burkhardt, C. (1950). *Annales Paediatrici* **175**, 274–283.

Hayden, G. F., Herrmann, K. L., Buimovici-Klein, E., Weiss, K. E., Nieburg, P. I. and Mitchell, J. E. (1980). *J. Pediatr.* **96**, 869–872.

Healy, M. J. R. (1971). *Med. Res. Coun. Spec. Rpt Ser.* **310**, 115–123.

Heiner, D. C. and Evans, L. (1967). *J. Pediatr.* **70**, 820–827.

Henney, C. S. and Ellis, E. F. (1968). *N. Engl. J. Med.* **278**, 1144–1146.

Hill, P. G. and John, T. J. (1979). *Lancet* **2**, 300–301.

Hill, L. E. and Mollison, P. L. (1971). *Med. Res. Coun. Spec. Rpt Ser.* **310**, 124–127.

Hollinger, F. B. (1979). *Gastroenterology* **77**, 187–189.

Hoofnagle, J. H. and Waggoner, J. C. (1980). *Gastroenterology* **78**, 259–263.

Hoofnagle, J. H., Aronson, D. and Roberts, H. (1975a). *Thromb. Diath. Haemorrh.* **33**, 606–609.

Hoofnagle, J. H., Gerety, R. J. and Barker, L. F. (1975b). *Transfusion* **15**, 408–413.

Hoofnagle, J. H., Seeff, L. B., Bales, Z. B., Wright, E. C., Zimmerman, H. J. and The Veterans Administration Cooperative Study Group (1979). *Ann. Intern. Med.* **91**, 813–818.

Hoppe, H. H., Mester, T., Hennig, W. and Krebs, H. J. (1973). *Vox Sang.* **25**, 308–316.

Hosea, S. W., Brown, E. J., Hamburger, M. I. and Frank, M. M. (1981). *N. Engl. J. Med.* **304**, 245–250.

Hughes-Davies, T. H. (1979). *Med. J. Austral.* **2**, 308.

Immunization Division, Bureau of State Services (1978). *Morbid. Mortal. Wkly Rpt* **27**, 379–381.

Iwarson, S., Ahlmén, J., Eriksson, E., Hermodsson, S., Kjellman, H., Ljunggren, C. and Selander, D. (1977). *J. Infect. Dis.* **135**, 473–477.

Iwarson, S., Norkrans, G., Hermodsson, S. and Nordenfelt, E. (1979). *Scand. J. Infect. Dis.* **11**, 167–169.

Janeway, C. A. (1970). *In* "Immunoglobulins. Biologic Aspects and Clinical Uses" (E. Merler, ed.) pp. 3–14, National Academy of Sciences, Washington.

Janeway, C. A. and Rosen, F. S. (1966). *N. Engl. J. Med.* **275**, 826–831.

Johnson, F. (1970). *In* "Immunoglobulins. Biologic Aspects and Clinical Uses" (E. Merler, ed.) pp. 380–384, National Academy of Sciences, Washington.

Johnson, K. M. (1979). *Ann. Intern. Med.* **91**, 117–119.

Johnson, K. M., Webb, P. A., Lange, J. V. and Murphy, F. A. (1977). *Lancet* **1**, 569–571.

Jones, R. J., Roe, E. A. and Gupta, J. L. (1979). *Lancet* **2**, 977–982.

Jones, R. J., Roe, E. A. and Gupta, J. L. (1980). *Lancet* **2**, 1263–1265.

Judelsohn, R. G., Meyers, J. D., Ellis, R. J. and Thomas, E. K. (1974). *Pediatrics* **53**, 476–480.

Karliner, J. S. and Belaval, G. S. (1965). *J.A.M.A.* **193**, 359–362.

Kay, H. E. M. and Maycock, W. d'A. (1974). *Lancet* **2**, 298–299.

Kempe, C. H. (1960). *Pediatrics* **26**, 176–189.

Kempe, C. H. (1979). *Vox Sang.* **36**, 123.

Kempe, C. H., Berge, T. O. and England, B. (1956). *Pediatrics* **18**, 177–188.

Kempe, C. H., Bowles, C., Meiklejohn, G., Berge, T. O., St Vincent, L., Sundara Babu, B. V., Govindarajan, S., Ratnakannan, N. R., Downie, A. W. and Murthy, V. R. (1961). *Bull. Wld Hlth Org.* **25**, 41–48.

Kishimoto, S., Tomino, S., Mitsuya, H., Fujiwara, H. and Tsuda, H. (1980). *J. Immunol.* **125**, 2347–2352.

Kleinknecht, D., Courouce, A. M., Delons, S., Naret, C., Adhemar, J. P., Ciancioni, C. and Fermanian, J. (1977). *Clin. Nephrol.* **8**, 373–376,
Kleinmann, P. K. and Weksler, M. E. (1973). *J. Pediatr.* **83**, 827–829.
Kneapler, D. and Cohen, P. (1977). *Vox Sang.* **32**, 159–164.
Knodell, R. G., Conrad, M. E., Ginsberg, A. L., Bell, C. J. and Flannery, E. P. (1976). *Lancet* **1**, 557–561.
Knodell, R. G., Conrad, M. E. and Ishak, K. G. (1977). *Gastroenterology* **72**, 902–909.
Koch, F. (1963). *Dtsch Med. Wochenschr.* **88**, 282–285.
Köhler, G. and Milstein, C. (1975). *Nature* **256**, 495–497.
Koprowski, H. and Witkor, T. (1980). *In* "Monoclonal Antibodies. Hybridomas: A New Dimension in Biological Analyses" (R. H. Kennett, T. J. McKearn and K. B. Bechtol, ed.) pp. 335–351, Plenum Press, New York.
Kornhuber, B. (1979). *Vox Sang.* **37**, 121.
Kornhuber, B. (1980). *In* "Immunoglobulins: Characteristics and Uses of Intravenous Preparations" (B. M. Alving and J. S. Finlayson, ed.) pp. 107–110, DHHS Publication No. (FDA)-80-9005, U.S. Government Printing Office, Washington.
Krugman, S. (1976). *J. Infect. Dis.* **134**, 70–74.
Krugman, S. (1979). *Gastroenterology* **77**, 187.
Krugman, S. and Giles, J. P. (1970). *J.A.M.A.* **212**, 1019–1029.
Krugman, S. and Giles, J. P. (1973). *N. Engl. J. Med.* **288**, 755–760.
Krugman, S., Giles, J. P. and Hammond, J. (1971). *J.A.M.A.* **218**, 1665–1670.
Kryzhanovsky, G. N. (1973). *Naunyn-Schmiedebergs Arch. Pharmacol.* **276**, 247–270.
Kuwert, E. K., Werner, J., Marcus, I. and Cabasso, V. J. (1978). *J. Biol. Stand.* **6**, 211–219.
Lane, R. S., Rankin, A. and Kay, H. E. M. (1980). *Lancet* **1**, 705–706.
Lang, G. E. and Veldhuis, B. (1973). *Amer. J. Clin. Pathol.* **60**, 205–207.
Levine, L., McComb, J. A., Dwyer, R. C. and Latham, W. C. (1966). *N. Engl. J. Med.* **274**, 186–190.
Lewis, G. E., Jr and Metzger, J. F. (1978). *Lancet* **2**, 634–635.
Lowbury, E. J. L., Kidson, A., Lilly, H. A., Wilkins, M. D. and Jackson, D. M. (1978). *J. Hygiene* **80**, 267–274.
Luiken, G. A. (1979). *Vox Sang.* **37**, 121–123.
McComb, J. A. and Dwyer, R. C. (1963). *N. Engl. J. Med.* **268**, 857–862.
McCracken, G. H., Jr, Dowell, D. L. and Marshall, F. N. (1971). *Lancet* **1**, 1146–1149.
McKhann, C. F. and Chu, F. T. (1933). *J. Infect. Dis.* **52**, 268–277.
McKhann, C. F., Green, A. A. and Coady, H. (1935). *J. Pediatr.* **6**, 603–614.
Magilavy, D. B., Cassidy, J. T., Tubergen, D. G., Petty, R. E., Chisholm, R. and McCall, K. (1978). *J. Allergy Clin. Immunol.* **61**, 378–383.
Maiztegui, J. I., Fernandez, N. J. and de Damilano, A. J. (1979). *Lancet* **2**, 1216–1217.
Makula, M.-F. and Plan, R. (1979). *Dev. Biol. Stand.* **44**, 75–81.
Masuho, Y., Tomibe, K., Matsuzawa, K. and Ohtsu, A. (1977). *Vox Sang.* **32**, 175–181.
Maynard, J. E. (1979). *Gastroenterology* **77**, 190–191.
Medical Research Council and Public Health Laboratory Service (1980). *Lancet* **1**, 6–8.
Meiklejohn, G. (1978). *Adv. Intern. Med.* **23**, 385–404.
Merchant, B. (1980). *In* "Immunoglobulins: Characteristics and Uses of Intravenous Preparations" (B. M. Alving and J. S. Finlayson, ed.) pp. 123–126, DHHS Publication No. (FDA)-80-9005, U.S. Government Printing Office, Washington.
Metzger, J. F. and Lewis, G. E., Jr (1979). *Rev. Infect. Dis.* **1**, 689–692.
Milstein, C. (1980). *Sci. Amer.* **243 (4)**, 66–74.

Mondorf, A. W. and Duswald, K. H. (1980). *In* "Immunoglobulins: Characteristics and Uses of Intravenous Preparations" (B. M. Alving and J. S. Finlayson, ed.) pp. 37–40, DHHS Publication No. (FDA)-80-9005, U.S. Government Printing Office, Washington.

Morell, A., Schürch, B., Ryser, D., Hofer, F., Skvaril, F. and Barandun, S. (1980). *Vox Sang.* **38**, 272–283.

Morris, D. and McDonald, J. C. (1957). *Arch. Dis. Childh.* **32**, 236–239.

Mosley, J. W. (1979a). *Gastroenterology* **77**, 189–190.

Mosley, J. W. (1979b). *Ann. Intern. Med.* **91**, 914–916.

Mozen, M. M., Schroeder, D. D. and Cabasso, V. J. (1980). *Arzneim.-Forsch.* **30(II)**, 1484–1486.

Nanning, W. (1962). *Bull Wld Hlth Org.* **27**, 312–324.

Nation, N. S., Pierce, N. F., Adler, S. J., Chinnock, R. F. and Wehrle, P. F. (1963). *California Med.* **98**, 305–307.

Neff, J. M. (1979). *Vox Sang.* **36**, 123–125.

Netter, R. (1979). *Vox Sang.* **36**, 125–126.

News Item (1980). *Lancet* **1**, 107.

Nicholson, K. G. and Turner, G. S. (1978). *Dev. Biol. Stand.* **40**, 115–120.

Nolte, M. T., Pirofsky, B., Gerritz, G. A. and Golding, B. (1979). *Clin. Exp. Immunol.* **36**, 237–243.

Nydegger, U. E. (ed.) (1981). "Immunohemotherapy. A Guide to Immunoglobulin Prophylaxis and Therapy." Academic Press, London and New York.

Oberst, F. W., Crook, J. W., Cresthall, P. and House, M. J. (1968). *Clin. Pharmacol. Ther.* **9**, 209–214.

Ochs, H. D. (1979). *Vox Sang.* **37**, 123–126.

Ochs, H. (1980). *In* "Immunoglobulins: Characteristics and Uses of Intravenous Preparations" (B. M. Alving and J. S. Finlayson, ed.) pp. 9–14, DHHS Publication No. (FDA)-80-9005, U.S. Government Printing Office, Washington.

Ochs, H. D., Buckley, R. H., Pirofsky, B., Fischer, S. H., Rousell, R. H., Anderson, C. J. and Wedgwood, R. J. (1980a). *Lancet* **2**, 1158–1159.

Ochs, H., Witherspoon, R. P., Storb, R. and Wedgwood, R. J. (1980b). *In* "Immunoglobulins: Characteristics and Uses of Intravenous Preparations" (B. M. Alving and J. S. Finlayson, ed.) pp. 99–106, DHHS Publication No. (FDA)-80-9005, U.S. Government Printing Office, Washington.

Olsson, L. and Kaplan, H. S. (1980). *Proc. Natl Acad. Sci. USA* **77**, 5429–5431.

Oncley, J. L., Melin, M., Richert, D. A., Cameron, J. W. and Gross, P. M., Jr (1949). *J. Amer. Chem. Soc.* **71**, 541–550.

Ordmann, C. W., Jennings, C. G., Jr and Janeway, C. A. (1944). *J. Clin. Invest.* **23**, 541–549.

Painter, R. H. and Minta, J. O. (1969). *Vox Sang.* **17**, 434–444.

Painter, R. H., Walcroft, M. J. and Weber, J. C. W. (1966). *Can. J. Biochem.* **44**, 381–387.

Painter, R. H., Weber, J. C. W. and Wardlaw, A. C. (1968). *Clin. Exp. Immunol.* **3**, 179–187.

Passwell, J., Rosen, F. S. and Merler, E. (1980). *In* "Immunoglobulins: Characteristics and Uses of Intravenous Preparations" (B. M. Alving and J. S. Finlayson, ed.) pp. 139–142, DHHS Publication No. (FDA)-80-9005, U.S. Government Printing Office, Washington.

Pirofsky, B. (1979). *Vox Sang.* **37**, 126–128.

Place, E. H., Keller, M. J. and Shaw, E. W. (1949). *J. Pediatr.* **34**, 699–710.

Plotkin, S. A. and Witkor, T. (1979). *Pediatrics* **63**, 219–221.

Polin, R. A. (1980). *In* "Monoclonal Antibodies. Hybridomas: A New Dimension in Biological Analyses" (R. H. Kennett, T. J. McKearn and K. B. Bechtol, ed.) pp. 353–359, Plenum Press, New York.

Pollack, M. (1980). *In* "Immunoglobulins: Characteristics and Uses of Intravenous Preparations" (B. M. Alving and J. S. Finlayson, ed.) pp. 73–79, DHHS Publication No. (FDA)-80-9005, U.S. Government Printing Office, Washington.

Pollack, M. and Young, L. S. (1979). *J. Clin. Invest.* **63**, 276–286.

Pollock, T. M. and Reid, D. (1969). *Lancet* **1**, 281–283.

Preblud, S. R., Zaia, J. A., Nieberg, P. I., Hinman, A. R. and Levin, M. J. (1979). *J. Pediatr.* **95**, 334–335.

Prince, A. M. (1978). *N. Engl. J. Med.* **299**, 198–199.

Prince, A. M., Szmuness, W., Mann, M. K., Vyas, G. N., Grady, G. F., Shapiro, F. L., Suki, W. N., Freidman, E. A., Avram, M. M. and Stenzel, K. H. (1978). *J. Infect. Dis.* **137**, 131–144.

Public Health Service Advisory Committee on Immunization Practices (1977a). *Morbid. Mortal. Wkly Rpt* **26**, 393–394.

Public Health Service Advisory Committee on Immunization Practices (1977b). *Morbid. Mortal. Wkly Rpt* **26**, 401–402, 407.

Public Health Service Advisory Committee on Immunization Practices (1977c). *Morbid Mortal. Wkly Rpt* **26**, 425–428, 441–442.

Public Health Services Advisory Committee on Immunization Practices (1978). *Morbid. Mortal. Wkly Rpt* **27**, 427–437.

Redeker, A. G., Mosley, J. W., Gocke, D. J., McKee, A. P. and Pollack, W. (1975). *N. Engl. J. Med.* **293**, 1055–1059.

Reed, D., Brown, G., Merrick, R., Sever, J. and Feltz, E. (1967). *J.A.M.A.* **199**, 967–971.

Reesink, H. W., Reerink-Brongers, E. E., Lafeber-Schut, B. J. T., Kalshoven-Benschop, J. and Brummelhuis, H. G. J. (1979). *Lancet* **2**, 436–438.

Richerson, H. B. and Seebohm, P. M. (1966). *Arch. Intern. Med.* **117**, 568–572.

Ring, J. and Duswald, K. H. (1980). *Klin. Wochenschr.* **58**, 797–809.

Rosen, F. S. (1970). *In* "Immunoglobulins. Biologic Aspects and Clinical Uses" (E. Merler, ed.) p. 183, National Academy of Sciences, Washington.

Ross, A. H. (1962). *N. Engl. J. Med.* **267**, 369–376.

Rubbo, S. D. (1966). *Lancet* **2**, 449–453.

Sadoff, J. C., Sidberry, H., Schilhab, J., Hirshfeld, D. and Cross, A. (1980). *In* "Immunoglobulins: Characteristics and Uses of Intravenous Preparations" (B. M. Alving and J. S. Finlayson, ed.) pp. 63–71, DHHS Publication No. (FDA)-80-9005, U.S. Government Printing Office, Washington.

Sandberg, H. E., ed. (1978). "Proceedings of the International Workshop on Technology for Protein Separation and Improvement of Blood Plasma Fractionation". DHEW Publication No. (NIH) 78-1422, U.S. Government Printing Office, Washington.

Scheiermann, N. and Kuwert, E. K. (1980). *Fortschr. Med.* **98**, 39–45.

Schiff, G. M. (1969). *Amer. J. Dis. Child.* **118**, 322–327.

Schiff, P. (1979). *Med. J. Austral.* **2**, 604.

Schless, A. P. and Harell, G. S. (1968). *Amer. J. Med.* **44**, 325–329.

Schultze, H. E. and Schwick, G. (1962). *Dtsch Med. Wochenschr.* **87**, 1643–1650.

Sedaghatian, M. R. (1979). *Arch. Dis. Childh.* **54**, 623–625.

Seeff, L. B. and Hoofnagle, J. H. (1979). *Gastroenterology* **77**, 161–182.

Seeff, L. B., Zimmerman, H. J., Wright, E. C., Finkelstein, J. D., Garcia-Pont, P., Greenlee, H. B., Dietz, A. A., Leevy, C. M., Tamburro, C. H., Schiff, E. R.,

Schimmel, E. M., Zemel, R., Zimmon, D. S. and McCollum, R. W. (1977). *Gastroenterology* **72**, 111–121.

Seeff, L. B., Wright, E. C., Zimmerman, H. J., Alter, H. J., Dietz, A. A., Felsher, B. F., Finkelstein, J. D., Garcia-Pont, P., Gerin, J. L., Greenlee, H. B., Hamilton, J., Holland, P. V., Kaplan, P. M., Kiernan, T., Koff, R. S., Leevy, C. M., McAuliffe, V. J., Nath, N., Purcell, R. H., Schiff, E. R., Schwartz, C. C., Tamburro, C. H., Vlahcevic, Z., Zemel, R. and Zimmon, D. S. (1978). *Ann. Intern. Med.* **88**, 285–293.

Selimov, M. A., Klyueva, E. V., Aksenova, T. A., Lebedeva, I. R. and Gribencha, L. F. (1978). *Dev. Biol. Stand.* **40**, 141–146.

Sgouris, J. T. (1967). *Vox Sang.* **13**, 71–84.

Sgouris, J. T., Volk, V. K., Angela, F., Portwood, L. and Gottshall, R. Y. (1969). *Vox Sang.* **16**, 491–495.

Siber, G. R. (1980). *Amer. J. Dis. Child.* **134**, 668–672.

Siber, G. R., Weitzman, S. A., Aisenberg, A. C., Weinstein, H. J. and Schiffman, G. (1978). *N. Engl. J. Med.* **299**, 442–448.

Singh, A. K., Bansal, A., Goel, S. P. and Agarwal, V. K. (1980). *Arch. Dis. Childh.* **55**, 527–531.

Skvaril, F. (1960a). *Nature* **185**, 475–476.

Skvaril, F. (1960b). *Folia Microbiol.* **5**, 264–271.

Smallwood, L. A., Tabor, E., Finlayson, J. S. and Gerety, R. J. (1980). *Lancet* **2**, 482–483.

Smallwood, L. A., Tabor, E., Finlayson, J. S. and Gerety, R. J. (1981). *J. Med. Virol.* **7**, 21–27.

Smith, G. N., Griffiths, B., Mollison, D. and Mollison, P. L. (1972). *Lancet* **1**, 1208–1212.

Smith, T. W., Haber, E., Yeatman, L. and Butler, V. P., Jr (1976). *N. Engl. J. Med.* **294**, 797–800.

Solmonova, K. and Vizev, S. (1973). *Z. Immunitätsforsch.* **146**, 81–90.

Soothill, J. F. (1971). *Med. Res. Coun. Spec. Rpt Ser.* **310**, 106–114.

Spiegelberg, H. L. (1970). *In* "Plasma Protein Metabolism. Regulation of Synthesis, Distribution, and Degradation" (M. A. Rothschild and T. Waldmann, ed.) pp. 307–319, Academic Press, New York and London.

Stephan, W. (1975). *Vox Sang.* **28**, 422–437.

Stiehm, E. R. (1979). *Pediatrics* **63**, 301–319.

Stiehm, E. R. (1980). *In* "Immunoglobulins: Characteristics and Uses of Intravenous Preparations" (B. M. Alving and J. S. Finlayson, ed.) pp. 232, DHHS Publication No. (FDA)-80-9005, U.S. Government Printing Office, Washington.

Stiehm, E. R. and Kobayashi, R. H. (1980). *In* "Immunoglobulins: Characteristics and Uses of Intravenous Preparations" (B. M. Alving and J. S. Finlayson, ed.) pp. 89–98, DHHS Publication No. (FDA)-80-9005, U.S. Government Printing Office, Washington.

Stokes, J. and Neefe, J. R. (1945). *J.A.M.A.* **127**, 531–540.

Stokes, J., Jr, Maris, E. P. and Gellis, S. S. (1944). *J. Clin. Invest.* **23**, 531–540.

Stollerman, G. H. (1978). *Adv. Intern. Med.* **23**, 405–434.

Sudre, Y., Becq-Giraudon, B. and Boutaud, P. (1975). *Sem. Hop. Paris* **51**, 807–810.

Sussman, S. and Grossman, M. (1965). *J. Pediatr.* **67**, 1168–1173.

Szmuness, W., Stevens, C. E., Harley, E. J., Zang, E. A., Oleszko, W. R., William, D. C., Sadovsky, R., Morrison, J. M. and Kellner, A. (1980). *N. Engl. J. Med.* **303**, 833–841.

Tabor, E. and Gerety, R. J. (1979a). *Lancet* **2**, 1293.

Tabor, E. and Gerety, R. J. (1979b). *Transfusion* **19**, 669–674.

Tabor, E. and Gerety, R. J. (1979c). *J. Pediatr.* **95**, 647–650.
Tabor, E., Aronson, D. L. and Gerety, R. J. (1980a). *Lancet* **2**, 68–70.
Tabor, E., Seeff, L. B. and Gerety, R. J. (1980b). *N. Engl. J. Med.* **303**, 139–143.
Tankersley, D. L., Alving, B. M., Yi, M., Blou, M. G., Mason, B. L. and Finlayson, J. S. (1980). *In* "Immunoglobulins: Characteristics and Uses of Intravenous Preparations" (B. M. Alving and J. S. Finlayson, ed.) pp. 173–178, DHHS Publication NO. (FDA)-80-9005, U.S. Government Printing Office, Washington.
Taylor, H. L., Bloom, F. C., McCall, K. B., Hyndman, L. A. and Anderson, H. D. (1956). *J. Amer. Chem. Soc.* **78**, 1356–1358.
Tong, M. J., McPeak, C. M., Thursby, M. W., Schweitzer, I. L., Henneman, C. E. and Ledger, W. J. (1979). *Gastroenterology* **76**, 535–539.
Turner, K. J., Bartholomaeus, W. N., Tribe, A. and Hobday, J. D. (1971). *Aust. N.Z. J. Med.* **1**, 76–82.
Urquhart, G. E. D., Crawford, R. J. and Wallace, J. (1978). *Br. Med. J.* **2**, 1331–1332.
Vakil, B. J., Armitage, P., Clifford, R. E. and Laurence, D. R. (1979). *Trans. Roy. Soc. Trop. Med. Hyg.* **73**, 579–583.
Vic Dupont, V., Vachon, F., Gaudebout, C., Manuel, C., Tremolieres, F. and Gibert, C. (1975). *In* "Proceedings of the Fourth International Conference on Tetanus", pp. 401–408. Fondation Mérieux, Lyon.
Vogel, L. C., Kretschmer, R. R., Padnos, D. M., Kelly, P. D. and Gotoff, S. P. (1980). *Pediatr. Res.* **14**, 788–792.
Vogelaar, E. F., d. Boer-v. d. Berg, M. A. G., Brummelhuis, H. G. J., Beentjes, S. P. and Krijnen, H. W. (1974). *Vox Sang.* **27**, 193–206.
Wadsworth, C. (1976). *Vox Sang.* **31**, 394–396.
Waldmann, T. A. and Strober, W. (1969). *Progr. Allergy* **13**, 1–110.
Walsh, J. J. (1974). *Dev. Biol. Stand.* **27**, 31–36.
Wehrle, P. F. (1979). *Vox Sang.* **36**, 128.
Weibel, R. E., Buynak, E. B., McLean, A. A., Roehm, R. R. and Hilleman, M. R. (1980). *Proc. Soc. Exp. Biol. Med.* **165**, 260–263.
Weiland, O., Berg, J. V. R., Bäck, E. and Lundbergh, P. (1979). *Infection* **7**, 223–225.
Welch, A. G., McClelland, D. B. L. and Watt, J. G. (1980). *In* "Immunoglobulins: Characteristics and Uses of Intravenous Preparations" (B. M. Alving and J. S. Finlayson, ed.) pp. 195–200, DHHS Publication No. (FDA)-80-9005, U.S. Government Printing Office, Washington.
WHO Expert Committee on Viral Hepatitis (1977). *Wld Hlth Org. Tech. Rpt Ser.* **602**, 1–62.
Winsnes, R. (1978). *Acta Paediatr. Scand.* **67**, 77–82.
Winsnes, R., Frøland, S. S. and Degré, M. I. (1978). *Scand. J. Infect. Dis.* **10**, 21–27.
Young, A. M., Aronson, D. L. and Finlayson, J. S. (1978). *J. Biol. Stand.* **6**, 27–43.
Zaia, J. A., Levin, M. J., Wright, G. G. and Grady, G. F. (1978). *J. Infect. Dis.* **137**, 601–604.
Zaia, J. A., Levin, M. J., Leszczynski, J., Wright, G. G. and Grady, G. F. (1979). *Transplantation* **27**, 66–67.
Zaia, J. A., Levin, M. J. and Preblud, S. R. (1980). *In* "Immunoglobulins: Characteristics and Uses of Intravenous Preparations" (B. M. Alving and J. S. Finlayson, ed.) pp. 111–121, DHHS Publication No. (FDA)-80-9005, U.S. Government Printing Office, Washington.
Ziegler, E. J. and Braude, A. I. (1980). *In* "Immunoglobulins: Characteristics and Uses of Intravenous Preparations" (B. M. Alving and J. S. Finlayson, ed.) pp. 55–62, DHHS Publication No. (FDA)-80-9005, U.S. Government Printing Office, Washington.

5 Immunological, immunochemical and structural studies of the types III and Ia group B streptococcal polysaccharides

DENNIS L. KASPER
and HAROLD J. JENNINGS

It will not be the purpose of this chapter to review clinical or epidemiological aspects of group B streptococcal (GBS) infections of humans or animals: these topics have recently been amply reviewed by Baker (1980). Rather, we shall emphasize the immunological and chemical aspects of the type-specific polysaccharides of these bacteria with special emphasis on our work with the types III and Ia antigens. These are capsular antigens which are responsible for serotype specificity; they comprise the major surface immunological determinants, appear to be responsible to a significant degree for group B streptococcal virulence, and offer potential for use as vaccines to prevent group B streptococcal infection.

Beta haemolytic streptococci belonging to group B were recognized as a distinct species called *Streptococcus agalactiae* prior to Lancefield's description of a common determinant ("C" substance) and the subsequent serological classification based on this determinant (Lancefield, 1933; Lancefield, 1934; Lancefield, 1938). These organisms have a somewhat distinctive colonial morphology and characteristically produce a narrow zone of beta haemolysis. A double zone of haemolysis has been reported to appear after the incubation of haemolytic colonies in a refrigerator for 12–16 hours (Brown, 1920; Brown, 1937). Unfortunately, for those of us wanting to simplify methods of classification, these characteristics are not unique to group B organisms. In particular, they can be morphologically confused with serogroups D, C and G streptococci. Also, not all group B strains are beta haemolytic, particularly those which are isolated from non-human sources which tend to be primarily alpha haemolytic. Regardless of haemolysis pattern, several useful biochemical characteristics serve to distinguish group B strains from other serogroups (Pollack and Dahlgren, 1974; Facklam et al., 1974; Christie et al., 1944; Wilkinson, 1977). Over 90% of strains are Bacitracin-resistant, over 99% of strains hydrolyse sodium hippurate, and over 98% of strains produce synergistic haemolysis with the beta lysin of *Staphylococcus aureus* (Camp factor). Despite all the morphological and biochemical tests that are routinely used to identify group B streptococci, it must be remembered that this is an antigenic classification based on the presence of a common immunodeterminant, the group B antigen ("C" substance), which is present in all strains. Definitive identification requires serological grouping of isolates with antiserum containing antibodies to the group B determinant. Lancefield's method of classification uses capillary immunoprecipitation between reference-group-specific antisera and pH neutralized supernatants of organisms boiled in 0.2 N HCl for 10 min. More recently, several other methods of identifying group B strains have been developed. These include counterimmunoelectrophoresis, immunofluorescence and staphylococcal coagglutination (Hill et al., 1975; Fenton and Harper, 1978; Romero and Wilkinson, 1974; Mason et al., 1976; Edwards and Larson, 1974; Rosner, 1972; Szilagyi et al., 1978).

Group B streptococci can be divided into 5 distinct serotypes based on the presence of type specific antigens which are immunologically distinct from the common group determinant (Table 1). Types Ia, Ib, II and III strains all have distinct carbohydrate determinants. Type Ic strains have the type Ia carbohydrate determinant and also another determinant thought to be a protein which it shares with type Ib strains, the Ibc protein (Wilkinson and Eagon, 1971). Strains designated type I were shown to share an additional common determinant, the Iabc minor carbohydrate (Lancefield et al., 1975). Less than 1% of strains isolated from human sources are not typable with this scheme which used capillary immunoprecipitation between neutralized acid extracts and type-specific antisera.

The scope of this review will be (1) to define the morphological location of these type-specific antigens; (2) to review the basis for the definition of the chemical structures of the types Ia–Ic and III polysaccharide antigens and the interrelation of chemistry and immunospecificity; (3) to define the role specific antibodies to type III antigens play in human disease; and (4) to discuss how type III organisms interact with the complement system.

Table 1 Major antigens of group B *Streptococcus*[a]

Serotype	Ia cHo[b]	Ib cHo	Ibc protein[c]	Iabc cHo	II cHo	III cHo	B cHo
Ia	+	−	−	+	−	−	+
Ib	−	+	+	+	−	−	+
Ic	+	−	+	+	−	−	+
II	−	−	±	−	+	−	+
III	−	−	−	−	−	+	+

[a] All antigens listed except the group B carbohydrate are related to protective antibodies in mouse models.
[b] cHo=carbohydrate.
[c] Some group B strains also contain streptococcal T and R proteins.

I. MORPHOLOGICAL LOCATION OF THE TYPE-SPECIFIC ANTIGEN

Electronmicrographs using ferritin-conjugated type-specific antibodies demonstrated that the location of the type-specific antigens was the surface of the GBS organism (Kasper and Baker, 1979). Type Ia strain 090 has large quantities of capsule on its surface (Ia carbohydrate) (Fig. 1). In contrast to the type Ia organism, the prototype Ib strain (H36B) had variable but smaller quantities of capsule (Ib carbohydrate) seen when stained with homologous ferritin-conjugated antibodies (Fig. 2). Type Ib cells exposed to ferritin-conjugated Ic typing serum which contained precipitating antibodies to the Ibc protein antigen also had ferritin-conjugated antibodies clustering on the outside of the cell (Fig. 3), indicating that the Ibc protein also had a surface location on the Ib cell. Ferritin-conjugated Ic typing sera localized on the surface at the outer lamina of type Ic cells (Fig. 4), indicating the surface location of the Ibc protein on this serotype as well. A small polysaccharide capsule was found on type Ic cells (Fig. 5) exposed to ferritin-conjugated type Ia antibodies, a finding that confirms the sharing of the Ia polysaccharide antigen by this serotype. Therefore, both the Ibc protein and the Ia polysaccharide antigens appear to have surface locations on type Ic cells. A large capsule was found when type II (Fig. 6) and type III (Fig. 7) cells were

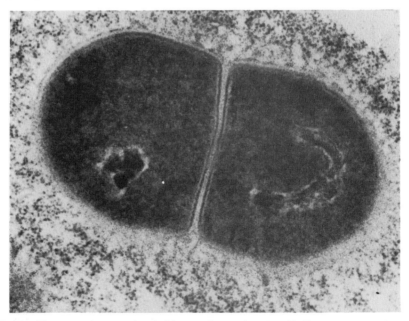

Fig. 1 Electronmicrograph of thin sections of group B *Streptococcus* type Ia (strain 090) stained with ferritin-conjugated type Ia antibodies. (Courtesy of Kasper and Baker, 1979.)

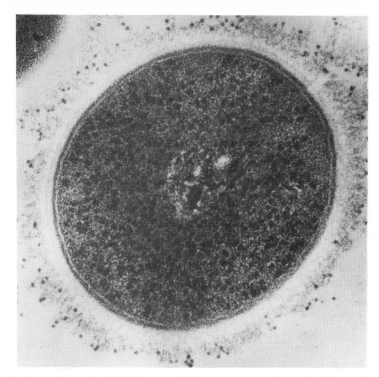

Fig. 2   Type Ib (strain H36B) group B *Streptococcus* shows ferritin-conjugated type Ib antibodies adhering to a capsular structure. (Courtesy of Kasper and Baker, 1979.)

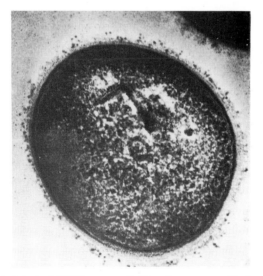

Fig. 3   Type Ib (strain H36B) group B *Streptococcus* with ferritin-conjugated antibodies to the Ibc protein adhering to the surface. (Courtesy of Kasper and Baker, 1979.)

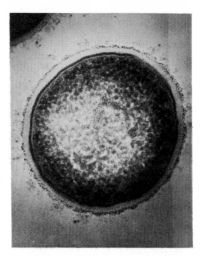

Fig. 4 Type Ic (strain A909) group B *Streptococcus* showing attachment of ferritin-conjugated type Ic antibodies at the outer lamina, indicative of the location of the Ibc protein antigen. (Courtesy of Kasper and Baker, 1979.)

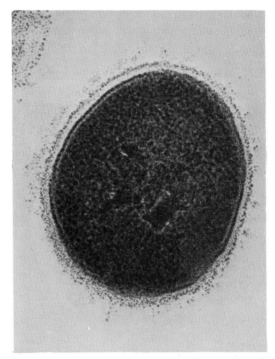

Fig. 5 Type Ic (strain A909) group B *Streptococcus* showing reaction with ferritin-conjugated type Ia serum, indicative of the location of the shared type Ia polysaccharide. (Courtesy of Kasper and Baker, 1979.)

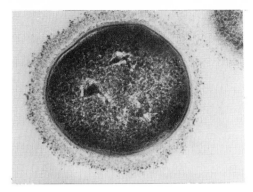

Fig. 6 Type II (strain 18RS21) group B *Streptococcus* shows reaction with ferritin-conjugated type II serum. (Courtesy of Kasper and Baker, 1979.)

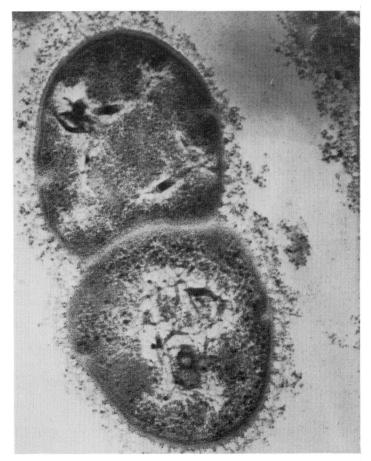

Fig. 7 Type III (strain M732) group B *Streptococcus* demonstrating a large concentration of ferritin particles outside the outer lamina when stained with ferritin-conjugated type III antibodies. (Courtesy of Kasper and Baker, 1979.)

exposed to homologous ferritin-labelled antibodies, confirming the capsular location of the type-specific antigens. Various control experiments with type III organisms treated with either ferritin-conjugated normal rabbit serum, unconjugated type III antiserum, or untreated type III cells revealed no non-specific binding of ferritin conjugated immunoglobulin. These morphological investigations of group B streptococci established the surface location of the type-specific polysaccharide antigens on each serotype strain and the Ibc protein antigen on types Ib and Ic strains.

II. STRUCTURAL ELUCIDATION OF THE TYPE-SPECIFIC POLYSACCHARIDE ANTIGENS OF GROUP B STREPTOCOCCI

The acid-extracted type-specific antigens (types Ia, Ib, Ic, II and III) of group B streptococci (Lancefield, 1933; Lancefield, 1934; Lancefield, 1938; Wilkinson and Eagon, 1971) all contain galactose, glucose and 2-acetamido-2-deoxy-glucose as exclusive components (Lancefield and Freimer, 1966; Wilkinson, 1975; Russel and Norcross, 1972; Kane and Karakawa, 1978; Tai et al., 1979; Kasper et al., 1979; Jennings et al., 1980a; Jennings et al., 1980b). For the type Ia (Jennings et al., 1980b) and type III (Jennings et al., 1980a) antigens, it has been demonstrated that all of these component sugars are present in the D-form. Galactose, glucose and 2-acetamido-2-deoxy-glucose occur in the molar ratio of 2:1:1, respectively, in the type Ia (Jennings et al., 1980b), type Ib (Tai et al., 1979), type Ic and type III (Jennings et al., 1980a) antigens; thus these antigens constitute a group of isomeric polysaccharides. The acid-extracted antigens are immunologically incomplete and form a lower molecular weight core to the native antigens which all contain additional terminal acid-labile sialic acid residues (Lancefield and Freimer, 1966; Wilkinson, 1975; Freimer, 1967; Baker and Kasper, 1976b; Kane and Karakawa, 1977; Kasper et al., 1978). The native type Ia (Jennings et al., 1980b), type Ib (Tai et al., 1979), type Ic and type III (Jennings et al., 1980a) polysaccharide antigens have also been shown to be an isomeric group of polysaccharides as they all contained galactose, glucose, 2-acetamido-2-deoxy-glucose and sialic acid in the molar ratio of 2:1:1:1, respectively. The complete structures of the types Ia–Ic and III antigens are discussed below.

The structure of the type III native antigen was determined by first elucidating the structure of the more simple incomplete core antigen obtained by either the direct acid (hot 1M HCl) extraction of the whole organism (Lancefield, 1934; Lancefield, 1938) or by the selective hydrolysis of the terminal sialic acid residues from the native type III antigen using milder conditions (Jennings et al., 1980a). The structure of the type III incomplete antigen (Jennings et al., 1980a) is shown in Fig. 8 and proved to be identical to

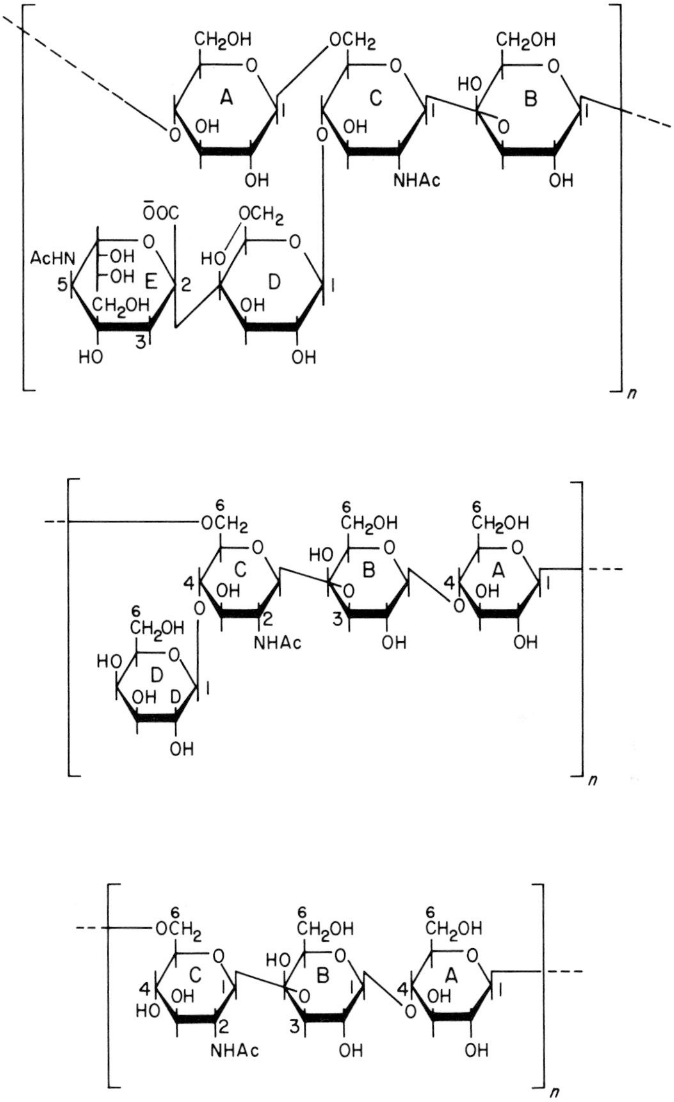

Fig. 8 The structures of the repeating units of the native (*upper*), core (*middle*), and backbone (*lower*) antigens from type III group B *Streptococcus*.

the structure proposed for the capsular polysaccharide of type 14 *S. pneumoniae* (Lindberg *et al.*, 1977). By methylation of the type III incomplete antigen, the individual specifically methylated component sugars were identified and quantified by gas chromomatographic–mass spectrographic (GC–MS) analysis and they are listed in Table 2. These components were consistent with the type III incomplete antigen having the above structure (Fig. 8), although sequence and linkage configuration data were still required. The sequence was determined using two degradation procedures (Jennings *et al.*, 1980a). The first involved a modified Smith degradation in which the polyalcohol obtained was permethylated and the product was partially hydrolysed. This yielded a partially methylated trisaccharide moiety having newly formed hydroxyl groups at the linkage position of its terminal residues which were then specifically labelled by methylation with trideuteriomethyl iodide. The resultant labelled trisaccharide is shown in Fig. 9 together with some of the major fragments formed when it was subjected to GC–MS analysis. The sequence of the individual methylated sugars in the trisaccharide could be determined from the larger fragments obtained in this analysis. This sequence represents the sequence of the original glucose components A, B and C of the incomplete type III antigen (Fig. 8); the erythritol residue of the methylated trisaccharide originating from the oxidized backbone glucopyranose residue (A). Because the 2-acetamido-2-deoxy-glucose residue (C) is a branch point in the incomplete type III antigen, a further degradation was required to elucidate its point of attachment to the terminal galactopyranose residue (D). This was achieved by the oxidation of this latter residue to β-D-galactopyranosyluronic acid residues and subjecting the modified polysaccharide to a uronic acid degradation (Jennings *et al.*, 1980a). This degradation involved the methylation of the modified polysaccharide, removal of the methylated galactopyranosyluronic acid residues, and remethylation of the polymeric material with trideuteriomethyl iodide. The identification by GC–MS analysis of 2-deoxy-3-*0*-methyl-4-*0*-trideuterio-methyl-2-(*N*-methyl-acetamino)-D-glucose in the hydrolysis products of the above polymer demonstrated unambiguously that the terminal β-D-galactopyranose residues (D) of the incomplete type III antigen were linked to *0*-4 of the backbone 2-acetamido-2-deoxy-glucopyranose residues (C). That all the sugar components were in the β-D-configuration was ascertained from the ^{13}C NMR spectrum of the incomplete type III antigen (see Fig. 13) which exhibited only one narrow signal in the anomeric region of the spectrum due to the coincidence of the anomeric signals of all the individual sugar residues. From previous studies on model compounds the low field chemical shift (104.2 p.p.m.) of this signal is only consistent with the β-D-configuration of all these residues (Jennings *et al.*, 1980a).

Table 2 Methylation analysis of the native and incomplete core type 1a and type III streptococcal polysaccharides

Methylated glucose derivatives	Molar ratios			
	Type III incomplete core polysaccharide	Type III native polysaccharide	Type 1a incomplete core polysaccharide	Type 1a native polysaccharide
2,3,4,6-Tetra-O-methyl-D-galactose	0.9	–	0.8	–
2,4,6-Tri-O-methyl-D-galactose	1.0	0.9	–	0.8
2,3,6-Tri-O-methyl-D-glucose	0.9	1.0	1.0	1.0
2,3,4-Tri-O-methyl-D-galactose	–[a]	0.9	–	–
2,6-Di-O-methyl-D-galactose	–	–	0.9	0.9
3,6-Di-O-methyl-N-methyl-N-acetyl-D-glucosamine	–	–	+	+
3-Mono-O-methyl-N-methyl-N-acetyl-D-glucosamine	+[b]	+	–	–
4,7,8,9-Tetra-O-methyl-N-methyl-N-acetyl-D-neuraminic acid	–	+	–	+

[a] Not detected.
[b] Nonquantitative response.

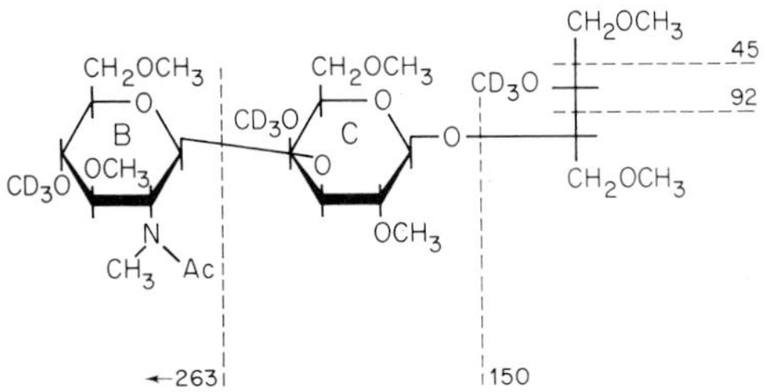

Fig. 9   Methylated oligosaccharide degradation product obtained from the incomplete type III streptococcal antigen.

The structure of the repeating unit of the native type III antigen (Jennings *et al.*, 1980a) is shown in Fig. 8. The structure was clearly established by differences in the individual methylated sugars yielded by the hydrolysis of its permethylated product as compared to those yielded on hydrolysis of the permethylated core antigen (Table 2). The detection of only 2,3,4-tri-*0*-methyl galactose in the former as compared to only 2,3,4,6-tetra-*0*-methyl galactose in the latter established that the sialic acid residues of the native type III antigen were linked to *0*-6 of all the terminal β-D-galactopyranose residues of the core antigen. In addition the detection of only the fully methylated derivative of sialic acid established that all these sialic acid residues were terminally located. The α-D-configuration of these sialic acid residues could be determined by the characteristic chemical shift (Jennings and Bhattacharjee, 1977) of their carboxylate carbons in the ^{13}C NMR spectrum of the native type III antigen.

The structure of the native type Ia antigen (Jennings *et al.*, 1980b) was determined using similar procedures to those previously described for the native type III antigen. Hydrolysis of the more simple methylated type Ia core antigen yielded individual specifically methylated component sugars which were identified and quantified by GC–MS analysis and are listed in Table 2. These methylated components were consistent with the alternative repeating unit structures shown in Figs 10a and b. The sequence of the individual sugar residues was determined by the methylation and partial hydrolysis of the periodate oxidized type Ia core antigen, as in the case of the type III core antigen. The resultant partially methylated trisaccharide derivative was then further methylated with trideuteriomethyl iodide to label the hydroxyl groups exposed in the breaking of the linkages to this trisaccharide. The trisaccharide is shown in Fig. 11, together with some of the major fragments formed when it was subjected to GC–MS analysis. These masses were only consistent with the sequence of sugars BCA as depicted, the erythritol residue being derived from the original glucopyranose residue (A) of the linear portion of the type Ia

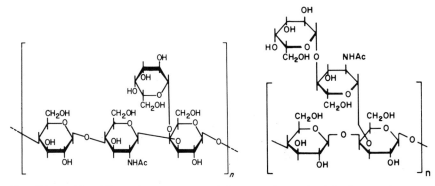

Figs 10a and b Alternative structures of the repeating unit of the incomplete core type Ia polysaccharide antigen of group B *Streptococcus*. (Recent chemical degradation analysis of this polysaccharide indicates that structure *b* is correct.)

antigen. Hydrolysis of the methylated oligosaccharide (Fig. 11) gave the individual methylated sugars (B and C) which were identified by GC–MS analysis. The detection of 2,4,5-tri-O-methyl-D-galactose with a trideuterimethyl group O-4 indicated that the terminal galactopyranose residue (D) was linked to O-4 of the branched β-D-galactopyranose residue (C), the latter residue thus having its interchain linkage at O-3. Also the detection of 2-deoxy-3,4,6,-tri-O-methyl-2-(N-methylacetamide)-glucose and 1,3,4-tri-O-methyl-erythritol, both residues having trideuteriomethyl groups on their respective O-4 and O-3 positions, confirmed the other interchain linkage assignments made from previous methylation data (Table 2). As in the case of the core type III antigen, the β-D-configuration of all the glucose constituents of the core type Ia antigen was ascertained by the characteristic chemical shift (104.2 p.p.m.) of the anomeric carbon signals in its ^{13}C NMR spectrum.

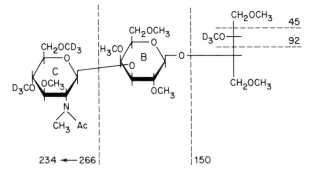

Fig. 11 Methylated oligosaccharide degradation product obtained from the incomplete type Ia streptococcal antigen.

Methylation analysis of the native type Ia antigen established that all the sialic acid residues were present as single non-reducing end-groups, because in the methanolysis of the permethylated antigen only fully methylated derivatives of sialic acid were detected (Jennings et al., 1980b). Hydrolysis of the methylated antigen yielded the individual specifically methylated component sugars which were identified and quantified by GC–MS analysis and are listed in Table 2. The difference between these partially methylated sugars and those yielded by the permethylated type Ia core antigen clearly reflect the structural relationship between the native and incomplete core type Ia antigens. In addition to the fully methylated sialic acid residue, the native antigen also yielded a 2,4,6-tri-0-methyl-galactopyranose residue which replaced the 2,3,4,6-tetra-0-methyl galactopyranose residue of the core antigen. This is indicative of the sialic acid residue (E) being linked to 0-3 of the peripheral end-group galactopyranose residues (D) of the type Ia core antigen. The fact that no 2,3,4,6-tetra-0-methyl galactopyranose was detected in the methylated type Ia native antigen is consistent only with it being composed of a repeating unit (Fig. 12) in which all the peripheral β-D-galactopyranose residues of the incomplete core antigen are substituted by sialic acid residues. As in the case of the type III native antigen, the α-D-configuration of the sialic acid residues was confirmed by the characteristic chemical shift of their carboxylate carbons (Jennings and Bhattacharjee, 1977) in the ^{13}C NMR spectrum of the native type Ia antigen.

Both the native and core type Ic antigens gave identical ^{13}C NMR spectra to the corresponding type Ia antigens thus corroborating the serological

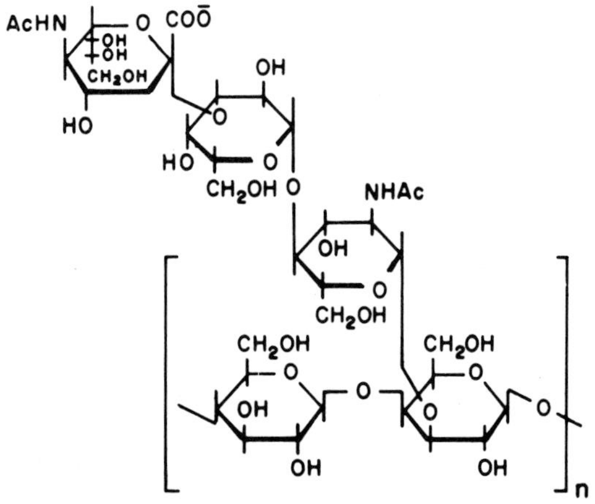

Fig. 12   Repeating unit of the native type Ia polysaccharide antigen of group B *Streptococcus.*

evidence (Wilkinson, 1975) for the structural identity of the native type Ia and type Ic antigens.

Despite many similarities in the structure of the native and core type Ia and type III streptococcal antigens, structural differences which account for their serological specificity were elucidated. While the type Ia and type III core antigens still retain two common structural features in the form of β-D-galactopyranose residues and a β-D-GlCNAcp-(1→3)-β-D-Galp-(1→4)-β-D-Glcp trisaccharide unit, they differ in that the terminal β-D-galactopyranose residues of the type Ia core antigen are linked to 0-4 of a side-chain β-D instead of 0-6 of the backbone 2-acetamido-2-deoxy-D-glucopyranose residues, as they are in the type III core antigen. The two native antigens also differ in the position of linkage of their terminal sialic acid residues to the branch β-D-galactopyranose residues of their respective core antigens. The sialic acid residues are linked to 0-6 of the β-D-galactopyranose residues in the native type III antigen (Jennings et al., 1980a) and to 0-3 of the same residues in the native type Ia antigen (Jennings et al., 1980b).

Despite the presence of terminal β-D-galactopyranose residues in both type Ia and type III core antigens, they maintain a high degree of serological specificity with respect to antisera raised to their respective whole organisms. This is at first surprising because although these residues could not be detected by chemical analysis in the isolated purified type Ia (Jennings et al., 1980b) or type III (Jennings et al., 1980a) antigens, they were thought to be present on the surface of the type Ia and type III organisms used as vaccines (Lancefield, 1934). These residues were probably generated by the loss of the masking terminal sialic acid residues from their respective cell-associated capsular polysaccharides (Kasper et al., 1979; Jennings et al., 1980a). The presence of these β-D-galactopyranose determinants was predicted on the basis of serological studies in which one of the major populations of antibodies produced by both the whole type Ia (Jennings et al., 1980b) and type III (Wilkinson, 1978; Hill et al., 1975) streptococcal organisms in rabbits was specific for their respective core antigens. Supportive evidence for the production of β-D-galactopyranose-specific antibodies in the type III anti-serum was also obtained from the observation that although the type III core antigen cross-reacted strongly with antibodies specific for the structurally identical type 14 pneumococcal polysaccharide, the type III native antigen did not. In addition, antisera produced by type 14 pneumococcal organisms in rabbits proved to be bactericidal against the type III streptococcal organisms (Fisher et al., 1978). However, more recent evidence consistent with the serological specificity of the type Ia and type III core antigens, was obtained in serological studies using the de-galactosylated type III backbone antigen (Fig. 8) when it was shown that while antibodies to terminal β-D-galactopyranose determinants are dominant in the type 14 antipneumococcal serum, they are not, in fact, prevalent in the type III antistreptococcal serum (Jennings *et al.*, in press). Although the presence of some antibodies in this latter antiserum, with β-D-galactopyranose-specificity, cannot be completely dismissed at this time, the principal determinant of the type III core-specific antibody population is, in fact, contained in the backbone of the type III core antigen (Jennings *et al.*, in press). Because of the structural identity of the type III core streptococcal antigen (Jennings *et al.*, 1980b) and the capsular polysaccharide of type 14 *S. pneumoniae* (Lindberg *et al.*, 1977), this backbone determinant is also common to both polysaccharides and is thus the basis of the major cross-reaction using antisera made to whole type III streptococcal organisms. This evidence implies that there is probably less degradation of the cell-associated type III native antigen than at first postulated and that while the antigenic specificity of this backbone determinant is independent of the presence of terminal sialic acid residues on the native type III antigen, the immunogenic expression of this determinant is not (Jennings *et al.*, in press). It is interesting to note that the other large population of antibodies in the antiserum produced by type III streptococcal organisms has an exclusive antigenic and immunogenic specificity for the native type III antigen which is dependent on the presence of the terminal sialic acid residues of the native antigen (Kasper *et al.*, 1979; Jennings *et al.*, 1980a). However, the sialic acid residues are not determinants themselves because the native type Ia antigen, having similar terminal sialic acid residues, did not cross-react with an antiserum to the type III streptococcal organisms and did not inhibit the homologous serological reaction using the same antiserum (Jennings *et al.*, in press). The fact that terminal sialic acid is not a determinant is probably due to the ubiquitous occurrence of this component sugar in human and animal systems (Jeanloz and Codington, 1976), thus resulting in its non-immunogenic properties. In fact the structural homology between both the type Ia and type III native antigens and these glycoproteins can be extended even further. The terminal α-D-NeuAcp-(2→3)-β-D-Galp unit of the type Ia antigen exists as an end-group in both the multiple 0- and N-tetrasaccharide units of fetuin (Spiro and Bhoyroo, 1974) and the important human M and N blood group substances (Sadler *et al.*, 1979), while the equivalent 2→6-linked disaccharide of the type III antigen is found as end-group in human (Spik *et al.*, 1975) and rabbit (Leger *et al.*, 1978) serotransferrin.

This creates an interesting dilemma in the fact that although the sialic acid residues of the type Ia and type III antigens are associated with the specificity of their respective native antigens, they are not immunodominant. One possible explanation for this could be that specificity is achieved via a much larger determinant of which sialic acid is only a part. However, this possibility was rejected when in classical inhibition studies (Kabat and Mayer, 1961) both serotransferrin and the core type III antigen, having all the additive and

Fig. 13 Linkage region of the Fourier-transformed ¹³C NMR spectra (300 MHz) of the native (*upper*), reduced native (*middle*), and incomplete core (*lower*) type III streptococcal polysaccharide antigens.

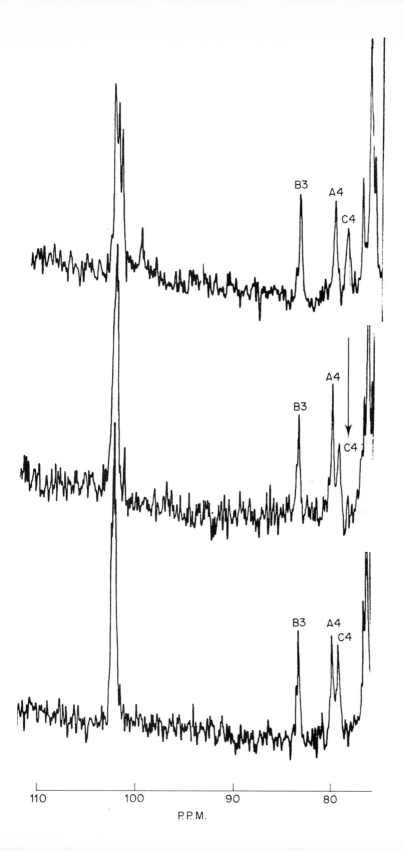

overlapping structural features of the native type III antigen, proved to be very poor inhibitors of the homologous serological reaction (Jennings *et al.*, in press).

Therefore the conformational dependence of this determinant was postulated (Jennings *et al.*, in press) in which the terminal sialic acid residues must play an important role. Confirmatory evidence for the occurrence of such a conformational change on the loss of the sialic acid residues can be obtained by a comparison of the chemical shifts of the linkage carbons in the ^{13}C NMR spectrum of the native, reduced native and core type III antigens (Fig. 13). Chemical shift displacements involving linkage carbons can be indicative of inter-glycose conformational change (Jennings and Smith, 1978) and in the ^{13}C NMR spectrum of the native type III antigen only one linkage signal at 78.3 p.p.m. not associated with the sialic acid residues, undergoes such a displacement on the reduction or removal of these sialic acid residues (Fig. 13). Using the de-galactosylated type III antigen (Fig. 13) as a model system in ^{13}C NMR spectroscopy studies, it was possible to assign this signal to C-4 of the backbone 2-acetamido-2-deoxy-β-D-glucopyranose (C) residues. A further concomitant unassigned chemical shift displacement observed in one of the anomeric signals at 103.6 p.p.m. could also be associated with the anomeric carbons of these latter residues. This evidence indicated a conformational change involving the branches of the native type III antigen rather than more extensive conformational changes in its backbone and is consistent with the serological evidence in which the antigenicity of the backbone determinant was found to be independent of the presence of terminal sialic acid residues. It is possible that this conformational control could involve interactions between the branches and backbone of the native antigen to form ring structures, and that hydrogen bonding through the carboxylate groups of the sialic acid residues could be a factor in their formation (Fig. 14). Certainly, reduction of these carboxylate groups to hydroxymethyl groups caused the reduced native type III antigen to behave both serologically and spectroscopically like the core antigen which is supportive of the above hypothesis and, in any event, demonstrates the importance of the charged carboxylate group to this conformational control (Jennings *et al.*, in press). Space-filling models (CPK) suggest that such a structure is plausible and that this hydrogen bonding might occur between the carboxylate group of the sialic acid residues (E) and the hydroxyl group at C3 of the 2-acetamido-2-deoxy-glucopyranose residue (C). However, the formation of such a ring type structure cannot be solely responsible for the specificity of the native type III antigen because in all probability the terminal oligosaccharide of serotransferrin could also form an identical structure and yet does not inhibit the homologous serological reaction of the native type III antigen. Obviously, this serological specificity must involve additional backbone sugar residues, although the fact that the

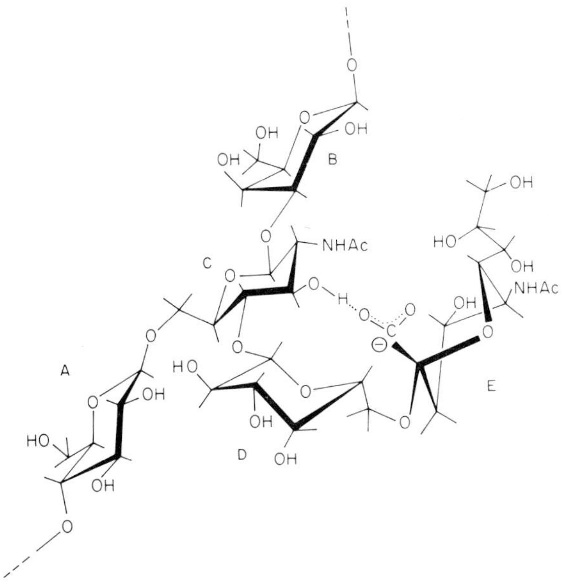

Fig. 14 Proposed conformation of the repeating unit of the type III poly-saccharide antigen of group B *Streptococcus*.

core antigen is also a poor inhibitor of the above serological reaction would suggest only a limited participation by these residues (Jennings *et al.*, in press). On this evidence it is conceivable that the determinant need not be too large to achieve specificity and in fact that sialic acid need not be directly involved in the determinant but simply function as an external factor in the confor-mational control of the determinant. This is certainly consistent with all the serological data and is supported by the inability of the removal of a large part of the glycol chain of all the sialic acid residues to change the specificity of the native type III antigen (Jennings *et al.*, in press). Space-filling models (CPK) suggest that the determinant is probably located at residues C and D with the possible involvement of residue A. It is interesting to note that the backbone determinant must also be located in the same general area as the type specificity of all the group B streptococcal core antigens and is probably derived from the variable linkages between their A and C backbone residues (Figs 8 and 10) (Jennings *et al.*, 1980a,b and unpublished results). The fact that the antigenicity of this determinant is independent of the branches of the native type III antigen means that it must be located on the opposite side of the native antigen to the sialic acid-dependent determinant (Jennings *et al.*, in press).

It is interesting to speculate on the role of this type of conformational control by sialic acid in other molecules. Certainly the isomeric type Ia antigen also has a specificity dependent on its terminal sialic acid residues (Jennings *et al.*, 1980b).

III. ANTIBODIES AGAINST GROUP B STREPTOCOCCAL POLYSACCHARIDES

Using a mouse lethality model, Lancefield defined the potential protective role of antibodies directed to various group B streptococcal antigens. Her studies demonstrated that the types Ia, Ib, Ic and II specific sera afforded passive protection to mice challenged with homologous mouse virulent strains (Table 1). Interestingly, the type III strain (D136C) used by Lancefield was not virulent. More recent studies have shown that the type III strains which are currently involved in human infection are mouse virulent if these organisms are inoculated when suspended in blood broth, Todd-Hewitt broth or given with oleic acid rather than in saline (Baltimore *et al.*, 1979; Kretschmer *et al.*, 1979). In this model, antibody to the type III polysaccharide was noted to be protective against challenge with serotype III organisms.

Within type I strains, Lancefield found cross-protection. She attributed this to a population of antibodies directed to another determinant, which she termed the Iabc carbohydrate. Her studies also demonstrated that antibody to the Ibc protein antigen, shared by serotypes Ib and Ic strains, protected against challenge with either of these 2 serotypes. Rabbit antibodies directed to the group B determinant failed to protect mice against fatal challenge with group B streptococcal strains of any serotype.

Based on these animal experiments, we felt that to study human immunity to group B streptococci, it was important to identify antibodies directed against the type specific surface antigens of these organisms. The antigens used for these studies have been those described in the chemistry section and are representative of the antigens as they exist in their native state on the surface of the organism. It was unnecessary to use these antigens, because the acid extraction methods used by others destroy terminal sialic acid residues and result in an antigen of altered immunospecificity (Kasper *et al.*, 1979; Jennings *et al.*, 1980a; Jennings *et al.*, 1980b). To extract these native antigens, we used neutral buffered solutions and also grew the organisms in conditions which maintained the pH neutrality. These conditions assured us that any acid labile sugar, such as sialic acid, would not be removed during the growth or extraction procedure. In 1976, Baker and Kasper (1976a) demonstrated that neonates at risk for the development of type III group B streptococcal infection are those whose mothers have low concentrations of antibody to the native type III capsular polysaccharide in their sera. Women who are vaginal carriers of type III organisms and whose children do not become infected have a significantly higher prevalence of antibody to the type III native polysaccharide when compared to the levels of serum antibody in mothers whose infants become infected with type III group B streptococci. A significant correlation existed between the antibody concentration of matched maternal-cord sera pairs ($r = 0.76$), indicating transplacental transfer of antibody (Baker *et al.*, 1977). These data indicated that neonatal antibody levels could be estimated from the maternal antibody level, but that additional factors such as immunoglobulin class may be important.

More recently, it has become evident that antibody specific to the native type III polysaccharide is of importance in understanding susceptibility to inspection. Wilkinson had reported that high levels of antibody to acid extracted antigens (hot HCl or cold TCA) existed in acute sera of infants infected with type III group B streptococci (Wilkinson, 1977). Fisher *et al.* (1978) had found that the type 14 capsular polysaccharide of *Streptococcus pneumoniae* cross-reacted immunologically with the core HCl-extracted antigens of type III GBS. Our chemical studies showed structural identity of the type 14 *S. pneumoniae* and HCl-extracted type III GBS polysaccharide (Kasper *et al.*, 1979; Jennings *et al.*, 1980a). This fortuitous relationship allowed exploration of the relative protective role of antibodies to the native and core polysaccharides. Antibody concentrations in the acute sera of mothers whose infants had invasive type III group B streptococcal infection was significantly higher to the type III core antigen than that found in the same sera to the native type III antigen (Table 3). Antibody to the core antigen is

Table 3 Antibody concentrations in sera from eleven mothers of infants with invasive, type III Group B streptococcal infection (Kasper *et al.*, 1979)

	Antibody to the type III desialated core antigen (µg antibody protein ml^{-1})	Antibody to the type III native antigen (µg antibody protein ml^{-1}
1	13.2	0.85
2	8.2	2.52
3	10.8	2.0
4	5.4	0.58
5	5.7	0.46
6	4.0	0.42
7	8.2	0.68
8	8.2	0.55
9	6.72	1.06
10	5.86	1.00
11	7.96	0.77

Table 4 Immunization of adult volunteers with low preimmunization levels of antibody to Type III Group B *Streptococcus* (GBS) with multivalent pneumococcal polysaccharide vaccine (Baker *et al.*, 1980)

	Antibody concentration to type 14 *Pneumococcus* (ng of antibody/ml)		Antibody concentration to type III GBS (µg antibody protein/ml)		Type III GBS opsonic titre[a]	
	Pre-immunization	4 wk Post-immunization	Pre-immunization	4 wk Post-immunization	Pre-immunization	4 wk Post-immunization
	79	163	0.4	0.4	<1:2	<1:2
	100	127	0.4	0.5	<1:2	<1:2
	133	288	0.4	0.5	<1:2	<1:2
	141	1154	0.4	0.9	<1:2	<1:2
	43	666	0.5	0.5	<1:2	<1:2
	63	156	0.5	0.5	<1:2	<1:2
	127	644	0.5	0.5	<1:2	<1:2
	140	273	0.5	0.5	<1:2	<1:2
	145	231	0.5	0.5	<1:2	<1:2
	217	1097	0.6	12.2	<1:2	<1:2
	551	227	0.6	0.6	<1:2	<1:2
	170	310	0.7	1.1	<1:2	<1:2
	1049	1189	0.7	1.2	<1:2	<1:2
	986	1695	0.8	0.8	<1:2	<1:2
	436	1180	0.9	1.2	<1:2	<1:2
	1132	1194	0.9	1.9	<1:2	<1:2
	129	1186	1.0	2.0	<1:2	<1:2
	228	444	1.0	0.9	<1:2	<1:2
	135	2690	1.6	8.1	<1:2	<1:2
	110	95	2.0	3.7	<1:2	<1:2
Geometric mean concentration	192	497.3	0.67	1.06		
95% confidence interval	34–150	192–803	0.5–0.9	0–2.42		
Significance of difference[b]	*t* = 3.17; *P* < 0.01		*t* = 1.8; *P* > 0.05			

unlikely to be protective because the concentration of antibodies of core specificity which is present in the acute sera of infected infants and their mothers is indistinguishable from those levels in normal healthy controls. Interestingly, the level of antibody to the core polysaccharide in the sera of mothers whose infants became sick with type III group B streptococcal infection in our studies was quite similar to levels found by Wilkinson using acid-extracted antigens. It is exceedingly important to understand the chemical composition of antigens when doing studies of immunity. In this case, the native and the core polysaccharides are quite similar structurally although clearly not identical and antibody directed to one antigen, the native, is responsible for human immunity and antibody directed to the other antigen, the core, apparently has little to do with human immunity to type III group B streptococci. To establish a protective basis for these observations, it was necessary to extend the studies to include studies of opsonophagocytosis because of the assumption that it is these opsonic antibodies which are important in human immunity. The basis of these studies were human volunteers immunized with the type III GBS polysaccharide or with the *S. pneumoniae* type 14 polysaccharide (Kasper *et al.*, 1979; Baker *et al.*, 1980). The target population for active immunoprophylaxis to prevent type III GBS disease in infants will consist of women with low concentrations of antibody to the native type III antigen. Therefore, volunteers for preliminary immunization studies were selected based on their pre-immunization antibody status.

Twenty volunteers who had low levels of antibody to the native type III polysaccharide of GBS in their pre-immunization serum samples were immunized with multivalent pneumococcal vaccine (MSD). Four and 26 weeks after immunization, a significant increase in antibody to the type 14 pneumococcal polysaccharide ($P < 0.01$) but not in antibody to the native type III polysaccharide resulted (Baker *et al.*, 1980) (Table 4). Only three subjects responded with over $1.0 \mu g \ ml^{-1}$ in antibody to type III GBS. None of these volunteers had a rise in opsonic antibody titres to type III GBS. In contrast, immunization of volunteers with type III GBS vaccines are usually associated with a rise in opsonic antibody. In these latter subjects, the opsonic rise correlated with a rise in antibody concentration to the native antigen ($r = 0.94$) rather than the core antigen ($r = 0.51$) (Table 5) (Kasper *et al.*, 1979; Baker *et al.*, 1978; Edwards *et al.*, 1979).

The importance of looking at the potentially susceptible population when studying vaccines was suggested when adults with moderate to high levels of antibody to native type III antigen in preimmunization serum were immunized with pneumococcal vaccine. In contrast to those with low pre-existing levels, these volunteers all responded with over $1.0 \mu g \ ml^{-1}$ of antibody to the type III GBS antigen four weeks later (Table 6). However, by 26 weeks after immunization, their antibody levels to the type III GBS antigen decreased to

Table 5   Antibody levels in sera from adult volunteers immunized with type III Group B streptococcal vaccine (Kasper *et al.*, 1979)

Antibody to type III group B streptococcal core antigen (µg/ml)		Antibody to type III group B streptococcal native antigen (µg/ml)		Type III group B *Streptococcus* opsonic titre (µg/ml)	
0	*2*	*0*	*2*	*0*	*2*
34.2	69.6	1.31	198.0	<1:2	1:80
15.1	15.1	1.91	4.58	<1:2	1:2
11.5	11.5	0.65	2.8	<1:2	1:2
7.4	27.8	1.63	314.0	<1:2	1:80
49.5	53.05	2.96	172.2	<1:2	1:20
11.2	12.78	0.72	33.8	<1:2	1:5
21.96	44.8	1.31	51.5	<1:2	1:10
34.2	69.6	1.46	167.0	<1:2	1:40
9.1	9.1	0.58	38.1	<1:2	1:2

Mean difference in antibody concentration between paired sera standard error. 13.24 ± 5.11 ($P<0.05$), $107.71 + 35.92$ ($P<0.02$).

pre-immunization levels. Again, the increase in serum antibody to type III GBS antigen correlated with a rise in opsonic antibody to GBS. Individuals with moderate or high levels of pre-existing antibody responded better to type III antigen than Pneumovax, and their levels persisted for longer than 6 months (Baker *et al.*, 1980).

These data strongly suggest that immunization with pneumococcal type 14 polysaccharide as a means of increasing maternal antibody to type III group B streptococci and thereby preventing infant disease caused by this organism has little promise. Women who deliver infected infants have low levels (<2 µg ml^{-1}) of antibody to native type III polysaccharide, and they would not be expected to respond to immunization with pneumococcal vaccine. In addition, these studies emphasize the importance of quantitatively assessing the role of pre-immunization antibody concentration in the immunogenicity of specific polysaccharide vaccines. This need is underscored by the interesting observation that an immunochemically distinct polysaccharide (type 14 pneumococcal antigen) induces a population of antibodies in persons who have been sensitized to the specific antigen (native type III group B streptococcal polysaccharide) but fails to induce antibody in persons who have not been sensitized. These data suggest that although specific antigens are necessary for priming B-cell function, structurally similar antigens may be adequate in eliciting a secondary B-cell proliferation. Although Francis's hypothesis (1960) concerning "original antigenic sin" was set forth more than two decades ago, these findings appear to validate this concept as it relates to human immunity to structurally defined bacterial polysaccharide antigens.

Table 6 Immunization of adult volunteers with moderate to high preimmunization levels of antibody to type III Group B *Streptococcus* (GBS) with multivalent pneumococcal polysaccharide vaccine (Baker *et al.*, 1980)

	Antibody concentration to type 14 *Pneumococcus* (ng of antibody/ml)		Antibody concentration to type III GBS (µg antibody protein/ml)		Type III GBS opsonic titre[a]	
	Pre-immunization	4 wk Post-immunization	Pre-immunization	4 wk Post-immunization	Pre-immunization	4 wk Post-immunization
	126	1044	2.1	10.4	<1:2	<1:2
	119	484	3.0	34	<1:2	1:2
	111	461	3.3	7.1	<1:2	<1:2
	466	967	4.8	64.8	<1:2	1:2
	33	438	8.3	18.8	<1:2	1:2
	949	1113	10.9	80	<1:2	1:5
	161	555	14.3	21	<1:2	1:2
	80	2755	21.0	55	1:2	1:5
	163	479	21.0	38	ND[c]	ND
	202	268	91.0	199	1:20	1:80
Geometric mean concentration	159	681.3	9.3	34.3		
95% confidence interval	0–346	187–1175	0–27.4	0–72.8		
Significance of difference[b]		t=2.6; P<0.05		t=3.2; P<0.01		

[a] Titre of serum is the highest dilution at which >90% reduction in colony-forming units occurs after one hour.
[b] Paired t-test on arithmetic differences.
[c] ND denotes not determined.

IV. INTERACTIONS WITH THE COMPLEMENT SYSTEM

It has been suggested that a major mechanism of natural immunity in the absence of specific antibody is activation of the alternative complement pathway by the surface of organisms (Fearon, 1978; Pangburn and Müller, 1978; Kazatchkine, 1979).

One surface moiety that has been found to modulate activation by the alternative pathway is sialic acid. Activating particles such as zymosan and erythrocytes are relatively deficient in surface-associated sialic acid, whereas non-activating particles such as sheep erythrocytes contain an abundance of sialic acid moieties (Fearon, 1978; Pangburn and Müller-Eberhard, 1978; Kazatchkine et al., 1979). Enzymatic removal of sialic acid residues with neuraminidase (Fearon, 1978; Pangburn and Müller-Eberhard, 1978) or conversion by mild oxidation with sodium periodate and reduction with borohydride to heptulosonic acid (Fearon, 1978) converts the sheep erythrocyte from a nonactivating to an activating surface for the alternative pathway. Activation by sheep erythrocytes requires removal or modification of at least 40% of membrane sialic acid, and increases proportionately when larger amounts are affected (Fearon, 1978). Surface-associated sialic acid modulates alternative pathway function by increasing the affinity of B1H relative to B for C3b. This results in blocking formation of the alternative pathway C3 convertase C3bBb (Fearon, 1978; Pangburn and Müller-Eberhard, 1978; Kazatchkine et al., 1979). If one could extrapolate to the sialic acid-rich capsule of type III GBS from mammalian erythrocytes, group B streptococci might be expected to function as a nonactivating surface for the alternative complement pathway.

A crucial role for type-specific antibody in host defence against group B streptococcal infection has been defined (Baker and Kasper, 1976a; Baker et al., 1977), but the role of type-specific antibody in an alternative pathway-mediated bactericidal activity for type III group B streptococci has not been investigated. Although efficient activators of the alternative pathway such as zymosan (Fearon and Austen, 1977b) and rabbit erythrocytes (Fearon and Austen, 1977a; Schreiber et al., 1978) require only C3, B, D, properdin, B1H, and the C3b inactivator (C3BINA) for cleavage of C3, immunoglobulin can have a facilitatory role (Polhill et al., 1978; Nelson and Ruddy, 1979). For example, IgG participates in the alternative-pathway-mediated opsonization of Streptococcus pneumoniae (Winkelstein et al., 1972; Winkelstein and Shin, 1974), Bacteroides fragilis and Bacteroides thetaiotaomicron (Bjornson and Bjornson, 1978), Shigella (Reed and Albright, 1974), Pseudomonas aeruginosa (Bjornson and Michael, 1973; Bjornson and Michael, 1974), group C meningococci (Nicholson and Lepow, 1978) and some strains of Staphylococcus aureus and Staphylococcus epidermidis (Verhoef et al., 1978).

Studies were designed to define the participation of the alternative complement pathway in opsonophagocytosis of type III group B streptococci and the role of specific antibody directed to the sialic-acid-rich native capsular polysaccharide antigen in facilitating alternative pathway activation (Edwards et al., 1980).

These studies show that complement is required for the opsonophagocytosis of type III group B streptococci. The effect of a critical concentration of antibody in promoting opsonophagocytosis was mediated by complement fixation and not by interaction of antibody with neutrophil Fc receptors, because additional antibody failed to influence opsonophagocytosis after complement was fixed. Low levels of antibody utilize the classical pathway, but higher levels of specific antibody, in the range correlated with in vivo protection in infants (Baker et al., 1977), recruit the alternative pathway (Table 7). Three possible mechanisms may be involved in antibody-dependent activation of the alternative pathway.

First, the role of immunoglobulin in the recruitment of the alternative pathway might depend on deposition of C3b (Root et al., 1972; Nicholson et al., 1974) by the classic complement pathway 142 convertase. C3b, the major cleavage fragment of C3, participates in the assembly of the alternative complement C3 cleaving convertase (Müller-Eberhard and Götze, 1972). In our studies using serum deficient in C2, we demonstrated that the classical pathway is not needed to recruit the alternative pathway for opsonization of group B streptococci when there is sufficient antibody.

Secondly, May and Frank (1973a and 1973b) described a C1-bypass mechanism of complement activation. The pathway depends on high concentrations of specific antibody, C1 and B for activation of C3. In our experiments, MgEGTA was used to dilute serum for chelation of Ca^{2+} and inactivation of C1, therefore preventing classical pathway activation. The MgEGTA-diluted serum was comparable to normal serum and C2D serum in supplying a complement source. These results rule out a critical role for the C1-bypass mechanism for the antibody-dependent activation of the alternative pathway for opsonization of group B streptococci.

Finally, the surface of an alternative pathway activator must capture the C3b generated by the Mg^{2+}-dependent fluid-phase C3 convertase formed by the interaction of native C3, B, properdin and D in the presence of B1H and C3bINA (Fearon and Austen, 1977a; Fearon and Austen, 1977b; Schreiber et al., 1978). The enzymatic activity of this convertase is held in check by B1H which accelerates the intrinsic decay of C3bBb (Weiler et al., 1976; Whaley and Ruddy, 1976) and augments the activity of the C3bINA in irreversibly destroying the binding site for B (Alper et al., 1972). Sialic acid is one membrane constituent that has been shown to modulate surface activation of the alternative pathway (Fearon, 1978; Pangburn and Müller-Eberhard,

Table 7 Mechanism of alternative-pathway-mediated opsonophagocytosis of type III Group B *Streptococcus* (Edwards *et al.*, 1980)

Type III, group B streptococcal antibody concentration to native polysaccharide (μg ml^{-1})	Complement source	Concentration of type III group B streptococcal antibody added after opsonization procedure (μg ml^{-1})	Bactericidal index[a]
2.8	Autologous	2.8	92
0.7	Autologous	2.8	77
2.8	None	2.8	0
0.7	None	2.8	0
2.8[b]	C2D	2.8	94
0.7[b]	C2D	2.8	3
0.4	C2D	2.8	0

[a] Bactericidal index $= 100 - \left[\dfrac{\text{CFU at 40 min}}{\text{CFU at 0 min}} \right] \times 100$

[b] Heat-inactivated at 56°C for 30 min.

1978). Surfaces of activating particles for the alternative pathway have little sialic acid. Surface-associated sialic acid greatly increases the binding affinity of B1H for C3b, thereby accelerating intrinsic decay of the convertase, whereas the decreased affinity of B1H for the surface of an activating particle favours formation of the convertase on bound C3b (Fearon, 1978; Pangburn and Müller-Eberhard, 1978; Kazatchkine et al., 1979).

The native polysaccharide antigen of type III group B streptococci contains an abundance of sialic acid residues that are all present as end-groups completely masking the peripheral galactopyranosyl residues of the repeating unit of the antigen (Kasper et al., 1979; Jennings et al., 1980a). Our experiments indicate that this particle functions as a non-activating surface for the alternative pathway in sera that contained low concentrations of specific antibody. However, in the presence of a critical concentration of antibody with specificity for the sialic-acid-containing immunodeterminant, alternative pathway activation occurs. The specificity of this antibody requirement was demonstrated by the complete inhibition of alternative-pathway-mediated opsonization after absorption of serum that contained 2.8 µg ml^{-1} of type-specific antibody with either whole type III organisms or native type III capsular polysaccharide (Table 8).

The role of terminal sialyl residues in creating an antibody-dependent requirement for activation of the alternative pathway was explored. Because enzymatic removal of sialic acid residues on sheep erythrocytes will convert this particle from a non-activating to an activating surface for the alternative pathway (Fearon, 1978), type III group B streptococcal terminal sialic acid residues were enzymatically cleaved to examine the effect that altering this surface moiety would have on the requirement for specific antibody. Bacteria grown in the presence of neuraminidase exhibited reduced agglutination with antibody to S. pneumoniae, type 14. Because the non-sialated core antigen of type III group B streptococci is structurally identical to the S. pneumoniae type 14 antigen (Kasper et al., 1979; Jennings et al., 1980a), these serological reactions indicated that neuraminidase had cleaved a portion of the terminal sialic acid residues. Antibody-deficient sera exhibited alternative-pathway-mediated bactericidal activity for the partially desialated organisms that was equal to that observed in sera with antibody concentrations sufficient for alternative pathway activation. Therefore, once sialic acid is removed, antibody is no longer required for activation of this pathway (Fig. 15).

These experiments did not elucidate the mechanism by which antibody directed at an immunodeterminant that contains a terminal sialic acid residue permits alternative pathway activation. One possibility is that the antibody binds and neutralizes the sialic acid residues, resulting in impaired B1H binding to C3b, which would allow the formation of a deregulated C3bBb convertase (Fearon, 1978). Alternatively, carbohydrate groups on the immuno-

Table 8 Role of antibody to the native capsular polysaccharide antigen in alternative-pathway-mediated opsono-phagocytosis of type III Group B *Streptococcus* (Edwards *et al.*, 1980)

Serum	Absorption	Final type III GBS antibody concentration to native antigen (μg/ml)	Complement	Bactericidal index[a]
NHS$_1$[b]	None	2.8	Autologous	98
ΔNHS$_1$[c]	None	2.8	None	0
ΔNHS$_1$	None	2.8	C2D	90
ΔNHS$_1$	Type III GBS cells	0.3	None	0
ΔNHS$_1$	Type III GBS polysaccharide	0.4	None	0
ΔNHS$_1$	Type III GBS cells	0.3	C2D	0
ΔNHS$_1$	Type III GBS polysaccharide	0.4	C2D	39
ΔNHS$_1$	Type 3 pneumococcal polysaccharide	2.8	C2D	95
C2D	None	0.4	Autologous	29

[a] Bactericidal index $= 100 - \dfrac{\text{CFU at 40 min}}{\text{CFU at 0 min}} \times 100$.

[b] NHS$_1$, Serum from normal donor containing the antibody concentration specified.

[c] ΔNHS$_1$, Normal human serum that was heat-inactivated at 56°C for 30 min.

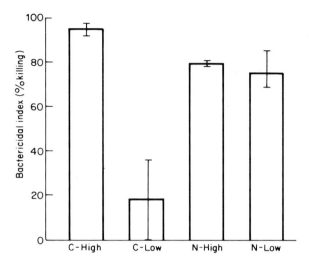

Fig. 15   Bactericidal index for alternative pathway-mediated opsonophago-cytosis of type III group B streptococci grown in pH-titrated media (C) or in the presence of neuraminidase (N) by sera that contain high or low concentrations of type specific antibody. Mean and range of four sera are shown (69). (Courtesy of Edwards *et al.*, 1980.)

globulin might provide a protected site for C3b deposition that is topically removed from the bacterial capsular sialic acid residues.

A receptor for activators of the alternative pathway that permits ingestion in the absence of exogenous proteins has been demonstrated for human blood monocytes (Czop *et al.*, 1980a,b). The possibility that specific antibody or neuraminidase cleavage created an activating particle that could be directly digested by monocytes in the opsonic reaction mixture was ruled out by including a serum-free control in each opsonophagocytosis test. Because bacterial growth was always observed, these findings confirmed the comple-ment dependence of bactericidal activity and excluded a significant role for leucocyte-mediated opsonization in the absence of exogenous proteins in this assay system.

These experiments have shown an essential role for complement in this opsonophagocytosis assay. The essential ligand is presumably C3b which is the most important opsonic ligand generated during complement activation (Gigli and Nelson, 1968). Potentially, fixation of C3b by the alternative pathway is a major factor in natural host defence because activation by this pathway can occur in the absence of antibody (Fearon and Austen, 1977a,b; Schreiber *et al.*, 1978), whereas activation of the classical complement pathway usually requires specific antibody (Mayer, 1978). Our experiments show that sialic acid residues on the type III, group B streptococcal capsule allow this pathogen to evade this natural host-defence mechanism. Only the presence of specific anti-capsular antibody, i.e., acquired immunity, will permit alternative complement pathway activation by the organism in its fully sialated state.

It is of interest that several virulent bacteria other than group B streptococci have sialic acid residues in their capsules. The type III group B streptococci presents itself to the host as a fully sialated surface as do serogroups B and C *Neisseria meningitidis* and K1 *Escherichia coli* (Jennings *et al.*, 1977; Robbins *et al.*, 1974). Interestingly, less pathogenic serogroups of meningococci and *E. coli* that have some sialic acid in their capsule have this present in a repeating unit, but it is not the exclusive terminal sugar.

ACKNOWLEDGEMENT

Supported by Contract No. AI-72538 and Grant No. AI-13249-05 from the National Institutes of Allergy and Infectious Diseases. We would like to thank Loreen Carr for assistance in the preparation of this manuscript.

REFERENCES

Alper, C. A., Rosen, F. S. and Lachmann, P. J. (1972). *Proc. Natl Acad. Sci., U.S.A.* **69**, 2910–2913.
Baker, C. J. (1980). *Adv. Int. Med.* **25**, 475–499.
Baker, C. J., Edwards, M. S. and Kasper, D. L. (1978). *J. Clin. Invest.* **61**, 1107–1110.
Baker, C. J. and Kasper, D. L. (1976a). *N. Engl. J. Med.* **294**, 753–756.
Baker, C. J. and Kasper, D. L. (1976b). *Infect. Immun.* **13**, 284–288.
Baker, C. J., Kasper, D. L., Edwards, M. S. and Schiffman, G. (1980). *N. Engl. J. Med.* **303**, 173–178.
Baker, C. J., Kasper, D. L., Tager, I. B., Paredes, A., Alpert, S., McCormack, W. M. and Goroff, D. (1977). *J. Clin. Invest.* **59**, 810–818.
Baltimore, R. S., Kasper, D. L. and Vecchitto, J. (1979). *J. Infect. Dis.* **140**, 81–88.
Bjornson, A. B. and Bjornson, A. S. (1978). *J. Infect. Dis.* **138**, 351–358.
Bjornson, A. B. and Michael, J. G. (1973). *J. Infect. Dis.* **128**, S182–S186.
Bjornson, A. B. and Michael. J. G. (1974). *J. Infect. Dis.* **130**, S119–S124.
Brown, J. H. (1920). *J. Exp. Med.* **31**, 35–47.
Brown, J. H. (1937). *J. Bacteriol.* **34**, 35–48.
Christie, R., Atkins, N. E., Munch-Petersen, E. (1944). *Aust. J. Exp. Biol. Med. Sci.* **22**, 197–200.
Czop, J. K., Fearon, D. T. and Austen, K. F. (1978a). *J. Immunol.* **120**, 1132–1138.
Czop, J. K., Fearon, D. T. and Austen, K. F. (1978b). *Proc. Natl Acad. Sci., U.S.A.* **75**, 3831–3835.
Edwards, E. A. and Larson, G. C. (1974). *Appl. Microbiol.* **28**, 972–976.

Edwards, M. S., Baker, C. J. and Kasper, D. L. (1979). *J. Infect. Dis.* **140**, 1004–1008.
Edwards, M. S., Nicholson-Weller, A., Baker, C. J. and Kasper, D. L. (1980). *J. Exp. Med.* **151**, 1275–1287.
Facklam, R. R., Padula, J. F., Thacker, L. G., Wortham, E. C., Scongers, B. J. (1974). *Appl. Microbiol.* **27**, 107–113.
Fearon, D. T. (1978). *Proc. Natl Acad. Sci., U.S.A.* **75**, 1971–1975.
Fearon, D. T. and Austen, K. F. (1977a). *J. Exp. Med.* **146**, 22–33.
Fearon, D. T. and Austen, K. F. (1977b). *Proc. Natl Acad. Sci., U.S.A.* **74**, 1683–1687.
Fenton, L. J. and Harper, M. H. (1978). *J. Clin. Microbiol.* **8**, 500–502.
Fisher, G. W., Lowell, G. H., Cumrine, M. H. and Bass, J. W. (1978). *J. Exp. Med.* **148**, 776–786.
Francis, T., Jr (1960). *Proc. Amer. Philos. Soc.* **104**, 572–578.
Freimer, E. H. (1967). *J. Exp. Med.* **125**, 381–392.
Gigli, I. and Nelson, R. A., Jr (1968). *Exp. Cell. Res.* **51**, 45–67.
Hill, H. R., Riter, M. E., Menge, S. K., Johnson, D. R. and Matsen, J. M. (1975). *J. Clin. Microbiol.* **1**, 188–191.
Jeanloz, R. W. and Codington, J. F. (1976) *In* "Biological Role of Sialic Acid" (Rosenberg and Schengrund, ed.) pp. 201–238, Plenum Press, New York.
Jennings, H. J. and Bhattacharjee, A. K. (1977). *Carbohydr. Res.* **55**, 105–112.
Jennings, H. J., Bhattacharjee, A. K., Bundle, D. R., Kenny, C. P., Martin, A. and Smith, I. C. P. (1977). *J. Infect. Dis.* **136**, S78–S83.
Jennings, H. J., Lugowski, C. and Kasper, D. L. (1981). *Biochemistry* (in press).
Jennings, H. J., Rosell, K.-G. and Kasper, D. L. (1980a). *Can. J. Biochem.* **58**, 112–120.
Jennings, H. J., Rosell, K.-G. and Kasper, D. L. (1980b). *Proc. Natl Acad. Sci., U.S.A.* **77**, 2931–2935.
Jennings, H. J. and Smith, I. C. P. (1978). *Methods Enzymol.* **50**, 39–50.
Kabat, E. A. and Mayer, M. M. (1961). *In* "Experimental Immunochemistry" (Thomas, ed.) pp. 241–267, Springfield, Ill.
Kane, J. A. and Karakawa, W. W. (1977). *J. Immunol.* **118**, 2155–2160.
Kane, J. A. and Karakawa, W. W. (1978). *Infect. Immun.* **19**, 983–991.
Kasper, D. L. and Baker, C. J. (1979). *J. Infect. Dis.* **139**, 147–151.
Kasper, D. L., Baker, C. J., Baltimore, R. S., Crabb, J. H., Schiffman, G. and Jennings, H. J. (1979). *J. Exp. Med.* **149**, 327–339.
Kasper, D. L., Goroff, D. K. and Baker, C. J. (1978). *J. Immunol.* **121**, 1096–1105.
Kazatchkine, M. D., Fearon, D. T. and Austen, K. F. (1979). *J. Immunol.* **122**, 75–81.
Kretschmer, R. R., Vogel, L. C., Kelly, P., Padnos, D., Goldman, M., Audch, W. M. and Gotoff, S. P. (1979). *In* "Pathogenic Streptococci" (Redbook Ltd) p. 160.
Lancefield, R. C. (1933). *J. Exp. Med.* **57**, 571–582.
Lancefield, R. C. (1934). *J. Exp. Med.* **59**, 441–458.
Lancefield, R. C. (1938). *J. Exp. Med.* **67**, 25–40.
Lancefield, R. C. and Freimer, E. H. (1966). *J. Hyg.* **64**, 191–203.
Lancefield, R. C., McCarty, M. and Everly, W. W. (1975). *J. Exp. Med.* **142**, 165–179.
Leger, D., Tordera, V., Spik, G., Dorland, L., Haverkamp, J. and Vliegenthart, J. F. G. (1978). *FEBS Lett.* **93**, 255–260.
Lindberg, B., Lönggren, J. and Powell, D. A. (1977). *Carbohydr. Res.* **58**, 177–186.
Mason, E. O., Wong, P. and Barrett, J. (1976). *J. Clin. Microbiol.* **4**, 429–431.
May, J. E. and Frank, M. M. (1973a). *J. Immunol.* **111**, 1661–1667.
May, J. E. and Frank, M. M. (1973b). *J. Immunol.* **111**, 1668–1676.
Mayer, M. M. (1978). *Harvey Lect.* **72**, 139.
Müller-Eberhard, H. J. and Götze, O. (1972). *J. Exp. Med.* **135**, 1003–1008.

Nelson, B. and Ruddy, S. (1979). *J. Immunol.* **122**, 1994–1999.

Nicholson, A., Brade, V., Lee, G. D., Shin, H. S. and Mayer, M. M. (1974). *J. Immunol.* **112**, 1115–1123.

Nicholson, A. and Lepow, I. H. (1978). Clin. Res. 26, 525A (abstract).

Pangburn, M. K. and Müller-Eberhard, H. J. (1978). *Proc. Natl Acad. Sci., U.S.A.* **75**, 2416–2420.

Polhill, R. B., Newman, S. L., Pruitt, K. M. and Johnston, R. B., Jr (1978) *J. Immunol.* **121**, 371–376.

Pollack, H. M. and Dahlgren, B. J. (1974). *Appl. Microbiol.* **27**, 141–143.

Reed, W. P. and Albright, E. L. (1974). *Immunology* **26**, 205–215.

Robbins, J. B., McCracken, G. H., Gotschlich, E. C., Ørskov, F., Ørskov, I. and Hanson, L. A. (1974). *N. Engl. J. Med.* **290**, 1216–1220.

Romero, R. and Wilkinson, H. W. (1974). *Appl. Microbiol.* **28**, 199–204.

Root, R. K., Ellman, L. and Frank, M. M. (1972). *J. Immunol.* **109**, 477–486.

Rosner, R. (1977). *J. Clin. Microbiol.* **6**, 23–26.

Russel, H. and Norcross, N. L. (1972). *J. Immunol.* **109**, 90–96.

Sadler, J. E., Paulson, J. C. and Hill, R. L. (1979). *J. Biol. Chem.* **254**, 2112–2119.

Schreiber, R. D., Pangburn, M. K., Lesavere, P. H. and Müller-Eberhard, H. J. (1978). *Proc. Natl Acad. Sci., U.S.A.* **75**, 3948–3952.

Spik, A., Bayard, B., Fournet, B., Streker, G., Bougelet, S. and Montreuil, J. (1975). *FEBS Lett.* **50**, 269–299.

Spiro, R. and Bhoyroo, V. D. (1974). *J. Biol. Chem.* **249**, 5704–5717.

Szilagyi, G., Mayer, E. and Eidelman, A. I. (1978). *J. Clin. Microbiol.* **8**, 410–412.

Tai, J. Y., Gotschlich, E. C. and Lancefield, R. C. (1979). *J. Exp. Med.* **149**, 58–66.

Verhoef, J., Peterson, P. K., Kim, Y., Sabath, L. D. and Quie, P. G. (1978). *Immunology* **33**, 191–197.

Weiler, J. M., Daha, M. R., Austen, K. F. and Fearon, D. T. (1976). *Proc. Natl Acad. Sci., U.S.A.* **733**, 3268–3272.

Whaley, K. and Ruddy, S. (1976). *J. Exp. Med.* **144**, 1147–1163.

Wilkinson, H. W. (1975). *Infect. Immun.* **11**, 845–852.

Wilkinson, H. W. (1977). *J. Clin. Microbiol.* **6**, 42–45.

Wilkinson, H. W. (1978). *J. Clin. Microbiol.* **7**, 194–201.

Wilkinson, H. W. and Eagon, R. (1971). *Infect. Immun.* **4**, 596–604.

Winkelstein, J. A. and Shin, H. S. (1974). *J. Immunol.* **122**, 1635–1642.

Winkelstein, J. A., Shin, H. S. and Wood, W. B., Jr (1972). *J. Immunol.* **108**, 1681–1689.

6 Legionellosis

ARTHUR L. REINGOLD
and JEFFREY D. BAND

I. INTRODUCTION

Legionellosis is a newly coined term that refers to human illness caused by any of the five known species of the genus *Legionella*. Currently recognized syndromes that fall into this category include Legionnaires' disease and Pontiac fever, which are caused by *Legionella pneumophila*, and pneumonia associated with the other four *Legionella* species. Although, in retrospect, human illness caused by *Legionella* has been occurring sporadically or in epidemics since at least 1943, recognition of these organisms as human pathogens, development of laboratory techniques for their isolation and characterization, and studies of their epidemiology have taken place predominantly since the investigation in 1976 of an outbreak of a mysterious febrile respiratory illness among those attending an American Legion convention in Philadelphia, Pennsylvania.

In the midst of the celebration of the United States bicentennial year, over 4400 delegates, family members, and other conventioneers gathered at the 58th annual convention of the American Legion's Pennsylvania Department in Philadelphia between July 21 and July 24, 1976. Over the ensuing two weeks, an illness characterized by fever, cough, and pneumonia developed in 149 of the conventioneers and 72 other individuals, all of whom had been in the vicinity of the Bellevue-Stratford Hotel. Thirty-four of the 221 cases resulted in death. Because of the large number of people affected, the severity of the illness, and the inability to identify a causative agent, an in-depth investigation of the epidemic was undertaken by the Center for Disease Control of the U.S. Public Health Service in collaboration with state and local public health agencies (Fraser *et al.*, 1977; McDade *et al.*, 1977). The joint epidemiological and laboratory investigation which followed was a model of modern medical detective work, and it paved the way for the subsequent studies whose results are summarized in this chapter.

II. MICROBIOLOGY

A. Taxonomy

Guanine-plus-cytosine content and deoxyribonucleic acid homology studies of bacteria isolated from patients studied during the Philadelphia outbreak indicated that they were unrelated to other known bacterial genera (Brenner *et al.*, 1978, 1979). On the basis of these studies, as well as of the biochemical reactions and growth characteristics of the organisms, the Legionnaires' disease bacterium was classified as a new family, genus, and species, *Legionella pneumophila*. Since 1976, six distinct serogroups of *L. pneumophila* have been identified.

Subsequent work has suggested that there are four additional members of the genus *Legionella*, three of which had been previously isolated from clinical specimens but could not initially be propagated on artificial media. The decision to classify these bacteria in the same genus as *L. pneumophila* is based on phenotypic similarities and nutritional requirements. Human isolates previously known as Tatlock, HEBA, and Pittsburgh pneumonia agent (PPA) have been shown to be strains of a single species, now known as *L. micdadei* (Hebert *et al.*, 1980). Similarly, other isolates from individuals with pneumonia have been demonstrated to be closely related, and the names *L. bozemanii* (strains WIGA, ALLO 1–2, MI–15) and *L. dumoffii* (strains TEX KL, ALLO–4, NY–23) have been proposed (Brenner *et al.*, 1980). An environmental isolate previously designated LS-13 has also been placed in this genus and the name *L. gormanii* has been proposed (Morris *et al.*, 1980). While this organism has never been isolated from clinical specimens, it has been observed in lung tissue from a patient with pneumonia (Morris *et al.*, 1980).

B. Microbiological features

Members of the genus *Legionella* are aerobic, non-spore forming, weakly staining Gram-negative bacilli measuring 0.3–0.4 μm in width and 2–3 μm in length, though much longer, filamentous forms are commonly seen after growth on artificial media (Fig. 1). Organisms grown on artificial media are not acid fast with the Ziehl-Neelsen stain, but on rare occasions organisms in tissue sections will stain weakly. Flagella are present, but motility has not been demonstrated (Fig. 2). The ultrastructure is similar to that of other Gram-

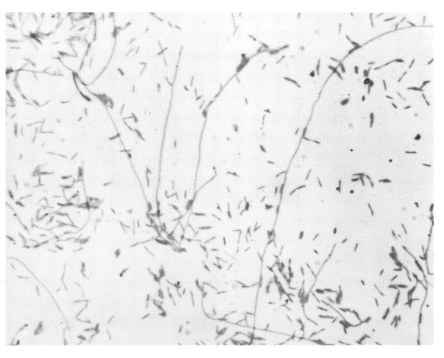

Fig. 1 Carbol fuschin stained *Legionella pneumophila* grown on CYE agar rods and filaments (×1000).
(From Weaver, R. E., and Feeley, J. C. (May 1979). *In* "Legionnaire's: the disease, the bacterium and methodology" (G. L. Jones and G. A. Hebert ed.), 20–25. CDC, Atlanta.)

negative bacteria, with two three-layer unit membranes separated by 75 Å. There is evidence of a thin cell wall composed of peptidoglycan. Lipid-containing vacuoles which stain with Sudan black B are present.

All of the *Legionella* species have a distinctive fatty acid composition in which branched-chain forms predominate (60% to 80% of the fatty acids, depending on the growth medium). *L. pneumophila* and *L. micdadei* each have a characteristic GLC pattern, while *L. gormanii*, *L. dumoffii*, and *L. bozemanii* share a common GLC pattern (Brenner *et al.*, 1980; Hebert *et al.*, 1980; Moss *et al.*, 1977; Moss and Dees, 1979). (See Table 1.)

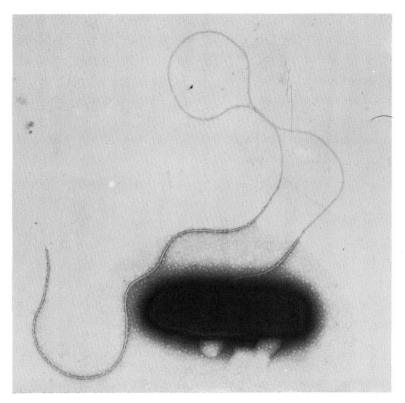

Fig. 2 Transmission electronmicrograph of a *Legionella pneumophila* grown on CYE agar with a single, probably lateral, flagellum (×61,712 magnification). (From Chandler, F. W. *et al.* (1980). *Ann. Intern. Med.* **93**, 711–14.)

C. Growth characteristics

L. pneumophila was first isolated by intraperitoneal inoculation of guinea pigs, followed by transfer of infected tissue (i.e. spleen) into embryonated hen's eggs, a method still used for testing some environmental and clinical samples (McDade *et al.*, 1977; Morris *et al.*, 1979). Failure of the organism to grow on commonly used bacteriological media such as blood agar and nutrient agar prompted a search for media that would support its growth. These include Mueller-Hinton agar supplemented with 1% haemoglobin and 1% IsoVitaleX,* Feeley-Gorman (FG) agar. (Mueller-Hinton agar enriched with

* Use of trade names is for identification only and does not constitute endorsement by the Public Health Service, U.S. Department of Health and Human Services.

Table 1 Cellular fatty acid composition of *Legionella pneumophila, L. micdadei, L. bozemanii, L. dumoffii,* and *L. gormanii*

Fatty acid[b]	Percentage of fatty acids in isolates[a]		
	L. pneumophila	*L. micdadei*[c]	*L. bozemanii. L. dumoffii,* and *L. gormanii*
i14:0	8	T[d]	4
a15:0	14	40	29
15:0	T	5	T
i16:1	3	T	T
i16:0	32	11	17
16:1	13	10	13
16:0	10	10	11
a17:1	T	3	T
a17:0	11	24	14
17:	3	T	7
17:0	2	T	2
18:0	2	T	2
19:0	T	T	T
20:0	2	T	T
Total branched-chain acids	68	78	64

[a] Percentage was determined from extracts of isolates grown on CYE agar.
[b] Number preceding colon refers to number of carbon atoms; number following colon refers to number of double bonds;
  i indicates methyl branch at the iso carbon atom;
  a indicates a methyl branch at the anteiso carbon atom;
  indicates a cyclopropane.
[c] Percentage is an average of values determined for HEBA and TATLOCK. PPA is identical to these strains and gives a similar profile.
[d] T = <2% (Trace).

ferric pyrophosphate and L-cysteine) (Feeley *et al.*, 1977), and charcoal yeast extract agar (CYE) (Feeley *et al.*, 1979).) Buffered CYE agar (BCYE), recently found to support maximally the growth of these organisms, has become the preferred medium (Pascule *et al.*, 1980). Although both FG and CYE media support the growth of four of the *Legionella* species after passage in the laboratory (*L. gormanii* does not grow on FG agar), only CYE supports primary isolation of these four species from clinical specimens. The growth characteristics of all of the *Legionella* species on artificial media may vary with the source of the isolate (i.e., previously agar-adapted strains, environmental isolates, and isolates from clinical specimens). *L. pneumophila* grows better than the other species on both FG and CYE media.

Antibiotic supplementation of CYE agar has been used to improve isolation of *L. pneumophila* from heavily contaminated lung specimens (Edelstein and Finegold, 1979). Other media which have been developed for growth of legionellae include enriched blood agar, selective blood agar, and a variety of broths (Greaves, 1980; Pine *et al.*, 1979; Ristroph *et al.*, 1980; Warren and Miller, 1979). A diphasic blood culture medium is currently being developed.

Optimal growth of *L. pneumophila* occurs under aerobic conditions in an atmosphere of 2.5% carbon dioxide at a temperature of 35°C and at pH 6.85 to 6.95. Growth on FG agar is characterized by small colonies which are visible in 4 to 10 days, a characteristic ground glass appearance, the production of a brown pigment, and yellow fluorescence with long-wave (356 mm) ultraviolet light. Growth on CYE agar produces more and larger colonies in a shorter period of time (2 to 4 days), but the brown pigment is absent and yellow fluorescence is usually absent. Most of the other *Legionella* species also produce a brown pigment when grown on FG agar, but ultraviolet light produces a blue-white fluorescence with *L. bozemanii*, *L. gormanii* and *L. dumoffii*, and dull yellow fluorescence with *L. micdadei*.

Many clinical microbiology laboratories possess the materials and expertise to make a preliminary identification of an organism as a *Legionella* sp. The absence of growth on common media and the development of typical colonies on CYE agar suggests that an organism may be a *Legionella* species. Further confirmation can be obtained by demonstrating absence of growth on CYE agar when L-cysteine is absent and by direct fluorescence antibody staining of the organisms (see below). Additional definitive methods, usually available only in reference laboratories, include gas liquid chromatography (GLC) analysis of the fatty acid composition and DNA homology studies.

D.   Biochemical properties

The cultural, biochemical, and staining properties of the various species are summarized in Table 2. *Legionella* species are relatively inert biochemically. All are catalase- and gelatinase-positive, and nitrate- and urease-negative. *L. pneumophila* and *L. micdadei* are weakly oxidase-positive. *L. pneumophila* has recently been shown to hydrolyse hippurate, while *L. bozemanii*, *L. dumoffii*, and *L. micdadei* do not (Hebert, 1981). All but *L. micdadei* produce beta-lactamase, although occasional strains of *L. bozemanii* seem to be variable in this regard.

E.   Antibiotic sensitivity

Legionella species are susceptible to a wide array of antibiotics when tested by

Characteristics examined	L. pneumophila	L. micdadei	L. bozemanii	L. dumoffii	L. gormanii
			Organisms and test results		
GROWTH					
Agars CYE[a]	primary[c]	primary[d]	primary	primary	primary
F–G	primary	adapted	adapted	adapted	no growth
MH–IH	primary	adapted	adapted	adapted	no growth
Others	no growth	no growth	no growth	no growth	no growth
FLUORESCENCE[b] ON CYE	dull yellow	dull yellow	blue–white	blue–white	blue–white
BROWNING OF F–G AGAR	+	+/−	+	+	NG
STAINS					
Gram[e]	−	−	−	−	−
Gimenez[f]	red rods	red rods	red rods	red rods	red rods
Ziehl–Neelsen[g]	−	+	−	−	−
Leifson[h]	+	+	+	+	+
FLAGELLA	+	+	+	+	+
BIOCHEMICALS					
hippurate hydrolysis	+	−	−	−	ND
catalase	+	+	+	+	+
gelatinase	+	+	+	+	+
oxidase	+	+	−	−	−
nitrate	−	−	−	−	ND*
urease	−	−	−	−	−
beta-lactamase[i]	+	−	+	+	+

[a] CYE = charcoal yeast extract, F–G = Feeley-Gorman, MH-IH = supplemented Mueller-Hinton, Others = agars without IsoVitaleX or L-cysteine. [b] Long-wavelength UV excitation. [c] Primary isolation. [d] Adapted after multiple transfers on CYE. [e] Faint pink rods from CYE. [f] Smears of infected yolk sac. [g] Rods are stained blue from CYE. [h] Flagella. [i] Chromogenic cephalosporin test for *Legionella*; 24 h growth from CYE agar tested and reported as negative (yellow, weak positive (orange) or positive (red) after 60 min.

NG, No growth on Feeley-Gorman agar. *L. gormanii* does grow and produce browning on media containing 1% yeast extract with 0.025% ferric pyrophosphate soluble, 0.04% L-cysteine HCl, 0.04% L-tyrosine, and 1.7% agar.

ND, Not determined. ND*, Not determined; does not grow in medium.

agar dilution on Mueller-Hinton-base media (Saravolatz *et al.*, 1980; Thornsberry *et al.*, 1978) (Table 3). The susceptibility of *L. dumoffii* and *L. gormanii* is similar to that shown for *L. pneumophila* (Thornsberry, personal communication). *L. micdadei*, which does not produce a beta-lactamase, is the only *Legionella* species highly susceptible to penicillin *in vitro*. The results of *in vitro* antibiotic susceptibility testing must be interpreted cautiously, however, because they are dependent on innoculum size, type of medium employed, and other factors, particularly when dealing with slow growing organisms.

F. Specimen handling

The *Legionella* species do not seem to present an extraordinary safety hazard in the laboratory. Only one case of laboratory-acquired illness has been observed with these organisms, and a prospective serosurvey of those working in and near a laboratory handling large numbers of samples containing *Legionella* has found no increase in antibody titres (Edelstein and Meyer, 1980). Proper safety precautions and good bacteriological technique should be used, however, including the use of protective clothing and prevention of aerosols. Samples should be handled in a safety cabinet, work surfaces decontaminated with hypochlorite or phenolic solutions, and glassware autoclaved.

Specimens should ideally be cultured within 2 hours of collection, but can be stored on wet ice or in a refrigerator for 2 days. Samples which cannot be cultured within 2 days of collection should be frozen at $-70°C$ or packed on dry ice.

III. DIAGNOSTIC TESTS

A. Serological tests

1. Indirect Immunofluorescence Assay (IFA)

The detection of antibody to *L. pneumophila* with the IFA has become the most common means of establishing a diagnosis of Legionnaires' disease, despite the fact that results are only available retrospectively. At present, a four-fold rise in antibody titre to ≥ 128 is considered diagnostic of recent infection with *L. pneumophila* when appropriately timed samples are examined (i.e. a sample taken within a week of onset of the illness and a second sample taken at least 3 weeks later). If seroconversion has not occurred by three weeks and Legionnaires' disease is considered the most likely diagnosis, additional serum samples should be examined, because delayed seroconversion in culture documented cases has been observed (Edelstein and Meyer,

Table 3 *In vitro* activity of eight antimicrobial agents on *Legionella* grown on charcoal yeast extract agar. Adapted from *Legionella Update*, p. 19

Antimicrobial Agent	Minimum inhibitory concentration (g ml^{-1}) for					
	L. pneumophila[a]			*L. micdadei*	*L. bozemanii*	Controls
	GM[b]	Mode	Range	Range	Range	S. aureus ATCC29213	S. aureus ATCC25923
Penicillin	8.0	4.0	4.00–16.0	≤0.12	2.0	0.5	≤0.12
Erythromycin	0.22	0.25	0.06–0.5	2.00–4.0	2.0–4.0	2.0[c]	2.0[c]
Rifampin	0.06	0.06	0.03–0.06	0.06	0.06	0.5[c]	1.0[c]
Cephalothin	16.0	16.0	16.00–32.0	1.00–2.0	8.0	≤0.25	≤0.25
Cefoxitin	0.4	0.5	0.12–0.5	0.12–0.25	0.25	2.0	1.0
Doxycycline	6.0	8.0	2.00–8.0[d]	2.0	8.0	2.0[c]	2.0[c]
Chloramphenicol	1.2	1.0	1.00–2.0	4.0	2.0	8.0	8.0
Sulfamethoxazole/ trimethoprim	9.5/0.5	9.5/0.5		9.5/0.5	1.2/0.6– 9.5/0.5	2.4/0.12	9.5/0.5[c]

[a] Philadelphia 1 and 2, Pontiac, and 9 other clinical isolates.
[b] Geometric mean.
[c] Values for the controls were higher on charcoal yeast extract agar than on conventional media.
[d] Only one strain (Pontiac 1) had an MIC of 2.0 g ml^{-1}; the others were 8 g ml^{-1}.

1980). A single titre of ≥ 256 is considered presumptive evidence of infection with *L. pneumophila*, but does not necessarily signify recent infection.

The criteria for making a serological diagnosis of infection with *L. pneumophila* with the IFA depend on the antigen preparation employed. The titres given above refer to the IFA method currently employed at CDC, using a polyvalent antigen prepared from heat-killed organisms grown on CYE agar. In England, where the antigen is prepared from formalin-killed organisms grown in embryonated hens' eggs, a four-fold or greater rise in antibody titre to ≥ 64 is considered diagnostic of recent infection and a single or standing titre of ≥ 128 is considered presumptive evidence of infection. Examination of multiple pairs of sera using both antigen preparations has demonstrated that they give comparable results when the stated criteria are employed.

It has been difficult to determine the sensitivity of the IFA test because the number of culture-positive patients with appropriately timed serum samples has been limited. Reproducible estimates of the test's sensitivity (for individual strains of *L. pneumophila*) have, however, resulted from investigations of outbreaks of Legionnaires' disease. In the Philadelphia outbreak of 1976, 87% of 111 patients who met clinical and epidemiological criteria for a case of Legionnaires' disease had convalescent titres ≥ 128, while at the Wadsworth Medical Center in Los Angeles, 75% of 8 culture-documented cases demonstrated seroconversion (Edelstein and Meyer, 1980; McDade *et al.*, 1979). The sensitivity of the IFA method currently employed at CDC has been estimated to be between 78 and 91% (Wilkinson *et al.*, 1981). Reducing the IFA titre considered diagnostic improves the sensitivity of the assay but at the cost of markedly reducing its specificity.

The specificity of the IFA assay for Legionnaires' disease has been questioned, in part because of reports of concomitant rises in titre against *L. pneumophila* and *M. pneumoniae* (Grady and Gilfillan, 1979; Oldenburger *et al.*, 1979). Additionally, there have been undocumented reports of individual patients with plague, tularaemia, and leptospirosis being incorrectly diagnosed as having Legionnaires' disease on the basis of IFA titre rises. The IFA method currently used at CDC has been tested against paired sera from culture-proven, epidemic-associated cases of *Mycoplasma* pneumonia, Q fever, tularaemia, and psittacosis, as well as culture-proven sporadic cases of plague (Wilkinson *et al.*, 1981; Wilkinson, personal communication). Four-fold or greater rises in titre to ≥ 128 against *L. pneumophila* were not found, indicating that specificity approaches or equals 100% and suggesting that occasional concomitant rises in titre against *L. pneumophila* and another organism in sporadic cases of respiratory illness may represent dual infection rather than the presence of cross-reacting antigens.

A recent study of 41 patients with culture-proven *B. fragilis* group infections, however, found that five had standing titres ≥128 and three showed a four-fold or greater rise in titre against *L. pneumophila* (Edelstein *et al.*, 1980). These results suggest that infection with *B. fragilis* can cause a false positive reaction in the IFA test, although dual infection of these patients cannot be ruled out. Fortunately, most patients with *B. fragilis* infections present with a clinical picture unlike that seen with infection caused by *L. pneumophila*, so such reactions will infrequently lead to confusion.

Sera from patients with Legionnaires' disease have been shown to react with antigens prepared from a number of heterologous Gram-negative bacteria (Wilkinson *et al.*, 1981). Pre-treatment of such sera with a crude extract of *E. coli* 013:K92:H4 will inhibit 97% of these cross reactions without substantially lowering the response to *L. pneumophila*. Routine use of this technique prior to testing sera against *L. pneumophila* antigens does not appear necessary, as long as the diagnostic criteria discussed above are employed.

The antibody response to *L. pneumophila* is complex (see Fig. 3). It can include antibodies in the IgG, IgA, and IgM classes, either singly or in various combinations, and can be directed against serogroup specific antigens, antigens common to various *Legionella* species and serogroups, and antigens found in multiple Gram-negative bacteria (White *et al.*, 1980). Unlike the situation with various viral diseases, no consistent relationship has been noted between immunoglobulin class and time elapsed since infection. Furthermore, no individual class has been found to be more sensitive or specific for diagnosing infection with *L. pneumophila*, so conjugates used in serological tests should react against all three classes in order to ensure maximal sensitivity.

Six serogroups of *L. pneumophila* have been defined on the basis of direct fluorescence antibody (DFA) testing of a large number of strains (England *et al.*, 1980; McKinney *et al.*, 1979, 1980). While approximately 50% of pairs of sera from suspected or culture-proven cases of Legionnaires' disease show either a titre rise against only one serogroup or a substantially greater titre rise against a single serogroup than against the others, comparable rises in titre to two or more serogroups can be seen.

Antigens from the other *Legionella* species have recently been prepared for use in the IFA test and preliminary evidence suggests that their specificity will approach or equal that of the IFA test for *L. pneumophila* (Wilkinson, personal communication). Their sensitivity, however, remains largely un-tested, due to the lack of culture-confirmed and/or epidemic-associated cases of human illness. Screening of paired sera submitted to CDC from patients with suspected Legionnaires' disease has demonstrated that a substantial proportion demonstrate a four-fold or greater increase in titre to ≥128 against one of these organisms, ranging from 5.8% for *L. gormanii* to 9.9% for *L. bozemanii* and *L. micdadeii* (Wilkinson, personal communication). Sero-

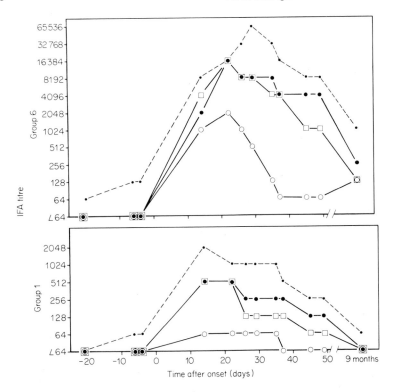

Fig. 3   Legionella pneumophila serogroup 6 antibody response.
Top   IFA titres against the autologous, serogroup 6 strain with antihuman IgG,
antihuman IgM, and antihuman IgA conjugates.
Bottom   IFA titres against the serogroup 1 strain represent the antibody
response against *Legionella* common antigen.
          •— — —• Poly Ig; ●—● IgG; □—□ IgM; ○—○ IgA
Permission has been granted by Hazel Wilkinson, Ph.D., Special Immunology
Laboratory Branch, Bacteriology Division, Bureau of Laboratories, and the
publisher to reprint figure from *Journal of Clinical Microbiology*, Volume 12,
1980.

positivity against at least one *Legionella* species was found in 27.6% of such
serum pairs. This finding suggests that pneumonia caused by the other
Legionella species may be more common than previously recognized and that
some suspected cases of Legionnaires' disease in which seroconversion was
absent may have been due to these organisms. When the sensitivity and
specificity of serological responses to these antigens have been defined, it may
be useful to expand the battery of antigens used to screen sera from patients
with pneumonia of undefined aetiology.

2. Other serological tests

A number of other methods which detect the presence of antibodies to *L. pneumophila* have been developed, including a microagglutination test (MAT) (Farshy *et al.*, 1979), a haemagglutination test (HAT) (Edson *et al.*, 1979), and an enzyme-linked immunoabsorbent assay (ELISA) (Farshy *et al.*, 1978). Although each of these methods has certain advantages over the IFA test, none has been sufficiently standardized to allow substitution for the IFA test.

B. Tissue stains

1. Direct Fluorescence Antibody Test (DFA)

The diagnosis of Legionnaires' disease can be made rapidly by examining secretions from the respiratory tract (sputum, bronchial washings, trans-tracheal aspirates, or pleural fluid) or lung tissue (fresh, fresh-frozen, paraffin-embedded, or formalin-fixed) by direct immunofluorescence (DFA), using hyperimmune rabbit sera to the various *L. pneumophila* serogroups conjugated with fluorescein isothiocyanate (Cherry *et al.*, 1978). DFA staining has proven to be highly specific when tested against pure cultures of a wide array of bacterial genera and species (Cherry *et al.*, 1978) and in clinical situations (Edelstein and Meyer, 1980). It has been noted, however, that one strain of *Pseudomonas fluorescens* was specifically stained by the serogroup 1 *L. pneumophila* conjugate (Cherry and McKinney, 1979) and that staphylo-cocci and streptococci may fluoresce due to binding of pre-existing antibodies in the rabbit serum. An experienced observer, however, can usually distin-guish *L. pneumophila* from these other bacteria on the basis of cell morphology. Early DFA conjugates also stained *Mycobacterium* species, but this artifact was eliminated by removal of Freund's adjuvant from the material used to immunize rabbits.

More recently, it has been reported that 3 of 53 strains of *B. fragilis* (and none of 271 strains of other anaerobic species) reacted with polyvalent and monovalent *L. pneumophila* serogroup 1 conjugate and appeared morphologi-cally similar to *L. pneumophila* (Edelstein *et al.*, 1980). Since *B. fragilis* has been found in transtracheal aspirates from patients with aspiration pneu-monia, this could be a source of confusion in making an aetiological diagnosis. Whether this cross reactivity is likely to lead to false positive results on clinical samples is unclear, because most patients with Legionnaires' disease do not have a history of aspiration and the frequency of positive DFA results on respiratory secretions from patients with aspiration pneumonia is unknown.

Estimates of the sensitivity of the DFA test on respiratory secretions have ranged from 24 to 70% of culture-positive cases (Broome *et al.*, 1979; Edelstein and Meyer, 1980; Gump *et al.*, 1980). The sensitivity of the test depends on: (1) the number of serogroups included in the polyvalent conjugated antiserum,

(2) the source and quality of the respiratory secretions submitted for analysis, and (3) the duration of previous antibiotic therapy. Since the test is highly serogroup-specific, the antiserum used should react against all of the six currently recognized serogroups to ensure maximal sensitivity. Examination of serial specimens from 13 culture positive patients receiving antibiotic therapy has shown that the DFA test becomes negative within four to six days (Edelstein and Meyer, 1980). The same authors reported that expectorated sputum contained larger numbers of fluorescent bacteria than specimens obtained by transtracheal aspiration or bronchoscopy from the same patients.

DFA reagents have been prepared against the other *Legionella* species. While their specificity appears equal to that of the DFA test for *L. pneumophila*, their sensitivity is unknown.

2. Other tissue stains

L. pneumophila and the other *Legionella* species can be demonstrated in lung tissue sections stained with a modified Dieterle silver impregnation stain, though this method is not specific. The organisms appear as brownish-black, short rods against a yellow background. Other common tissue stains such as the Brown-Benn or Brown Hopps modifications of the Gram stain and haematoxylin and eosin do not stain these organisms. An immunohistochemical staining technique employing glucose oxidase and antiserum prepared against *L. pneumophila* serogroup 1 has recently been described (Suffin *et al.*, 1980).

C. Antigen detection

An enzyme-linked immunoabsorbent assay (ELISA) specific for antigen from *L. pneumophila* has been developed and detection of antigen in the urine of patients with Legionnaires' disease has been reported (Tilton, 1979). Use of this test has been limited, however, and there have been reports of failure to detect the antigen in the urine of patients with culture-proven cases (Edelstein and Meyer, 1980).

IV.   CLINICAL FEATURES

A.   Pneumonia

Infection with *L. pneumophila* can produce a variety of clinical pictures, ranging from no illness through an acute, self-limiting illness (Pontiac fever), to severe, rapidly fatal pneumonia. Although "Legionnaires' disease" is considered by many to be synonymous with clinical and radiographic evidence of pneumonia, individuals studied in outbreaks and found to demonstrate seroconversion to *L. pneumophila* have also presented with mild systemic symptoms (fever, chills, malaise, anorexia, and myalgias) alone, severe non-bloody diarrhoea alone, and encephalopathy suggestive of a primary neurological problem. Among 15 patients in the Wadsworth Medical Center who had seroconversion to *L. pneumophila*, only seven developed pneumonia; the others had subclinical or mild illnesses (Haley *et al.*, 1979).

A patient infected with *L. pneumophila* typically develops a prodrome of malaise, anorexia, fever, chills, and myalgias after a two- to ten-day incubation period. Non-bloody diarrhoea, occasionally severe, and non-productive cough are frequently present at this stage, and pleuritic chest pain, headache, dyspnoea, and confusion may also occur. Fever, chills, rigors, and pulmonary symptoms progress over the ensuing three to five days and hospitalization frequently becomes necessary. Coryza, rash, sore throat, conjunctivitis, mucous membrane lesions, and photophobia are not features typical of Legionnaires' disease.

Physical findings include fever, tachycardia (though the heart rate is often relatively slow for the observed temperature), tachypnoea, râles, and rhonchi. Signs of consolidation are less frequently present, while hepatosplenomegaly and lymphadenopathy are not commonly seen.

Laboratory findings include leucocytosis with an increased percentage of early forms, an increased erythrocyte sedimentation rate, and hypoxaemia with an accompanying respiratory alkalosis. Proteinuria, microscopic haematuria, azotaemia, hypophosphataemia, elevated serum transaminases, and hyponatraemia, occasionally associated with inappropriate secretion of antidiuretic hormone, have also been commonly observed. Gram stain examination and routine culture of sputum, as well as standard blood, urine, and stool cultures are unrevealing. Radiological abnormalities can include patchy, occasionally nodular, segmental, or lobar alveolar infiltrates, either unilateral or bilateral in distribution (Storch *et al.*, 1981). Interstitial infiltrates are not a feature of Legionnaires' disease. Pleural effusions are not uncommon, but are usually small in size and limited to one side of the thorax. Abscess formation and cavitation have been observed infrequently.

Pneumonia due to *L. micdadei*, *L. bozemanii*, and *L. dumoffii* is similar to the pneumonia caused by *L. pneumophila*, although only a small number of cases have been observed (Cordes *et al.*, 1979; Lewallen *et al.*, 1979; Myerowitz *et al.*, 1979; Rogers *et al.*, 1979; Thomason *et al.*, 1979). As with *L. pneumophila*, the other species seem to have a predilection for causing illness in individuals with underlying conditions associated with immunosuppression (i.e. lymphoma, leukaemia) and in those receiving immunosuppressant drugs (i.e. renal transplant patients). Whether other factors recognized to predispose to infection with *L. pneumophila* such as, age, male sex, alcohol consumption, cigarette smoking, recent travel, and proximity to excavation sites also predispose to infection with the other *Legionella* species remains to be determined.

B. Pontiac Fever

L. pneumophila is the cause of Pontiac fever, a non-pneumonic, acute, self-limited, febrile illness which has only been recognized in two epidemics (Fraser *et al.*, 1979; Glick *et al.*, 1978). Pontiac fever is characterized by a short incubation period (mean of 36 hours) and abrupt onset of symptoms, including fever, malaise, myalgias, and headache. Nausea, dizziness, upper respiratory symptoms, and non-productive cough may be present. Elevated leucocyte counts have been observed, but chest radiographs have been normal. The illness resolves in two to five days without treatment, and long-term sequelae have not been observed.

C. Course and complications

Most cases of Legionnaires' disease have been recognized in patients sufficiently ill to require hospitalization. Among hospitalized cases, various degrees of respiratory insufficiency have been observed, with ventilatory assistance frequently necessary. Renal failure requiring dialysis is occasionally seen. Fatality rates among those not receiving specific therapy range between 15 and 40%, compared to a 5 to 10% fatality rate among those receiving erythromycin. Resolution of clinical symptoms among survivors is gradual, and return of the chest radiograph to normal is frequently delayed. Patients who recover may continue to complain of dyspnoea, chest pain, and weakness for several months, and diminished pulmonary diffusing capacity may persist for years.

D. Therapy

Although *L. pneumophila* has been shown to be sensitive to antibiotics on the basis of *in vitro* tests of minimal inhibitory concentrations (see above), only rifampin and erythromycin prevent death of infected embryonated eggs and guinea pigs (Fraser *et al.*, 1978; Lewis *et al.*, 1978). Controlled prospective clinical trials of antimicrobial therapy have not been performed, but retrospective studies of the outcome of cases treated with a variety of antibiotic regimens show that erythromycin was associated with the lowest fatality rates (Broome *et al.*, 1979; Fraser *et al.*, 1977). Oral or intravenous erythromycin at a dose of 2 to 4 grams per day for 14 to 21 days is the usual regimen employed. Rifampin has generally been reserved for use in patients responding poorly to erythromycin and those with associated lung abscess.

The treatment of pneumonia caused by the other *Legionella* species has not been studied in a systematic fashion, either in animals or man. The use of erythromycin as described above would appear to be the most reasonable choice at the moment, although the absence of beta-lactamase production by *L. micdadei* suggests that penicillin might be effective in patients infected with this organism.

V. PATHOLOGY

Early reports on the pathological findings in Legionnaires' disease dealt primarily with the changes found in the lung (Carrington, 1979; Winn *et al.*, 1978, 1979). Pathological changes in the lungs of patients with pneumonia caused by the other *Legionella* species are similar to those described for *L. pneumophila* (Cordes *et al.*, 1979; Lewallen *et al.*, 1979; Myerowitz *et al.*, 1979; Rogers *et al.*, 1979; Thacker *et al.*, 1978). Gross findings typically include congestion and bronchopneumonia with areas of consolidation. Although significant haemorrhage is uncommon, abscess formation and cavitation have been observed. Microscopically, prominent features include intra-alveolar infiltrates composed of neutrophils, macrophages, and fibrin, as well as fibrinous pleuritis. Disruption of neutrophils and macrophages is frequently seen. Lymphocytes and granuloma formation are not features of Legionnaires' disease. All of these findings are similar to those observed in bacterial pneumonia of other aetiologies and are not distinctive.

L. pneumophila has been found in extrapulmonary sites including hilar and thoracic lymph nodes, kidney, spleen, and liver (Watts *et al.*, 1980; White *et al.*, 1980; Weisenburger *et al.*, 1979). It has also been isolated from blood cultures (Edelstein *et al.*, 1979; McDade *et al.*, 1979). Focal myocarditis associated with DFA-staining bacteria has recently been reported (White *et al.*, 1980).

VI. PATHOGENESIS

A variety of toxins from *L. pneumophila* have been demonstrated, but their role in human illness remains undetermined. *L. pneumophila* produces haemolysis *in vitro*, and the plasma and urine of experimentally infected rabbits have haemolytic activity (Baine, 1979). *L. pneumophila* also produces an endotoxin which demonstrates activity in the Limulus assay and causes fever in rabbits (Highsmith *et al.*, 1978), as well as a cytotoxin (Friedman *et al.*,

1980), and a protease (Muller, 1980). *L. pneumophila* has been demonstrated to be capable of intracellular multiplication in cultured human embryonic lung fibroblasts and monocytes (Horwitz and Silverstein, 1980; Wong *et al.*, 1978).

VII. EPIDEMIOLOGY

The epidemiology of legionellosis has been the subject of intense study since the discovery of Legionnaires' disease in 1976. It is now clear that Legionnaires' disease occurs sporadically and in explosive point-source epidemics; between these two extremes are situations in which Legionnaires' disease and/or serological evidence of exposure to the bacterium are so strikingly common that infection seems to be "hyperendemic". More than 23 clusters of cases of illness due to *L. pneumophila* (21 of Legionnaires' disease, 2 of Pontiac fever), either epidemic or hyperendemic in pattern, have been identified to date; 20 in the U.S., 1 in Spain, 1 in Italy, and several in the U.K. These clusters have ranged in size from 2 to over 200 cases, with more than 1100 individuals being affected overall. Two clusters of cases of pneumonia due to *L. micdadei* have also been recognized (Myerowitz, 1980; Rogers *et al.*, 1979).

Epidemics have usually been associated with exposure to a building (hospital, office building, hotel, convention centre, or factory) and in four outbreaks, heat rejection systems (cooling towers, evaporative condensers, steam turbine condensers) have been epidemiologically implicated as the source (Cordes *et al.*, 1980; Dondero *et al.*, 1980; Fraser *et al.*, 1979; Glick *et al.*, 1978). Other epidemics have occurred, however, where no such systems existed. Point-source epidemics have usually occurred in late summer and autumn (August–November).

L. pneumophila is a cause of nosocomial pneumonia, both in sporadic cases, hyperendemic situations, and point-source epidemics (Broome *et al.*, 1979; Cohen *et al.*, 1979; Dondero *et al.*, 1980; Haley *et al.*, 1979; Marks *et al.*, 1979; Tobin *et al.*, 1980). One study has shown that 10 (3.8%) of 263 patients with fatal nosocomial pneumonia from 40 hospitals in 24 states had Legionnaires' disease (Cohen *et al.*, 1979). Patients with underlying illnesses or receiving medications which are associated with immunosuppression are at greatest risk, but male sex, increasing age, and history of alcohol or cigarette use are predisposing factors.

Over 1800 cases of sporadic Legionnaires' disease have been reported to the Centers for Disease Control from virtually every state in the U.S. Cases have also been recognized in Australia, Austria, Belgium, Canada, Denmark, Israel, Italy, Japan, the Netherlands, New Zealand, South Africa, Spain, Sweden, Switzerland and the U.K. Sporadic Legionnaires' disease occurs throughout the year, but more commonly in the summer and autumn. It is associated with the same underlying risk factors as those mentioned above, in addition to a history of recent travel and living near excavation sites (Storch *et al.*, 1979). Legionnaires' disease has been reported in children and infants, but is uncommon in this age group (Orme *et al.*, 1980; Ryan *et al.*, 1979).

Studies of paired sera and tissue samples submitted for testing from patients with pneumonia of uncertain aetiology have shown that from 1 to 5% of these patients had Legionnaires' disease, though more cases would probably have been found if a wider array of serogroups had been included in the testing battery (Foy *et al.*, 1979; Grady and Gilfillan, 1979; Renner *et al.*, 1979). Frequency of prior exposure to *L. pneumophila*, as measured by detection of antibodies with the IFA method, has been examined among non-ill individuals in a variety of geographic settings and occupational groups. Titres ≥ 128 have been found in 1.3 to over 20% of those tested in various geographical areas (Broome *et al.*, 1979; Cordes *et al.*, 1980; Dondero *et al.*, 1979; Haley *et al.*, 1979; Politi *et al.*, 1979). Employees at a hospital experiencing an epidemic of Legionnaires' disease have been shown to have a higher prevalence of antibody titres ≥ 128 to *L. pneumophila* compared with a nearby control population (Haley *et al.*, 1979), and hospital employees who have worked with patients with Legionnaires' disease have been demonstrated to have a higher rate of seropositivity than employees without patient contact (Saravolatz *et al.*, 1979). It should be noted that the latter study used a haemagglutination assay to measure antibodies, a test of uncertain specificity and sensitivity, that no correlation between amount of patient contact and seropositivity was found, and that other studies have failed to confirm this finding. A serosurvey of air-conditioning maintenance personnel found no increased prevalence of antibodies to *L. pneumophila* compared to control populations (Goldman and Marr, 1980).

The epidemiology of illness caused by the other *Legionella* species is unknown, but it appears that there will be similarities to that described for *L. pneumophila*. The underlying risk factors which predispose to infection, the clinical findings, and the distribution of the organisms in the environment appear to be similar to those of *L. pneumophila*. The potential for nosocomial acquisition of infection with *L. micdadei* has already been well demonstrated.

VIII. MODE OF TRANSMISSION

Airborne transmission via aerosols of contaminated water has been the presumed manner of spread in a number of epidemics. Generation of such aerosols has been caused by air-conditioning and heat-rejection systems. Airborne spread via dust from an excavation site has been implicated in one outbreak (Thacker *et al.*, 1978), as has the use of compressed air to clean mud from a steam turbine condenser (Fraser *et al.*, 1979). Potable water has also been suggested as a source of infection, though the evidence to date is circumstantial (Cordes *et al.*, 1981; Tobin *et al.*, 1980). Finally, it is worth noting that two patients with pneumonia caused by other *Legionella* species experienced immersion in fresh water prior to their illness (Cordes *et al.*, 1981; Thomason *et al.*, 1979). Person-to-person spread of the organism has not been demonstrated.

IX. ENVIRONMENTAL ASPECTS

Legionella species have been isolated from a variety of sites in the environment, including lakes, streams, mud, cooling towers, evaporative condensers, and potable water (Cordes *et al.*, 1981; Fliermans *et al.*, 1979, 1981; Morris *et al.*, 1979; Tobin *et al.*, 1980). *L. pneumophila* has been shown to survive in distilled water for over four months and in tap water for over a year (Skaliy, 1979). It has been demonstrated that *L. pneumophila* grows well in the presence of blue-green algae, and that under these conditions, its temperature, pH, and nutritional requirements are less stringent than when grown on artificial media (Tison *et al.*, 1980). It has also been suggested that free-living amoebae may contribute to the growth of *Legionella* species in aquatic environments (Rowbotham, 1980).

Preliminary work has been done on the effectiveness of biocidal agents against *L. pneumophila* (Grace *et al.*, 1981; Skaliy, 1980). Suspensions of *L. pneumophila* in tap water have been tested against a variety of biocides frequently used in cooling towers and evaporative condensers; chlorine, 2,2-dibromo-3-nitrilopropionamide, and a compound containing didecyl dimethyl ammonium chloride and isopropanol were effective in destroying concentrations of 10^5–10^6 viable cells ml^{-1}. Other compounds, including phenolics, were less effective. Similar studies on the effectiveness of these compounds in cooling towers and evaporative condensers have not yet been performed.

REFERENCES

Baine, W. B., Rasheed, J. K., Maca, H. W. and Kaufmann, A. F. (1979). *Rev. Infec. Dis.* **1**, 912–916.

Brenner, D. J., Steigerwalt, A. G., Weaver, R. E. *et al.* (1978). *Curr. Microbiol.* **1**, 71–75.

Brenner, D. J., Steigerwalt, A. G. and McDade, J. E. (1979). *Ann. Intern. Med.* **90**, 656–658.

Brenner, D. J., Steigerwalt, A. G., Gorman, G. W., Weaver, R. E., Feeley, J. C., Cordes, L. G., Wilkinson, H. W., Patton, C., Thomason, B. M. and Sasseville, K. R. (1980). *Curr. Microbiol.* **4**, 111–116.

Broome, C. V., Cherry, W. B. and Winn, W. C., Jr *et al.* (1979). *Ann. Intern. Med.* **90**, 1–4.

Broome, C. V. and Fraser, D. W. (1979). *Epidemiol. Rev.* **1**, 1–16.

Broome, C. V., Goings, S. A. J., Thacker, S. B. *et al.* (1979). *Ann. Intern. Med.* **90**, 573–577.

Carrington, C. B. (1979). *Ann. Intern. Med.* **90**, 496–499.

Cherry, W. B. and McKinney, R. M. (1979). Detection of Legionnaires' disease bacteria in clinical specimens by direct immunofluorescence. *In* "Legionnaires', the disease, the bacterium and methodology" (G. L. Jones and G. A. Hebert, ed.), pp. 99–103. Center for Disease Control, Atlanta, Georgia.

Cherry, W. B., Pittman, B., Harris, P. P. *et al.* (1978). *J. Clin. Microbiol.* **8**, 329–338.

Cohen, M. L., Broome, C. V., Paris, A. L. *et al.* (1979). *Ann. Intern. Med.* **90**, 611–613.

Cordes, L. G., Goldman, W. D., Marr, J. S. *et al.* (1980). *Bull. N.Y. Acad. Med.* **56**, 467–482.

Cordes, L. G., Wilkinson, H. W., Gorman, G. W. *et al.* (1979). *Lancet* **2**, 927–930.

Cordes, L. G., Fraser, D. W., Skaliy, P., Perlino, C. A., Elsea, W. R., Mallison, G. F. and Hayes, P. S. (1980). *Amer. J. Epidemiol.* **111**, 425–431.

Cordes, L. G., Wiesenthal, A. M., Gorman, G. W. *et al.* (1981). *Ann. Intern. Med.* **94**, 195–197.

Dondero, T. J., Jr, Clegg, H. W., Tsai, T. F. *et al.* (1979). *Ann. Intern. Med.* **90**, 569–573.

Dondero, T. J., Rendtorff, R. C., Mallison, G. F., Weeks, R. M., Levy, J. S., Wong, E. W. and Schaffner, W. (1980). *N. Engl. J. Med.* **302**, 365–370.

Edelstein, P. H. and Finegold, S. M. (1979). *J. Clin. Microbiol.* **10**, 141–143.

Edelstein, P. H., Meyer, R. D. and Finegold, S. M. (1979). *Lancet* **1**, 750–751.

Edelstein, P. H. and Meyer, R. D. (1980). *Amer. Rev. Resp. Dis.* **121**, 317–327.

Edelstein, P. H., McKinney, R. M., Meyer, R. D., Edelstein, M. A. C., Krause, C. A. and Finegold, S. M. (1980). *J. Infect. Dis.* **141**, 652–655.

Edson, D. C., Stiefel, H. E., Wentworth, B. B. *et al.* (1979). *Ann. Intern. Med.* **90**, 691–693.

England, A. C., III, McKinney, R. M., Skaliy, P. and Gorman, G. W. (1980). *Ann. Intern. Med.* **93**, 58–59.

Farshy, C. E., Cruce, D. D., Klein, G. C. *et al.* (1979). *Ann. Intern. Med.* **90**, 690.

Farshy, C. E., Klein, G. C. and Feeley, J. C. (1978). *J. Clin. Microbiol.* **7**, 327–331.

Feeley, J. C., Gorman, G. W., Weaver, R. E. *et al.* (1978). *J. Clin. Microbiol.* **8**, 320–325.

Feeley, J. C., Gibson, R. T. J., Gorman, G. W. *et al.* (1979). *J. Clin. Microbiol.* **10**, 437–441.

Fliermans, C. B., Cherry, W. B., Orrison, L. H. *et al.* (1979). *Appl. Environ. Microbiol.* **37**, 1239–1242.

Fliermans, C. B., Cherry, W. B., Orrison, L. Y., Smith, S. J., Tison, D. L. and Pope, D. H. (1981). *Appl. Environ. Microbiol.* **4**, 9–16.

Foy, H. M., Broome, C. V., Hayes, P. S. *et al.* (1979). *Lancet* **1**, 767–770.

Fraser, D. W., Tsai, T. F., Orenstein, W. *et al.* (1977). *N. Engl. J. Med.* **297**, 1189–1197.

Fraser, D. W., Wachsmuth, I. K., Bopp, C. *et al.* (1978). *Lancet* **1**, 175–177.

Fraser, D. W., Deubner, D. C., Hill, D. L. *et al.* (1979). *Science* **205**, 691–692.

Friedman, R. L., Iglewski, B. H., Miller, R. D. (1980). *Infect. Immun.* **29**, 271–274.

Glick, T. H., Gregg, M. D., Berman, B. *et al.* (1978). *Amer. J. Epidemiol.* **107**, 149–160.

Goldman, W. D. and Marr, J. S. (1980). *Appl. Environ. Microbiol.* **40**, 114–116.

Grace, R. D., Dewar, H. E., Barnes, W. G. and Hodges, G. R. (1981). *Appl. Environ. Microbiol.* **41**, 233–236.

Grady, G. F. and Gilfillan, R. F. (1979). *Ann. Intern. Med.* **90**, 607–610.

Greaves, P. W. (1980). *J. Clin. Path.* **33**, 581–584.

Grist, N. R., Reid, D. and Hamera, R. (1979). *Ann. Intern. Med.* **90**, 563–564.

Gump, D. W., Frank, R. O., Winn, W. C., Jr *et al.* (1979). *Ann. Intern. Med.* **90**, 538–542.

Haley, C. E., Cohen, M. L., Halter, J. *et al.* (1979). *Ann. Intern. Med.* **90**, 583–586.

Hebert, G. A., Steigerwalt, A. G. and Brenner, D. J. (1980). *Curr. Microbiol.* **3**, 255–257.

Hebert, G. A. (1981). *J. Clin. Microbiol.* **13**, 240–242.

Highsmith, A. K., Mackel, D. C., Baine, W. B., Anderson, R. L. and Fraser, D. W. (1978). *Curr. Microbiol.* **1**, 315–317.

Horwitz, M. A. and Silverstein, S. C. (1980). *J. Clin. Invest.* **66**, 441–450.

Lattimer, G. L., Ormsbee, R. A., Peacock, M. G. and Rhodes, L. V. (1979). *Scand. J. Infect. Dis.* **11**, 271–273.

Lewallen, K. R., McKinney, R. M., Brenner, D. J., Moss, C. W., Kail, D. H., Thomason, B. M. and Bright, R. A. (1979). *Ann. Intern. Med.* **91**, 831–834.

Lewis, V. J., Thacker, W. L., Shephard, C. C. *et al.* (1977). *Antimicrob. Agents Chemother.* **13**, 419–422.

McDade, J. E., Shepard, C. C., Fraser, D. W. *et al.* (1977). *N. Engl. J. Med.* **297**, 1197–1203.

McDade, J. E., Brenner, D. J. and Bozeman, F. M. (1979). *Ann. Intern. Med.* **90**, 659–661.

McKinney, R. M., Thacker, L., Harris, P. P. *et al.* (1979). *Ann. Intern. Med.* **90**, 621–624.

McKinney, R. M., Wilkinson, H. W., Sommers, H. M. *et al.* (1980). *J. Clin. Microbiol.* **12**, 395–401.

Marks, J. S., Tsai, T. F., Martone, W. J. *et al.* (1979). *Ann. Intern. Med.* **90**, 565–569.

Morris, G. K., Patton, C. M., Feeley, J. C. *et al.* (1979). *Ann. Intern. Med.* **90**, 664–666.

Morris, G. K., Steigerwalt, A., Feeley, J. C. *et al.* (1980). *J. Clin. Microbiol.* **12**, 718–721.

Moss, C. W., Weaver, R. D. and Dees, S. B. (1977). *J. Clin. Microbiol.* **6**, 140–143.

Moss, C. W. and Dees, S. B. (1979). *J. Clin. Microbiol.* **9**, 648–649.

Muller, H. E. (1980). *Infect. Immun.* **27**, 51–53.

Myerowitz, R. L., Pasculle, A. W., Dowling, J. W., Pazin, G. J., Puerzer, M., Yee, R. B., Rinaldo, G. R. and Hakala, T. R. (1979). *N. Engl. J. Med.* **301**, 953–958.

Oldenburger, D., Carson, J. P., Gundlach, W. J., Ghaly, F. I. and Wright, W. H. (1979). *J.A.M.A.* **241**, 1269–1270.

Orme, R. L. E., Haas, L., Cruickshank, J. G., Hart, R. J. C. and Anderson, A. W. (1980). *Lancet* **2**, 1027.

Ormsbee, R. A., Peacock, M. G., Lattimer, G. L., Page, L. A. and Fiset, P. (1978). *J. Infect. Dis.* **138**, 260–264.

Pasculle, A. W., Feeley, J. C., Gibson, R. J. *et al.* (1980). *J. Infect. Dis.* **141**, 727–732.

Pine, L., George, J. R., Reeves, M. W. and Harrell, W. K. (1979). *J. Clin. Microbiol.* **9**, 615–626.

Politi, B. D., Fraser, D. W., Mallison, G. F. *et al.* (1979). *Ann. Intern. Med.* **90**, 587–591.

Renner, E. D., Helms, C. M., Hierholzer, W. J., Jr *et al.* (1979). *Ann. Intern. Med.* **90**, 603–606.

Ristroph, J. D., Hedlund, K. W. and Allen, R. G. (1980). *J. Clin. Microbiol.* **11**, 19–21.

Rogers, B. W., Donowitz, G. R., Walker, G. H., Harding, S. A. and Sande, M. A. (1979). *N. Engl. J. Med.* **301**, 959–961.

Rowbotham, T. J. (1980). *Lancet* **2**, 969.

Ryan, M. E., Feldman, S., Pruitt, B. and Fraser, D. W. (1979). *Pediatrics* **64**, 951–953.

Saravolatz, L., Arking, L., Wentworth, B. *et al.* (1979). *Ann. Intern. Med.* **90**, 601–603.

Saravolatz, L. D., Pohlod, D. J. and Quinn, E. L. (1980). *Scand. J. Infect. Dis.* **12**, 215–219.

Skaliy, P. and McEachern, H. V. (1979). *Ann. Intern. Med.* **90**, 662–663.

Skaliy, P., Thompson, T. A., Gorman, G. W., Morris, G. K., McEachern, H. V. and Mackel, D. C. (1980). *Appl. Environ. Microbiol.* **40**, 697–700.

Storch, G., Baine, W. B., Fraser, D. W. *et al.* (1979). *Ann. Intern. Med.* **90**, 596–600.

Storch, G., Hayes, P. S., Hill, D. L. *et al.* (1979). *J. Infect. Dis.* **140**, 784–788.

Storch, G., Sagel, S. S. and Baine, W. B. (1981). *J.A.M.A.* **245**, 587–590.

Suffin, S. C., Kaufmann, A. F., Whitaker, B., Muck, K. B., Prince, G. A. and Porter, D. D. (1980). *Arch. Pathol. Lab. Med.* **104**, 283–286.

Thacker, S. B., Bennett, J. V., Tsai, T. F. *et al.* (1978). *J. Infect. Dis.* **138**, 512–519.

Thomason, B. M., Harris, P. P., Hicklin, M. D., Blackmon, J. A., Moss, W. and Matthews, F. (1979). *Ann. Intern. Med.* **91**, 673–676.

Thornsberry, C., Baker, C. N. and Kirven, L. A. (1978). *Antimicrob. Agents Chemother.* **13**, 78–80.

Tilton, R. C. (1979). *Ann. Intern. Med.* **90**, 697–698.

Tison, D. L., Pope, D. H., Cherry, W. B. and Fliermans, C. B. (1980). *Appl. Environ. Microbiol.* **39**, 456–459.

Tobin, J. O'H., Dunhill, M. S., French, M. *et al.* (1980). *Lancet* **2**, 118–121.

Warren, W. J. and Miller, R. D. (1979). *J. Clin. Microbiol.* **10**, 50–55.

Watts, J. C., Hicklin, M. D., Thomason, B. M., Callaway, C. S. and Levine, A. J. (1980). *Ann. Intern. Med.* **92**, 186–188.

Weisenburger, D. D., Helms, C. M., Viner, J. P. *et al.* (1979). *Arch. Path. Lab. Med.* **103**, 153.

White, H. J., Felton, W. W. and Sun, C. N. (1980). *Arch. Pathol. Lab. Med.* **104**, 287–289.

Wilkinson, H. W., Farshy, C. E., Fikes, B. J. *et al.* (1979). *J. Clin. Microbiol.* **10**, 685–689.

Wilkinson, H. W., Cruce, D. D. and Broome, C. V. (1981). *J. Clin. Microbiol.* **13**, 139–146.

Winn, W. C., Jr, Glavin, F. L., Perl, D. P. *et al.* (1979). *Ann. Intern. Med.* **90**, 548–551.

Winn, W. C., Jr, Glavin, F. L., Peri, D. P. *et al.* (1978). *Arch. Path. Lab. Med.* **102**, 344–350.

Wong, M. C., Ewing, E. P., Callaway, C. S. and Peacock, W. L. (1980). *Infect. Immun.* **28**, 1014–1018.

7 Staphylococcal alpha-toxin as a biological tool

IWAO KATO

I. INTRODUCTION

Staphylococcus aureus is known to produce a number of extracellular toxic proteins (Jeljaszewicz, 1978). One of these, staphylococcal alpha-toxin, has been the most intensely studied of the staphylococcal toxins. Alpha-toxin has been considered to play a significant role in the pathogenesis of staphylococcal infection and has been reported to affect numerous cells and tissues both *in vivo* and *in vitro*. The biological properties most typical of this toxin are its lethal effect for laboratory animals, its marked haemolytic effect for rabbit erythrocytes, its ability to cause dermonecrosis, and its ability to cause contraction and paralysis of smooth muscle, which has been termed "spastic paralysis". Apart from being haemolytic, alpha-toxin is cytotoxic and cytolytic to a wide variety of cell types. Therefore, it has been suggested that the toxin be called a membrane-damaging toxin (McCartney and Arbuthnott, 1978) or a cytolytic toxin (Bernheimer, 1974), rather than a haemolysin, in order to use a term that provides a more accurate description of the toxin's biological activity. Many strains of *S. aureus* produce four known cytolysins (α-, β-, γ-, and δ-toxins) each of which is capable of exerting profound effects on cell membranes. Thus it is mandatory to exclude trace amounts of the other cytolytic toxins in studies of the mode of action of alpha-toxin. Failures to meet the criteria for purity led to some of the conflicting reports published in the 1960s. In the past decade several groups have reported purification of alpha-toxin. These purification procedures have been summarized and discussed in two recent reviews (Arbuthnott, 1970 and Wiseman, 1975). Watanabe and Kato (1974) utilized a novel procedure to obtain crystallized toxin by zone-electrophoresis and studied its physicochemical and biological properties.

This review will only devote a limited amount of discussion to the structure of staphylococcal alpha-toxin protein and to the toxic action of the alpha-toxin at the molecular level.

II. STRUCTURE AND MODE OF ACTION OF STAPHYLOCOCCAL ALPHA-TOXIN

A. Structure

1. Purification and crystallization

The Wood 46 strain of *Staphylococcus aureus* used is considered to produce much more alpha-toxin than most staphylococcal strains. A highly purified staphylococcal alpha-toxin was obtained by a combination of procedures, such as precipitation with zinc chloride, gel-filtration on Sephadex G-25, zone-electrophoresis on starch and pevikon, and column chromatography on CM-Sephadex C-50. A 435-fold increase in the specific activity was attained and approximately 24% of the alpha-toxin in the crude material was recovered in the pure form. Several attempts were made to obtain the highly purified alpha-toxin in a crystalline form, among which dialysis against concentrated ammonium sulphate solution at 4°C gave the most satisfactory result.

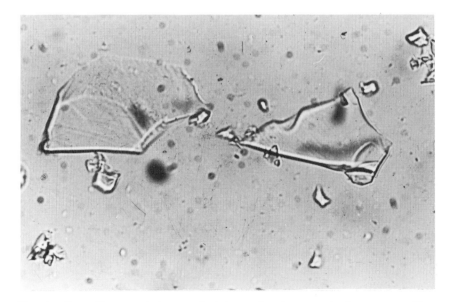

Fig. 1 Crystalline staphylococcal alpha-toxin photographed at a magnification of ×360.

Crystallization of alpha-toxin was achieved by dialysing the highly purified toxin preparation against a saturated ammonium sulphate solution (pH 7.0) at 4°C for 3 days. The crystallized alpha-toxin protein showed the plate or rhomboidal form (Fig. 1). The purified alpha-toxin preparation showed a single band in electrophoresis in polyacrylamide gel at various concentrations containing 0.1% sodium dodecylsulphate and in agar gel immunodiffusion. It proved to be homogeneous.

2. Physical nature

Estimates for the molecular weight of the alpha-toxin protein vary from 22 000 to 39 000, depending on the methods used for isolation and determination of molecular weight. Nearly all investigators used strain Wood 46, so variation in molecular weight due to strain differences is not a factor. Two stable forms of alpha-toxin, designated A and B, were isolated from broth cultures of Wood 46 strain of *S. aureus* by Six and Harshman (1973). The sedimentation coefficient of alpha-toxin is 2.8–3.14 S. However, the toxin can also exist in a 12 S form. The 3 S form aggregates or polymerizes into the 12 S form. Approximately 8–15% of purified alpha-toxin preparation consists of the 12 S component (Bernheimer and Schwartz, 1963; Lominski *et al.*, 1963). In Ouchterlony double diffusion tests, purified 12 S material gave a line of partial identity with the main alpha-toxin line of precipitation. The purified 12 S material also had a strikingly uniform appearance when examined by negative staining in the electron microscope. It consisted of small rings having an outside diameter of approximately 9 nm, which appeared to consist of a hexagonal arrangement of six subunits each measuring 2–2.5 nm in diameter. McNiven and Arbuthnott (1972) estimated the molecular weight of the 12 S material to be 170 000. This indicated that each of the six subunits was a 3 S monomer with an approximate molecular weight of 28 000. By electrofocussing, the highly purified alpha-toxin had isoelectric point (pI) values of 7.2–8.5 and our crystalline toxin had a pI of 8.0.

3. Isolation of lethal toxic and haemolytic fragments from alpha-toxin by tryptic digestion

The crystallized alpha-toxin, one polypeptide chain with a molecular weight of approximately 36 000, has been proved to be endowed with diverse biological properties, such as lethal, dermonecrotic, and haemolytic activities (Watanabe and Kato, 1976). However, the relationship between its chemical structure and its mechanism of action at the molecular level is not fully understood. Since the purified alpha-toxin is devoid of free SH-groups and disulphide bridges, the toxin was subjected to proteolytic treatment with the aim of obtaining split products which might be more amenable to structural studies. Watanabe and Kato (1978) reported that the purified alpha-toxin treated with trypsin yielded two components by sodium dodecyl sulphate (SDS)-polyacrylamide gel electrophoresis. A heavy chain fragment (molecular weight 17 000) had lethal activity in mice but lacked haemolytic and dermonecrotic activities, whereas a light fragment (molecular weight 14 000) had unstable haemolytic activity which was reduced to 10% of the original values. The time course of the digestion of the purified alpha-toxin by trypsin was followed by a SDS-slab polyacrylamide gel electrophoresis (Fig. 2). The position of the heavy and light chain fragments of alpha-toxin was established by staining a few gels. The relevant regions of the unstained gels were removed, pooled, homogenized with 0.03% SDS and extracted overnight with the detergent. The extracts were lyophilized and used for the analyses of amino acid compositions and N-terminal amino acid residues. Both the lethal toxic (heavy chain) fragment and haemolytic (light chain) fragment were separated. Trypsin-digested alpha-toxin (2h-digest) was applied to a column of Sephadex G-200 and starch zone-electrophoresis. The purified lethal toxic fragment had a lethal activity (LD_{50}) of 8 μg for mice. However, the purified

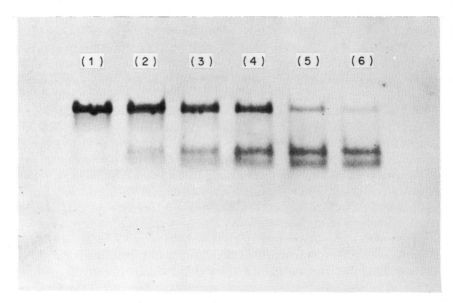

Fig. 2 Electrophoresis of trypsin-treated alpha-toxin on slab SDS-poly-acrylamide gels.
The purified alpha-toxin (2 mg ml^{-1} in 0.05 M sodium phosphate buffer, pH 7.0) was incubated for the indicated time in the presence of trypsin (40 μg ml^{-1}) at 25°C. Each sample was then treated at 100°C for 3 min in 1% SDS, and 15 μg of each were electrophoresed on 0.1% SDS gels. The gels show samples treated for (1) 0 min, (2) 10 min, (3) 30 min, (4) 1 h, (5) 3 h, and (6) 6 h with trypsin. H-chain: heavy chain subunit (lethal toxic fragment). L-chain: light chain subunit (haemolytic fragment).

lethal toxic fragment had no haemolytic activity in contrast with the high haemolytic activity (1×10^5 HU mg^{-1}) of native alpha-toxin, and had only traces of dermonecrotic activity; more than 123 µg had to be injected to give a positive reaction in rabbit skin in contrast with 0.03 µg of native alpha-toxin. The light chain fragment had a haemolytic activity of 1×10^4 haemolytic unit (HU) mg $^{-1}$ for rabbit erythrocytes and had a dermonecrotic activity of 0.4 µg. Immunodiffusion analyses, using antitoxin raised against alpha-toxin, showed that lethal toxic and haemolytic fragments were antigenically distinct from each other but were partially identified with native alpha-toxin. Purified lethal toxic fragment ($200 \, \text{LD}_{50}$) were completely neutralized by 1 ml of specific rabbit antiserum against the purified lethal toxic fragment. When neutralization of haemolytic activity of alpha-toxin by specific antiserum to purified lethal toxic fragment was investigated, the anti-haemolytic titre of antiserum to purified lethal toxic fragment was only 1:32. On the contrary, both antiserum to native alpha-toxin and commercial (Wellcome) antitoxin showed high neutralizing titres of 1024 and 512, respectively. These findings indicate that the specific antiserum to the lethal toxic fragment was strongly antitoxic but only weakly antihaemolytic.

4. Chemical nature of alpha-toxin and its fragment

The amino acid composition of alpha-toxin and its heavy and light chain fragments are summarized in Table 1. Amino acid analyses indicate different contents of lysine, histidine, threonine, methionine, and tyrosine in the two fragments. The lethal toxic fragment is distinctive in containing only one histidine residue. In experiments where we wanted to examine the effects of photo-oxidation of the histidine residue (Weil and Buchert, 1951), exposure of the lethal toxic fragment to visible light in the presence of methylene blue at pH 8.0 resulted in a 60% loss of lethal activity in mice. The total molecular weight and number of amino acid residues in the two fragments are 31 000 and 268, respectively (Table 1). When the alpha-toxin molecule is cleaved simultaneously in more than one position by trypsin, one or several small peptide(s) of no more than ten amino acids each (e.g. 26 amino acid residues in Table 1) are lost during fragment isolation procedures. Amino-terminal analysis of alpha-toxin and its lethal toxic and haemolytic fragments, performed by the dansyl chloride method (Gray, 1972), indicated alanine, isoleucine, and alanine residues, respectively. The sequences of the carboxy-methylated alpha-toxin and its lethal toxic fragment were determined by the method of Edman and Begg (1967). The results of the first ten cycles are summarized as follows:

$$
\begin{array}{ccccccccccc}
 & 1 & 2 & 3 & 4 & 5 & 6 & 7 & 8 & 9 & 10 \\
\text{Alpha-toxin: } \text{NH}_2- & \text{Ala} & \text{Asp} & \text{Ser} & \text{Asp} & \text{Ile} & \text{Leu} & \text{Asn} & \text{Ile} & \text{Lys} & \text{Pro} & \text{Gly}-
\end{array}
$$

$$
\begin{array}{ccccccccccc}
 & 1 & 2 & 3 & 4 & 5 & 6 & 7 & 8 & 9 & 10 \\
\text{Lethal toxic fragment: } \text{NH}_2- & \text{Ile} & \text{Leu} & \text{Val} & \text{Leu} & \text{His} & \text{Val} & \text{Arg} & \text{Ala} & \text{Val} & \text{Val}-
\end{array}
$$

Table 1   Amino acid composition of alpha-toxin and its heavy chain and light chain subunits from SDS-polyacrylamide gels[a]

	Residues per molecule		
Amino acid	Alpha-toxin (MW 36 000)	Heavy chain (MW 17 000)	Light chain (MW 14 000)
Lysine	31	13	18
Histidine	9	1	8
Arginine	8	6	3
Aspartic acid	43	25	15
Threonine	24	11	11
Serine	21	13	7
Glutamic acid	20	12	9
Proline	10	6	4
Glycine	36	16	12
Alanine	17	7	4
Half-cystine	—	—	—
Valine	19	9	7
Methionine	8	2	4
Isoleucine	16	8	6
Leucine	16	8	6
Tyrosine	7	3	4
Phenylalanine	9	6	3
Total	294	146	122

[a] A 6 hour-digest of the alpha-toxin with trypsin was analysed in a 10% slab polyacrylamide gel in the presence of 0.1% SDS. The stained bands of heavy chain and light chain and undigested alpha-toxin (see Fig. 2) were carefully collected and extracted. Hydrolysis was carried out for 20 h at 110°C in 3 ml 6 N HCl and 0.08 M β-mercaptoethanol to prevent the degradation of tyrosine and histidine. Hydrolysate was analysed by a JEOL model JLC-6AH amino acid analyser.

The sequence of the first 10 amino acid residues from the amino terminal of our crystallized alpha-toxin is in good agreement with that obtained by Six and Harshman (1973) using their alpha-toxin A and B preparations. It has not been possible to subunit the haemolygic fragment to the same degradation because of its poor solubility in the quadrol buffer at 55°C.

The carboxyl-terminal residues of alpha-toxin and its lethal toxic and haemolytic fragments are determined by digestion with carboxypeptidase Y, according to the procedure of Hayashi *et al.* (1973). Similar peptide sequences were isolated from both alpha-toxin and its lethal toxic fragment; –Tyr–Val–Lys–COOH and –Thr–Tyr–Val–Lys–COOH, respectively, while the C-terminal sequence of the haemolytic fragment was –Gly–Arg–COOH. These observations allow the localization of the lethal toxic fragment at the C-terminal moiety of the intact alpha-toxin molecule.

B.   Toxic action

1.   Interaction of alpha-toxin with rabbit erythrocytes

(a)   Kinetics of haemolysis

Haemolytic activity against rabbit erythrocytes was determined by measurement of 50% haemolysis at 541 nm, using Hitachi spectrophotometer. One haemolytic unit of crystalline alpha-toxin was equivalent to 0.01 µg of protein. A spectrophotometric assay of the kinetics of haemolysis of alpha-toxin was introduced by Mangalo and Raynaud (1959) and Kato *et al.* (1975a), who determined a mathematical relationship between the time taken to reach 50% haemolysis and the concentration of alpha-toxin. The S-shaped curves typical of haemolysis by alpha-toxin can be seen in Fig. 3. There is a characteristic prelytic lag phase, followed by a period of rapid haemolysis, taking the slopes of the curves at the time of maximum rate of haemolysis as an index of the velocity of the reaction. The sensitivity of erythrocytes to lysis by alpha-toxin varies greatly. A concentration of alpha-toxin capable of lysing completely

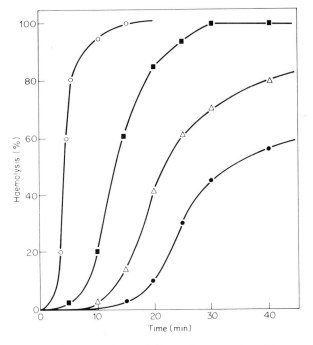

Fig. 3   Kinetics of haemolysis of rabbit erythrocytes by different concentrations of alpha-toxin.
○ =0.5 µg ml^{-1}; ■ =0.1 µg ml^{-1}; △ =0.05 µg ml^{-1}; ● =0.01 µg ml^{-1}.

rabbit erythrocytes will lyse rat, human, or guinea pig erythrocytes less efficiently. The ability of erythrocytes from different animal species to bind [^{125}I]-labelled toxin correlates with cellular haemolytic sensitivity (Table 2). It appears possible that cells with low sensitivities may differ in their receptors for alpha-toxin or may differ in their relative distribution or composition of membrane protein and lipid compared to rabbit erythrocytes.

Table 2 Relative binding of [^{125}I]-labelled alpha-toxin by erythrocytes of different species

Erythrocytes	Haemolytic activity[a] (HU μg^{-1})	[^{125}I]-labelled alpha-toxin bound to erythrocytes (c.p.m. per cell)
Rabbit, maturity	0.019 (100%)	2360 (100%)
Rabbit, reticulocytes	0.038 (50%)	1478 (62%)
Rat	0.437 (4.4%)	204 (8.6%)
Human	2.09 (1.1%)	40 (1.7%)
Guinea pig	6.84 (0.4%)	12 (0.5%)

[a] Haemolytic assays were performed by the method of Bernheimer and Schwartz (1963) utilizing alpha-toxin and an erythrocyte suspension (1×10^9 cells ml^{-1}).

A comparison of the concentrations needed for 50% haemolysis inhibition shows that flavin mononucleotide (FMN) is an order of magnitude more active than riboflavin or alloxazine (Kato *et al.*, 1975b). Riboflavin (vitamin B$_2$) is at least an order of magnitude more active than the phospholipids such as phosphatidylcholine, phosphorylcholine and phosphatidylethanolamine. Treatment of alpha-toxin with alloxazine did not change its haemolytic activity and [^{14}C]-labelled alloxazine did not bind the alpha-toxin. Furthermore, alloxazine, known as an inhibitor of phospholipase A$_2$, inhibited the haemolytic activity of alpha-toxin.

(b) Binding of alpha-toxin to the cell membranes
The binding of [^{125}I]-labelled alpha-toxin to rabbit erythrocytes (1×10^9 cells ml^{-1}) was examined quantitatively at various concentrations from 0.01 to 1 HU ml^{-1}. The maximum binding of [^{125}I]-alpha-toxin to the cells was reached between 5 and 10 min at 20°C. It was calculated that approximately 3.5×10^3 toxin molecules bind to a mature rabbit erythrocyte, which is in close agreement with results obtained by Cassidy and Harshman (1973) who estimated the number of sites to be 5×10^3 per cell. The number of binding sites per rabbit reticulocytes, prepared by the injection of acetylphenylhydrazine, was calculated as 1.6×10^3 per cell. Erythrocytes of different species were assayed for their abilities to bind [^{125}I]-alpha-toxin to find

whether the known haemolytic specificity for rabbit erythrocytes is correlated with specificity of toxin binding (Table 2). At a final concentration of one HU per cell, [^{125}I] alpha-toxin was incubated for the 5 min with each of suspensions of equivalent numbers of rabbit, rat, human, and guinea pig erythrocytes to bind iodinated toxin paralleled to their relative haemolytic sensitivities to unlabelled alpha-toxin. It appears possible that specific receptor substances for alpha-toxin exist in rabbit erythrocyte membranes. Results of the effect of native toxin and concanavalin A on the binding of [^{125}I] alpha-toxin to the cells are presented in Fig. 4. Iodinated toxin binds very effectively to rabbit erythrocytes. This indicates that the total non-specific binding in

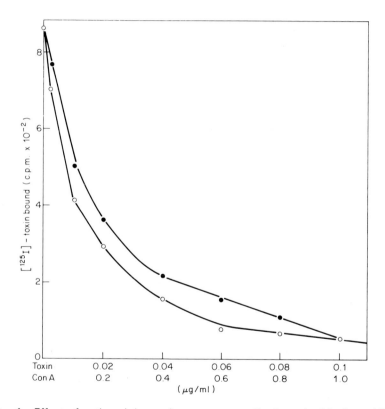

Fig. 4 Effect of native alpha-toxin or concanavalin A on the binding of [^{125}I]-labelled alpha-toxin to rabbit erythrocytes.

Increasing concentrations of native alpha-toxin (unlabelled) or con A were each added to 1 ml of rabbit erythrocyte suspension (6×10^8 cells) in 0.1 M phosphate-buffered saline, pH 7.0. After incubation for 5 min at 20°C, [^{125}I]-labelled alpha-toxin (7×10^4 counts min^{-1} ml^{-1} was added and samples were further incubated for 15 min at 20°C. (○), native alpha-toxin; (●), con A.

relation to the total quantity of radioactive uptake is very small, since virtually all of the bound radioactivity can be selectively blocked by prior addition of native toxin.

(c) Rabbit erythrocyte membrane receptor for alpha-toxin

Rabbit erythrocytes appear to contain approximately 3.5–5×10^3 binding sites per cell compared to no detectable binding sites for human erythrocyte. The chemical nature of the binding site for staphylococcal alpha-toxin has been postulated to exist on erythrocyte membranes by Kato *et al.* (1975b) and Kato and Naiki (1976). However, the exact nature of the receptor remains uncertain. Evidence presented by Kato *et al.* (1975b) demonstrated that alpha-toxin binding and haemolytic sensitivity were considerably reduced when rabbit erythrocytes, 2% v/v final concentration, in 0.05 M phosphate-buffered saline, pH 7.0, were incubated with purified pronase (1 mg ml^{-1}) at 37°C for 60 min with periodic shaking. Furthermore, Kato *et al.* (1975b) obtained some glycoprotein fractions from Bio-gel filtration with the supernatant, soublized by Tween X-100, from pronase treated rabbit erythrocyte ghosts. One of main fractions with molecular weight of about 20 000 containing sialic acid (38%), hexose (23%), hexosamine (24%), and peptides (24%) was found to reduce both haemolytic sensitivity and binding of the alpha-toxin. Kato and Naiki (1976) demonstrated that prior incubation of alpha-toxin with an N-acetylglucosamine-containing ganglioside (GlcNAc-ganglioside, obtained from human erythrocytes) inhibited, in parallel, the ability of the toxin to bind to rabbit erythrocytes and to activate the haemolytic response in the cells and provided evidence that, at least for the erythrocytes, the GlcNAc-ganglioside might resemble, or be part of, the receptor site for the alpha-toxin.

Table 3 shows that the relative order of inhibitory potency of the glycosphingolipids studied, in addition to the approximate concentration required to obtain 50% inhibition of the haemolysis and the specific binding of [125I]-labelled alpha-toxin to rabbit erythrocytes. The most potent inhibitor of both haemolysis by alpha-toxin and of the binding of [125I]-labelled alpha-toxin to the erythrocytes is GlcNAc-ganglioside (NAN), which is effective in final concentrations as low as 10 ng ml^{-1}. Quantitative analyses indicated that 10 ng of GlcNAc-ganglioside (NAN) inactivated approximately 10 HU of alpha-toxin, compared with 10 ng of crystallized preparation which inactivated 1 HU (Watanabe and Kato, 1976). Thus, 1 weight unit of the ganglioside could inactivate up to approximately 10 weight units of toxin. This corresponds to a molar proportion of 2:1 since the molecular weight of GlcNAc-ganglioside (NAN) is 1600 and that of toxin is 36 000. The gangliosides and related neutral glycosylceramides were tested by the double-diffusion-in-agar technique for the capacity to fix and precipitate alpha-toxin.

Only the GlcNAc-ganglioside (NAN) was reactive with toxin, giving a specific fine precipitation line, since the precipitate formed between the toxin and the ganglioside was not due to unspecific precipitation of protein.

Even minor changes in these glycolipid structures severely affected the inhibitory capacities of haemolysis and toxin binding. Both GlcNAc-ganglioside (NGN), in which the terminal galactose is linked to an N-glycolylneuraminic acid (NGN), and paragloboside, which is devoid of the terminal N-acetylneuraminic acid (NAN), had an affinity for alpha-toxin about 500- and 1700-fold, respectively, lower than that of GlcNAc-ganglioside (NAN). It may be concluded, therefore, that the position NANα2-3Galβ1-4GlcNAc-containing ganglioside and/or glycoprotein of rabbit erythrocyte membranes is the critical region for fixation and inactivation of alpha-toxin.

(d)   Effects of lectins on haemolytic activity of alpha-toxin

Further evidence implicating NAN–Gal–GlcNAc– containing glycolipid and/or glycoprotein as the receptor for alpha-toxin was derived from studies with lectins. Lectins, which are cell-agglutinating proteins that recognize specific saccharide sequences in oligosaccharides, have been used widely as molecular probes for determining cell surface structure and dynamics (Sharon and Lis, 1972; Nicolson, 1974). Four purified lectins with different sugar specificities were used: concanavalin A (specific for D-glucose and D-mannose), *Phaseolus vulgaris* phytohaemagglutinin-P (N-acetyl-D-galactosamine), soybean agglutinin (N-acetyl-D-galactosamine and D-galactose), and wheat germ agglutinin (1–4 linked oligosaccharides of N-acetyl-D-glucosamine). Among the lectins used, relatively low concentrations of concanavalin A (con A) and wheat germ agglutinin greatly inhibited the lysis of rabbit erythrocytes by alpha-toxin, while the two other lectins were twenty times less active than con A in inhibiting the lytic activity of the toxin (Table 4). Con A (1 μg ml^{-1}) completely inhibited haemolysis of rabbit erythrocytes by alpha-toxin, and the fact that 0.1 M of α-methyl-D-glucoside and α-methyl-D-mannoside reversed this inhibition of the haemolysis by con A concomitantly with its removal, might indicate that this reversal of the inhibitory effect of con A was rather specific, since neither α-methyl-D-glucoside nor α-methyl-D-mannoside directly inhibited alpha-toxin haemolytic activity. Under the conditions of these experiments, the reason is not yet clear, but it can be considered that the interference with the lytic activity of alpha-toxin produced by these lectins may be due to the specific sugars of different lectins having a partial common structure in the alpha-toxin receptor (NANα2-3Galβ1-4GlcNAc-containing glycolipid and/or glycoprotein), because different lectins have different sugars or surface receptor specificities. Lineweaver Burk plots of alpha-toxin haemolytic activity in the presence and

Table 3 Effect of various glycosphingolipids and other glycolipids on the inhibition of haemolysis by alpha-toxin

Glycolipid[a]	Chemical structure	Concentration in preincubation mixture (μg ml^{-1})	Haemolysis of rabbit erythrocytes[b] (%)
None	—	—	100
GlcNAc-ganglioside (NAN)	NANα2–3GAlβ1–4GlcNAcβ1–3Galβ1–4Glc–Cer	0.05 0.025 0.01 0.005	8 16 48 62
GlcNAc-ganglioside (NGN)	NGNα2–3Galβ1–4GlcNAcβ1–3Galβ1–4Glc–Cer	10 5 1	28 52 76
G$_{M1}$	Galβ1–3GalNAcβ1–4(NANα2–3)Galβ1–4Glc–Cer	20 10 5	32 54 82
G$_{M2}$	GalNAcβ1–4(NANα2–3)Galβ1–4Glc–Cer	25 15 5	30 54 92
G$_{D1a}$	NANα2–3Galβ1–3GalNAcβ1–4(NANα2–3)Galβ1–4Glc–Cer	25 15 5	34 56 94

Glycolipid	Structure		
Paragloboside	Galβ1–4GlcNAcβ1–3Galβ1–4Glc–Cer	25	42
		15	60
		5	98
GlcNAc-CTS	GlcNAcβ1–3Galβ1–4Glc–Cer	40	34
		20	52
		10	76
Globoside	GalNAcβ1–3Galα1–4Galβ1–4Glc–Cer	50	32
		25	48
		15	68
Forssman	GalNAcβ1–3GalNAcβ1–3Galα1–4Galβ1–4Glc–Cer	80	26
		50	48
		25	78
Haematoside(NAN)	NANα2–3Galβ1–4Glc–Cer	100	32
		60	50
Haematoside(NGN)	NGNα2–3Galβ1–4Glc–Cer	100	40
		75	54

[a] Cer, ceramide; CTS, ceramide trisaccharide; Gal, galactose; GalNAc, N-acetylgalactosamine; Glc, glucose; GlcNAc, N-acetylglucosamine; NAN, N-acetylneuraminic acid and NGN, N-glycolylneuraminic acid.

[b] Each glycolipid preparation was incubated with 10 Hu ml⁻¹ of alpha-toxin for 30 min at 37°C. Rabbit erythrocytes (2%) were then added and incubated for 30 min at 28°C. Haemolytic assays were performed by the method of Bernheimer and Schwartz (1963).

Table 4 Effects of lectins on haemolysis by alpha-toxin and on binding of $[^{125}I]$-labelled alpha-toxin to rabbit erythrocytes

Addition	Concentration (μg ml^{-1})	Haemolysis (%)	$[^{125}I]$-labelled toxin bound to cells (c.p.m.)
None	0	100	1230
Concanavalin A	1	72	—
	3	34	479
	5	4	26
	8	3	25
	5+α-MDG (0.1 M)	98	1206
	5+α-MDM (0.1 M)	97	1210
WGA	3	91	1188
	5	69	—
	7	38	512
	10	5	33
	15	3	21
	10+GlcNAc (0.05 M)	97	1220
Lens culinaris agglutinin	50	96	—
	100	44	563
PHA-P	50	90	—
	100	31	439
Soybean agglutinin	50	95	—
	100	40	517
Staphylococcal protein A	100	98	1232
GlcNAc-ganglioside	0.5	6	22
Anti-alpha-toxin serum 2 (units ml^{-1})		2	22

2% of rabbit erythrocytes were preincubated with the indicated concentrations of lectins and their specific sugar haptens at 20°C. After absence of con A suggest that the mode of action of this lectin is based on competitive inhibition. Recently, Maharaj and Fackrell (1980) have also confirmed that con A inhibits the haemolytic activity of alpha-toxin as a result of the blocking of a receptor site on the erythrocyte membrane for the toxin, since the presence of mannose or glucose reduced the protective effect of con A. Kato et al. (1975b) reported that pronase treatment rendered erythrocytes more resistant to alpha-toxin and decreased the number of toxin molecules bound. Pronase has been shown to cleave only two polypeptides on the erythrocyte membrane, band 3 and glycophorin (Bender et al., 1971). Maharaj and Fackrell (1980) demonstrated that rabbit erythrocyte band 3 obtained from pronase treated ghosts inhibited both the haemolytic activity of alpha-toxin and the binding of the toxin to the cell membranes. Finally they postulated that the purified erythrocyte band 3 was the receptor for alpha-toxin. Their purified band 3 component had a molecular weight of 1×10^5 and consisted of polypeptides and sugar residues including mannose, galactose, glucose, fucose, N-acetylglucosamine, and sialic acid residues. The band 3 component is a ubiquitous component of the erythrocyte membrane and there are about 5×10^5 copies of this receptor per erythrocyte in man and rabbits (Bretscher, 1973; Maharaj et al., 1980). However, human erythrocytes are resistant to lysis by the alpha-toxin, whereas rabbit erythrocytes are very sensitive. Furthermore, Kato et al. (1975a) and Cassidy and Harshman (1976) reported 3500 and 5000 receptors per rabbit erythrocyte, respectively, whereas Barei and Fackrell (1979) has estimated as many as 12.5×10^4 per cell. Together the data of Maharaj and Fackrell (1980) did not provide sufficient evidence to show that the reaction between rabbit erythrocyte band 3 and alpha-toxin was specific.

2.   Action of alpha-toxin on isolated cells in vitro

Staphylococcal alpha-toxin damages not only intact or isolated erythrocyte membranes but also primary or established cell line cultures of various origin, which include HeLa cells, human diploid fibroblast, polymorphonuclear leucocytes, platelets, mouse kidney epithelial cells, and Ehrlich ascites tumour cells. In contrast, bacterial membranes or spheroplasts and mycoplasmas are unaffected by the toxin. To determine the susceptibility of specific membranes to alpha-toxin, Kato et al. (1977) demonstrated leakages of [^{86}Rb]-Cl and non-metabolizable [^{14}C]-labelled α-aminoisobutyric acid from preloaded SV_{40} transformed epithelial cells after exposure to the crystallized alpha-toxin. The date from these leakage experiments provided some insight into the kinetics of the toxin–membrane interaction. A significant release of [^{86}Rb] and α-aminoisobutyric acid label occurred after 10 min of exposure to the toxin and reached 90% after 30 min. The SV_{40} epithelial cells remained viable, and light microscopy revealed no morphological changes in cells releasing up to 100% of the leakage markers (Kato *et al.*, 1977). Changes observed in isolated cells cultured *in vitro* with the purified alpha-toxin can be explained by disturbance of membrane permeability and lysosome membrane labilization. However, there is no direct evidence for the demonstration of primary damage to the sodium–potassium pump in somatic cells, and Na^+–K^+-dependent ATPase activity in isolated cell systems does not change the influence of the alpha-toxin (Cassidy *et al.*, 1974). Kato *et al.* (1979a) showed that the cytotoxic effects of alpha-toxin might be caused by the stimulation of the active transport of Ca^{2+} ions into the cell resulting from the inactivation of cyclic AMP-dependent protein kinase in the membrane by the toxin.

Freer *et al.* (1968) and Bernheimer *et al.* (1972) showed that 3 S alpha-toxin disrupted lipid spherules with the formation of a ring structure characteristic of 12 S alpha-toxin, which is formed upon the addition of 3 S toxin to liposomes composed of many different individual lipids. Extended studies by Arbuthnott *et al.* (1973) showed that polymerization could be induced by diglyceride, phosphatidylcholine, cholesterol or lysolecithin. Kato *et al.* (1975a, 1977) found that the haemolytic and cytolytic activities of alpha-toxin were inhibited after treatment of rabbit erythrocytes and SV_{40} transformed epithelial cells with alloxazine or indomethacin, an inhibitor of phospholipase A_2 activity. This finding implies that the 12 S ring polymers are formed upon the interaction of 3 S alpha-toxin with membrane lipids split by phospholipase A_2, which may be activated by the binding of alpha-toxin on the cell membranes.

3. Effect of alpha-toxin on the activities of cellular membrane associated enzymes

Alpha-toxin is probably the most studied of the staphylococcal membrane-damaging toxins. Much of the earlier work can be criticized on the grounds that the alpha-toxin preparations employed were contaminated with other membrane-damaging toxins, especially with delta-toxin. For instance, Cassidy *et al.* (1974) reported that three activities previously attributed to alpha-toxins — disruption of mitochondrial membrane fraction, lysis of bacterial protoplasts, and inhibition of the Na^+–K^+-dependent ATPase activity of guinea pig kidney — were not in fact properties of alpha-toxin.

With respect to the interaction of alpha-toxin with biological membranes, the haemolytic and cytolytic activities, and probably also the lethal effect of alpha-toxin, are closely associated with biological membrane damage (McCartney and Arbuthnott, 1978). However, there is no evidence indicating the specificity of this toxin for any identifiable substrate in the cell membrane or enzymic activity. Among the enzymes associated with rabbit erythrocyte membranes, Na^+–K^+- and Mg^{2+}-ATPase, adenylate cyclase, and cyclic AMP phospodiesterase activities, were unaffected by alpha-toxin and its lethal toxic fragment (Kato, 1979a). The $Ca^{2+}-Mg^{2+}$-dependent ATPase activity of the rabbit erythrocyte membrane was, however, stimulated to a considerable extent by the lethal toxic fragment (Kato, 1979b).

(a)   Inhibitory effect of alpha-toxin and its lethal toxic fragment on cyclic AMP-dependent protein kinase activity
Kato et al. (1979a,b) and Kato (1979a) reported that alpha-toxin inhibited cyclic AMP-dependent protein kinase activity in membranes from rabbit erythrocyte ghosts. Further detailed evidence demonstrated that a lethal toxic fragment of alpha-toxin inhibited the activity of a soluble cyclic-AMP-dependent protein kinase by its interaction with the cyclic-AMP-binding site of regulatory subunit in the holoenzyme molecule (Table 5). Cyclic-AMP-dependent protein kinase contains a dimeric regulatory subunit and two catalytic subunits which dissociate when cyclic AMP binds to the regulatory subunit (2 mol cyclic AMP per mol of subunit monomer) (Corbin et al., 1978) and the protein kinase inhibitor specifically binds to the dissociated catalytic subunits (Demaille et al., 1977). Concerning the effective concentrations of alpha-toxin and its lethal toxic fragment on the cyclic-AMP-dependent protein kinase, Kato et al. (1979a) and Kato (1979a) found that the lethal toxic fragment produced a dose-dependent decrease in both the binding of cyclic AMP activity to the regulatory subunit and the phosphorylating activity of the protein kinase, the latter reaching a plateau at a 50% inhibitory effect. The lethal toxic fragment had no effect on the catalytic subunit activity. On studying the kinetics obtained from linear double-reciprocal plots, the Lineweaver-Burk plot showed competitive inhibition of substrate (cyclic AMP) kinetics by the lethal toxic fragment. Because a complex of enzyme–toxin protein which appeared in the gel filtration corresponded to a molar ratio proportion of 2:1 and cyclic $[^3H]$-AMP binds neither the alpha-toxin nor its lethal toxic fragment, the mechanism proposed for the inhibitory effect of the lethal toxic fragment on the binding of cyclic AMP to the protein kinase is the interaction of the lethal toxic fragment with one of two cyclic AMP-binding sites in the regulatory subunit molecule. Furthermore, Kato (1979b) demonstrated stimulation of calcium ion permeability in rabbit heart muscle membrane by the alpha-toxin, the result of the inhibition of the cyclic AMP-dependent protein kinase activity in the membrane.

(b)   Inhibitory effect of alpha-toxin and its lethal toxic fragment on acetylcholinesterase activity
The contractile effect of alpha-toxin on smooth muscle has been reported by Brown and Quilliam (1965) and Wuezel et al. (1966). The type of contraction of isolated smooth-muscle preparations is known as spastic paralysis. Cassidy et al. (1974) found that alpha-toxin (B) at a concentration of 1 µg ml^{-1} causes

Table 5 Effect of staphylococcal alpha-toxin on cyclic AMP binding and activity of cyclic-AMP-dependent protein kinase

Addition to assay mixture	Concentrations	[³H]cAMP bound (pmol μg protein⁻¹)[a]		Protein kinase activity (units)[b]	
			%		%
None	—	0.71	(100)	21.4	(100)
Alpha-toxin	0.5 μM	0.60	(85)	18.8	(88)
Alpha-toxin	1 μM	0.36	(50)	11.4	(53)
Alpha-toxin	5 μM	0.37	(52)	11.1	(52)
Alpha-toxin (1 μM) + Antiserum	40 μg ml⁻¹	0.70	(99)	20.8	(97)
Lethal toxic fragment	1 μM	0.35	(49)	10.0	(47)
Protein kinase inhibitor	50 μg ml⁻¹	0.89	(127)	4.1	(19)
Ribonuclease A	50 μg ml⁻¹	0.68	(95)	21.6	(101)
Lysozyme	50 μg ml⁻¹	0.72	(101)	21.8	(102)
Histone II	10 μg ml⁻¹	0.99	(133)	—	
Protamine	50 μg ml⁻¹	0.80	(113)	—	
Cyclic GMP	5 μM	0.35	(50)	19.5	(91)
GTP	50 μM	0.64	(90)	19.2	(90)
ATP	50 μM	0.70	(98)	285.2	(1330)

[a] The standard binding reaction mixture contained, in a final volume of 0.2 ml, 50 mM sodium acetate buffer (pH 4.0) and 0.1 μM [³H]-cyclic AMP. Reactions were initiated by the addition of 5 μg of protein kinase and were incubated for 100 min at 0°C.
[b] The standard assay contained, in a final volume of 0.2 ml, 50 mM sodium acetate buffer (pH 6.0), 40 μg of histone II, 5 μM [γ-³²P]-adenosine 5'-triphosphate containing 1.4×10⁶ c.p.m., 10 mM magnesium acetate, and 5 μg of protein kinase in the absence or presence of 5 μM cyclic AMP. Incubations were carried out at 30°C for 10 min.

a pig smooth-muscle preparation which remains responsiveness to acetyl-choline. Edelwejn et al. (1968) and Jeljaszewicz et al. (1969) reported that the lethal effect of alpha-toxin is associated with its primary action on the central nervous system, with disturbances in the polarization and depolarization of neuron membranes. These activities of alpha-toxin are closely related in the biological and pharmacological activities of acetylcholine or serotonin. Since serotonin was found to inhibit human erythrocyte acetylcholinesterase and serum cholinesterase activities (Gilboa-Garber et al., 1978) and erythrocyte acetylcholinesterase is a membrane-bound enzyme with its catalytic activity directed entirely towards the outside of the cell membrane (Heller and Hanahan, 1972), alpha-toxin is considerable to response to the acetylcholin-esterase activity in the cell membranes. The acetylcholinesterase activity of both rabbit erythrocyte membranes and serum was assayed spectrophotometri-cally by measuring the conversion of acetylcholine to thiocholine using 5,5'-dithiobis-(2-nitrobenzoic acid) (DTNB) (Ellman, 1959; Weber, 1966). The activity of acetylcholinesterase in intact rabbit erythrocytes and membranes was reduced by alpha-toxin and its lethal toxic fragment to 30–40% of normal, cholinesterase activity of rabbit serum was also being inhibited to the same degree. However, the inhibitory mechanism of the enzymic activity by alpha-toxin is not entirely clear.

4. The site for the lethal action of alpha-toxin and its lethal toxic fragment in vivo

Kato (1979a) reported that when [^{125}I]-labelled alpha-toxin was injected intravenously in sublethal amounts into mice, even 24 hours later the label from heart, small intestine, brain, kidney, and lung continually remained at a high level, while the rapid disappearance of the label from the other tissues paralleled its rate of disappearance from the blood stream. The effects of alpha-toxin and its lethal toxic fragment, acetylcholine, and epinephrine on cyclic AMP and cyclic GMP levels and the cyclic-AMP-dependent protein–kinase activity ratio were investigated in rabbit heart (Kato, 1979a). The perfused normal rabbit heart was cut into slices approximately 1 mm thick using a tissue slicer. About 10 mg of sliced tissue was placed in a 10-ml conical tube containing 1 ml of each reaction mixture. After incubation at 37°C, the incubated tissue was homogenized and centrifuged. As shown in Table 6, epinephrine, a cardioactive agent, produced increases in cyclic AMP and in the cyclic-AMP-dependent protein kinase activity ratio. Acetylcholine, while producing a three-fold increase in cyclic GMP, marginally suppressed epinephrine stimulation of the cyclic AMP and the protein–kinase activity ratio. The lethal toxic fragment reduced the protein–kinase activity ratio by approximately 40% compared with that of the control and also suppressed epinephrine stimulation of the protein–kinase activity ratio. The toxic lethal

Table 6 Effects of staphylococcal lethal toxic fragment, epinephrine and acetylcholine on cAMP content, cAMP-dependent protein–kinase activity ratio and cyclic GMP content in rabbit heart slices

Treatment[a]	cAMP (nmol g^{-1})	Protein kinase activity ratio (−cAMP/+cAMP)	Cyclic GMP (pmol g^{-1})
(1) Control	0.63 (0.44–0.82)	0.17±0.05	82 (69–93)
(2) Lethal toxic fragment	0.74 (0.55–0.93)	0.10±0.02	83 (70–96)
(3) Epinephrine	1.20 (0.94–1.46)	0.38±0.02	120 (103–137)
(4) Acetylcholine	0.55 (0.48–0.62)	0.15±0.04	299 (278–320)
(5) Epinephrine+acetylcholine	0.89 (0.67–1.10)	0.24±0.04	364 (332–396)
(6) Lethal toxic fragment+acetylcholine	0.58 (0.50–0.66)	0.09±0.02	290 (262–318)
(7) Lethal toxic fragment+epinephrine	1.10 (0.88–1.32)	0.18±0.03	120 (101–139)

[a] Rabbit heart slices were incubated with each reaction mixture containing (1) no additions, (2) 0.1 μM lethal toxic fragment, (3) 0.1 μM epinephrine, (4) 5 μM acetylcholine, (5) 0.1 μM epinephrine plus 5 μM acetylcholine, (6) 0.1 μM lethal toxic fragment plus 5 μM acetylcholine, (7) 0.1 μM lethal toxic fragment plus 0.1 μM epinephrine. The incubated slices were homogenized and centrifuged. Each value represents the mean of 5 heart slices.

fragment, however, slightly elevated the cyclic AMP levels resulting from the inhibition of binding of cyclic AMP to the protein kinase. The stimulation of protein kinase activity by cyclic AMP has been shown to mediate the effects of cardioactive agents on both heart metabolism and function (Dobson, 1978). An attempt was made to relate the demonstrated effect to a known physiological action of the alpha-toxin: the lethal toxic fragment attenuated the stimulation of the cyclic-AMP-dependent protein–kinase activity ratio in the isolated heart by addition of epinephrine (Table 6), since epinephrine stimulates contractile force and antagonizes the action of acetylcholine which decreases cardiac contractile force and produces an increase in the cyclic GMP level (George et al., 1970).

On injection of sublethal doses of alpha-toxin, De Navasquez (1938) observed a typical symmetrical cortical necrosis of the kidney, and Cassidy et al. (1974) reported the induction of spastic paralysis of smooth muscle of the guinea pig ileum or blood vessels, possibly resulting in the fatal drop in blood pressure. This phenomenon might be due to inhibition of the cell-membrane-associated acetylcholinesterase and serum cholinesterase activity (Kato et al., 1979b). Weigershausen (1962) observed that alpha-toxin caused constriction of coronary arteries and systolic arrest in perfused heart muscle from the rabbit, cat, and chicken. Furthermore, Kato (1979a) demonstrated stimulation of calcium ion permeability in the rabbit heart muscle membrane by alpha-toxin as a result of the inhibition of cyclic-AMP-dependent protein kinase activity in the membrane. Work in other laboratories indicated that the lethal target might be localized at a site other than the heart muscles. Appreciable amounts of $[^{125}I]$-labelled alpha-toxin were also detected in the brain. Edelwejn et al. (1976) reported that the primary lethal effect of the toxin in rabbits was triggered in the hypothalamus reticular system and in the visual-sensory region of the cerebral cortex and death was caused by a rapid collapse of brain bioelectric activity. Finally, there is no unified concept that the site for the lethal action of alpha-toxin appears to be located in either the circulatory system or the central nervous system.

III. PROTECTION OF STAPHYLOCOCCAL INFECTION BY TOXOIDS OF ALPHA-TOXIN AND LEUCOCIDIN

Kato et al. (1974, 1980) reported that the crystallized staphylococcal alpha-toxin and leucocidin were readily detoxified by overnight incubation at 37°C in the presence of 0.4% formaldehyde solution at pH 7.4. Staphylococcal leucocidin consists of two components (F and S components) which were isolated and crystallized from broth culture of V8 strain of S. aureus (Noda et al., 1980a). Toxoids of staphylococcal alpha-toxin and leucocidin are antigenic in most experimental animals. Subcutaneous injection of each toxoid with adjuvant elicits the formation of circulating IgG antibody, which neutralizes the toxic activities of alpha-toxin and leucocidin (Noda *et al.*, 1980b). Kato *et al.* (1974, 1980) reported that acquired or passive immunity to a mixture of toxoids of alpha-toxin and leucocidin protected against staphylococcal infection in man (e.g. acne pustulosa, acne vulgaris, purulent abscess, sycosis vulgaris, and carbuncle).

In order to produce a subcutaneous abscess in a mouse, it is necessary to inject as few as 100 staphylococci in the presence of a cotton-dust (Agarwal, 1967). Twenty mice were injected intramuscularly twice in 3 days with a mixture of toxoids of alpha-toxin and leucocidin. After 2 days, the mice were injected subcutaneously with 200 cells of *S. aureus* strains of Wood 46 and V8, which produce large quantities of alpha-toxin and leucocidin *in vitro*, in the presence of cotton-dust. The mice were observed for 20 days and produced no subcutaneous abscesses, whereas within 24 hours of staphylococcal injection 20 mice not given toxoids showed both abscess formation and dermonecrosis (Kato *et al.*, 1980).

Many different vaccines—cell fractions (Stamp, 1961), surface polysaccharide (Fisher *et al.*, 1963), and leucocidin toxoid (Mudd *et al.*, 1965)—have been tested with varying degrees of success. However, assessment of the relative value of these vaccines is difficult, since different experimental strains of staphylococci produce various cellular and extracellular products and may participate in various phases of staphylococcal infection. Finally, the author firmly believes that among the membrane-damaging toxins, alpha-toxin and leucocidin are the most likely play an important role in the initial stage of staphylococcal infection as a result of localized tissue damage. In future, it will be an important research to develop adequate experimental animal model systems to study toxin–disease relationships.

IV. SUMMARY

Staphylococci produce multiple cellular and extracellular toxic substances. The biological properties of staphylococcal membrane-damaging toxins (haemolysins and leucocidin) and their possible participation in the pathogenesis of staphylococcal infection have attracted the attention of several investigators. Alpha-toxin is a potent and selective cytotoxin and therefore may be considered an important probe in cell biology as well as a potential virulence factor for *Staphylococcus aureus*. Recently, the cytolytic activity of cell-membrane damage by alpha-toxin was taken as indicating a likely enzymatic mode of action for alpha-toxin. This chapter has dealt mainly with the activation of cell-membrane-associated enzymes by alpha-toxin. With regard to the interaction of rabbit erythrocyte with alpha-toxin, the following sequence of events is proposed. The haemolytic fragment of alpha-toxin preferentially binds to NAN–Gal–GlcNAc-containing ganglioside and/or glycopeptide in the surface membrane of the erythrocyte, resulting in the stimulation of phospholipase A_2 in the membrane. Pretreatment of rabbit erythrocytes with alloxazine or indomethacin, an inhibitor of phospholipase A_2, causes the inhibition of haemolysis by alpha-toxin. Phosphatidylcholine, acting as a substrate for phospholipase A_2 in the double layer membranes, is split to lysolecithin and fatty acid by activated phospholipase A_2. The interaction of these split fatty acids with 3 S alpha-toxin results in the formation of alpha-toxin in the 12 S polymer with lysolecithin in the membrane. This seems to cause perturbation of the cell-membrane surface and the lethal toxic fragment, devoid of haemolytic and necrotic activity, then inhibits the activity of cyclic-AMP-dependent protein kinase, resulting in the stimulation of Ca^{2+} permeability. An alteration of ion permeability of the membrane is thus effected. The outcome of alpha-toxin–membrane interaction, in terms of the binding to the receptor, polymerization of alpha-toxin molecules by the split membrane lipids and alternation of ion permeability, is to induce an increase in the fluidity and stability of the bilayer membrane. Recently, aspects of cellular membrane structure and function have been the subject of intense interest among biologists, and it is encouraging that many of these studies have involved the use of bacterial toxins, including membrane-damaging toxins, as tools in membrane research. Considerable progress has been made in the past decade in understanding the mode of action of the staphylococcal alpha-toxin *in vitro* and *in vivo*, but some aspects of the process still remain to be elucidated.

The study of the role of either individual highly purified alpha-toxin, its lethal toxic fragment, or the other cytolytic toxins (e.g. haemolysins and leucocidin) in staphylococcal pathogenesis, will entail *in vivo* studies in experimental animal models aimed at determining the role of the toxin in tissue damage and impairment of host defence systems.

In conclusion, recent progress from studies with alpha-toxin has done much to enhance our understanding of bacterial toxinology and the alpha-toxin, as a membrane-damaging toxin, will compose a highly significant aspect of the microbiological research in the future.

REFERENCES

Agarwal, D. S. (1967). *Brit. J. Exp. Path.* **48**, 436–449.
Arbuthnott, J. P. (1970). *In* "Microbial Toxins" (T. C. Montie, S. Kadis and S. J. Ajl, ed.), Vol. III, pp. 189–236. Academic Press, New York and London.

Arbuthnott, J. P., Freer, J. H. and Billcliff, B. (1973). *J. Gen. Microbiol.* **75**, 309–319.
Barei, G. M. and Fackrell, H. B. (1979). *Can. J. Microbiol.* **25**, 1219–1226.
Bender, W. W., Hasan, G. and Berg, H. C. (1971). *J. Mol. Biol.* **58**, 783–797.
Bernheimer, A. W. (1974). *Biochim. Biophys. Acta* **344**, 27–50.
Bernheimer, A. W., Kim, K. S., Remsen, C. C., Antan vage, J. and Watson, S. W. (1972). *Infect. Immun.* **6**, 636–642.
Bernheimer, A. W. and Schwartz, L. L. (1963). *J. Gen. Microbiol.* **30**, 455–468.
Bretsher, M. S. (1973). *Science* **181**, 622–629.
Brown, D. A. and Quilliam, J. P. (1965). *Br. J. Pharmacol.* **25**, 781–789.
Cassidy, P. S. and Harshman, S. (1973). *J. Biol. Chem.* **284**, 5545–5546.
Cassidy, P. S. and Harshman, S. (1976). *Biochemistry* **15**, 2348–2355.
Cassidy, P. S., Six, H. R. and Harshman, S. (1974). *Biochim. Biophys. Acta* **332**, 413–423.
Corbin, J. D., Sugden, P. H., West, L., Flockhart, D. A., Lincoln, T. M. and McCarthy, D. (1978). *J. Biol. Chem.* **253**, 3997–4003.
Demaille, J. G., Peters, K. A. and Fischer, E. H. (1977). *Biochemistry* **16**, 3080–3086.
De Navasquez, S. (1938). *J. Pathol. Bacteriol.* **46**, 47–58.
Dobson, J. G., Jr (1978). *Amer. J. Physiol.* **234**, H638–H645.
Edelwejn, Z., Jeljaszewicz, J., Szmigielski, S. and Zak, C. (1968). *Toxicol. Appl. Pharmacol.* **13**, 133–145.
Edelwejn, Z., Jeljaszewicz, J., Wadstrom, T., Mollby, R. and Pulverer, G. (1976). *In* "Staphylococci and Staphylococcal Diseases" (J. Jeljaszewicz, ed.), pp. 747–754, S. Karger, Basel.
Edman, P. and Begg, G. (1967). *Eur. J. Biochem.* **1**, 80–91.
Ellman, G. L. (1959). *Arch. Biochem. Biophys.* **82**, 70–77.
Fisher, M. W., Devlin, H. B. and Erlandson, A. L. (1963). *Nature* **199**, 1074–1075.
Freer, J. H., Arbuthnott, J. P. and Bernheimer, A. W. (1968). *J. Bacteriol.* **95**, 1153–1168.
George, W. J., Wilkerson, R. D. and Kadowitz, P. J. (1970). *Proc. Natl Acad. Sci. U.S.* **66**, 398–403.
Gilboa-Garber, N., Katz-Bergman, Y. and Pinsky, A. (1978). *Experientia* **34**, 992–993.
Gray, W. R. (1972). *In* "Methods in Enzymology" (S. P. Colowick and N. O. Kaplan, ed.), Vol. 25, pp. 121–138, Academic Press, New York and London.
Hayashi, R., Moore, S. and Stein, W. H. (1973). *J. Biol. Chem.* **248**, 2296–2302.
Heller, M. and Hanahan, D. J. (1972). *Biochim. Biophys. Acta* **255**, 251–272.
Jeljaszewicz, J., Szmigielski, S. and Hryniewicz, W. (1978). *In* "Bacterial Toxins and Cell Membrane" (J. Jeljaszewicz and T. Wadstrom, ed.), pp. 185–197, Academic Press, New York and London.
Jeljaszewicz, J., Szmigielski, S. and Zak, C. (1969). *Zbl. Bakt. I. Abt.* **209**, 310–313.
Kato, I. (1979a). *Biochim. Biophys. Acta* **570**, 388–396.
Kato, I. (1979b). *Jpn J. Bacteriol.* **34**, 59.
Kato, I. and Naiki, M. (1976). *Infect. Immun.* **13**, 289–291.
Kato, I., Noda, M. and Sanai, Y. (1980). *Protein, Nucleic Acid and Enzyme* **25**, 693–706.
Kato, I., Saito, M., Sakoda, K. and Suzuki, Y. (1977). *Jpn J. Bacteriol.* **32**, 53.
Kato, I., Saito, M. Sato, I., Suzuki, Y., Watanabe, M., Ishii, T., Fukuda, H. and Sakoda, K. (1974). *Med. Biol.* **88**, 323–327.
Kato, I., Sakoda, K., Saito, M., Suzuki, Y. and Watanabe, M. (1975a). *Jpn J. Med. Sci. Biol.* **28**, 332–334.

Kato, I., Sakoda, K., Saito, M., Suzuki, Y. and Watanabe, M. (1975b). *Infect. Immun.* **12**, 696–697.
Kato, I., Watanabe, M. and Kumazawa, N. H. (1979a). *Infect. Immun.* **24**, 286–288.
Kato, I., Watanabe, M. and Kumazawa, N. H. (1979b). Abstracts of the Annual Meeting 1979, American Society for Microbiology, B(H)25.
Lominski, I., Arbuthnott, J. P. and Spence, J. B. (1963). *J. Pathol. Bacteriol.* **86**, 258–262.
Maharaj, I. and Fackrell, H. B. (1980). *Can. J. Microbiol.* **26**, 524–531.
Mangalo, R. and Raynaud, M. (1959). *Ann. Inst. Pasteur* **97**, 188–197.
McCartney, C. A. and Arbuthnott, J. P. (1978). *In* "Bacterial Toxins and Cell Membrane" (J. Jeljaszewicz and T. Wadstrom, ed.), pp. 89–127, Academic Press, New York and London.
McNiven, A. C. and Arbuthnott, J. P. (1972). *J. Med. Microbiol.* **5**, 123–127.
Mudd, S., Gladstone, G. P. and Lenhart, N. A. (1965). *Brit. J. Exp. Path.* **66**, 455–459.
Nicolson, G. L. (1974). *Int. Rev. Cytol.* **39**, 89–190.
Noda, M., Hirayama, T., Kato, I. and Matsuda, F. (1980a). *Biochim. Biophys. Acta* **633**, 33–44.
Noda, M., Kato, I., Hirayama, T. and Matsuda, F. (1980b). *Infect. Immun.* **29**, 678–684.
Sharon, N. and Lis, H. (1972). *Science* **177**, 945–959.
Six, H. R. and Harshman, S. (1973). *Biochemistry* **12**, 2672–2676.
Stamp, L. (1961). *Brit. J. Exp. Path.* **42**, 30–37.
Watanabe, M. and Kato, I. (1974). *Jpn J. Exp. Med.* **44**, 165–178.
Watanabe, M. and Kato, I. (1976). *In* "Animal, Plant and Microbial Toxins" (A. Ohsaka, K. Hayashi and Y. Sawai, ed.), Vol. 1, pp. 437–454, Plenum, New York.
Watanabe, M. and Kato, I. (1978). *Biochim. Biophys. Acta* **535**, 388–400.
Weber, H. (1966). *Dtsch Med. Wschr* **43**, 1927–1932.
Weigershausen, B. (1962). *Acta Biol. Med. Ger.* **9**, 517.
Weil, L. and Buchert, A. R. (1951). *Arch. Biochem. Biophys.* **34**, 1–15.
Wiseman, G. M. (1975). *Bacteriol. Rev.* **39**, 317–344.
Wuezel, M., Bernheimer, A. W. and Zweiface, B. W. (1966). *Amer. J. Physiol.* **210**, 360–364.

8 Urinary tract infection in adults: selective clinical, microbiological and therapeutic considerations

RICHARD A. GLECKMAN

Urinary tract infections, the all-inclusive term denoting the pathological presence of micro-organisms in the urinary tract, are the most prevalent bacterial infections in the U.S. and Europe. For specific segments of the adult population — pregnant women and patients with obstruction — urinary tract infections constitute a particularly serious problem. In fact, acute, bacterial pyelonephritis has been identified as the source of the majority of community-acquired bacteraemias experienced by elderly patients (Esposito et al., 1980).

The incidence of "significant bacteriuria", defined as the persistent isolation of more than 100 000 colony-forming units ml^{-1} from clean-voided urine, in young, non-pregnant women is approximately 1–3%. In elderly women the incidence of "significant bacteriuria" approaches 30%. It is a rare disease in men less than 40 years of age, but its incidence in elderly men has been estimated to be in excess of 15%. Factors predisposing to urinary tract infections include instrumentation of the bladder, renal stones, prostatic calculi, and vesico-ureteral reflux.

Escherichia coli, Klebsiella pneumoniae, Proteus mirabilis, and *Staphylococcus saprophyticus* cause most community-associated urinary tract infections. These organisms (excluding *S. saprophyticus*), *Pseudomonas aeruginosa, Serratia marcescens, Enterobacter* sp., and enterococci are most frequently isolated from patients who develop their infection within the hospital, usually in association with catheterization of the bladder. Prediction of the causative micro-organism of a urinary tract infection, however, is impossible, thereby making cultures of the urine and blood mandatory to identify the aetiological agent.

I. TERMINOLOGY AND CLASSIFICATION

The primary tissue source of a urinary tract infection can reside in the kidney (pyelonephritis), bladder (cystitis), prostate (prostatitis), or urethra (urethritis). Chronic bacterial pyelonephritis, a vague term at best, conveys to the clinician the concept of persistent, bacterial kidney infection involving the pelvo-calyceal system and the renal substance, but the term has eluded precise definition (Beeson, 1965). Radiologists and pathologists apply the expression "chronic pyelonephritis" when describing the end result of bacterial ravages on the kidney, namely, calyceal dilatation and focal parenchymal reduction.

A clinical classification of urinary tract infections that provides the physician with invaluable guidance in formulating diagnostic evaluations and therapeutic programmes has been developed (Kaye, 1972). This system recognizes four categories of urinary tract infections: symptomatic infection, asymptomatic bacteriuria, relapse (also known as bacterial persistence), and reinfection. *Symptomatic urinary tract infection* refers to the initial episode of a symptomatic infection and this designation pertains exclusively to a new urinary tract infection, one believed not to have been preceded by a recurrent infection. *Asymptomatic bacteriuria* indicates a bacterial urinary tract infection unassociated with symptoms. Detection of the bacteriuria would represent a new finding and not constitute a manifestation of a recurrent infection. In *relapse* the pretreatment pathogen is temporarily eliminated from the urine in response to chemotherapy, survives within the urinary tract, and subsequently initiates a recurrent infection. Relapse can be considered a measure of drug ineptitude. *Reinfection*, which develops after chemotherapy has eliminated the original, pretreatment organism from the urine, occurs after medication has been discontinued and represents a recurrent, bacterial infection caused by an organism different from that initiating the original infection. This classification, however, fails to identify the tissue site of the urinary tract infection, as this determination requires additional data derived from the medical history, physical examination, and laboratory investigations.

II. DIAGNOSIS

Quantitative analysis of mid-stream, "clean-voided" urine has emerged as the preferred method to support the clinical impression of a symptomatic urinary tract infection and to establish the diagnosis of an asymptomatic urinary tract infection (Kass, 1956). A number of quantitative techniques, such as the poured plate dilution method, the calibrated, bacteriological loop, and the agar-coated dip slide test, appear to provide reliable and comparable results.

The poured plate method consists in adding 0.1 ml well-mixed urine to 9.9 ml sterile water, discharging 0.1 ml diluted urine into a sterile petri dish, mixing the urine with 10–20 ml nutrient agar maintained at 45°C, and incubating the contents of the plate. Each colony identified on the agar represents 1000 viable units in the original urine sample. The poured plate method is considered the standard quantitative method against which all other methods of urine quantitation are compared. Alternative quantitative techniques, such as the streak plate method and the agar-coated dip slide test, appear to provide reliable information and are technically less demanding (Hoeprich, 1960; McGeachie, 1963). The streak plate method uses a 0.001 ml calibrated, platinum, bacteriological, dilution loop to surface streak medium. Each colony identified represents 1000 organisms ml^{-1} in the original urine specimen. The dip slide test uses a glass or plastic slide coated with an agar medium. Results are interpreted by comparison with drawings of bacterial cultures of defined quantities (Cohen and Kass, 1967). A maintenance fluid, consisting of a boric acid–glycerol–sodium formate preservative, has recently become commercially available and appears to be capable of preserving a stable bacterial population in urine for 24 hours, thus obviating the problem of spuriously "high" bacterial counts attributed to delays in urine transport or inoculation (Lauer *et al.*, 1979).

Automated techniques that permit rapid processing of urine specimens have been developed (Isenberg *et al.*, 1979; Jenkins *et al.*, 1980; Nicholson and Koepke, 1979). Screening, identification, and antimicrobial susceptibility testing of urine cultures can be accomplished within one day. These automated screening procedures require expensive instrumentation, however, and on occasion fail to provide accurate information. Conventional urine processing remains essential when patients receive antibiotics, harbour polymicrobic bacteriuria, are subjected to suprapublic bladder aspiration or diagnostic catheterization, or are being assessed for evidence of chronic bacterial prostatitis.

Numerous laboratory tests have been evaluated as alternatives to urine quantitation to detect urinary tract infections. Microscopy examination of fresh urine, both centrifuged and uncentrifuged, stained and unstained, to identify bacteria has become a ritual in many laboratories. However, until standard criteria for a "positive" or "negative" test have been developed and the sensitivities and the specificities of this screening technique are defined, the validity of the procedure remains unknown, and it should not replace quantitative urine cultures as the preferred method of establishing the diagnosis of a urinary tract infection. The detection of pyuria from centrifuged, urine sediment fails to correlate with the presence of bacteriuria identified by quantitative urine cultures. Quantitative analysis of pyuria performed on uncentrifuged urine, as determined by a haemocytometer, does appear to provide valid data, and this method seems capable of excluding the diagnosis of a urinary tract infection in men (Musher *et al.*, 1976), but the determination of white blood cells in uncentrifuged urine with the haemocytometer has not been widely adopted as a screening test to detect urinary tract infections.

Chemical methods have been developed as screening techniques to identify "significant" bacteriuria in voided urine. Procedures that measure the ability of bacteria in the urine to reduce nitrate to nitrite (the Griess test), metabolize urinary glucose (glucose oxidase), reduce triphenyltetrazolium to a triphenyl formazan (TTC test), and produce catalase (the urinary catalase test) and endotoxin have been evaluated, but the value of these techniques remains uncertain and as yet they fail to provide an acceptable alternative to quantitative urine cultures (Craig *et al.*, 1973).

The last five years have witnessed an explosion of new, rapid screening tests to detect bacteriuria. The development of rapid, accurate, inexpensive screening tests for bacteriuria could reduce the time, effort, and expense consumed by inoculating plates that fail to grow organisms, encourage screening of asymptomatic, high-risk populations (i.e. pregnant women), and provide invaluable information to the clinician. A chemical test of the bioluminescent reaction of bacterial adenosine 5′-triphosphate (ATP) with luciferin and luciferase has not proven to be sufficiently accurate to merit introduction into the clinical laboratory (Conn *et al.*, 1975; Alexander *et al.*, 1976). Gas liquid chromatography has been used as a technique to detect microbial metabolites in urine and quantitate bacteriuria. This procedure appears incapable of detecting some urinary pathogens, however, and fails to provide a sensitive indication of bacteriuria (Barrett *et al.*, 1978; Coloe, 1978). Measurement of impedance (change in the resistance to the flow of an alternating current) of urine, resulting from bacterial alteration of nutrients and production of metabolic products, can be applied to urine quantitation. Initial reports suggest that this determination can provide reliable screening for bacteriuria within three hours (Throm *et al.*, 1977; Cady *et al.*, 1978). Detection of bacteriuria by electrical impedance monitoring can be applied in laboratories that process large numbers of urine samples.

Combining the features of rapid, multiple techniques, including detection and quantitation by direct Gram stain evaluation of uncentrifuged urine, identification of urinary isolates with reagent strips, and antibiotic susceptibility testing by disk-elution, laboratories can provide reasonable accuracy on those urine specimens considered clinically urgent by the physician and issue a presumptive report within four to six hours (Heinze, 1979).

Urinary tract infection merits diagnostic consideration when a patient experiences fever accompanied by or unassociated with irritative voiding symptoms. The absence of significant pyuria in routine analysis of urine virtually excludes urinary tract infection as the explanation for the febrile state, but there are three exceptions to this general rule: patients with leucopenia, resulting from drugs, aplastic anaemia or leukaemia, are incapable of developing an inflammatory response, and some patients with obstructive uropathy and others with infectious process remote from the kidney's collecting system, such as renal cortical abscess, may fail to manifest pyuria.

Blood cultures provide invaluable diagnostic assistance in the assessment of the febrile patient with a presumptive diagnosis of acute, symptomatic, bacterial pyelonephritis or catheter-trauma-induced urosepsis. Multiple blood cultures should be obtained because evidence exists that Gram-negative bacteraemia occurs as an inconstant event, thus, in contrast to the bacteraemia characteristic of infective endocarditis (Kreger et al., 1980). When patients have received prior antibiotics, blood cultures should be processed through an antimicrobial removal device that has recently become commercially available. The antimicrobial removal device, consisting of a cationic and polymeric resin, permits more rapid identification of bacteraemias and increases the incidence of their detection (Wallis et al., 1980).

It must be emphasized, however, that no absolute bacterial count precisely identifies or excludes the diagnosis of a urinary tract infection and that quantitation of the urine depends on a number of factors, including the collection and processing of the sample, state of hydration and frequency of urination, the presence of obstruction, and the administration of antimicrobial agents (Roberts et al., 1967).

Although providing more accurate information, bladder aspiration and catheterization, two invasive diagnostic techniques, should be performed only when clean-voided urine cannot be obtained or interpreted, or when a research study requires precise data. Bladder aspiration, regarded as *the* definitive diagnostic procedure, appears to be a safe and invaluable manoeuvre to identify a urinary tract infection. The practice of forcing fluids prior to the performance of the suprapubic bladder aspiration will, however, reduce the bacterial count in the urine. The isolation of a recognized, urinary, bacterial pathogen, regardless of bacterial count in the bladder urine, indicates a urinary tract infection (Stamey et al., 1965). The existence of a resident, urethral bacterial flora diminishes the diagnostic validity of urine obtained by catheterization. In addition, diagnostic catheterization can evoke a urinary tract infection (Kaye et al., 1962).

A single, clean-void urine sample containing more than 100 000 colony-forming units (CFU) per ml should be anticipated in the man or woman with acute symptomatic urinary tract infection, particularly when pyelonephritis occurs (Rantz and Keefer, 1940). Failure of the colony count to achieve a concentration of 10^5 CFU ml^{-1} does not, however, refute the diagnosis

(Gleckman, 1978). Clinical history, physical findings, urine analysis, and blood cultures contribute essential information in formulating the diagnosis of acute symptomatic bacterial pyelonephritis. Bacteriuria of $>10^5$ CFU ml^{-1} can also be an insensitive criterion to exclude the diagnosis of acute symptomatic bacterial cystitis in women, particularly when suprapubic discomfort, gross haematuria, and pyuria exist (Stamm, 1980).

In the elderly, the diagnosis of acute symptomatic pyelonephritis often provides a diagnostic challenge (Esposito *et al.*, 1980). Neurological damage can obscure the classical findings of irritative voiding symptoms, and the development of altered mental status, tachypnoea, and vague abdominal pain often raises the possibility of alternative infectious disorders, such as meningitis, pneumonitis, and diverticulitis. The findings of pyuria, "significant" bacteriuria, and bacteraemia lend invaluable support to the clinical diagnosis of acute symptomatic pyelonephritis in the geriatric patient.

For the non-catheterized, asymptomatic man, the detection of more than 10 000 CFU ml^{-1} of clean-void urine establishes the diagnosis of a urinary tract infection. The results obtained from a single urine culture appear to be valid, if the patient co-operates in obtaining the urine and the specimen is processed expeditiously. The persistent recovery of more than 10^5 CFU ml^{-1} from a clean-void, mid-stream urine establishes the diagnosis of a urinary tract infection in the asymptomatic woman. Quantitation of a single, mid-stream, clean-void urine obtained from a woman requires confirmation, contrary to the situation with men. Unfortunately, however, no absolute count exists that decisively differentiates infection from contamination, and mid-stream urine concentrations of less than 10^5 CFU ml^{-1}, particularly when the isolates are Gram-negative aerobic bacilli, should not be summarily dismissed as contaminants.

There is ample evidence that enterococci, other streptococci, *Staphylococcus saprophyticus*, and, rarely, *Staphylococcus aureus* cause urinary tract infections. Nevertheless, when they are recovered in the urine of asymptomatic patients, physicians often regard these organisms as urethral contaminants. Although no clear statement appears in the literature that the arbitrary quantitative criteria that establish the diagnosis of urinary tract infection caused by Gram-negative bacilli (namely, persistent recovery of the organism in a count that exceeds 10^5 CFU ml^{-1}) apply to Gram-positive cocci, limited published data do seem to imply this (Gower and Roberts, 1975).

Polymicrobic bacteriuria often represents an inadequate collection technique; alternatively, it often develops in patients with indwelling Foley or suprapubic catheters. Often dismissed as a result of "contaminated" urine, polymicrobic bacteriuria, when consistently confirmed, would signal the possibility of a structural abnormality of the urinary tract, such as a stone or a bladder diverticulum. Polymicrobic bacteriuria merits serious consideration, as it can antedate Gram-negative bacteraemia (Gross *et al.*, 1976).

Anaerobic bacteria are components of the normal urethral flora and rarely cause urinary tract infections; attempts by clinical laboratories to isolate these organisms from clean-void, mid-stream urine samples have been discouraged (Kuklinca and Gavan, 1969). Anaerobic urinary tract infections occur in the setting of structural abnormalities. Diagnosis of an anaerobic urinary tract infection, as suggested by analysis of clean-void urine, requires confirmation by bladder aspiration or blood cultures.

There are no criteria to establish the diagnosis of renal candidiasis by quantitation of mid-stream, clean-void urine. The detection of pseudohyphae in the urine fails to provide conclusive evidence of tissue invasion by *Candida* sp. It has been suggested that the isolation of $> 10\,000$ *Candida* ml^{-1} from a catheterized specimen provides a useful criterion to distinguish colonization from infection (Kozinn, 1978). The diagnostic accuracy of this procedure can be supported by immunological studies and blood cultures. The problem remains, however, of establishing the diagnosis of renal candidiasis in the patient without a Foley catheter. Currently, the practising physician does not have access to immunological tests that reliably detect evidence of invasive urinary tract candidiasis, and these diagnostic tests, limited to a small number of research laboratories, are undergoing continuous refinement and improvement.

III.   LOCALIZATION OF URINARY TRACT INFECTIONS

The introduction, evaluation, and refinement of laboratory procedures capable of establishing the tissue focus of a urinary tract infection continue at a frantic pace. A number of observations explain the rationale for this intensive effort.

(1) Signs and symptoms fail to localize accurately the tissue source of a urinary tract infection (Boutros *et al.*, 1971).

(2) Knowledge of the site of a urinary tract infection provides a powerful epidemiological instrument to study the pathogenesis of disease (Gonick *et al.*, 1975; Forland *et al.*, 1977).

(3) A reliable method to determine the tissue site of infection can influence decisions about the duration and intensity of therapy (Ronald *et al.*, 1976; Fang *et al.*, 1978; Gleckman *et al.*, 1979).

(4) Identification and subsequent treatment of patients at increased risk, presumably patients with a renal site of infection, can prevent serious complications, such as bacteraemia (Rubin *et al.*, 1979).

(5) A technique to identify asymptomatic patients at minimum risk of serious morbidity or mortality, patients with cystitis and no structural abnormalities of the urinary tract, could guide the physician in withholding antibiotic therapy, thereby eliminating unnecessary expense and potential for side-effects (Gleckman, 1976).

(6) A procedure that could accurately establish the tissue site of a urinary tract infection could identify those asymptomatic bacteriuric pregnant women destined to develop symptomatic pyelonephritis, a disease requiring hospitalization and associated with considerable morbidity.

Current techniques to localize the site of a urinary tract infection (Table 1) can be classified into two categories: direct (or invasive) and indirect (or non-invasive) methods.

Table 1   Tests to identify the site of a urinary tract infection

DIRECT
1. Kidney biopsy
2. Ureteral catheterization
3. Bladder washout technique
4. Culture of prostatic secretions

INDIRECT
1. Clinical signs and symptoms
2. Microscopic examination of urine
3. Maximum urine osmolality
4. Water-loading test
5. Measurement of urinary fibrin degradation products
6. Measurement of urinary B_2-microglobulin and muramidase
7. Measurement of urinary enzymes
8. Serum antibody determinations
9. Pattern of response to therapy
10. Radiographic techniques
11. Antibody-coated-bacteria (ACB) immunofluorescence

A.   Direct techniques

Cultures of kidney specimens obtained by percutaneous biopsies provide an unequivocal diagnosis of bacterial pyelonephritis, but the risks engendered by this invasive procedure render this method obsolete for demonstrating a renal source of infection. The focal nature of bacterial pyelonephritis restricts the capacity of a percutaneous renal biopsy to provide bacteriological confirmation.

Quantitative bacteriology performed on urine obtained from the ureters effectively differentiates bacterial pyelonephritis from bacterial cystitis (Stamey et al., 1965). Investigators have successfully carried out this localization procedure on defined populations of patients with urinary tract infections (Stamey et al., 1965; Turck, 1978), and ureteric catheterization has become established as the definitive technique for establishing the tissue source of a urinary tract infection. This technique has been relegated exclusively to a research procedure, however, because cystoscopy with retrograde bilateral ureteral catheterization of the infected urinary tract requires the expertise of a skilled urologist and entails the risk of bacteraemia. In addition, this lengthy, uncomfortable, and expensive procedure cannot readily be repeated when patients experience a recurrent infection. Isolation of organisms from the ureters implies bacterial pyelonephritis, not simply "pyelitis" (Whitworth et al., 1974).

In 1967 Fairely and his associates developed a bladder-washout method to differentiate the site of a urinary tract infection (Fairley et al., 1967), and confirmed its validity when compared with the earlier ureteric catheterization procedure of Stamey, Govan, and Palmer (Stamey et al., 1965). The bladder-washout method fails to localize the infection to an individual kidney but does not require the expertise of a urologist. The procedure consists in the insertion of a Foley catheter and the introduction of 0.1% neomycin (to sterilize the bladder contents) with Elase (to remove fibrinous exudate from the bladder wall). The bladder is washed with two litres of sterile water, and urine samples, obtained immediately after catheterization of the bladder, immediately after the bladder-washout, and each 10 min over a period of 30 min after the bladder-washout, are collected and quantitated. Patients with bacterial cystitis demonstrate sterile urines in all collection periods that follow the washout, and patients with bacterial pyelonephritis manifest bacteriuria in each of the post-washout samples. The bladder-washout technique has recently been modified by the substitution of 0.5% gentamicin sulphate for 0.1% neomycin and the adoption of new criteria for a renal focus of infection (Ronald et al., 1976). These investigators require an increase of a power of 10 between the bladder-wash culture and the subsequent post-washout specimens and bacteria counts greater than 100 ml $^{-1}$ in virtually all post-washout specimens to establish the diagnosis of bacterial pyelonephritis.

The bladder-washout technique has proved to be a safe and reliable procedure in the evaluation of women with recurrent urinary tract infections (Fairley et al., 1967; Ronald et al., 1976), bacteriuria of pregnancy, and diabetes mellitus and has occasionally eradicated the infection when cystitis existed (Fairley et al., 1967). However, some objections to the bladder-washout procedure have been raised. Investigators contend that this technique could provide misleading information—false-positive results, when bacterial infection caused transient vesico-ureteral reflux. In addition, other researchers cite the problem that the valid counting of bacteria in post-washout urine samples requires a constant outflow of organisms from the renal pelvis. However, an intermittent discharge of infected urine from the renal parenchyma, which would explain a false-negative test result, has been documented (Fairley and Butler, 1971). Despite these shortcomings, the bladder-washout technique remains an invaluable procedure to localize the site of a urinary tract infection.

When urethral or prostatic infection is suspected in the male, partitioned urine collections should be performed and subjected to quantitative bacteriological analysis (Stanley *et al.*, 1965). The first voided 10 ml of urine ("urethral urine"), a mid-stream portion of urine ("bladder urine"), the prostatic expressate (expressed prostatic secretions obtained by prostatic massage), and a third aliquot of urine (obtained immediately after prostatic massage) are surface streaked on to agar (Meares and Stamey, 1968). A significant titre of bacteria in the urethral urine, but not in the bladder urine, indicates urethritis. The diagnosis of chronic bacterial prostatitis is confirmed when quantitative bacterial colony counts of the prostatic secretions exceed those of the urethral and bladder specimens by at least a power of 10. The presence of a urinary tract infection precludes the performance of this localizing technique. Precise performance of this procedure requires considerable patience and co-operation by the patient, as he is subjected to a time-consuming and uncomfortable experience. When prostatic secretions cannot be obtained, quantitative cultures of the ejaculate appear adequate to establish the diagnosis of chronic bacterial prostatitis (Mobley, 1975).

B. Indirect techniques

It is traditional practice to base a diagnosis of cystitis or acute pyelonephritis on the patients' medical history and physical findings. Researchers have classified patients as having cystitis when irritative voiding symptoms, such as urgency, dysuria, nocturia, and suprapubic discomfort, occurred in the absence of fever and costovertebral-angle pain (Vosti *et al.*, 1965). However, when women with symptomatic urinary tract infections were studied by the ureteric catheterization or bladder-washout procedures (Fairley *et al.*, 1965), it was noted that a poor correlation existed between the site of an infection established by the direct techniques and the patients' symptoms and physical findings. Symptoms usually considered consistent with bacterial cystitis (urinary frequency, urgency, suprapubic pain) also occur in patients with proven bacterial pyelonephritis (Fairley *et al.*, 1967). The presence of fever, however, should direct attention to the kidneys (Fairley *et al.*, 1967).

Tests measuring the excretion rates, staining properties, cast formation, and response of urinary white blood cells to provocative stimuli, have failed to identify accurately the tissue site of a urinary tract infection and have been abandoned.

A number of studies have associated bacterial pyelonephritis with a defect in maximal urinary concentrating ability. Concentrating capacity is evaluated in patients who receive an intramuscular injection of 5 units of vasopressin in oil, are subjected to 36 hours of fluid deprivation, and ingest a 50–80 g protein diet. During the last 24 hours of fluid restriction, all urine is collected at six-hour intervals, and the aliquot with the highest osmolality is considered the maximum osmolality. In this procedure, a maximum urinary osmolality of less than 700 mOsm kg^{-1} is considered abnormal. Women with urinary tract infections localized by the ureteral catheterization or bladder-washout procedure have been subjected to tests of urine-concentrating ability. Measurement of maximum urinary osmolality failed to provide a sensitive method of localizing the site of the urinary tract infection (Ronald *et al.*, 1969).

A water-loading test which analyses bacterial excretion rates was introduced in 1972 (Papanayioutou and Dontas, 1972) and eventually modified in 1974 and has been labelled by one expert as a "useful test" to establish the presence of asymptomatic pyelonephritis (Kass, 1972). Measurements of bacterial excretion rates (urine flow per min × the bacterial concentration per ml) are performed in subjects who have been hydrated with intravenous saline. In the initial studies, a correlation was noted between increased bacterial excretion rates following hydration and renal function abnormalities, and it was suggested that the water-loading test could identify "occult" bacterial pyelonephritis (Papanayioutou and Dontas, 1972). The researchers failed, however, to define the site of infection by any direct technique. Subsequently, a team of investigators did compare the water-loading test with the bladder-washout procedure in patients with recurrent urinary tract infections (Prat *et al.*, 1977). They identified limitations of the water-loading test as a technique to determine the site of a urinary tract infection. The future position of the water-loading test remains unknown, and its value has been questioned (Prat *et al.*, 1977).

Increased concentrations of urinary fibrin degradation products (FDP) have been detected in multiple renal diseases, including bacterial pyelonephritis (Whitworth *et al.*, 1973). Increased concentrations of urinary FDP appear to be a rare event in women with bacterial cystitis (Whitworth *et al.*, 1973). The detection of increased concentrations of urinary FDP could provide an effective test to help exclude bacterial cystitis as the site of a urinary tract infection. Kits for the measurement of urinary FDP are commercially available. Failure to demonstrate increased concentrations of urinary FDP in a patient with a urinary tract infection does not exclude a renal source of the infection.

Measurements of the urinary concentrations of two low molecular weight proteins, B_2-microglobulin and lysozyme, have recently been performed in patients with urinary tract infections (Bonadio et al., 1979; Schardijn et al., 1979). The sites of infection were established definitively in most patients. The initial reports, which require confirmation, suggest that measurement of urinary B_2-microglobulin and lysozyme can distinguish bacterial cystitis from bacterial pyelonephritis. Increased B_2-microglobulin and lysozyme excretion have been reported to occur in association with numerous renal diseases characterized by tubular injury, as well as shock, fever, and administration of nephrotoxic agents such as gentamicin.

Bank and Bailine (1965) reported finding elevated urinary concentrations of beta-glucuronidase activity in patients with pyelonephritis but not cystitis. These investigators defined the site of infection primarily upon clinical parameters, however, rather than precise localization techniques. Studies using the ureteric catheterization technique concluded that no correlation existed between urinary beta-glucuronidase activity and the anatomical site of the infection (Ronald et al., 1971).

Carvajal et al. (1975) reported that measurement of urinary LDH isoenzymes accurately defined the site of urinary tract infections in children subjected to the bladder-washout procedure. Analysis of isoenzyme patterns revealed significant differences in the urinary concentration of LDH isoenzyme-5 in patients with bacterial pyelonephritis and bacterial cystitis. Two studies performed in children have confirmed the findings that measurement of urinary LDH isoenzyme-5 provides a powerful instrument to localize the site of an infection (Devaskar and Montgomery, 1978; Lorentz and Resnick, 1979). It has been suggested that the elevated concentrations of isoenzyme-5 originate from renal cortical tissue damaged by pyelonephritis or acute tubular necrosis.

Only one report of the measurement of urinary LDH isoenzyme-5 in adults with urinary tract infections has been published (Fries et al., 1977). Although they failed to subject their patients to the more definitive invasive localization procedures, their study also suggests that elevation of urinary LDH isoenzyme-5 occurs in bacterial pyelonephritis and not bacterial cystitis. A number of factors must be considered when interpreting the result of the LDH assay. Nitrofurantoin, repeated slow freezing and thawing of the urine, and exposure of the urine for hours at room temperature will interfere with the determination of LDH activity. Initial reports of this non-invasive test appear so promising that further studies performed in adults, whose infection sites have been identified by definitive techniques, are indicated.

Brumfitt and colleagues studied the immune response in defined groups of women with urinary tract infections and concluded that an immunological technique – the direct bacterial agglutination method – identified patients with bacterial pyelonephritis (Brumfitt and Percival, 1965). Other investigators, who analysed serum antibody titres, using indirect haemagglutination and direct bacterial agglutination tests in patients whose site of a urinary tract infection was defined, have determined that measurements of these antibodies provide limited useful information to identify the site of infection (Brenner *et al.*, 1969; Scarpelli *et al.*, 1979). Alternative tests of immune response in urinary tract infection, including indirect immunofluorescence and solid-phase radioimmunoassay, are currently being refined (Sanford *et al.*, 1978).

Recently, considerable attention has focussed on the measurements of Tamm-Horsfall protein, a renal glycoprotein and primary constituent of urinary casts. Elevated serum IgG antibodies to Tamm-Horsfall protein has been identified in girls with acute pyelonephritis. Further studies have suggested that detection of elevated serum levels of antibody to Tamm-Horsfall protein should raise the suspicion of infection superimposed on obstruction to urine flow (Marier *et al.*, 1978).

Two studies performed in women who had experienced recurrent urinary tract infections and were subjected to direct techniques to establish the tissue source of the infection have demonstrated that the pattern of recurrence accurately identifies the site of infection in approximately 80% (Turck *et al.*, 1968; Ronald *et al.*, 1976). Relapses that occur within two weeks of the cessation of drug treatment usually signify bacterial pyelonephritis. Recurrences due to reinfections usually originate from bacterial cystitis. These studies were, however, conducted among selective women who appeared free of renal stones, obstructive uropathy, and azotaemia.

Radiographic techniques offer no advantage in the localization of urinary tract infections. Excretory urography (Fries *et al.*, 1977) and gallium citrate scanning often fail to identify accurately the sites of infection in patients experiencing recurrent disease.

The antibody-coated-bacteria immunofluorescence test (ACB) has emerged as the preferred technique to determine the tissue source of a urinary tract infection (Jones *et al.*, 1974; Thomas *et al.*, 1974). The test consists in the detection of bacteria coated with human antibody directed against bacterial surface antigens which has been synthesized in the kidney or prostate (Smith *et al.*, 1977). Direct immunofluorescence permits visualization of the antibody complexed with the bacteria in the urine. With tissue invasion, as occurs in bacterial pyelonephritis or prostatitis, antibody is synthesized and a positive antibody-coated-bacteria test results. In most cases of cystitis, the infection appears limited to the mucosa and tunica propria and a negative ACB test results (Jones *et al.*, 1974; Thomas *et al.*, 1974). Using animal models of ascending pyelonephritis, 10–16 days elapse before a positive ACB test result occurs with an initial infection (Smith *et al.*, 1977; Rubin *et al.*, 1980). Reinfection, however, will result in a positive ACB assay within 2–5 days.

The advantages of the ACB test have established it as one of the techniques of choice among the indirect studies to localize a urinary tract infection (Jones, 1979). The test is non-invasive, inexpensive, and reproducible. Results are available within hours and can influence therapy (Rubin *et al.*, 1980). The test can be performed on urine previously stored in the frozen state, and the administration of immunosuppressive drugs fails to influence results. The ACB test appears more sensitive than serum antibody titrations for distinguishing pyelonephritis from cystitis (Jones *et al.*, 1974; Thomas *et al.*, 1974).

The ACB test will not define accurately the site of a urinary tract infection when the infection is caused by yeast, Gram-positive cocci (Jones, 1979), or mucoid *Pseudomonas aeruginosa*. In the interpretation of the ACB test, it should be emphasized that heavy proteinuria, contamination of the specimen by antibody-coated-bacteria from a mucosal surface other than the bladder (Jones, 1979), prostatitis, or epididymitis can evoke a positive ACB assay.

The last five years have witnessed an explosion of reports extolling the virtues of the ACB test. The procedure has been applied to the study of urinary tract infections in children, adults, pregnant women, diabetics, catheterized patients, renal transplant recipients, and patients with ileal conduits (Gleckman, 1979a). Two questions remain to be answered before physicians embrace the ACB test as the decisive procedure to localize the tissue source of a urinary tract infection and permit the results of this determination to influence decision making. What constitutes a positive test? How accurately does the ACB test determine the site of infection?

The investigators who introduced the ACB test considered the test positive when more than 25% of the bacteria in the urinary sediment fluoresced (Thomas *et al.*, 1974). Other researchers appear to have arbitrarily selected a different criterion (Rumans and Vosti, 1978). Evidently, the standards for interpreting the ACB test established by a laboratory can only be determined after prior studies in that institution had correlated the test with definitive direct procedures, such as ureteral catheterization or bladder-washout. One laboratory appears to have verified its interpretation this way (Jones, 1976).

Rumans and Vosti (1978) sounded the alarm that the ACB test should not be considered an infallible index of the tissue site of the infection and emphasized a previous observation (Jones, 1976) that a number of falsely negative ACB test results occur among patients with acute bacterial pyelonephritis. Recently, investigators have attempted to establish the value of the ACB test by subjecting patients to direct localization with ureteric catheterization or bladder-washout (Jones *et al.*, 1974; Thomas *et al.*, 1974;

Prat et al., 1977; Lorentz and Resnick, 1979). Their results form the basis for two contemporary critical reviews of the ACB test (Gleckman, 1979a; Mundt and Polk, 1979).

Studies performed in children demonstrate the unreliability of the ACB test to localize the site of a urinary tract infection (Lorentz and Resnick, 1979). Some studies performed in adults confirm the reliability of the ACB assay to define accurately the tissue source of infection (Jones et al., 1974; Thomas et al., 1974), but other investigators failed to establish the accuracy of the ACB test, particularly when applied to women with recurrent urinary tract infections (Prat et al., 1977). As a result of the controversies that have arisen because of the ACB test (Gleckman, 1979a), this procedure continues to have supporters (Jones, 1979) and detractors (Mundt and Polk, 1979). Undoubtedly, the value of the ACB test to localize the site of a urinary tract infection in adults will remain unsettled until uniform standards have been accepted.

IV. PATTERNS OF THERAPEUTIC RESPONSE

Following the onset of drug treatment, patients with urinary tract infections demonstrate one of five patterns of therapeutic response: cure (synonymous with therapeutic success), unresolved (continuous) bacteriuria, superinfection, relapse (also referred to as bacterial persistence), and reinfection. The patient is considered cured if less than 10 000 CFU ml^{-1} are isolated from the urine on each occasion the urine is quantitated during therapy and for a minimum of six weeks after cessation of the course of therapy. Failure of drug treatment to achieve eradication of the bacteriuria, known as unresolved or continuous bacteriuria, can be explained by the following causes: non-compliance occurred, the organism was resistant to the medication prescribed, renal insufficiency or obstructive uropathy existed, or chemotherapy was directed against only one of the pathogens involved in a polymicrobic infection (Lindemeyer et al., 1963; Stamey, 1975). Superinfection is the emergence, during therapy, of significant bacteriuria caused by an organism different from the pretreatment urinary pathogen.

Colonial morphology, biochemical tests, antimicrobial susceptibility patterns, colicine typing, and, most importantly, serotyping have traditionally been the methods used by researchers to differentiate bacterial relapse from a reinfection. The technique of serotyping E. coli, based on the presence of O, K, and H antigens, has proven an invaluable epidemiological tool to study urinary tract infections (Turck et al., 1962). However, this procedure fails to identify a relatively large number of isolates that are untypable. In addition, access to high quality, diagnostic grade, E. coli antisera has been restricted.

The commercially available Analytab (API 20E) system has been used for biotyping *E. coli* (Davies, 1977), and this technique has been applied to an investigation of patients who experienced recurrent urinary tract infections (Cicmanec and Evans, 1980). Biotyping and resistotyping techniques provide additional highly acurate methods for the precise discrimination of urinary strains of *E. coli*, and these procedures can be performed in conventional diagnostic laboratories (Buckwold *et al.*, 1979; Old *et al.*, 1980). Efforts should be extended to differentiate bacterial relapse from reinfection; however, it should be appreciated that reinfections caused by the same organism cannot be distinguished from relapses and, rarely, infection is caused by multiple serotypes of the same organism, each of which possesses different antimicrobial susceptibility patterns (Gower and Tasker, 1976).

V. RECURRENT URINARY TRACT INFECTIONS IN MEN

Men with recurrent urinary tract infections present a formidable therapeutic challenge. Sterility of the urine for a minimum of six weeks after therapy, an arbitrary definition of successful treatment ("cure"), occurs in only 20–30% of those men subjected to the conventional ten-day or two-week course of chemotherapy (Gleckman *et al.*, 1979; Smith *et al.*, 1979; Gleckman *et al.*, 1980a). This response stands in marked contrast to the greater than 90% cure rates experienced by women with acute, symptomatic, bacterial cystitis who have received single-dose or ten-day treatment (Rubin *et al.*, 1980).

Recurrent urinary tract infections are detected almost exclusively in men over 50 years of age. Coexisting medical diseases include diabetes mellitus and essential hypertension. Radiographic studies identify structural abnormalities in approximately half of the patients. The anatomical and physiological alterations most often revealed by excretory urograms include pyelonephritic scarring and prostatic calculi; postvoid bladder residual *E. coli* causes the lion's share of those recurrent urinary tract infections that develop in men without urethral catheters or ileal-loop bladders.

When drug treatment is prescribed in accordance with the *in vitro* susceptibility pattern of the pretreatment organism, patients with recurrent urinary tract infections invariably demonstrate a bacteriological response. The urine becomes sterile immediately after the onset of treatment and remains sterile during the course of therapy. Superinfection appears to be an infrequent occurrence.

Cure of recurrent invasive infection of the urinary tract with a renal or prostatic focus does not depend exclusively on appropriate antibiotic selection (Stamey and Pfau, 1963). Structural abnormalities contribute to the inability of drugs to eradicate infections, but these processes are not the sole determinants of therapeutic success for men with recurrent invasive urinary tract infections; poorly defined host factors undoubtedly explain some therapeutic failures (Stamey and Pfau, 1963).

Recent investigations have identified bacterial relapse ("bacterial persistence"), rather than reinfection, as the more prevalent pattern of recurrence experienced by men with recurrent urinary tract infections (Gleckman *et al.*, 1979; Smith *et al.*, 1979; Gleckman *et al.*, 1980a). The bacterial relapses experienced by men with recurrent urinary tract infections exposed to drug therapy are usually asymptomatic and occur predominantly within a month of the discontinuation of medication. The organisms associated with bacterial relapse remain susceptible to the antimicrobial agent exhibited, thus excluding the development of drug resistance as the cause of therapeutic failure.

Numerous explanations (Table 2), some documented and others conjectural, have been offered in an attempt to understand why bacterial relapses occur so frequently in men with recurrent invasive urinary tract infections (Gleckman, 1979b).

Table 2   Causes of bacterial relapse (persistence)

1. "Infection" stones
   (a) Kidneys
   (b) Prostate
2. Chronic bacterial prostatitis
3. Inadequate duration of therapy
4. Cell-wall-defective bacteria

Infection stones, known also as "triple phosphate" or struvite urinary stones, are a mixture of struvite (magnesium ammonium phosphate) and carbonate-apatite. They form only as a consequence of urease-induced hydrolysis of urea and are invariably infected, primarily with *Proteus mirabilis* (Griffith, 1978). Infection stones contain bacteria incorporated within the stone substance, thereby explaining the inability of antibiotics to sterilize the urine in their presence and the high relapse rate. Chronic urea-splitting urinary tract infection recalcitrant to eradication with antimicrobial agents poses a great risk for recurrent or persistent calculogenesis. Patients with infected staghorn calculi who receive no therapy have a 50% chance of losing the kidney (Singh *et al.*, 1973). Treatment of infection stones consists of removal or dissolution of the stone, antibiotic therapy directed at the urease-producing bacteria, and perhaps the administration of acetohydroxamic acid, an effective inhibitor of urease (Griffith *et al.*, 1979).

Investigators have noted an association between bacterial relapse and the presence of a prostatic calculus (Freeman *et al.*, 1975; Gleckman *et al.*, 1980a).

In fact, on rare occasions, bacteria become embedded within the substance of a prostatic calculus and create a situation analogous to the renal infection stone (Eykyn *et al.*, 1974; Meares, 1974). Infected prostatic calculi, however, are usually caused by *E. coli* rather than *Proteus mirabilis*. Antibiotics fail to cure permanently infections that originate from infected prostatic calculi, and these patients experience recurrent urinary tract infections following discontinuation of drug therapy. Total prostatectomy offers the best opportunity to eradicate recurrent urinary tract infections that arise from infected prostatic calculi.

Meares and Stamey (1968) stated that chronic bacterial prostatitis explains most bacterial relapses experienced by men with recurrent urinary tract infections. Presumably drug therapy fails because currently available medications are incapable of penetrating the infected prostate and eradicating the bacterial infection. A recently published study appears to support these observations (Smith *et al.*, 1979). Smith and his colleagues identified evidence of chronic bacterial prostatitis in 22 of 42 men evaluated for recurrent urinary tract infections. Their study also confirms the inability of drug treatment to cure most recurrent urinary tract infections arising from the infected prostate. Currently, on the basis of limited data, recurrent urinary tract infections, secondary to chronic bacterial prostatitis, should be treated with an extended course of therapy (Meares, 1975). Recent investigations have provided new insights on the pathophysiology of the infected prostate, and undoubtedly these findings will pave the way for the development of future treatment strategies (Pfau *et al.*, 1978; Fair *et al.*, 1979).

A. Prophylaxis

The optimum duration of therapy for patients with recurrent urinary tract infections has remained the subject of controversy for years. Numerous flaws in protocol design have precluded critical assessment of the value of extended courses of therapy. Studies have failed to define the patient population, evaluate a homogeneous population, predefine outcome criteria, distinguish bacterial relapse from reinfection, randomly assign drug therapies, identify structural abnormalities, determine the tissue site of the infection, and prospectively assess treatment results in accordance with a double-blind technique. Two developments have provided the opportunity to compare the conventional course of therapy with an extended course for men with recurrent urinary tract infections. In 1975 the U.S. Food and Drug Administration issued guidelines to evaluate drug efficacy for the therapy of urinary tract infections. These guidelines precisely defined the terms cure, superinfection, relapse, and reinfection. The introduction of the antibody-coated bacterial immunofluorescence (ACB) test provided an inexpensive, reproducible, non-invasive, valid procedure to measure tissue invasion of the urinary tract, a marker for evidence of a urinary tract infection associated with pyelonephritis or prostatitis. The ACB test has proved to be a reliable indicator of tissue invasion in men with recurrent urinary tract infections.

Two groups of investigators have reported the results of their prospective, double-blind study performed on a homogeneous population of elderly men with recurrent invasive urinary tract infections (Gleckman et al., 1979; Smith et al., 1979). These studies were designed to determine whether an extended course of therapy would be more effective than the conventional ten-day to two-week course of treatment. Treatments were randomly assigned, urinary localization studies were performed, structural abnormalities were defined, and drug compliance was monitored. Trimethoprim-sulphamethoxazole was selected as the study medication because it had proved to be a safe and effective treatment of recurrent urinary tract infections and chronic bacterial prostatitis.

The studies showed convincingly that the customary practice of prescribing a ten-day to two-week course of therapy to men with recurrent invasive urinary tract infections fell far short of the desired treatment goal — sterility of the urinary tract. The studies did, however, demonstrate that the extended course of therapy resulted in fewer relapses and no more adverse reactions than the conventional course of therapy.

Neither group of investigators offered an explanation as to why the extended course of therapy resulted in fewer relapses. One researcher has suggested that an analogy exists between invasive recurrent urinary tract infections and subacute bacterial endocarditis (Turck, 1972), which requires prolonged therapy to achieve a cure because a brief course of antibiotics invariably results in a relapse. Alternatively, the increased cure rates associated with the extended course of therapy could represent a confirmation of the observation that prolonged drug administration enhances therapeutic efficacy for the treatment of chronic bacterial prostatitis (Meares, 1975).

These studies did not address a more fundamental issue: the need to treat asymptomatic men who have experienced recurrent urinary tract infections.

No evidence exists that asymptomatic urinary tract infections in men produce renal insufficiency in the absence of renal papillary damage or obstruction. The ultimate determinant of renal failure has not been persistent infection but obstruction to the flow of urine (Kunin, 1975).

It has been postulated that bacterial relapse results from the ability of microbial variants, known as cell-wall-defective bacteria, to remain in the kidney during chemotherapy and then revert to the parent, classical bacteria following discontinuation of medication. Wall-defective bacterial variants have been recovered from the urine and renal tissue of patients who have experienced recurrent urinary tract infections. Isolation of cell-wall-defective bacteria from the urine or kidney does not, however, constitute proof that the organism recovered existed in an aberrant bacterial form in the kidneys or was related to recurrent urinary tract infections. Criteria for attributing a pathophysiological role to cell-wall-defective bacteria have been developed (McGee *et al.*, 1971). Data have emerged to support and refute the concept that cell-wall-defective bacteria contribute to persistent pyelonephritis and provide an explanation for the relapses that occur after drug therapy. Other researchers are more cautious and consider that the importance attached to the recovery of these aberrant bacterial forms has been exaggerated (Watanakunakorn, 1979). A group of investigators recently performed a prospective study of men with recurrent invasive urinary tract infections to determine the impact provided by cell wall-defective bacteria (Gleckman *et al.*, 1980b). With the techniques employed, no cell wall-defective bacteria were isolated from the urine, although patients received antibiotics capable of inducing aberrant bacterial forms and the research laboratory specializing in the study of cell wall-defective bacteria has had considerable experience in the isolation of these organisms. Two notes of caution, however. The study group included only 11 patients, and the subjects consisted exclusively of elderly men with asymptomatic recurrent urinary tract infections. In addition, the patients were not cautioned to restrict fluids before voiding, and the possibility exists that failure to insure a high osmolality precluded survival or recovery of aberrant bacterial forms. To date, studies have failed to prove conclusively that cell wall-defective bacteria provide an explanation for bacterial relapses.

Prolonged, continuous prophylactic treatment has been recommended as a measure to reduce the incidence of recurrent urinary tract infections, decrease symptomatic exacerbations, eliminate bacteraemia and haematogenous dissemination originating from the urinary tract, and prevent the development of progressive renal failure in patients who experience either persistent or recurrent urinary tract infections. There exists only one study that has addressed the question of the value of prolonged prophylaxis in men with recurrent urinary tract infections (Freeman *et al.*, 1975). This study, performed through a co-operative effort by physicians of the U.S. Public Health Service, evaluated the clinical and microbiological response of 249 men with urinary tract infections who were subjected to two years of continuous therapy. Therapeutic agents administered for prophylaxis included sulphamethizole, nitrofurantoin, and methenamine mandelate. Prophylaxis was offered after antibiotics eradicated the infection. The following conclusions were reached: continued drug therapy results in significantly fewer microbiologically confirmed bacterial recurrences; prolonged prophylaxis invariably fails when calculi (renal, prostatic) or radiographic abnormalities characteristic of pyelonephritis exist;

the propensity for bacterial recurrences re-emerges after two years of prophylaxis or sooner, if continuous prophylaxis is prematurely discontinued. The study data suggested that persistent bacteriuria, unaccompanied by obstructive uropathy, did not result in any deterioration of renal function. Of equal importance was the observation that an increased mortality rate occurred in recipients of sulphamethizole, raising the possibility that sulphamethizole accelerated vascular death. In fact, the investigators recommended that sulphonamides not be considered the agents of choice for prolonged prophylaxis. As important as these study results are, it should be emphasized that a number of design problems tended to detract from the value of the investigation. Therapeutic criteria were arbitrary and failed to meet contemporary standards; drug compliance was not documented; bacterial relapse was not differentiated from a reinfection; no tests were performed to define the tissue source of the infection; and symptomatic exacerbations were treated with antibiotics but not defined or microbiologically confirmed.

The U.S. Public Health Service co-operative study group have provided a necessary background for formulating guidelines for prolonged prophylaxis. Three essential questions, however, require exploration. What is the natural course of persistent bacteriuria? What is the prophylactic "agent of choice"? Which specific men with recurrent urinary tract infections are candidates for prolonged chemoprophylaxis?

The natural course of persistent bacteriuria has not been defined. On rare occasions metastatic infection can arise from the urinary tract and result in vertebral osteomyelitis, septic arthritis, endocarditis, septic pulmonary emboli, meningitis, subdural empyema, and endophthalmitis. In men, however, these events invariably have followed in the wake of urological procedures performed on the bladder, prostate, and urethra (Siroky et al., 1976). Spontaneous haematogenous dissemination undoubtedly occurs in men with asymptomatic bacteriuria, but fortunately this sequence of events appears to be exceedingly infrequent, even in patients with prosthetic devices.

A number of observations influence the physician before he embarks on a course of prolonged prophylactic therapy.

(1) Unless prior bacteriuria is eradicated by antimicrobial agents, prophylactic therapy will fail.
(2) Recurrent urinary tract infections occur when medication has been discontinued.
(3) Prophylactic drugs have not demonstrated consistent efficacy.
(4) Continuous drug therapy is expensive and entails the possibilities of drug interactions and serious untoward events. Chronic administration of nitrofurantoin has resulted in life-threatening illness, including

irreversible pulmonary fibrosis, chronic active hepatitis, and polyneuropathy (Gleckman *et al.*, 1979). Sulphonamides have been incriminated as
possibly causing accelerated vascular death (Freeman *et al.*, 1975).

(5) The U.S. Food and Drug Administration has not sanctioned the use of
trimethoprim or trimethoprim-sulphamethoxazole as prophylactic
agents, although they have proved highly effective in preventing recurrent urinary tract infections in women (Stamm *et al.*, 1980).

(6) The presence of renal insufficiency places a severe restriction on
therapeutic options. Nitrofurantoin and methenamine mandelate are
contra-indicated for the patient with renal failure. When renal
insufficiency occurs, therapeutic urinary concentrations of nitrofurantoin are not achieved and drug-induced toxicity is enhanced. Limited
data have confirmed the value of trimethoprim as a prophylactic agent
for the patient with renal insufficiency who experiences recurrent,
symptomatic urinary tract infections (Kunin *et al.*, 1978).

No medication has emerged as the "drug of choice" for the prevention of
recurrent urinary tract infections in men. Limited clinical studies have
precluded endorsing any specific agent. One expert recommends the administration of the methenamine compounds (Kass, 1979), but no study has
established it as the preferred prophylactic drug.

Certainly, most men who experience recurrent urinary tract infections
should not be considered candidates for prolonged, continuous prophylactic
medication. Prolonged prophylaxis appears appropriate for those men who
experience multiple, recurrent, symptomatic urinary tract infections in the
absence of surgically remediable lesions, such as infection stones.

VI. RECURRENT URINARY TRACT INFECTIONS IN WOMEN

Women with urinary tract infections often experience recurrent bacteriuria in
spite of apparently adequate antimicrobial therapy (Mabeck, 1972). Most
recurrences are caused by *E. coli* and appear to be reinfections rather than
relapses (Harrison *et al.*, 1974) when the bladder is the site of the infection
(Turck *et al.*, 1968). Recurrences usually occur within six months of the
previous infection and are invariably accompanied by symptoms
(McGeachie, 1966; Kraft and Stamey, 1977; Stamm *et al.*, 1980). Factors
associated with recurrent urinary tract infections in women have included
infrequent voiding, uninhibited neurogenic bladder, persistent colonization of
the introitus and vaginal vestibule with Enterobacteriaceae, enhanced adherence of organisms to the mucosal cells of the introitus, and absence of
cervicovaginal antibody (Lapides *et al.*, 1968; Stamey *et al.*, 1978; Addato *et*

al., 1979). However, there is no consensus that patients with recurrent urinary tract infections are more likely to be colonized over prolonged periods of time with enteric, Gram-negative bacteria or that sexual intercourse contributes to the acquisition of urinary tract infections (Cattell *et al.*, 1974; Kunin *et al.*, 1980). The importance of oral contraception as a risk factor for the development of bacteriuria also remains undetermined (Evans *et al.*, 1978).

No convincing evidence exists that extending the duration of therapy or increasing the intensity of drug treatment will reduce the incidence of reinfections experienced by women with recurrent urinary tract infections, particularly when the infection is confined to the bladder (Fair *et al.*, 1980). In addition, with the present climate of stringent cost containment of medical procedures, the role of excretory urography and cystoscopy in the evaluation of the woman with recurrent urinary tract infections must be reassessed (Fair *et al.*, 1979; Engel *et al.*, 1980). Cystoscopy appears indicated only when unexplained haematuria occurs or the possibility of a colonic fistula or neurogenic bladder is raised. When a patient experiences a bacterial relapse rather than a reinfection, unexplained haematuria occurs, the patient admits to excessive analgesic ingestion or obstructive symptoms or the diagnostic considerations include renal calculi, papillary necrosis or neurogenic bladder, excretory urography appears indicated.

Studies indicate that women who develop a urinary tract infection are more likely to harbour subsequent infections than women who have never experienced a urinary tract infection. In addition, it appears that urinary tract infections tend to occur in clusters, and the longer the interval between infections, the less likely that recurrences will develop (Kraft and Stamey, 1977).

A. Prophylaxis

Prophylactic, low-dosage antimicrobial therapy reduces the incidence of recurrent urinary tract infections in susceptible women. Presumably, antimicrobial agents interfere with the sequence of events consisting of colonization of the vaginal vestibule by faecal flora and the subsequent development of bacteriuria. Antimicrobial prophylaxis is reserved for those women who experience multiple, disabling symptomatic flare-ups, because drug treatment entails an expense as well as the risk of adverse events and medication fails to eradicate the biological defect that predisposes to recurrent infections.

The efficacy and safety of antimicrobial prophylaxis of recurrent urinary tract infections have been consistently demonstrated (Bailey *et al.*, 1971; Harding and Ronald, 1974; Stamey *et al.*, 1977; Harding *et al.*, 1979). Numerous agents, including nitrofurantoin, methenamine mandelate, trimethoprim, and trimethoprim-sulphamethoxazole, have been shown to be well tolerated and capable of significantly reducing the incidence of recurrent urinary tract infections (Stamm *et al.*, 1980). Prophylaxis is initiated after drug therapy has eradicated the established infection. Antimicrobial prophylaxis, consisting of nitrofurantoin (100 mg), sulphamethoxazole (500 mg), trimethoprim-sulphamethoxazole (40 mg/200 mg), trimethoprim (100 mg) or methenamine mandelate (2 g) together with ascorbic acid (2 g), can be administered once daily. In fact, trimethoprim-sulphamethoxazole, thrice weekly, has been demonstrated to be effective for the prophylaxis of recurrent urinary tract infections (Harding *et al.*, 1979). A randomized, double-blind, controlled study has failed to detect any therapeutic difference between nitrofurantoin, a drug which does not alter rectal carriage of *E. coli* and produces only modest reduction of *E. coli* in vaginal and periurethral cultures, and trimethoprim or trimethoprim-sulphamethoxazole, compounds that eliminate *E. coli* from the rectum, urethra, and vagina (Stamm *et al.*, 1980). In the U.S., however, neither trimethoprim nor trimethoprim-sulphamethoxazole has yet been approved by the Food and Drug Administration for the antimicrobial prophylaxis of recurrent urinary tract infections in women.

All studies confirm that within a month of the discontinuation of antimicrobial prophylaxis the preventative effect of drug treatment has dissipated. The history of the number of previous urinary tract infections appears to identify those women who will experience recurrent infections following discontinuation of antimicrobial prophylaxis. Seventy-five per cent of those patients who experienced three or more infections during the year prior to prophylaxis sustained recurrences in the six months following discontinuation of antimicrobial prophylaxis. All patients who sustained four or more infections during the year prior to antimicrobial prophylaxis had recurrence of infection after prophylaxis was terminated (Stamm *et al.*, 1980). Although the record of frequency of infection appears capable of predicting the infection-prone patient, whether these "high risk" patients should be subjected to prolonged (defined as greater than six months) antimicrobial prophylaxis remains an unsettled issue. Prolonged administration of nitrofurantoin and sulphonamides have been incriminated in the initiation of life-threatening, untoward events (Freeman *et al.*, 1975; Gleckman *et al.*, 1979; Sharp *et al.*, 1980; Holmberg *et al.*, 1980). Chronic administration of nitrofurantoin has resulted in peripheral neuropathy, interstitial pneumonitis, and irreversible liver damage. Concern has been expressed that prolonged ingestion of a sulphonamide could result in accelerated coronary artery disease and subsequent death.

Antimicrobial prophylaxis with nitrofurantoin and trimethoprim-sulphamethoxazole does not predispose patients to recurrent infections caused by drug-resistant Enterobacteriaceae, but trimethoprim-sulphamethoxazole prophylaxis has been associated with recurrences caused by resistant enterococci. This observation should serve as a warning that trimethoprim-sulphamethoxazole administration should be reserved for the "high risk" patient (Stamey et al., 1977).

Topical antimicrobial therapy, applied directly to the urethra and vagina, has been prescribed to women with recurrent urinary tract infections (Motzkin, 1972). The rationale for this treatment is that colonization of the vaginal vestibule and urethra precedes recurrent bacteriuria. Nitrofurazone, a drug with cosmetic acceptability and minimal sensitization, has been regarded as the preferred treatment. No controlled study, however, has established the value of this practice, and the role of topical antimicrobial therapy in the prevention of recurrent urinary tract infections remains unknown.

Multiple procedures, including urethral dilatation and internal urethrotomy, have been performed on women to prevent recurrent urinary tract infections. An assumption has existed that obstruction invariably accompanies and enhances the development of recurrent infections. However, no data have emerged to support this contention and continued performance of these procedures appears unwarranted. Women with recurrent urinary tract infections experience long infection-free periods. This observation could explain some of the successes attributed to the invasive procedures (Kraft and Stamey, 1977).

Studies performed on a selective group of women experiencing recurrent urinary tract infections have identified an imperfect relationship between the tissue site of the infection and the pattern of therapeutic response. A trend exists for women with pyelonephritis to develop a relapsing infection rather than a reinfection following discontinuation of drug therapy (Gutman et al., 1978). There remains a difference of opinion, however, as to whether the relapses represent bacterial persistence in the kidney or the emergence of a new infection caused by the same organism residing in the urethra or vaginal introitus. E. coli serotyping fails to differentiate these two events. Relapses occurring within two weeks of the discontinuation of treatment have been considered persistent renal parenchymal infections, whereas relapses that develop more than a month after the cessation of drug therapy probably indicate reinfection from Enterobacteriaceae situated in the urethra and vaginal introitus (Levinson and Kaye, 1972). Radiographic abnormalities identified in women experiencing persistent bacterial pyelonephritis include renal calculi, renal scarring, and papillary necrosis (Nanra et al., 1970; Cattell et al., 1973; Gutman et al., 1978).

The conventional two-week course of chemotherapy for women with bacterial pyelonephritis often results in a relapsing infection (Nanra et al., 1970; Gutman et al., 1978). Some patients, however, experience a cure when an extended course of treatment is prescribed (Turck *et al.*, 1966; Motzkin, 1972).

The phenomenon of bacterial relapse can occur following treatment of bacterial cystitis (Cattell *et al.*, 1973; Gutman *et al.*, 1978), thereby reducing the value of this therapeutic response as a means of localizing the site of a urinary tract infection. No evidence has established the role or cell-wall-defective bacteria as the cause of bacterial relapses in women with recurrent urinary tract infections (Gutman *et al.*, 1978).

VIII. THERAPEUTIC PRINCIPLES

Forty years ago, Charles Marple formulated therapeutic principles for the treatment of patients with urinary tract infections (Marple, 1941). Marple stressed the importance of confirming the diagnosis, developing an organized therapeutic programme, identifying recurrent infections, and detecting anatomical abnormalities amenable to surgical correction. The general and specific principles of therapy advocated by contemporary experts merely represent a "fine tuning" of the recommendations enunciated by Marple.

A.   General principles

1. Establish the diagnosis
Urine should be Gram-stained and cultured prior to the onset of therapy, because symptoms are not a reliable indicator of infection (Dans and Klaus, 1976). In addition, some patients experience no symptoms, and others develop complaints that do not immediately direct attention to the urinary tract (Esposito *et al.*, 1980). Bacteriuria constitutes the only accurate indicator of a bacterial urinary tract infection. Multiple, clean-voided, mid-stream, pre-treatment urines should be processed from the asymptomatic patient. If the patient appears toxic or experiences severe symptoms, only one urine culture need be processed.

2. Determine who merits therapy
All symptomatic adults with a bacterial urinary tract infection require therapy. Therapy is also indicated for the pregnant woman who harbours an asymptomatic urinary tract infection: these infections have serious con-sequences for the patient and her pregnancy. No convincing evidence exists to treat asymptomatic bacteriuria in men or nonpregnant women (Gleckman, 1976). In the absence of obstructive uropathy, these patients do not appear to develop progressive impairment of renal function. In addition, treatment of

these infections often fails to achieve the desired result — cure of the infection (Asscher *et al.*, 1969; Gleckman *et al.*, 1980a).

3. Hydration and frequent voiding

Traditionally, physicians have advised patients with urinary tract infections to drink copious fluids and void frequently. The kinetics of urinary flow and bladder evacuation appear to provide adequate justification for these recommendations. Hydration contributes to the dilution of the bacteriuria, and bladder contraction exerts a "washout" effect. Water diuresis diminishes medullary hypertonicity, thereby increasing leucocytic migration activity in the renal medulla, as well as inhibiting the formation of cell-wall-defective bacteria. Forcing fluids could prove detrimental, however. Larger urinary flows would dilute urinary antibacterial substances, such as urea, and reduce renal medullary concentrations of antimicrobial agents. Although some experts recommend that patients with urinary tract infections ingest copious amounts of fluids, no conclusive evidence has documented the value of this ancillary form of treatment.

4. Impaired urinary flow

Altered urodynamics, accompanied by abnormal bladder residual, vesico-ureteral reflux or obstruction, impedes successful eradication of a bacterial urinary tract infection, and antimicrobial therapy is not likely to be effective unless impediments to urinary flow are relieved. Renal stones obstruct urinary flow and on occasion provide a focus for persistent infection. When patients experience recurrent urinary tract infections, urological consultation should be obtained to identify those urodynamic abnormalities amenable to surgical correction.

5. Influence of urinary pH

Urinary pH manipulation influences the antimicrobial activity of some of the compounds prescribed for the therapy and prevention of urinary tract infections (Brumfitt and Percival, 1962). Alkalinization of the urine will enhance the activity of the aminoglycoside antibiotics and erythromycin. The prophylactic action of methenamine depends on its conversion in the urine to formaldehyde. The generation of formaldehyde is pH dependent, and detectable quantities are not produced at a pH of 7 (Musher and Griffith, 1974).

6. Pregnancy

When treating a urinary tract infection in a pregnant woman, the physician should select an antimicrobial agent known to be effective for the disease and safe for both patients and fetus. Limited data are available, but it does appear that penicillin, ampicillin, cephalexin, erythromycin, nitrofurantoin, and sulphonamides are safe compounds for the pregnant woman (Perry *et al.*, 1967; Hirsh, 1971). The unsubstantiated theoretical risk exists that administration of sulphonamide during the third trimester of pregnancy could result in the development of kernicterus. Efforts should be extended not to prescribe streptomycin or tetracyclines to pregnant women with urinary tract infections.

7. *Renal insufficiency*
The presence of renal insufficiency restricts the physician's therapeutic options in treating a urinary tract infection by the oral route. Cephalexin, ampicillin, nalidixic acid, oxolinic acid, and trimethoprim-sulphamethoxazole are excreted in the urine in therapeutic concentrations in patients with reduced glomerular filtration, are non-nephrotoxic, and have a record of proven efficacy for patients with renal insufficiency and a urinary tract infection (Kunin and Finkleberg, 1970). Tetracycline, sulphonamides, and nitrofurantoin should be avoided in the patient with impairment of renal function and a urinary tract infection. Parenteral administration of aminoglycosides has successfully eradicated urinary tract infections in patients with renal insufficiency (Christensson *et al.*, 1973). This treatment programme, however, predisposes patients to irreversible auditory and vestibular toxicity in spite of careful sequential monitoring of aminoglycoside serum concentrations. Recently published guidelines provide a framework for prescribing antibiotics to patients with renal insufficiency (Bennett, 1980; Whelton, 1980).

B. Specific principles of drug therapy

(1) A strong correlation exists between immediate eradication of bacteriuria and *in vitro* antibiotic susceptibility. Without initial sterilization of the urine, successful therapy fails to occur. However, cure of a urinary tract infection depends upon a number of factors in addition to the antibiotic susceptibility of the pretreatment organism (Lindemeyer *et al.*, 1963).

(2) The therapeutic goal has been achieved when symptoms resolve, the organism has been eradicated, and the urine remains sterile for a minimum of six weeks after the cessation of drug therapy. Symptomatology, if used exclusively, constitutes an inadequate indicator of therapeutic cure. Symptoms can recede spontaneously or even when inappropriate therapy has been prescribed.

(3) Many infectious disease experts prefer to administer a bactericidal compound to patients with urinary tract infections. No evidence exists, however, that bactericidal drugs produce more cures than bacteriostatic

agents. In fact, the drug trimethoprim, a bacteriostatic compound, compares favourably with bactericidal antibiotics, such as ampicillin and cephalexin, for the therapy of women with acute, symptomatic and recurrent urinary tract infections caused by *E. coli* (Brumfitt and Pursell, 1972).

(4) No evidence has emerged to support the policy of prescribing multiple antimicrobials simultaneously to patients with urinary tract infections. Co-administration of unselected, antimicrobial drugs fails to produce a higher cure rate than does an effective single agent (McCabe and Jackson, 1960; Acar and Brisset, 1975). In fact, no study has conclusively demonstrated that trimethoprim-sulphamethoxazole is a more effective chemotherapeutic agent than trimethoprim for the treatment of women with acute, symptomatic, or recurrent urinary tract infections. A novel approach to the treatment of patients with urinary tract infections caused by ampicillin- or amoxycillin-resistant strains is to prescribe the antibiotic with a penicillin derivative, such as cloxacillin or methicillin, that resists degradation by B-lactamase from Gram-negative urinary pathogens (Sabath *et al.*, 1967) or with a potent inhibitor of bacterial B-lactamase, known as clavulanic acid (Ball *et al.*, 1980). The future role of this therapeutic programme remains unknown. (The combination of potassium clavulanate and amoxycillin (Augmentin) is now available in the U.K.)

(5) Since the areas of bacteriological activity in pyelonephritis are the medullary and papillary zones of the kidney, the attainment of "effective" chemotherapeutic concentrations at these sites of infection have evolved as the cardinal principle of drug therapy (Naumann, 1978). Some researchers have championed the concept that the high concentrations of antibiotics present in the collecting ducts are transferred into the interstitial tissue water of the medulla and so urine concentrations rather than serum concentrations determine the outcome of urinary tract infections (Stamey *et al.*, 1974). Other researchers have confirmed the importance of antibiotic activity in the urine as a prerequisite for eradication of bacteriuria (McCabe and Jackson, 1965). The demonstration that the administration of oral nitrofurantoin and penicillin G cures documented bacterial pyelonephritis appears to provide strong support for the importance of urinary drug concentrations (Stamey *et al.*, 1965). Recently, however, the concept that the urinary concentration of an antibiotic reflects the coexistent drug concentration in the renal medulla or papilla has been challenged, particularly for the patient with profound renal insufficiency (Chisholm, 1974; Whelton, 1974). When severe degrees of renal impairment exist, serum, rather than urinary, drug concentrations may assume increased importance in therapy of urinary tract infections, or additional factors, such as the inability of drugs to penetrate infected renal medulla, may dictate therapeutic results.

It has been suggested that adopting a single principle of therapy based exclusively on achievable drug serum or urinary concentrations is too restrictive and it would be preferable to prescribe treatment according to the tissue source of the infection and the nature of the complications (Naumann, 1978). Patients with acute, uncomplicated bacterial cystitis should be treated with drugs that achieve therapeutic concentrations in the urine; patients with acute, symptomatic, and recurrent pyelonephritis and patients experiencing bacteraemia should be treated with medications that result in therapeutic concentrations in urine and serum; and patients with recurrent pyelonephritis, associated with structural abnormalities or renal insufficiency, should be treated with agents that achieve effective serum and tissue concentrations. This approach tends to resolve the dispute of the relative therapeutic importance of serum and urinary antibiotic concentrations for the treatment of urinary tract infections. Attractive as this concept appears, however, a number of obstacles remain before it can be accepted: reliable methods of determining medullary tissue concentrations of antibiotics are not readily available, antimicrobial agents often fail to penetrate infected renal medullary tissue in patients with renal insufficiency, and prospective, controlled studies of homogeneous patients would be required to confirm the theory proposed.

(6) Soon after the initiation of therapy, the physician can be confident that appropriate medication has been prescribed. After two days of therapy, Gram staining of the urine should no longer demonstrate bacteria, and sterility of the urine should occur for the vast majority of patients (Stamey, 1967). Failure of the urine to achieve sterility usually warns that the patient is receiving incorrect therapy.

(7) The optimum length of drug treatment depends on the nature of the infection. One-day therapy is adequate for the woman with acute, symptomatic, community-acquired, bacterial cystitis (Fang *et al.*, 1978). An extended course of therapy, at least six weeks, achieves a higher cure rate in men with recurrent, invasive urinary tract infections with a renal or a prostatic tissue source of infection (Gleckman *et al.*, 1979; Smith *et al.*, 1979). The practice of prescribing a two-week course of therapy to men with recurrent invasive urinary tract infections often falls far short of the desired treatment goal. The optimum duration of therapy for women with recurrent urinary tract infections remains to be defined. Some patients who experience bacterial relapse appear to benefit from an extended course of therapy (Turck *et al.*, 1968). The present suggested course of therapy for patients experiencing acute, symptomatic, community-acquired, bacterial pyelonephritis is 10–14 days, but this has not evolved from prospective, controlled studies and it remains an arbitrary decision. Desperate measures, such as the administration of excessive doses of antibiotics, have failed to enhance the cure rates of patients with acute pyelonephritis (Ode *et al.*, 1980).

(8) The patient with an indwelling Foley catheter and an asymptomatic

urinary tract infection requires no therapy. Treatment often results in the emergence of organisms resistant to the agent prescribed. If, however, systemic signs or symptoms of a urinary tract infection develop, there should be no reluctance to confirm the patency of the catheter, obtain blood and urine cultures, Gram-stain the aspirated urine, and initiate drug treatment with appropriate antimicrobials, as defined by the susceptibility patterns in the hospital.

(9) When a patient develops pyelonephritis and suspected bacteraemia, characterized by shaking chills, sweats, fever, and tachypnoea, blood and urine cultures should be obtained and parenteral antibiotics administered. Antibiotic selection will depend upon the findings of Gram-stain evaluation of the urine, the patient's history of drug allergies, and the nature of the patient's concomitant diseases. For the young woman with community-acquired, acute, symptomatic pyelonephritis caused by a Gram-negative aerobic bacillus, parenteral administration of a cephalosporin antibiotic would appear to be appropriate therapy because these compounds possess activity against those organisms, such as *E. coli*, *Proteus mirabilis*, and *Klebsiella* sp., which initiate most of the infections in this patient population. When acute pyelonephritis caused by a Gram-negative aerobic bacillus develops in a patient who has recently been catheterized, subjected to a urological procedure, or has experienced recurrent urinary tract infections, therapy should be initiated with an aminoglycoside antibiotic. Gentamicin, tobramycin, and amikacin appear equally effective drug treatments for the therapy of urinary tract infections caused by susceptible organisms. A recent double-blind, prospective, controlled, randomized study demonstrated, however, that tobramycin caused less incidence of nephrotoxicity than gentamicin (Smith *et al.*, 1980). When the infecting organism and its susceptibility have been established, a potentially less toxic drug should be prescribed, if possible.

(10) Urological and radiological evaluation is indicated for those patients with acute pyelonephritis who experience bacteraemia or remain febrile more than 96 hours after the onset of antibiotic treatment. Persistent fever suggests obstructive uropathy or a perinephric abscess (Thorley *et al.*, 1974). Resolution of fever in patients treated for acute pyelonephritis cannot be equated with disappearance of bacteriuria.

VIII. SPECIFIC MEDICATIONS

Contemporary antimicrobial therapy of urinary tract infections requires considerably more sophistication than simply "matching a bug with a drug" in accordance with laboratory susceptibility reports. No drug has emerged as the agent of choice for the treatment of all urinary tract infections, and

Table 3   Factors influencing drug selection

Host	Drug	Organism
1. Knowledge of natural history of untreated disease	Spectrum of activity	Prior susceptibility pattern
2. History of drug sensitivity	Pharmacological properties	Community-acquired v. nosocomial
3. Severity of infection	Route of administration	Bacteraemia
4. Pregnancy	Potential for adverse reactions	Recent antimicrobial exposures
5. Concomitant diseases	Therapeutic "track record"	
6. Presence of foreign bodies	Potential for drug interactions	
7. Pre-existing renal insufficiency or auditory abnormality	Access to assay; cost	
8. Site of infection	Prior drug therapies	

numerous factors that should influence antimicrobial selection have been identified (Table 3).

This section focuses attention on those medications most frequently prescribed for the prevention and therapy of urinary tract infections.

1. Sulphisoxazole

Sulphisoxazole, the prototype of the short-acting sulphonamide, the sulphonamide widely used most in the U.S. for the therapy of urinary tract infections. A sulphonamide is a general name for the thousands of derivatives of the compound para-aminobenzene-sulphonamide, or sulphanilamide. Sulphonamides serve as competitive substrates for the enzyme that converts p-aminobenzoic acid to folic acid, thus blocking bacterial production of folic acid and preventing the generation of the tetrahydrofolate cofactors that are vital for the synthesis of methionine, purines, and thymine.

Sulphisoxazole is a bacteriostatic compound that possesses limited activity for most Gram-negative urinary pathogens that cause urinary tract infections. Organisms usually susceptible to sulphisoxazole are those *E. coli* that are isolated from patients with community-acquired urinary tract infections. Sulphonamide resistance develops by several mechanisms. Some bacteria can synthesize enough p-aminobenzoic acid to antagonize sulphonamides. Other bacteria appear to alter the enzyme dihydropteric acid synthetase and effectively reduce its affinity for sulphonamides. R factor may mediate sulphonamide resistance by excluding sulphonamides from susceptible bacteria, a mechanism that resembles tetracycline resistance.

Sulphisoxazole is rapidly and completely absorbed, mostly in the small intestine. Peak plasma levels achieved two hours after administration of 2 g range from 121 to 210 g ml^{-1} of the intact drug. From 28 to 35% of sulphisoxazole is present in the blood in the acetylated form. The acetyl derivative is bacteriologically inactive but can contribute to toxicity. Sulphisoxazole is eliminated exclusively by urinary excretion through the mechanisms of glomerular filtration and tubular secretion, Sulphisoxazole also undergoes tubular reabsorption. The urinary recovery of intact sulphonamide ranges from 40 to 65% of the administered dose. The solubility of sulphisoxazole is enhanced with alkalinization of the urine. In patients with renal insufficiency an accumulation of both intact and conjugated drug occurs and elevated serum concentrations, enhanced toxicity, and reduced urinary concentrations of intact sulphisoxazole are observed.

The recommended adult dose for the treatment of urinary tract infections is 1 g every six hours. If it is essential to achieve therapeutic urinary concentrations of free sulphisoxazole in the azotaemic patient, the medication will have to be administered as frequently as every six hours. This strategy, however, increases the likelihood of drug toxicity due to increased serum levels of both intact and acetylated derivative. Whenever sulphisoxazole is prescribed, adequate hydration should be maintained.

Sulphisoxazole is appropriate therapy for women with acute, symptomatic urinary tract infections or recurrent urinary tract infections caused by susceptible E. coli (Hughes et al., 1975). It has been advised that sulphonamides be avoided in the later stages of pregnancy because of the theoretical possibility that these compounds may cross the placenta and displace bilirubin from its conjugation with glucuronic acid. No cases of sulphonamide-induced kernicterus have been described.

The list of untoward reactions attributed to the sulphonamides is substantial. Which of the adverse reactions are actually caused by the sulphonamides and how often they develop remains unknown. Table 4 depicts the untoward events attributed to the sulphonamides. The potential for these drugs to cause deaths, through the development of aplastic anaemia or agranulocytosis, places an obligation on the physician to justify their administration (Bottiger and Westerholm, 1977).

In prospective surveillance studies on hospitalized patients who received sulphisoxazole, the rate of adverse reactions severe enough to require discontinuation of treatment was very low (Koch-Weser et al., 1971). The most common untoward events attributed to sulphonamides include skin reactions (macular, maculopapular, uriticarial), drug fever, and gastrointestinal intolerance (anorexia, nausea, vomiting). There is good evidence

Table 4   Adverse reactions attributed to sulphonamides

GASTRO-INTESTINAL	RENAL
Anorexia	Haematuria
Nausea	Crystalluria
Vomiting	Oliguria
Abdominal pain	Anuria
Diarrhoea	Toxic nephrosis
Pancreatitis	Glomerulonephritis
Hepatitis	Interstitial nephritis
	Acute tubular necrosis
	Necrotizing angiitis
NEUROLOGICAL	HAEMATOLOGICAL
Headache	Haemolytic anaemia in patients with
Lassitude	glutathione peroxidase deficiency,
Confusion	glucose-6-phosphate dehydro-
Depression	genase deficiency, and unstable
Nightmares	haemoglobins (haemoglobino-
Insomnia	pathy Zurich)
Psychosis	Granulocytopenia
Sterile meningitis	Agranulocytosis
Ataxia	Aplastic anaemia
Vertigo	Thrombocytopenia
Tinnitus	Methaemoglobinaemia
Benign intracranial hypertension	
Convulsions	
Peripheral neuropathy	
Myalgia	
SKIN	MISCELLANEOUS
Macular, papular, urticarial eruptions	Fever
Phototoxic drug eruptions	Bechet's syndrome
Erythema multiforme and	Serum sickness
Stevens-Johnson syndrome	Anaphylaxis
Erythema nodosum	Arthralgia
Generalized exofoliative dermatitis	Myocarditis
Toxic epidermal necrolysis	Conjunctivitis
("scalded skin syndrome")	Diffuse granuloma of organs
	Asthma
	Pulmonary infiltrates with
	eosinophilia
	Lupus erythematosus
	Periarteritis nodosa
	Accelerated vascular disease

that fever and skin eruptions caused by sulphonamides increase in direct proportion to the quantity of medication prescribed. The adverse reaction that may prove to be the most significant is accelerated vascular disease. One published study cites an increased mortality among patients who received prolonged therapy with a sulphonamide to prevent recurrent urinary tract infections (Freeman *et al.*, 1975). The authors suggested that the sulphonamide accelerated coronary artery disease. Until the significance of this observation is clarified, sulphonamides should not be considered the agents of choice for prolonged therapy to prevent recurrent urinary tract infections.

Sulphonamides have the potential to displace tolbutamide, methotrexate, and warfarin from protein-binding sites, and this can result in transient hypoglycaemia, methotrexate toxicity, and bleeding. Phenylbutazone, acetylsalicylic acid, and probenecid can displace sulphonamides from serum carrier states and, thereby, cause increased sulphonamide toxicity. Sulphonamides inhibit hepatic biotransformation of tolbutamide, chlorpropamide, and phenytoin with the potential for causing hypoglycaemia and phenytoin toxicity. Sulphonamides compete with tolbutamide and methotrexate for renal tubular secretion, and this results in the potential for hypoglycaemia and methotrexate toxicity. Sulphonamides will frequently cause an interference in the urinary glucose test performed by Benedict's method, resulting in a false positive result. Rarely, sulphonamides cause a positive LE cell test.

2. Trimethoprim-sulphamethoxazole

The trimethoprim-sulphamethoxazole combination is the result of research efforts to develop specific enzyme inhibitors of bacterial folate synthesis. Three advantages have been claimed for combining the two components: synergistic activity, bactericidal effect, and reduction in the rate of emergence of resistance to the individual chemotherapeutic agents. The validity of these claims remains unproven.

The combination of trimethoprim-sulphamethoxazole produces a sequential blockage (or perhaps simultaneous binding to bacterial dihydrofolate reductase) that reduces the microbial cell pool of tetrahydrofolate cofactors that are essential for bacterial growth and survival. Tetrahydrofolate cofactors are carriers of one-carbon fragments and are vital for the synthesis of purines, thymine, serine, and methionine.

Trimethoprim-sulphamethoxazole susceptibility testing requires careful attention to detail, because the quantity and dispersal of the inoculum, as well as the constituents of the culture media, will influence markedly the test results. Among the common Gram-negative aerobic bacilli that cause urinary tract infections, virtually all *E. coli*, *Klebsiella* sp., *Citrobacter* sp., *Enterobacter* sp., and *Acinetobacter* sp. are susceptible to trimethoprim-sulphamethoxazole. Approximately 50% of strains of *Serratia* sp., *Pro-*

videncia sp., and *Proteus* sp. are susceptible, but *Pseudomonas aeruginosa* is invariably resistant.

Trimethoprim and sulphamethoxazole are absorbed rapidly after oral administration, achieving peak trimethoprim blood levels of 0.6–1.8 µg ml^{-1} within one to four hours and peak sulphamethoxazole levels of 30–54 µg ml^{-1} within two to four hours after two single-strength tablets are ingested. Trimethoprim exists in the plasma primarily as the intact drug. Sulphamethoxazole circulates in the blood as the intact, conjugated, and acetylated forms. Renal impairment is not associated with augmented plasma concentrations of intact (non-metabolically altered) sulphamethoxazole, but there is an elevation of serum trimethoprim and sulphamethoxazole metabolites. Urinary excretion of trimethoprim declines when the creatinine clearance is reduced below 20 ml min^{-1}. Even with advanced renal disease, urinary concentrations of trimethoprim exceed the minimum inhibitory concentrations for most urinary pathogens. Therapeutic urinary concentrations of sulphamethoxazole, however, do not invariably occur in the presence of marked renal insufficiency.

The adult dosage for the treatment of an established urinary tract infection is 160 mg trimethoprim and 800 mg sulphamethoxazole twice daily for 10–14 days. Two recent studies performed in men with recurrent invasive urinary tract infections have established the value of an extended course (6 or 12 weeks) of trimethoprim-sulphamethoxazole therapy (Gleckman *et al.*, 1979; Smith *et al.*, 1979). Trimethoprim-sulphamethoxazole is effective treatment for women with acute symptomatic urinary tract infections and is therapeutically comparable to conventional agents, such as ampicillin, amoxycillin, sulphonamides, cephalexin, tetracycline, nitrofurantoin and pivmecillinam. A single dose of trimethoprim-sulphamethoxazole appears to be adequate therapy for women with acute symptomatic bacterial cystitis. The combination drug is not recommended for the management of acute symptomatic bacterial urinary tract infection because it is no more effective than the individual components. Furthermore, most patients who experience acute symptomatic bacterial infections are young women who could be pregnant, and the safety of trimethoprim-sulphamethoxazole for pregnant women has not been established.

Trimethoprim-sulphamethoxazole is effective therapy for patients with recurrent urinary tract infections. In studies comparing trimethoprim-sulphamethoxazole to other agents (ampicillin, cephalexin, and nitrofurantoin) a clear superiority for one drug has not emerged. Some reports have suggested that trimethoprim-sulphamethoxazole is more effective than its components for the therapy of recurrent urinary tract infections, but this observation has not been confirmed (Brumfitt and Pursell, 1972; Harding *et al.*, 1975). Trimethoprim-sulphamethoxazole has successfully treated urinary tract infections in patients with severe renal functional impairment. The compound has been prescribed for patients with chronic bacterial prostatitis. It has been suggested that this combination antimicrobial agent is the most effective drug available for the therapy of chronic bacterial prostatitis and that the likelihood of success is enhanced by prolonged therapy (Meares, 1975). Trimethoprim-sulphamethoxazole reduces the incidence of symptomatic reinfections in women who experience recurrent urinary tract infections, presumably by interfering with colonization of the vaginal vestibule by faecal flora (Stamm et al., 1980). Trimethoprim-sulphamethoxazole does in fact attain therapeutic concentrations in vaginal fluid following oral ingestion and eradicates Enterobacteriaceae from the faecal flora.

Gastro-intestinal intolerance and skin eruptions appear as the most prevalent adverse reactions to trimethoprim-sulphamethoxazole. Toxicity is seldom, if ever, life-threatening and is almost always completely reversible. The incidence of untoward events from trimethoprim-sulphamethoxazole compares favourably with that from other agents administered for the same indications, and most untoward events develop within two weeks of the onset of therapy (Lawson and Jick, 1978). Gastro-intestinal intolerance develops in 3–8% of patients who receive trimethoprim-sulphamethoxazole. It is usually manifested as nausea with or without vomiting and frequently does not require discontinuation of therapy. Diarrhoea, glossitis, and stomatitis occur more rarely. Pseudomembranous colitis has been attributed to trimethoprim-sulphamethoxazole. Skin reactions develop in approximately 3% of cotrimoxazole recipients. The reactions consist of erythema, urticaria, or maculopapular, purpuric, or morbilliform lesions. The Stevens-Johnson syndrome and toxic epidermal necrolysis have developed from trimethoprim-sulphamethoxazole administration, and nodules, papules, and pustules have resulted from a necrotizing vasculitis. Untoward dermatological reactions are not caused exclusively by the sulphonamide component of the combination. Hepatic damage is a very rare manifestation of trimethoprim-sulphamethoxazole toxicity.

Deterioration of renal function has been observed in patients receiving trimethoprim-sulphamethoxazole. It has developed in patients with and without previous renal function impairment and is usually reversible. The reduction in serum creatinine apparently is not caused by an altered glomerular filtration rate. The rise in serum creatinine induced by trimethoprim-sulphamethoxazole may be caused by competitive inhibition of tubular secretion of creatinine (Berglund et al., 1975). Concern that trimethoprim-sulphamethoxazole would initiate frequent and serious haematological toxicity has not been borne out. Life-threatening haematological reactions, including anaemia (haemolytic, macrocytic, aplastic, hypoplastic), thrombocytopenia, granulocytopenia, and agranulocytosis do occur and, rarely, have been fatal, but these events are extraordinarily rare. Previous or simultaneous administration of diuretics with trimethoprim-sulphamethoxazole appears to enhance the likelihood of thrombocytopenia. This occurs most frequently in elderly patients with chronic, congestive heart failure.

Trimethoprim-sulphamethoxazole can potentiate the anticoagulant effect of warfarin and the hypoglycaemic response to tolbutamide, as well as impair the renal excretion of methotrexate.

3. Nitrofurantoin

Nitrofurantoin, a broad-spectrum chemotherapeutic compound of the nitro-furan family, inhibits bacterial growth by interfering with the translation process of protein synthesis. The compound is currently prescribed for two indications: as definitive therapy for an established urinary tract infection and as a prophylactic agent for patients with recurrent urinary tract infections.

The vast majority of *E. coli, Citrobacter* sp., group B streptococci, enterococci, *Staphylococcus aureus*, and *Staphylococcus epidermidis*, that cause urinary tract infections, are susceptible, *in vitro*, to nitrofurantoin. Virtually all *Pseudomonas aeruginosa* are resistant. Most *Klebsiella pneumoniae* and *Enterobacter* sp. are susceptible. The susceptibilities of *Proteus* (*mirabilis, vulgaris, rettgeri*), *Morganella morganii, Providencia* sp., and *Serratia* sp. are non-predictable, with the percentage of susceptible strains varying markedly in different laboratories. This is partly explained by a lack of standardization; microbiologists use different discs, inocula, and interpretations. Most strains of *Acinetobacter* sp. are resistant. Susceptible organisms do not readily develop resistance during treatment.

Nitrofurantoin is commercially available as an oral suspension, tablets, and parenteral liquid — the latter is virtually never prescribed, and its place in the therapeutic armamentarium has never been defined. The conventional dosage of nitrofurantoin for an established urinary tract infection is 50 or 100 mg four times a day. One study suggests that these doses produce comparable clinical and bacteriological response rates (Welling *et al.*, 1957). There are conflicting data on the influence of urinary pH on the therapeutic activity of nitrofurantoin. Patients should be advised that nitrofurantoin be ingested with meals, because the bio-availability of nitrofurantoin is enhanced when the drug is taken with food; the amount of drug absorbed and the duration of therapeutic urinary concentrations are increased substantially. Also, patients will experience less nausea and vomiting if nitrofurantoin is ingested with meals.

Approximately 40% of ingested drug is recovered intact in the urine. Urinary excretion results from glomerular filtration, tubular secretion, and tubular reabsorption. Patients with mild reduction of glomerular filtration fail to excrete nitrofurantoin in therapeutic concentrations, so it is contra-indicated in renal insufficiency.

Nitrofurantoin has proved effective for women with acute symptomatic community-acquired urinary tract infections caused by *E. coli* and it compares favourably with ampicillin (Brumfitt *et al.*, 1962). The therapeutic response is considerably worse when *Proteus mirabilis* is the aetiological agent, however. Nitrofurantoin does not appear to exert any untoward effects on the fetus when administered to the pregnant female (Perry *et al.*, 1967). Acute symptomatic urinary tract infections in men often are associated with structural abnormalities and accompanied by bacteraemia. Oral nitrofuran-toin fails to achieve therapeutic concentrations in serum and should not be administered to these men.

Nitrofurantoin treatment resulted in an 80–100% immediate cure rate of urinary tract infections in women without obstructive uropathy who have asymptomatic bacteriuria or recurrent urinary tract infections caused by *E. coli* (Ormonde *et al.*, 1969), but substantial recurrences occur when med-ication is discontinued. Therapeutic efficacy is not enhanced when alternative standard agents are prescribed. Limited data suggest that nitrofurantoin is not very effective for recurrent urinary tract infections in men.

Recurrent urinary tract infections in women have been prevented by a single dose of nitrofurantoin administered after sexual intercourse (Vosti, 1975) and by continuous single nightly doses taken over a prolonged time (Stamey *et al.*, 1977). Nitrofurantoin is a more effective prophylactic agent than a placebo and compares well with other chemotherapeutic agents used for prophylaxis (Stamm *et al.*, 1980). When continuous nitrofurantoin prophylaxis is discontinued, however, the recurrence rate over the next months is considerable. This is not unique to nitrofurantoin but characteristic of women with recurrent urinary tract infections. Continuous prophylactic treatment with nitrofurantoin has resulted in a decreased incidence of recurrences in men with recurrent urinary tract infections (Freeman *et al.*, 1975). For adult women, a single nightly dose of 50 mg nitrofurantoin is effective prophylaxis for recurrent urinary tract infections. For adult men a dose of 50 mg nitrofurantoin, four times a day, is effective prophylaxis, but a lower dose might be equally effective.

Adverse reactions to nitrofurantoin are frequent. A survey of untoward events experienced by hospitalized patients revealed an incidence of 9.2% (Koch-Weser *et al.*, 1971). Adverse reactions have included gastro-intestinal disturbances, skin eruptions, haematological disorders, neurological defects, pulmonary complications, hepatotoxicity, and miscellaneous abnormalities. Gastro-intestinal disturbances (anorexia, nausea, vomiting) are the most common side-effects. Nausea and vomiting usually develop during the first week of therapy, are experienced more often by women than men, and appear to be related to the daily drug dose and the patient's weight. An initial study suggested that patients were able to tolerate the macrocrystalline form better than crystalline nitrofurantoin, and a subsequent double-blind comparison confirmed this finding (Kaslowski *et al.*, 1974). Skin eruptions, consisting of macular, maculopapular, or urticarial lesions, are the second most common side-effect of nitrofurantoin. Haemolytic anaemia developing in patients with red blood cells deficient in the enzyme glucose-6-phosphate dehydrogenase (G6PD) is a well-documented haematological complication of nitrofurantoin. Nitrofurantoin has also precipitated haemolytic anaemia in patients who are deficient in other erythrocytic enzymes, namely enolase and glutathione peroxidase.

A serious and frequent adverse reaction to nitrofurantoin is peripheral polyneuropathy (Toole and Parish, 1973). Nitrofurantoin-induced poly-neuritis usually develops in a setting of azotaemia. The onset of the polyneuropathy is insidious and symmetrical, occurring after days to years of either continuous or intermittent nitrofurantoin therapy. The initial symp-toms include paraesthesiae and dysaethesiae, and arise more often in the lower than the upper extremities. Polyneuropathy progresses in a matter of days to include a number of sensory deficits, including impairment of pain, light touch, and vibration. Weakness and muscle wasting ensue and result in a flaccid paresis. The severity of symptoms is not related to the total amount of drug ingested. The polyneuritis may resolve completely, incompletely, or not at all. Resolution of the polyneuropathy varies inversely with the severity of the muscle weakness.

Nitrofurantoin-induced pulmonary reactions have been arbitrarily classified into acute, subacute, and chronic (Sovijarvi *et al.*, 1977). The classical acute pulmonary reaction syndrome consists in the sudden onset of fever, chills, cough, myalgia, and dyspnoea (with or without cyanosis), râles at the lung bases, lower-lobe infiltrates on chest X-ray (with or without effusion), rapid resolution of clinical and radiological abnormalities following discon-tinuation of the medication, an elevated erythrocyte sedimentation rate, delayed onset of peripheral blood eosinophilia, and recurrence of similar clinical manifestations, with a shortened incubation period, on subsequent exposure. This reaction develops within hours to weeks of the ingestion of the drug and can be accompanied by headache, rash, generalized pruritus, chest discomfort, sputum production, and shock. The syndrome has been mistaken for congestive heart failure, pulmonary embolism, bacterial pneumonia, an asthmatic attack, anaphylaxis, pericarditis, and myocardial infarction. The reaction almost always resolves completely, although at least one fatality has been reported. The value of steroid therapy in accelerating recovery remains unproven.

Subacute pulmonary reactions from nitrofurantoin usually develop after one month of drug exposure and are characterized by persistent and progressive cough, dyspnoea, orthopnoea, and fever. Radiographically, there is interstitial pneumonitis. There may be an associated lupus-like syndrome consisting in arthralgia, pleural effusions, peripheral lymphadenopathy, impaired liver function, elevated erythrocyte sedimentation rate, polyclonal hypergammaglobulinaemia, positive latex agglutination test, antinuclear antibodies and antibodies to thyroid, glomeruli, and smooth muscle. Discontinuation of nitrofurantoin is followed by complete resolution of all abnormalities. The chronic nitrofurantoin pulmonary reaction is associated with the insidious development of non-productive cough and dyspnoea. Fever is not a consistent finding, and peripheral blood eosinophilia is absent. The erythrocyte sedimentation rate is usually elevated, and there may be abnormalities of liver function tests. The chronic nitrofurantoin pulmonary reaction develops after six months of drug treatment. Usually, but not always, regression of the syndrome follows discontinuation of nitrofurantoin therapy. Treatment with steroid may improve symptoms, but there is no firm evidence that pulmonary function or radiographs are improved. Irreversible pulmonary fibrosis culminating in respiratory failure and death has resulted from long-term treatment with nitrofurantoin.

Nitrofurantoin-induced hepatotoxicity is rare and is usually readily reversible with cessation of the medication. Recent reports, however, have focussed on nitrofurantoin-induced chronic active hepatitis, a disease that can result in death (Black *et al.*, 1980; Sharp *et al.*, 1980). The patients are invariably women who have taken the medication for months to years. These reports of hepatoxicity and death should force physicians to justify prolonged administration of nitrofurantoin.

Nitrofurantoin interferes with the determination of urinary LDH and yields a false-positive urine glucose determination when Benedict's qualitative reagent is used.

The frequency and potential severity of reactions attributed to nitrofurantoin, combined with its inability to achieve therapeutic blood concentrations, relegate this compound to a position of secondary importance (Holmberg *et al.*, 1980). Nitrofurantoin should not be administered to patients with acute bacterial pyelonephritis (this disease can be accompanied by bacteraemia) or to men with recurrent urinary tract infections, and it should not be an agent of first choice for patients with acute, symptomatic bacterial cystitis. Indications for nitrofurantoin could include the following: treatment of the penicillin- or cephalosporin-sensitive patient who has acute, symptomatic bacterial cystitis or a recurrent urinary tract infection unassociated with bacteraemia and caused by a nitrofurantoin-susceptible organism, chronic prophylaxis for the adult who experiences multiple disabling symptomatic exacerbations of recurrent urinary tract infections.

4. Nalidixic acid

Nalidixic acid (1-ethyl-1,4-dihydro-7-methyl-4-oxo-1,8-naphthyridine-3-carboxylic acid) is a synthetic antimicrobial agent that inhibits bacterial growth by interfering with DNA synthesis. Nalidixic acid possesses *in vitro* activity for most Gram-negative, aerobic urinary tract pathogens, including *E. coli, Citrobacter* (*diversus* and *freundii*), *Klebsiella* sp., *Enterobacter* sp., *Morganella morganii, Proteus* (*mirabilis, vulgaris, rettgeri*), and *Providencia* sp. *Pseudomonas aeruginosa* isolates are invariably resistant.

The usual adult dosage for the treatment of an established urinary tract infection is 1 g four times daily. The selection of resistant mutants and treatment failures occur when a less than a full therapeutic dosage of 4 g daily is administered (Stamey and Bragonje, 1976).

Alkalinization of the urine increases excretion of nalidixic acid, as well as the ratio of intact drug to inactive metabolites. However, adjustment of urinary pH has not been shown to enhance the microbiological response. Renal insufficiency increases serum concentrations and decreases the urinary concentrations of the patient compound, but urinary levels continue to exceed the minimum inhibitory concentrations for most urinary tract pathogens. Guidelines for dosage modifications in patients with renal failure have not been developed.

Adverse reactions to nalidixic acid develop frequently, occur more readily with prolonged administration, and have potentially serious consequences. The most common untoward reactions include gastro-intestinal disturbances, skin lesions, and neurological events. Nausea is the most frequent gastro-intestinal adverse effect of nalidixic acid. Epigastric pain, abdominal discomfort, vomiting, and diarrhoea have also occurred. Skin reactions have included pruritus, urticaria, purpuric and maculopapular eruptions, exfoliative lesions, and erythema multiforme. The most prevalent adverse skin reactions are the photosensitive bullous eruptions. These bullous lesions tend to occur on the hands, feet, and legs, usually sparing the face. The bullae generally develop days to weeks after the start of treatment. Although the lesions usually resolve within two weeks of the discontinuation of therapy, blisters and increased skin friability can persist for months after nalidixic acid is discontinued or sun exposure is avoided. Neurological reactions attributed to nalidixic acid are among the most common and the most serious. These reversible reactions include tremulousness, confusion, drowsiness, headache, and dizziness. Visual abnormalities — photophobia, halo formation, sensations of flashing lights, inability to focus, change in colour perception, diplopia, blurring of outlines, and visual hallucinations — have been reported in approximately 9–20% of patients. They appear to be dose related and can disappear with continued treatment. Convulsions, with or without hyperglycaemia, most commonly develop in patients with an underlying seizure disorder.

Numerous studies involving thousands of patients confirm the therapeutic efficacy of nalidixic acid for patients with acute, symptomatic urinary tract infections and recurrent urinary tract infections caused by *E. coli, Proteus* sp. and *Enterobacter* sp. The compound is neither more efficacious nor better tolerated than accepted standard agents, such as sulphonamides or ampicillin. Nalidixic acid is an alternative to ampicillin, amoxycillin, cephalixin, a sulphonamide, or trimethoprim-sulphamethoxazole when patients are hypersensitive to penicillins or sulphonamides. Nalidixic acid could be considered appropriate treatment for the patient with renal insufficiency who experiences a recurrent urinary tract infection. The drug should not be prescribed to patients who may be pregnant or have bacteraemia.

5. Cinoxacin

Cinoxacin is a new synthetic compound (1-ethyl-1,4-dihydro-4-oxo-(1,3)-dioxolo-(4,5-g)cinnoline-3-carboxylic acid) which has recently been approved by the U.S. Food and Drug Administration (FDA) for clinical use. Most Enterobacteriaceae, including *E. coli, Klebsiella* sp., Enterobacter sp., Proteus sp. and *Serratia marcescens* are susceptible *in vitro* to concentrations of cinoxacin readily achieved in the urine after oral administration. *Pseudomonas aeruginosa* and Gram-positive organisms remain resistant to this agent.

Limited published data have confirmed the therapeutic efficacy of cinoxacin for patients with acute symptomatic bacterial cystitis and recurrent urinary tract infections. In addition cinoxacin has been demonstrated to have substantial prophylactic effectiveness. The compound compares favourably with other agents prescribed for the treatment or prevention of bacterial urinary tract infections.

Cinoxacin shares with trimethoprim-sulphamethoxazole the advantage of infrequent administration. A dosage of 0.5 g twice a day is effective. Adverse events attributed to the drug occur infrequently and consist predominantly in gastro-intestinal intolerance, central nervous system derangements, and hypersensitivity reactions.

6. Oxolinic acid

Oxolinic acid (5-ethyl-5,8-dihydro-8-oxo-1,3 dioxolo[4,5-g] quinoline-7-carboxylic acid) is a synthetic antimicrobial agent which inhibits bacterial growth by interfering with DNA synthesis. The compound has been approved by the U.S. FDA exclusively for the treatment of adults with established bacterial urinary tract infections unassociated with bacteraemia. Oxolinic acid possesses *in vitro* activity for most Gram-negative, aerobic urinary tract pathogens, including *E. coli, Klebsiella* sp., *Enterobacter* sp., and *Proteus* sp. *Pseudomonas aeruginosa* and *Acinetobacter calcoaceticus* (var. *wolffi* and var. *anitratum*) are uniformly resistant, however.

Therapeutic concentrations of oxolinic acid can be maintained by dosing only twice a day. The drug has a propensity to evoke resistant mutants when the daily dose is less than 2 g. Urinary concentrations of unconjugated drug range of 15–155 µg ml $^{-1}$ in patients with normal renal function. Therapeutic urinary concentrations are achieved even in the presence of severe renal impairment, and excessive drug accumulation has not been observed in patients with renal insufficiency (Madsen and Rhodes, 1971).

Adverse reactions are experienced by 10–45% of oxolinic acid recipients. The most common are central nervous system and gastro-intestinal disturbances. These untoward events are usually mild and resolve with the discontinuation of treatment. Central nervous system toxicity has included insomnia (the most frequent), restlessness, dizziness, headache, drowsiness, and visual disturbances. An association with seizures has not been clearly established, but oxolinic acid has a stimulatory effect on the central nervous system and should not be prescribed for patients with known seizure disorders. Gasto-intestinal reactions include nausea (the most frequent), vomiting, abdominal discomfort, and diarrhoea. These reactions can be reduced by concurrent administration of food or antacids.

Data derived from a limited number of published studies indicate that oxolinic acid is effective therapy for adult patients with acute, symptomatic, and recurrent urinary tract infections caused by *E. coli* and *Proteus mirabilis*. Oxolinic acid is neither more efficacious nor better tolerated than other antimicrobial agents, such as trimethoprim-sulphamethoxazole, ampicillin, and nalidixic acid, which are prescribed for patients with urinary tract infections. Oxolinic acid is an effective prophylactic agent for adult women with recurrent symptomatic urinary tract infections (Monnisoto, 1976), but the U.S. FDA has not approved this indication.

Oxolinic acid should be considered an alternative form of therapy for the penicillin-, cephalosporin-, or sulphonamide-sensitive adult who experiences recurrent urinary tract infections caused by susceptible *E. coli* and *Proteus mirabilis*, nor should it be prescribed for patients with acute symptomatic urinary tract infections, patients experiencing bacteraemia, or pregnant women.

7. *Methenamine mandelate and methenamine hippurate*

The antimicrobial action of methenamine depends upon its conversion in the urine to formaldehyde. The generation of formaldehyde is contingent upon urinary pH, the urinary concentration of methenamine, and the duration that the urine is retained in the bladder. Peak concentrations of formaldehyde are achieved in the urine at a pH of 5.6, whereas detectable quantities are not produced at a pH of 7. An effective concentration of formaldehyde must persist in the urine for a minimum of two hours for bacterial killing to occur.

Mandelic and hippuric acids exert weak antibacterial activity that correlates with the number of undissociated acid molecules present in the urine. These organic acids have been combined with methenamine, not for their anti-bacterial effect, but because they reduce the urinary pH and thus enhance the generation of formaldehyde from methenamine.

Formaldehyde has a spectrum of activity that encompasses all bacteria that cause urinary tract infections. When the urinary pH exceeds 6.5, free formaldehyde is not generated and antimicrobial activity is negligible. When infection is caused by a urease-producing organism, such as *Proteus* sp., the relative alkalinity of the urine retards formaldehyde formation and anti-microbial activity. However, acetohydroxamine acid, an inhibitor of urease, can re-establish urinary acidity and promote the therapeutic efficacy of methenamine salts (Musher *et al.*, 1976b).

The mandelate and hippurate salts of methenamine undergo rapid and complete absorption following oral ingestion. The influence of renal insufficiency on the pharmacological action of methenamine compounds is unknown.

Methenamine mandelate and hippurate are effective prophylactic drugs for adults who experience recurrent urinary tract infections. These compounds compare favourably with other standard prophylactic agents (e.g. sulpho-namides, nitrofurantoin, trimethoprim-sulphamethoxazole). Methenamine mandelate and hippurate are not indicated for patients with indwelling Foley catheters or those who require intermittent catheterization (Varrub and Musher, 1977). Methenamine mandelate and methenamine hippurate are equally effective in preventing recurrent urinary tract infections. Adults should receive methenamine hippurate 1 g twice daily or methenamine mandelate 1 g four times daily. There is a need to reassess the common practice of co-administering acidifying agents, such as ascorbic acid, with methenamine derivatives, because there is no evidence that this enhances the therapeutic activity of the methenamine compounds. Limited data suggest that methenamine compounds can be administered safely to pregnant women during the second and third trimester.

The manufacturer recommends methenamine mandelate as appropriate therapy for an established bacterial urinary tract infection, but the consensus of the published data does not support this view. This issue will remain unresolved, however, until prospective studies are performed which include defined patient populations and valid objective criteria of therapeutic efficacy.

A review of published reports suggests that 1–7% of patients who receive these compounds experience untoward effects. Adverse reactions are mild and reversible. Common untoward events are gastro-intestinal intolerance (nausea, vomiting, and abdominal cramps) and skin reactions (pruritus, urticaria, and erythematous eruption). One study suggests that nausea occurs more frequently with the mandelate than with the hippurate (Gow, 1974). Stomatitis, anorexia, headache, dyspnoea, and generalized oedema are rare adverse reactions. Very large doses of the methenamine compounds have produced urological abnormalities (dysuria, urgency, urinary frequency, and haematuria) and intensified gastro-intestinal symptomatology. The concurrent administration of methenamine mandelate with sulphathiazole has resulted in asymptomatic precipitation of the sulphonamide.

The effect of methenamine administration in patients with renal insufficiency and metabolic acidosis is not established. Methenamine derivatives might exacerbate the acidotic state, but this has not been confirmed. Until this information becomes available, an alternative drug probably should be used in patients with renal insufficiency.

8. Tetracyclines

Tetracyclines are bacteriostatic antibiotics which inhibit bacterial growth by blocking ribosomal protein synthesis. The ability of bacteria to resist the activity of tetracycline depends upon the presence of an altered ribosome, or more frequently, the presence of a plasmid which causes decreased uptake of the antibiotic. The activity of the tetracyclines (tetracycline, oxytetracycline, chlortetracycline) against those Gram-negative, aerobic bacilli, such as *E. coli*, *Klebsiella* sp., *Proteus mirabilis*, and *Enterobacter* sp. which cause most urinary tract infections, can be best described as "variable". The frequency of resistant strains varies from community to community and hospital to hospital. As a general statement, hospital-acquired strains are more resistant than those acquired in the community. Because such widespread resistance exists, the tetracyclines cannot be relied upon as initial therapy of infections caused by Gram-negative facultative bacilli. The newer tetracyclines, minocycline, and doxycycline, also fail to possess *in vitro* activity for those Enterobacteriaceae resistant to the more established tetracyclines. Most strains of *Serratia* sp. and *Pseudomonas aeruginosa* are resistant to the tetracyclines, as are enterococci.

All tetracyclines are well absorbed when taken orally, except chlortetracycline. Food, antacids, milk, and iron tablets impair absorption of these antibiotics. Cimetidine does not interfere with absorption. Chlortetracycline and the newest compounds, minocycline and doxycycline, are eliminated largely by non-renal routes, while tetracycline and oxytetracycline are mainly excreted in the urine. Tetracycline antibiotics should be avoided in pregnant women and patients with renal insufficiency, as these compounds can exacerbate renal dysfunction and produce a catabolic state, increasing acidosis, liver toxicity, and death. For the patient with renal insufficiency who requires a tetracycline, doxycycline can be administered in conventional doses without fear of drug accumulation, enhanced renal dysfunction, or catabolic acidosis.

Tetracycline, oxytetracycline, and chlortetracycline are administered orally as 250–500 mg four times a day. Tetracyclines are effective therapy of acute symptomatic bacterial cystitis in women (Mogabgab and Pallock, 1977), but the possibility of pregnancy should preclude their use in this patient population. No recent study has critically evaluated the efficacy of the tetracycline compounds for the treatment of recurrent urinary tract infections, and their role in the therapy of these infections remains undefined. The newer tetracyclines, minocycline and doxycycline, have received considerable attention as drug therapy of chronic bacterial prostatitis, but at present in the U.S., these compounds have not been approved by the Food and Drug Administration for this indication.

Adverse reactions caused by the oral administration of tetracycline include gastro-intestinal disturbances (nausea, vomiting, anorexia, unpleasant taste, glossitis, proctitis), oral candidiasis and vulvovaginitis, and skin eruptions (rash, phototoxicity). Minocycline possesses a unique capability for inducing vestibular toxicity in recipients.

Tetracyclines can cause a false-positive urine glucose test with Clinitest reagents and a false-negative test with Tes-Tape, a glucose oxidase reagent. The half-life of doxycycline is significantly shortened by co-administration of phenobarbital, phenytoin, and carbamazepine.

9. Carbenicillin

Carbenicillin indanyl sodium, the sodium salt of the indanyl ester of carbenicillin, is a bactericidal, semi-synthetic penicillin which inhibits the synthesis of the bacterial-cell-wall peptidoglycan component by selectively blocking the transpeptidase enzyme involved in the final crosslinking step. In the U.S., the Food and Drug Administration approved indications for this antibiotic include acute, symptomatic, and recurrent bacterial urinary infections and acute and chronic bacterial prostatitis.

In vitro drug susceptibility tests reveal a consistent pattern for those bacteria that cause most urinary tract infections. The majority of strains of *E. coli, Proteus mirabilis, Proteus vulgaris, Proteus rettgeri, Morganella morganii, Enterobacter* sp., *Acinetobacter calcoaceticus, Pseudomonas aeruginosa,* and enterococci are susceptible to the concentrations of carbenicillin achieved in the urine. *Klebsiella* sp. are invariably resistant to carbenicillin indanyl sodium, as are many strains of *Serratia* sp. The emergence of resistance during therapy, although described, has not evolved as a major problem with administration of carbenicillin indanyl sodium.

Gastro-intestinal absorption of carbenicillin indanyl sodium approximates 24–52% of the administered dose. Following absorption, the compound is immediately and completely hydrolysed to 5-indanol and carbenicillin. Carbenicillin is excreted intact in the urine. Excretion of the indanol moiety occurs as the microbiologically inert glucuronide or sulphate conjugate.

Peak serum concentrations of carbenicillin, achieved 1–2 hours after the drug has been ingested, are 2–14 μg ml $^{-1}$ respectively, following a 500 mg or 1 g dose. These concentrations preclude oral administration of carbenicillin indanyl sodium for the therapy of bacteraemia or deep-seated tissue infections. Recovery of 22–40% of the administered dose in the urine during the 24 hours following drug administration occurs in patients with normal renal function. Patients with glomerular filtration rates of < 20 ml min $^{-1}$ fail to excrete carbenicillin indanyl sodium in therapeutic concentrations.

The adult dosage for the treatment of an established urinary tract infection due to susceptible organisms is 500 mg to 1 g carbenicillin indanyl sodium administered four times daily. For treatment of acute or chronic bacterial prostatitis, the dose is 1 g four times daily.

The data indicate that carbenicillin indanyl sodium has not precipitated an inordinate number of adverse reactions. As a general statement, untoward events attributed to this antibiotic have been more of a nuisance, rather than life-threatening and are invariably completely reversible with discontinuation of the medication. As with all penicillin derivatives, however, the risk of immediate and accelerated reactions exist and a history of penicillin-hypersensitivity precludes administration of this drug.

The actual incidence of adverse reactions attributed to carbenicillin indanyl sodium remains unknown. One investigator cites an incidence of 9.9%, a number derived from surveillance performed on 782 patients (Hernandez, 1974). Gasto-intestinal intolerance and hypersensitivity events appear as the most prevalent adverse reactions to carbenicillin indanyl sodium. Gastro-intestinal intolerance usually is manifested as nausea, with or without vomiting, diarrhoea, and abdominal cramps. Hypersensitivity reactions have included rash, consisting of urticaria, acneiform or maculopapular lesions, pruritus, drug fever, and peripheral blood eosinophilia.

Carbenicillin indanyl sodium has been evaluated extensively in adults with recurrent urinary tract infections. When compared to other standard agents, such as ampicillin, cephalexin, and nitrofurantoin, a clear therapeutic superiority has not emerged (Ries *et al.*, 1973). Carbenicillin indanyl sodium currently remains the only antibiotic that can be prescribed as an oral agent for patients with recurrent urinary tract infections caused by *Pseudomonas aeruginosa*. Therapy of these infections with carbenicillin indanyl sodium has not proven highly successful, however, undoubtedly reflecting the fact that the vast majority of these infections occur in patients with structural defects.

Following the recent completion of a multi-clinic study, the U.S. Food and Drug Administration approved the use of oral carbenicillin indanyl sodium for the therapy of acute and chronic bacterial prostatitis (Oliveri *et al.*, 1979). Although it has a number of design problems, this investigation has established carbenicillin indanyl sodium as the only medication currently approved by the Food and Drug Administration for the therapy of chronic bacterial prostatitis.

In the U.S. parenteral carbenicillin and ticarcillin have emerged as preferred agents to treat acute symptomatic pyelonephritis caused by susceptible strains of *Pseudomonas aeruginosa*, particularly when bacteraemia is suspected or known to be occurring. For the therapy of the leucopenic host carbenicillin and ticarcillin are often prescribed with an aminoglycoside in order to achieve a synergistic bactericidal effect.

Appropriate intravenous dosages for adult patients with life-threatening *Pseudomonas aeruginosa* pyelonephritis and normal renal function are carbenicillin (2–3 g every 2 hours) and ticarcillin (3 g every 4 hours).

Carbenicillin and ticarcillin can cause sodium overload for patients with cardiac, liver or renal failure, hypokalaemia, granulocytopenia, platelet dysfunction and bleeding.

Penicillin compounds with enhanced *in vitro* activity for *Pseudomonas aeruginosa*, such as azlocillin, mezlocillin and piperacillin, are currently being investigated in the U.S. These compounds have demonstrated efficacy in selected patients with pyelonephritis but have not been released by the U.S. Food and Drug Administration for general clinical use. They are, however, available in other countries.

10. Cephalexin

Cephalosporins, like penicillins, are bactericidal antibiotics that inhibit the enzymatic reactions necessary for the production of a stable bacterial cell wall, but the sites of action of the penicillins and the cephalosporin antibiotic, cephalexin, on the bacterial cell wall do not appear to be identical (Greenwood and O'Grady, 1973). The beta-lactum ring is vital to the antibacterial action of both penicillins and cephalosporins. Structurally, cephalexin, a cephalosporin, differs from members of the penicillin family of drugs, because the five-membered thiazolidine ring so characteristic of the penicillins has been replaced by the six-membered dihydrothiazine ring, a hallmark of the cephalosporins. In general, the Enterobacteriaceae that cause most urinary tract infections (*E. coli*, *Proteus mirabilis*, and *Klebsiella* sp.) are susceptible to cephalexin, particularly when associated with community-acquired infections. *Enterobacter* sp., *Serratia* sp., *Proteus vulgaris*, *Proteus rettgeri*, and *Morganella morganii* are usually resistant to cephalexin, as are all strains of *Pseudomonas aeruginosa* and enterococci. Most strains of *Staphylococcus aureus* and *Staphylococcus epidermidis* are susceptible *in vitro* to cephalexin.

Cephalexin is well absorbed following oral administration, reaching peak serum concentrations of 13–18 µg ml^{-1}. The presence of food in the stomach delays and reduces by about one-third, the peak serum levels. It is excreted in the urine by glomerular filtration and tubular secretion. Unlike cephalothin and cephapirin, it fails to undergo biotransformation. It achieves therapeutic urinary concentrations in patients with profound renal insufficiency.

Gastro-intestinal intolerance (nausea, vomiting, diarrhoea), hypersensitivity reactions (maculopapular rash, urticaria, fever), and vulvovaginitis are the most common adverse effects of cephalexin. Cephalexin can produce a positive Coombs' test and, more rarely, antibiotic-related pseudomembranous colitis caused by *Clostridium difficile*. Patients who have experienced an immediate or accelerated hypersensitivity reaction to a member of the penicillin family of drugs should not receive cephalexin. Whether patients who have demonstrated non-life-threatening, delayed hypersensitivity reactions to penicillins should receive cephalexin remains unresolved. Cephalexin appears to be as well tolerated as ampicillin and trimethoprim-sulphamethoxazole, when these medications are prescribed to patients with acute symptomatic bacterial urinary tract infections, asymptomatic bacteriuria, or recurrent urinary tract infections (Davies *et al.*, 1971).

No study has defined the optimum daily dose of cephalexin for patients with urinary tract infections. Investigators have prescribed 1–3 g daily in divided dose. It has been noted, however, that cephalexin, like other chemotherapeutic agents, often fails to cure urinary tract infections in patients with structural abnormalities. Limited data suggest that cephalosporins are safe for pregnant women.

Cephalexin is effective for patients with acute symptomatic bacteriuria and recurrent urinary tract infections and appears therapeutically comparable to conventional medications (sulphonamides, ampicillin, trimethoprim-sulphamethoxazole) prescribed for these infections.

11. Ampicillin

Ampicillin is an extended-spectrum, semisynthetic penicillin. This antibiotic exerts a bactericidal effect as it binds to B-lactam receptor proteins involved in cell division.

Ampicillin is active against *E. coli* and *Proteus mirabilis*, the Gram-negative bacilli that cause most community-acquired urinary tract infections, and also possesses *in vitro* activity for enterococci. The majority of hospital-acquired strains of *Staphylococcus aureus* and *Staphylococcus epidermidis* are resistant. *Klebsiella pneumoniae*, *Enterobacter colacae*, *Enterobacter aerogenes*, *Acinetobacter* sp., *Proteus rettgeri*, *Proteus vulgaris*, *Morganella morganii*, *Serratia* sp., and *Pseudomonas aeruginosa* are resistant to ampicillin.

From 30–50% of the oral ampicillin dose is absorbed, primarily in the duodenum, and serum and urinary concentrations of the medication are not significantly reduced when the antibiotic is ingested with food. The co-administration of probenecid increases the serum ampicillin concentration through blockage of renal tubular excretion. Approximately 30–45% of the drug is excreted in the urine, primarily as the intact compound.

The most common adverse reactions that develop after the ingestion of ampicillin include diarrhoea and skin eruptions (maculopapular rash, urticaria). Ampicillin has precipitated pseudomembranous colitis—fortunately, however, rarely. Ampicillin skin rashes have been reported to occur in 5% of drug recipients (Shapiro et al., 1969). The most prevalent, the maculopapular rashes, have developed with striking incidence in patients with cytomegalovirus, infectious mononucleosis, lymphocytic leukaemia, and in hyperuricaemic patients receiving allopurinol. The rash occurs 1–28 days after initiation of drug therapy and, on occasion, has its onset days after the antibiotic has been discontinued. In contrast to the urticarial reactions that follow ampicillin exposure, the maculopapular rash does not appear to have an allergic basis.

Ampicillin is effective therapy for community-acquired, acute symptomatic pyelonephritis and cystitis caused by susceptible E. coli, and it appears therapeutically comparable to other agents prescribed for these infections, such as nitrofurantoin, cephalexin, trimethoprim-sulphamethoxazole, and amoxycillin. In studies comparing ampicillin to other agents (cephalexin, trimethoprim-sulphamethoxazole) administered for the therapy of asymptomatic bacteriuria or recurrent urinary tract infections, a clear superiority of one medication has not emerged. Ampicillin has proved to be effective therapy for patients with urinary tract infections and concomitant severe renal failure.

12. Amoxycillin

Amoxycillin is a semisynthetic penicillin structurally related to ampicillin but differing by the addition of an hydroxyl group to the phenyl side-chain of ampicillin. Amoxycillin exerts a bactericidal effect by binding to B-lactam receptor proteins that are involved in cell wall synthesis and destruction. Against some Gram-negative bacteria, amoxycillin appears to have a greater affinity for an enzyme involved in shape, because bacterial cells exposed to it rupture rather than make long filaments as occurs with exposure to ampicillin.

Amoxycillin possesses in vitro activity for community-acquired E. coli and Proteus mirabilis, as well as enterococci. Klebsiella pneumoniae, Enterobacter colacae, Enterobacter aerogenes, Acinetobacter sp., Proteus rettgeri, Proteus vulgaris, Morganella morganii, Serratia sp., Citrobacter freundii, and Pseudomonas aeruginosa are resistant to amoxycillin. The majority of hospital- and many community-acquired isolates of Staphylococcus aureus and Staphylococcus epidermidis are resistant.

Amoxycillin is better and more rapidly absorbed than ampicillin and achieves mean serum concentrations twice those of ampicillin. Ingestion of food does not appreciably reduce its absorption. After absorption, it is not changed to ampicillin. Concomitant administration of probenecid blocks tubular secretion of the antibiotic, resulting in elevated and prolonged blood concentrations of amoxycillin. Urinary excretion of amoxycillin exceeds that of ampicillin, and it is excreted in the urine primarily in the active form. In patients with profound renal insufficiency (creatinine clearance <5 ml) the urinary concentrations of amoxycillin are less than 100 µg ml^{-1}.

Adverse reactions caused by amoxycillin occur in approximately 5% of recipients. Untoward events consist of gastro-intestinal intolerance (nausea, vomiting, diarrhoea) and skin rashes (maculopapular eruptions, urticaria). Diarrhoea appears to develop less frequently with amoxycillin than with ampicillin. Rare side-effects following administration of amoxycillin have included pseudomembranous colitis and neutropenia. It should never be given to a patient who has sustained an immediate or accelerated hypersensitivity-reaction to any penicillin.

Amoxycillin is effective therapy for women with community-acquired bacterial cystitis and pyelonephritis and no structural abnormalities of the urinary tract (Ronald *et al.*, 1977). Comparable results occur when women with symptomatic bacterial cystitis receive amoxycillin, ampicillin, or trimethoprim-sulphamethoxazole. Single-dose therapy (3 g) has proven highly successful treatment for women with symptomatic cystitis, and the cure rates have not been enhanced by the conventional ten-day course of medication.

13. Trimethoprim

Trimethoprim (2,4-diamino-5-(3,4,5-trimethoxy benzyl) pyrimidine) is a competitor inhibitor of dihydrofolic acid. Trimethoprim binds to the enzyme dihydrofolate acid reductase, thereby preventing bacteria from converting dihydrofolic acid to tetrahydrofolic acid. Blockade of tetrahydrofolic acid production results in inhibition of the formation of DNA and amino acids.

Trimethoprim possesses *in vitro* activity against *E. coli*, *Proteus mirabilis*, and *Staphylococcus aureus*. Most strains of *Klebsiella* sp., *Enterobacter* sp., *Citrobacter* sp., *Proteus rettgeri*, *Proteus vulgaris*, and *Morganella morganii* are susceptible, as are some enterococci and *Serratia* sp. *Pseudomonas aeruginosa* are invariably resistant.

The amount of trimethoprim excreted in the urine as intact drug shows considerable individual variation but on average approximates 50% of the dose. Renal insufficiency is associated with augmented plasma concentrations of trimethoprim and reduced urinary excretion of the compound. Urinary excretion of trimethoprim declines when the creatinine clearance is reduced below 20 ml min^{-1}. Even with advanced renal insufficiency, however, urinary concentrations of trimethoprim exceed the minimum inhibitory concentrations for most urinary pathogens.

Until recently, trimethoprim was prescribed as the trimethoprim-sulphamethoxazole fixed-dose antimicrobial combination, but within the last two years has been administered as the sole agent for the treatment of patients with acute, symptomatic, and recurrent urinary tract infections. Considerable scientific data appear to support the decision to prescribe trimethoprim as single component therapy because the prior arguments for preferentially administering the combination for the management of urinary tract infections have been repudiated. Some patients fail to tolerate sulphonamides, and these compounds have, infrequently, caused serious untoward events. Trimethoprim, in its own right, exerts antimicrobial activity and possesses a record of proven efficacy and safety for the therapy of urinary tract infections (Brumfitt and Pursell, 1972). Published studies have failed to confirm any enhanced clinical efficacy when trimethoprim-sulphamethoxazole was compared to trimethoprim for the therapy of acute, symptomatic, or recurrent urinary tract infections. In addition, the supposition that combining trimethoprim with a sulphonamide would prevent emergence of resistant organisms and create a bactericidal combination remains to be documented. Lastly, trimethoprim should be less expensive than the combination, trimethoprim-sulphamethoxazole.

Trimethoprim is prescribed as 100-mg tablets two times a day. Of concern is the possibility that a pregnant woman could inadvertently receive trimethoprim: the safety of this drug for the pregnant woman has not been established, although one investigator failed to demonstrate evidence of teratogenicity (Williams *et al.*, 1960). An unacceptable risk would exist for the pregnant woman exposed to trimethoprim, and often neither the patient nor the physician is aware of the pregnancy.

Trimethoprim appears to be as effective as ampicillin and cephalexin for the therapy of women with recurrent urinary tract infections, and this chemotherapeutic agent compares favourably with nitrofurantoin and trimethoprim-sulphamethoxazole when administered to women for the prevention of recurrent symptomatic urinary tract infections (Stamm *et al.*, 1980). Trimethoprim seems to provide considerable relief for patients with renal insufficiency who experience multiple disabling infections (Kunin *et al.*, 1978).

Adverse reactions attributed to trimethoprim include nausea, vomiting, and rash. Untoward events caused by trimethoprim resolve with discontinuation of drug administration, and it has not produced life-threatening toxicities. A concern exists that drug-resistant Enterobacteriaceae will emerge with the increasing administration of trimethoprim. This problem has already been recognized in some hospitals in the U.K.

14. Aminoglycosides

Gentamicin, tobramycin, and amikacin are invaluable antibiotics for the therapy of serious nosocomial and complicated, community-acquired, symptomatic bacterial pyelonephritis caused by Gram-negative, aerobic bacilli resistant to the penicillins and cephalosporins. The aminoglycoside antibiotics are bactericidal compounds that irreversibly bind to bacterial ribosomes and interfere with protein synthesis. As a general statement, these antibiotics possess *in vitro* activity for virtually all Enterobacteriaceae and *Pseudomonas aeruginosa* that cause life-threatening urinary tract infections. Amikacin often demonstrates *in vitro* activity for gentamicin-resistant *Proteus* sp., *Providencia* sp., *Serratia* sp., and *Pseudomonas aeruginosa.*

Bacterial resistance to the aminoglycosides occurs by three mechanisms: enzymatic inactivation of the antibiotic, failure of the antibiotic to penetrate to its site of activity, and alteration of the antibiotic binding site.

For the therapy of life-threatening urinary tract infections, the aminoglycosides should be administered parenterally. Numerous dosage schedules for the aminoglycosides have been developed. One acceptable programme for the patient with normal renal function consists in the infusion of a loading dose of $2 \, \text{mg kg}^{-1}$ of gentamicin or tobramycin followed by $1.75 \, \text{mg kg}^{-1}$ administered every eight hours. An effort should be made to achieve a peak serum concentration of $8–10 \, \mu\text{g ml}^{-1}$ and a trough serum concentration of $< 3.0 \, \mu\text{g ml}^{-1}$. When the patient has renal insufficiency, the gentamicin or tobramycin maintenance dose would consist of $0.8–1 \, \text{mg kg}^{-1}$, and this amount of drug would be administered at an interval in hours that is equal to four times the serum creatinine value. The standard initial dosage of amikacin has been $7.5 \, \text{mg kg}^{-1}$ exhibited every 12 hours. Desirable peak and trough serum concentrations for amikacin are $30–35 \, \mu\text{g ml}^{-1}$ and $< 8 \, \mu\text{g ml}^{-1}$ respectively.

Gentamicin, tobramycin, and amikacin appear equally effective drug treatments for the therapy of urinary tract infections caused by susceptible organisms. Amikacin has successfully treated life-threatening urinary tract infections caused by gentamicin- and tobramycin-resistant organisms (Yu *et al.*, 1977).

Allergic reactions, including rash and fever, occur in approximately 1–3% of patients receiving aminoglycosides. The most important adverse events caused by the aminoglycoside antibiotics include auditory-vestibular toxicity and nephrotoxicity. The prevalence of these reactions can be roughly correlated with the length of treatment, the age of the patient, and pre-existing renal impairment. A difference of opinion exists whether toxicities are related to excessive peak or trough serum concentrations of the aminoglycosides. Nephrotoxicity occurs more commonly in patients with contracted intravascular volume or who receive concomitant cephalosporin antibiotics (Wade *et al.*, 1978). Nephrotoxicity develops in 10–35% of patients receiving aminoglycosides. A recent double-blind, prospective, controlled, randomized study demonstrated that tobramycin caused less nephrotoxicity than gentamicin (Smith *et al.*, 1980). In most circumstances, aminoglycoside-induced nephrotoxicity appears to be reversible following discontinuation of the medication. Serial measurements of creatinine can, however, demonstrate continued deterioration of glomerular filtration after cessation of drug administration, and return of renal function to normal can take months.

Aminoglycosides can induce two forms of ototoxicity: cochlear damage, manifested by varying degrees of hearing loss, particularly for high tones, and vestibular impairment resulting in disequilibrium, nystagmus, nausea, vomiting, and vertigo. Auditory toxicity develops in approximately 10% of recipients of the aminoglycosides, and the incidence that occurs after the administration of gentamicin, tobramycin, and amikacin appears similar. Aminoglycoside-induced ototoxicity appears to be irreversible and progressive after the discontinuation of therapy. The ototoxic effects of the aminoglycosides are potentiated by co-administration of ethacrynic acid, furosemide, and mannitol. Monitoring of patients by performing caloric testing, electronystagmography and serial audiograms has been suggested but is not practical. The physician should attempt to reduce aminoglycoside-related toxicity by monitoring serum levels, discontinuing concomitant potentially ototoxic medications, evaluating renal function, and limiting patients from repetitive aminoglycoside exposures.

IX. SUMMARY

Selective aspects of bacterial urinary tract infections are examined. A terminology and classification are presented, the process of diagnosis is outlined, and contemporary concepts relating to the determination of the site of infection, the patterns of therapeutic response and the prevention of recurrent infections are described. General and explicit guidelines for the management of urinary tract infections are reviewed, and the indications, doses, routes of administration and potential for adverse reactions of specific drug regimens are detailed.

REFERENCES

Acar, J. F. AND Brisset, J. M. (1975). *In* "Clinical Use of Combinations of Antibiotics" (J. Klastersky, ed.) pp. 126–134. Wiley and Sons, New York.
Addato, K., Doebele, K. G., Galland, L. *et al.* (1979). *J.A.M.A.* **241**, 2525–2526.
Alexander, D. N., Ederer, G. M. and Matsen, J. M. (1976). *J. Clin. Micro.* **3**, 42–46.
Asscher, A. W., Sussman, M., Waters, W. E. *et al.* (1969). *Br. Med. J.* **1**, 804–806.
Bailey, R. R., Roberts, A. P., Gower, P. E. *et al.* (1971). *Lancet* **2**, 1112–1114.
Bailey, R. R. and Abbott, G. D. (1978). *Can. Med. Assoc. J.* **118**, 551–552.
Ball, A. P., Geddes, A. M., Davey, P. G. *et al.* (1980). *Lancet* **1**, 620–623.
Bank, N. and Bailine, S. H. (1965). *N. Engl. J. Med.* **272**, 70–75.
Barrett, E., Lynam, G. and Trustey, S. (1978). *J. Clin. Path.* **31**, 859–865.

Beeson, P. B. (1965). *In* "Progress in Pyelonephritis" (E. H. Kass, ed.) pp. 367–387. F. A. Davis, Co., Philadelphia.

Bennett, W. M., Muther, R. S., Parker, R. A. *et al.* (1980). *Ann. Intern. Med.* **93**, 62–89.

Berglund, F., Killander, J. and Pompeius, R. (1975). *J. Urol.* **114**, 802–808.

Black, M., Rabin, L. and Schatz, N. (1980). *Ann. Intern. Med.* **92**, 62–64.

Bonadio, M., Donadio, C., Catania, B. *et al.* (1979). *N. Engl. J. Med.* **301**, 1065–1066.

Bottiger, L. E. and Westerholm, B. (1977). *Europe J. Clin. Pharmacol.* **11**, 439–442.

Boutros, P., Mourtada, H. and Ronald, A. R. (1971). *In* "Antimicrobial Agents and Chemotherapy" (G. L. Hobby, ed.) pp. 114–116. American Society for Microbiology, Bethesda.

Brenner, D. A., Fairley, K. F. and Kincaid-Smith, P. (1969). *Med. J. Aust.* **1**, 1069–1071.

Brumfitt, W. and Percival, A. (1962). *Lancet* **1**, 186–190.

Brumfitt, W. and Percival, A. (1965). *In* "Progress in Pyelonephritis" (E. H. Kass, ed.) pp. 118–128. F. A. Davis Co., Philadelphia.

Brumfitt, W. and Pursell, R. (1972). *Br. Med. J.* **2**, 673–676.

Brumfitt, W., Percival, A. and Carter, M. J. (1962). *Lancet* **1**, 130–132.

Buckwold, F. J., Ronald, A. R., Harding, G. K. M. *et al.* (1979). *J. Clin. Micro.* **10**, 275–278.

Cady, P., Dufour, S. W., Lawless, P. *et al.* (1978). *J. Clin. Micro.* **7**, 273–278.

Carvajal, H. F., Passey, R. B., Berger, M. *et al.* (1975). *Kidney Int.* **8**, 176–184.

Cattell, W. R., Charlton, C. A. C., McSherry, A. *et al.* (1973). *In* "Urinary Tract Infection" (W. Brumfitt and A. W. Asscher, ed.) pp. 206–214, Oxford University Press, London.

Cattell, W. R., McSherry, M. A., Northeast, A. *et al.* (1974). *Br. Med. J.* **4**, 136–139.

Chisholm, G. D. (1974). *Postgrad. Med. J.* **50** (suppl.), 23–30.

Christensson, P., Ekberg, M. and Denneberg, T. (1973). *Acta Path. Microbiol. Scand.* **241** (suppl.), 69–72.

Cicmanic, J. F. and Evans, A. T. (1980). *J. Urol.* **124**, 68–69.

Clark, H., Ronald, A. R. and Turck, M. (1971). *J. Infect. Dis.* **123**, 539–543.

Cohen, S. N. and Kass, E. H. (1967). *N. Engl. J. Med.* **277**, 176–180.

Coloe, P. J. (1978). *J. Clin. Path.* **31**, 365–369.

Conn, R. B., Charache, P. and Chappelle, E. W. (1975). *Amer. J. Clin. Path.* **63**, 493–501.

Craig, W. A., Kunin, C. M. and DeGroot, J. (1973). *Appl. Microbiol.* **26**, 196–201.

Dans, P. E. and Klaus, B. (1976). *Johns Hopkins Med. J.* **138**, 13–18.

Davies, B. I. (1977). *J. Med. Microbiol.* **10**, 293–298.

Davies, J. A., Strangeways, J. E. M., Mitchell, R. G. *et al.* (1971). *Br. Med. J.* **2**, 215–217.

Devaskar, U. and Montgomery, W. (1978). *J. Pediatr.* **93**, 789–791.

Engel, G., Schaeffer, A. J., Grayhack, J. T. *et al.* (1980). *J. Urol.* **123**, 190–191.

Esposito, A. L., Gleckman, R. A., Cram, S. *et al.* (1980). *J. Amer. Geriatrics Soc.* **28**, 315–319.

Evans, D. A., Hennekens, C. H., Miao, L. *et al.* (1978). *N. Engl. J. Med.* **299**, 536–537.

Eykyn, S., Bultitude, M. I., Mayo, M. E. *et al.* (1974). *Br. J. Urol.* **46**, 527–532.

Fair, W. R., Crane, D. B., Schiller, N. *et al.* (1979). *J. Urol.* **121**, 437–441.

Fair, W. R., Crane, D. B., Peterson, L. J. *et al.* (1980). *J. Urol.* **123**, 717–721.

Fairley, K. F. and Butler, H. (1971). *In* "Renal Infection and Renal Scarring" (P. Kincaid-Smith and K. F. Fairley, ed.) pp. 51–67. Mercedes Publishing, Melbourne.

Fairley, K. F., Bond, A. G., Brown, R. B. *et al.* (1967). *Lancet* **2**, 427–428.

Fang, L. S. T., Rubin, N. E. T. and Rubin, R. H. (1978). *N. Engl. J. Med.* **298**, 413–416.

Freeman, R. B., Smith, W. M., Richardson, J. A. *et al.* (1975). *Ann. Intern. Med.* **83**, 133–147.
Fries, D., Delavelle, F., Simonet, M. *et al.* (1977). *Nouv. Presse. Med.* **6**, 3815–3818.
Gleckman, R. (1976). *J. Urol.* **116**, 776–777.
Gleckman, R. (1979a). *J. Urol.* **122**, 770–771.
Gleckman, R. A. (1979b). *Postgrad. Med.* **65**, 156–159.
Gleckman, R., Shannon, R. J. and Crowley, M. (1978). *J. Urol.* **120**, 645–646.
Gleckman, R., Crowley, M. and Natsios, G. A. (1979). *N. Engl. J. Med.* **301**, 878–880.
Gleckman, R., Crowley, M. and Natsios, G. A. (1980a). *Amer. J. Med. Sci.* **279**, 31–36.
Gleckman, R. A., Crowley, M. M., Natsios, G. A. *et al.* (1980b). *J. Clin. Micro.* **11**, 650–653.
Gonick, P., Falkner, B., Schwartz, A. *et al.* (1975). *J.A.M.A.* **233**, 253–255.
Gow, J. G. (1974). *Practitioner* **213**, 97–101.
Gower, P. E. and Roberts, A. P. (1975). *Clin. Nephrol.* **3**, 10–13.
Gower, P. E. and Tasker, P. R. W. (1976). *Br. Med. J.* **1**, 684–686.
Greenwood, D. and O'Grady, F. (1973). *J. Infect. Dis.* **128**, 791–794.
Griffith, D. P. (1978). *Kidney Int.* **13**, 372–382.
Griffith, D. P., Moskowitz, P. A., Carlton, C. E., Jr (1979). *Trans. Amer. Assoc. Genito-Urinary Surg.* **70**, 25–29.
Gross, P. A., Flower, M. and Borden, G. (1976). *J. Clin. Micro.* **3**, 246–250.
Gutman, L. T., Holmes, K. K., Wiesner, P. J. *et al.* (1978). *In* "Infections of the Urinary Tract" (E. H. Kass and W. Brumfitt, ed.) pp. 171–176, University of Chicago Press, Chicago.
Harding, G. K. M. and Ronald, A. R. (1974). *N. Engl. J. Med.* **291**, 597–601.
Harding, G. K. M., Ronald, A. R., Bontros, P. *et al.* (1975). *Can. Med. Assoc. J.* **112** (suppl.), 9–12.
Harding, G. K. M., Buckwold, F. J., Marrie, T. J. *et al.* (1979). *J.A.M.A.* **242**, 1975–1977.
Harrison, W. O., Holmes, K. K., Belding, M. E. *et al.* (1974). *Clin. Res.* **22**, 125A.
Heinze, P. A., Thrupp, L. D. and Anselmo, C. R. (1979). *Amer. J. Clin. Path.* **71**, 178–183.
Hernandez, O. G. (1974). *Curr. Med. Res. Opin.* **2**, 334–341.
Hirsh, H. A. (1971). *Postgrad. Med. J.* **47** (suppl.), 90–93.
Hoeprich, P. D. (1960). *J. Lab. Clin. Med.* **56**, 899–907.
Holmberg, L., Boman, G., Bottiger, L. E. *et al.* (1980). *Amer. J. Med.* **69**, 733–738.
Hughes, J., Roberts, L. C. and Coopridge, A. J. (1975. *J. Urol.* **114**, 912–914.
Isenberg, H. D., Gavan, T. L., Sonnenwirth, A. *et al.* (1979). *J. Clin. Micro.* **10**, 226–230.
Jenkins, R. D., Hale, D. C. and Matsen, J. M. (1980). *J. Clin. Micro.* **11**, 220–225.
Jones, S. R. (1976). *N. Engl. J. Med.* **295**, 1380.
Jones, S. R., Smith, J. W. and Sanford, J. P. (1974). *N. Engl. J. Med.* **290**, 591–593.
Jones, S. R. (1979). *In* "Infectious Diseases: Current Topics" (D. N. Gilbert and J. P. Sanford, ed.) pp. 97–106. Grune and Stratton, New York.
Kaslowski, S., Radford, N. and Kincaid-Smith, P. (1974). *N. Engl. J. med.* **280**, 385–387.
Kass, E. H. (1956). *Trans. Assn Amer. Physicians* **69**, 56–64.
Kass, E. H. (1972). *N. Engl. J. Med.* **287**, 563–564.
Kass, E. H. (1979). *Kidney Int.* **16**, 204–212.
Kaye, D. (1972). *In* "Urinary Tract Infections and Its Management" (D. Kaye, ed.) pp. 1–5. C. V. Mosby, St Louis.
Kaye, M., deVries, J. and MacFarlan, K. T. (1962). *Can. Med. Ass. J.* **86**, 9–14.

Koch-Weser, J., Sidel, V. W., Dexter, M. *et al.* (1971). *Arch. Intern. Med.* **128**, 399–404.
Kozinn, P. J., Faschdjian, C. L., Goldberg, P. K. *et al.* (1978). *J. Urol.* **119**, 184–187.
Kraft, J. K. and Stamey, T. A. (1977). *Medicine* **56**, 55–60.
Kreger, B. E., Craven, D. E., Carling, P. C. *et al.* (1980). *Amer. J. Med.* **68**, 332–343.
Kuklinca, A. G. and Gavan, T. L. (1969). *Cleve. Clin. Q.* **36**, 133–136.
Kunin, C. M. (1975). *Ann. Intern. Med.* **83**, 273–274.
Kunin, C. M. and Finkelberg, Z. (1970). *Ann. Intern. Med.* **72**, 349–356.
Kunin, C. M., Craig, W. A. and Uehling, D. T. (1978). *J.A.M.A.* **239**, 2588–2590.
Kunin, C. M., Polyak, F. and Postel, E. (1980). *J.A.M.A.* **243**, 134–139.
Lapides, J., Costello, R. T., Jr, Zierdt, D. K. *et al.* (1968). *J. Urol.* **100**, 552–555.
Lawson, D. H. and Jick, H. (1978). *Amer. J. Med. Sci.* **275**, 53–57.
Levinson, M. E. and Kaye, D. (1972). *In* "Urinary Tract Infections and Its Management" (D. Kaye, ed.) pp. 188–226. C. V. Mosby, St Louis.
Lindemyer, R. I., Turck, M. and Petersdorf, R. G. (1963). *Ann. Intern. Med.* **58**, 201–216.
Lorentz, W. B., Jr and Resnick, M. I. (1979). *Pediatrics* **64**, 672–677.
Mabeck, C. E. (1972). *Postgrad. Med. J.* **48**, 69–75.
Madsen, P. O. and Rhodes, P. R. (1971). *J. Urol.* **105**, 870–872.
Mannisoto, P. T. (1976). *Curr. Ther. Res.* **20**, 645–654.
Marier, R., Fong, E., Jansen, M. *et al.* (1978). *J. Infect. Dis.* **138**, 781–790.
Marple, C. D. (1941). *Ann. Intern. Med.* **14**, 2220–2239.
McCabe, W. R. and Jackson, G. G. (1960). *Amer. J. Med. Sci.* **240**, 754–763.
McCabe, W. R. and Jackson, G. G. (1965). *N. Engl. J. Med.* **272**, 1037–1044.
McGeachie, J. (1966). *Br. Med. J.* **1**, 952–954.
McGeachie, J. and Kennedy, A. C. (1963). *J. Clin. Path.* **16**, 32–38.
McGee, Z. A., Wittler, R. G., Gooder, H. *et al.* (1971). *J. Infect. Dis.* **123**, 433–438.
Meares, E. M., Jr (1974). *Urology* **4**, 560–566.
Meares, E. M. (1975). *Can. Med. Ass. J.* **112** (suppl.), 22–27.
Meares, E. M. and Stamey, T. A. (1968). *Invest. Urol.* **5**, 492–518.
Mobley, D. F. (1975). *J. Urol.* **114**, 83–85.
Mogabgab, W. J. and Pallock, B. (1977). *Curr. Therap. Res.* **22**, 172–177.
Motzkin, D. (1972). *J. Urol.* **107**, 454–457.
Mundt, K. A. and Polk, B. F. (1979). *Lancet* **2**, 1172–1175.
Musher, D. M. and Griffith, D. P. (1974). *Antimicrob. Agents Chemother.* **6**, 708–711.
Musher, D. M., Thorsteinsson, S. B. and Airola, V. M., III (1976a). *J.A.M.A.* **236**, 2069–2072.
Musher, D. M., Griffith, D. P. and Templeton, G. B. (1976b). *J. Infect. Dis.* **133**, 564–567.
Nanra, R., Friedman, A., O'Keefe, C. *et al.* (1970). *In* "Renal Infection and Renal Scarring" (P. Kincaid-Smith and K. F. Fairley, ed.) pp. 175–179, Mercedes Publishing, Melbourne.
Naumann, P. (1978). *J. Antimicrob. Chemother.* **4**, 9–17.
Nicholson, D. P. and Koepke, J. A. (1979). *J. Clin. Micro.* **10**, 823–833.
Ode, B., Broms, M., Walder, M. *et al.* (1980). *Acta Med. Scand.* **207**, 305–307.
Old, D. C., Crichton, P. B., Maunder, A. J. *et al.* (1980). *J. Med. Microbiol.* **13**, 437–444.
Oliveri, R. A., Sachs, R. M. and Caste, P. G. (1979). *Curr. Ther. Res.* **25**, 415–421.
Ormonde, N. W. H., Gray, J. A., McMurdoch, J. *et al.* (1969). *J. Infect. Dis.* **120**, 82–86.
Papanayiotou, P. and Dontas, A. S. (1972). *N. Engl. J. Med.* **287**, 531–534.
Perry, J. E., Toney, J. D. and LeBlanc, A. C. (1967). *Tex. Rep. Biol. Med.* **25**, 270–272.

Pfau, A., Perlberg, S. and Shapira, A. (1978). *J. Urol.* **119**, 384–387.
Prat, V., Bohuslav, M., Hatala, M. *et al.* (1977). *Zschr. Urol.* **70**, 25–31.
Rantz, L. A. and Keefer, C. S. (1940). *Arch. Intern. Med.* **65**, 933–956.
Ries, K. M., Cobbs, C. G., Gillenwater, J. Y. *et al.* (1973). *Antimicrob. Agents Chemother.* **4**, 593–596.
Roberts, A. P., Robinson, R. E. and Beard, R. W. (1967). *Br. Med. J.* **1**, 400–403.
Ronald, A. R., Cutler, R. E. and Turck, M. (1969). *Ann. Intern. Med.* **70**, 723–733.
Ronald, A. R., Silverblatt, F., Clark, H. *et al.* (1971). *Appl. Microbiol.* **21**, 990–992.
Ronald, A. R., Boutros, P. and Mourtada, H. (1976). *J.A.M.A.* **235**, 1854–1856.
Ronald, A. R., Jagdis, F. A., Harding, G. K. M. *et al.* (1977). *Antimicrob. Agents Chemother.* **11**, 780–784.
Rubin, R. H., Fang, L. S. T., Cosimi, A. B. *et al.* (1979). *Transplantation* **27**, 18–20.
Rubin, R. H., Fang, L. S. T., Jones, S. R. *et al.* (1980). *J.A.M.A.* **244**, 561–564.
Rumans, L. W. and Vosti, K. L. (1978). *Arch. Intern. Med.* **138**, 1077–1081.
Sabath, L. D., Elder, H. A., McCall, C. E. *et al.* (1967). *N. Engl. J. Med.* **277**, 232–238.
Sanford, B. A., Thomas, V. L., Forland, M. *et al.* (1978). *J. Clin. Micro.* **8**, 575–579.
Scarpelli, P. T., Lamanna, S., Bigioli, F. *et al.* (1979). *Clin. Nephrol.* **12**, 7–13.
Schardijn, G., Statius Van Eps, L. W. and Swaak, A. J. G. (1979). *Lancet* **1**, 805–807.
Shapiro, S., Sloane, D., Siskine, V. *et al.* (1969). *Lancet* **2**, 969–972.
Sharp, J. R., Ishak, K. G. and Zimmerman, H. J. (1980). *Ann. Intern. Med.* **92**, 14–19.
Singh, M., Chapman, R., Tresidder, G. C. *et al.* (1973). *Br. J. Urol.* **45**, 581–585.
Siroky, M. B., Moylan, R. A., Austen, G., Jr *et al.* (1976). *Am. J. Med.* **61**, 351–360.
Smith, C. R., Lipsky, J. J., Laskin, O. L. *et al.* (1980). *N. Engl. J. Med.* **302**, 1106–1109.
Smith, J. W., Jones, S. R. and Kaijser, B. (1977). *J. Infect. Dis.* **135**, 577–581.
Sovijarvi, A. R. A., Lemola, M., Stenius, B. *et al.* (1977). *Scand. J. Respir. Dis.* **58**, 41–50.
Stamey, T. (1967). *J. Urol.* **97**, 926–934.
Stamey, T. A. (1975). *South Afr. Med. J.* **68**, 934–939.
Stamey, T. A. and Pfau, A. (1963). *Invest. Urol.* **1**, 162–172.
Stamey, T. A., Govan, D. E. and Palmer, J. M. (1965). *Medicine* **44**, 1–36.
Stamey, T. A., Fair, W. R., Timothy, M. M. *et al.* (1974). *N. Engl. J. Med.* **291**, 1159–1163.
Stamey, T. A. and Bragonje, J. (1976). *J.A.M.A.* **236**, 1857–1860.
Stamey, T. A., Condy, M. and Mihara, G. (1977). *N. Engl. J. Med.* **296**, 780–783.
Stamey, T. A., Wehner, N., Mihara, G. *et al.* (1978). *Medicine* **57**, 47–56.
Stamm, W. E., Wagner, K. F., Amsel, R. *et al.* (1980). *N. Engl. J. Med.* **303**, 409–415.
Thomas, V., Shelkov, A. and Forland, M. (1974). *N. Engl. J. Med.* **290**, 588–590.
Thorley, J. D., Jones, S. R. and Sanford, J. P. (1974). *Medicine* **53**, 441–451.
Throm, R., Specter, S., Strauss, R. *et al.* (1977). *J. Clin. Micro.* **6**, 271–273.
Toole, J. F. and Parish, M. L. (1973). *Neurology* **23**, 554–559.
Turck, M. (1972). *Adv. Intern. Med.* **18**, 141–152.
Turck, M., Petersdorf, R. G. and Fournier, M. R. (1962). *J. Clin. Invest.* **41**, 1760–1765.
Turck, M., Ronald, A. R. and Petersdorf, R. G. (1968). *N. Engl. J. Med.* **278**, 422–427.
Vosti, K. L. (1975). *J.A.M.A.* **231**, 934–940.
Vosti, K. L., Goldberg, L. M. and Rantz, L. A. (1965). *In* "Progress In Pyelonephritis" (E. H. Kass, ed.) pp. 103–110. F. A. Davis Co., Philadelphia.
Wade, J. C., Smith, C. R., Petty, B. G. *et al.* (1978). *Lancet* **2**, 604–606.
Wallis, C., Melnick, J. L., Wende, R. D. *et al.* (1980). *J. Clin. Micro.* **11**, 462–464.
Watanakunakorn, C. (1979). *J. Antimicrob. Chemother.* **5**, 239–247.
Welling, A., Watkins, W. W. and Raines, S. L. (1957). *J. Urol.* **77**, 773–776.

Whelton, A. (1974). *Kidney Int.* **6**, 131–137.
Whelton, A. (1980). *Obstet. Gynecol.* **55** (suppl.), 128–137.
Whitworth, J. A., Fairley, K. F., McIvor, M. A. *et al.* (1973). *Lancet* **1**, 234–235.
Whitworth, J. A., Fairley, K. F., O'Keefe, C. M. *et al.* (1974). *Clin. Nephrol.* **2**, 9–12.
Williams, J. D., Brumfitt, W., Condie, A. P. *et al.* (1960). *Postgrad. Med. J.* **45**, 71–76.
Yu, V. L., Rhame, F. S., Pesanti, E. L. *et al.* (1977). *J.A.M.A.* **238**, 943–947.

9 Rapid diagnosis by the detection of microbial antigens

RICHARD B. KOHLER, L. JOSEPH WHEAT and ARTHUR WHITE

I. INTRODUCTION

In 1909 Vincent and Bellot discovered the presence of substances in the spinal fluid of patients with meningococcal meningitis which precipitated anti-meningococcal antiserum. Eight years later Dochez and Avery (1917) reported finding a soluble substance in the blood and urine of patients with pneumococcal pneumonia which specifically precipitated antipneumococcal antisera. Furthermore, a relationship existed between the presence of high quantities of the material, later determined to be capsular polysaccharide (Cruickshank, 1938), and a poor clinical outcome. In 1951 Neill *et al.* reported the presence of specific soluble antigens in spinal fluid, blood, and urine from a patient with cryptococcal meningitis, detected by immunoprecipation and complement fixation. Soluble microbial antigens are now known to be present in the majority of patients with many types of infections. With sensitive immunological techniques developed in the past twenty years, detection of these substances can lead to rapid, specific aetiological diagnoses. This chapter will review the technical aspects and applications of counter-immunoelectrophoresis, latex agglutination, radioimmunoassays, and enzyme immunoassays for this purpose.

II. COUNTERIMMUNOELECTROPHORESIS

A. General aspects

There have been several recent reviews of the use of counterimmunoelec-trophoresis (CIE) for the rapid diagnosis of bacterial, viral, fungal, and protozan infections (Anhalt *et al.*, 1978; Tilton, 1978; Rytel, 1979; Hill, 1981). This section will discuss the use of CIE for the rapid diagnosis of bacterial infections only.

The principle of precipitation in CIE is similar to double diffusion in agar in that a precipitin line is formed by the migration of antibody and antigen. In CIE, the antigen, which must be negatively charged under the conditions of the test, migrates rapidly toward the antibody well (anode), whereas the uncharged antibodies drift toward the cathode by electroendosmosis, the flow of buffer from the anode to the cathode. CIE, therefore, detects antigens and antibodies more rapidly and with greater sensitivity than double diffusion. Items of equipment typically used for performing CIE are shown in Fig. 1. A close-up view of CIE plate with positive and negative reactions is shown in Fig. 2. Sensitivities for a variety of antigens have varied from as low as 0.05 µg ml^{-1} for *Haemophilus influenzae* type b to 0.8 µg ml^{-1} for type 7 *Streptococcus pneumoniae*.

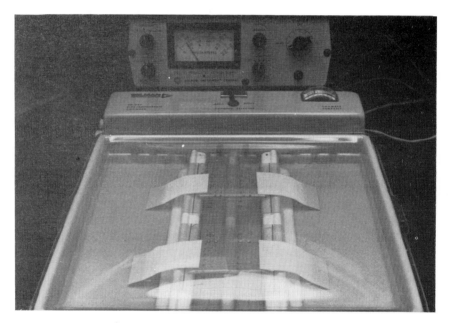

Fig. 1 Counterimmunoelectrophoresis equipment. It is simple and relatively inexpensive. Above is a variable DC power supply with amp and volt meters. Below is a chamber containing buffer reservoirs (right and left) which receive the electrodes attached to the power supply. The buffer wells are connected to the CIE plates by filter paper wicks. The cover is to prevent desiccation during electrophoresis and must be in place before the power can reach the electrodes —an important safety feature to protect the operator from serious electrical shocks due to inadvertent contact with the buffer, wicks, or slides.

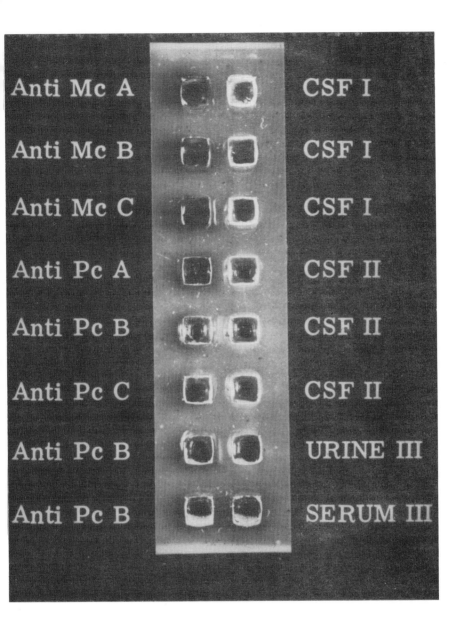

Fig. 2 Counterimmunoelectrophoresis slide. (*Left*) antiserum wells, (*Right*) patient specimens. Specimen CSF I is from a patient with group C *N. meningitidis* meningitis. A precipitin line is seen only with the anti-group C *N. meningitidis* antiserum (Anti McC). Specimen CSF II is from a patient with *S. pneumoniae* meningitis; a precipitin line is seen with anti-*S. pneumoniae* antiserum serotype pool B (anti PcB) but not with pools A or C. Urine III and Serum III are from a patient with bacteraemic pneumococcal pneumonia; a precipitin line is seen with the urine, but not the serum specimen.

B. Technical aspects

Both agar and agarose have been used as the supporting medium; the major advantage of agarose is its relative lack of negatively charged sulphate groups that adversely affect electrophoresis due to electroendosmosis. Barbital buffers are normally used with a pH range of 8.2 to 8.6 and a concentration of 0.05 mol 1^{-1}. The pH should not fall below this range; otherwise the antibodies acquire a negative charge and migrate away from the antigen well. Certain bacterial antigens, such as the pneumococcal types 7 and 14, do not migrate with barbital buffer but are active in systems using a boric acid derivative such as sulphonated phenylboronic acid or *m*-carboxy-phenylboronic acid (Anhalt *et al.*, 1978). Although electrophoresis for 30 min detects almost all positive reactions, an additional 30 min of electrophoresis followed by cooling to 4°C and observation for several hours slightly increases the maximum number of positive results (Anhalt *et al.*, 1978). In most patients, this allows the rapid detection of bacterial antigens or antibodies within one hour.

The sources of antibody for antigen detection have varied. Many investigators have prepared their own antisera while others have used commercially available antisera from such suppliers as Difco Laboratories, Hyland Laboratories, or the Statens Seruminstitute in Copenhagen.

C. Problems

CIE requires an electrical source and electrophoresis equipment (Fig. 1). In comparison latex agglutination is simpler, faster, and cheaper. The agarose gels used as the electrophoresis support medium must be used within several weeks of preparation unless stored in humidified or airtight bags; otherwise, they dry and are useless for CIE. In our experience weak precipitin lines are occasionally difficult to distinguish from the artifacts often seen close to the antiserum well. As a rule, however, these difficulties are not serious, and, as shown later in this section, CIE has been widely and successfully applied.

D. Applications

1. Meningitis (Table 1)

Counterimmunoelectrophoresis has been used to detect antigens in meningitis due to *Neisseria meningitidis*, *Streptococcus pneumoniae*, *Haemophilus influenzae* type b, group B *streptococci*, and K-1 *E. coli*. In most studies, CIE was positive in untreated patients less frequently than cultures, but CIE allowed the diagnosis to be established in one to two hours whereas cultures required one to three days. Results of published studies are summarized in Table 1. In

	No. patients	No. positive Gram stain	No. positive culture	No. positive culture or Gram stain	No. positive CIE	Reference
N. meningitidis	68	17	42	45	47	Greenwood et al. (1971)
	191	NS[a]	NS	162	129	Whittle et al. (1971)
	20	NS	17	NS	16	Edwards et al. (1979)
	69	NS	35	NS	25	Hoffman and Edwards (1972)
	135	101	135	135	121	Higashi et al. (1974)
	64	50	64	64	35	Colding and Lind (1977)
	4	2	4	1	1	Naiman and Albritton (1980)
	35	NS	34	NS	27	Severin (1972)
	34	33	30	34	20	Ende et al. (1977)
	126	NS	NS	108	112	Whittle et al. (1975)
S. pneumoniae	7	6	7	7	7	Coonrod and Rytel (1972)
	32	29	32	32	14	Colding and Lind (1977)
	6	4	6	6	5	Fossieck et al. (1973)
	55	44	40	NS	54	Denis et al. (1977)
	87	NS	NS	58	85	Whittle et al. (1974)
	32	26	30	NS	19	Webb and Baker (1980)
	22	21	21	22	16	Ende et al. (1977)
	5	4	4	NS	5	Naiman and Albritton (1980)
H. influenzae	19	17	17	19	17	Coonrod and Rytel (1972)
	14	NS	NS	NS	11	Ingram et al. (1972)
	30	25	30	30	23	Colding and Lind (1977)
	26	NS	26	NS	22	Ward et al. (1978)
	132	108	125	NS	113	Feigen et al. (1976a)
	31	20	30	NS	24	Naiman and Albritton (1980)
	15	14	13	15	12	Ende et al. (1977)
Gr. B. *Streptococcus*	16	NS	16	NS	16	Kaplan and Feigen (1979)
	28	NS	28	NS	23	Webb and Baker (1980)
	4	NS	4	NS	3	Naiman and Albritton (1980)
	27	NS	27	NS	17	Stechenbert et al. (1979)
	12	NS	12	NS	11	Feigen et al. (1966)

[a] NS: not stated.

addition, CIE may allow the diagnosis to be established in patients with negative culture who have been previously treated with antibacterial agents. Although the Gram stain and CIE detect similar numbers of patients, approximately 10% of patients detected by CIE are not detected by the Gram stain.

Testing concentrated urine as well as spinal fluid may improve the sensitivity of CIE for establishing a diagnosis in bacterial meningitis. This has improved the sensitivity of antigen detection in *H. influenzae*, pneumococcal and group B streptococcal infections by as much as 60%. By performing CIE on concentrated urines, spinal fluid, and sera, Kaplan and Feigin (1979) found specific antigens in essentially 100% of patients with *H. influenzae* meningitis, in 60% with pneumococcal meningitis, but in fewer than 50% with meningococcal meningitis.

The concentration of bacterial antigen detected by CIE is closely correlated with the concentration of bacteria in the spinal fluid (Naik and Duncan, 1978). In addition, the concentration of antigen correlates with both the severity and prognosis of the illness (Robbins *et al.*, 1974; Kaplan and Feigin, 1979). In patients with *H. influenzae* type b meningitis, the incidence and severity of sequelae increased dramatically when the concentration of polyribitolphosphate antigen exceeded 1.28 µg ml^{-1}.

In neonates *E. coli* neonatal meningitis is usually caused by strains carrying the K1 capsular serotype (Robbins *et al.*, 1974). The K1 polysaccharide is itself poorly immunogenic in animals. Antiserum against the group B meningococcus has been used in CIE to detect *E. coli* K1 antigens because of the cross-reaction between such antisera and the antigen. Antigen was detected in 71% of spinal fluids and 42% of sera from infected infants (McCracken *et al.*, 1974). A significant correlation was also noted between the maximum concentration of K1 antigen in spinal fluid and survival.

2. Pulmonary infections

The evaluations of CIE for detecting pneumococcal antigens in serum, urine, or sputum from patients with pneumococcal pneumonia is complicated by the frequent uncertainty that the pneumonia is due to the pneumococcus. In most studies, the aetiology has been established by Gram stain, sputum culture, and/or blood culture. However, Gram stains may be difficult to interpret, and because of asymptomatic carriage in the nasopharynx, pneumococci can be cultured from the sputum of patients infected with other organisms. In addition, positive blood cultures probably select the most severely ill patients with the highest antigenic load.

Pneumococcal polysaccharides can be detected in serum from 45–80% of patients with pneumococcal pneumonia and/or bacteraemia (Table 2). In patients with pneumonia without bacteraemia, antigens have been detected in

Table 2 Counterimmunoelectrophoresis in pneumococcal pneumonia

Specimen	Blood culture	No. patients	Percentage positive, CIE	Reference
Serum	Pos.[a]	51	45	Rytel (1979)
	Pos.	50	60	Kenny *et al.* (1972)
	Pos.	26	65	Coonrod and Drennan (1976)
	Pos.	10	80	Bartram *et al.* (1976)
	Neg.[a]	13	15	Rytel (1979)
	Neg.	25	0	Kenny *et al.* (1972)
	Neg.	12	33	Bartram *et al.* (1974)
	Neg.	20	10	Coonrod and Drennan (1976)
Urine	Pos.	11	63	Rytel (1979)
	Pos.	7	57	Bartram *et al.* (1974)
	Pos.	4	25	Naiman and Albritton (1980)
	Neg.	19	37	Rytel (1979)
	Neg.	4	25	Bartram *et al.* (1974)
	Neg.	5	100	Naiman and Albritton (1980)
Sputum	—	25	76	Leach and Coonrod (1977)
	—	19	95	Perlino and Shulman (1976)
	—	25	84	Trollfors *et al.* (1979)

[a] Pos.: positive, Neg.: negative.

as many as 33% in some studies and in none in other studies. Testing concentrated urines in bacteraemic patients has improved the detection rate by CIE from 45% to 64%. Tugwell and Greenwood (1975) studied 98 patients with lobar pneumonia and detected pneumococcal polysaccharide in the sera of 29% of patients and in the urine of 54%.

Pneumococcal polysaccharide has also been detected in sputum from 89–100% of patients with bacteraemic pneumococcal pneumonia and in a high proportion of patients with presumed pneumococcal pneumonia (Table 2). However, pneumococcal antigen can also be detected in 19% of patients with chronic bronchitis without pneumonia (Perlino and Shulman, 1976; Leach and Coonrod, 1977; Trollfors *et al.*, 1979). Some investigators have shown a good correlation between detection of pneumococci in the sputum by culture and detection of pneumococcal antigens by CIE. Others have pointed out that CIE is positive much more frequently than cultures in patients with pneumococcal bacteraemia and pneumococcal pneumonia (Perlino and Shulman, 1976; Leach and Coonrod, 1977). Other groups which reported on antigen detection in the sputum either did not list their diagnostic criteria for pneumococcal pneumonia or based the diagnosis primarily upon sputum cultures (El-Refaie and Dulake, 1975; Spencer and Savage, 1975; Michaels and Poziviak, 1976; Congeni and Nankervis, 1978; Wiernik *et al.*, 1978). In many patients from whom the pneumococcus was not isolated, pneumococcal antigens were detected in sputum. Whether or not these represented falsely positives is difficult to determine. In studies in which a definite aetiology other than the pneumococcus has been established for the pneumonia, the frequency of detection of pneumococcal antigens by CIE has been low.

Antigens have also been detected in pleural fluid by CIE in pneumonia due to *S. pneumoniae*, *Staphylococcus aureus*, or *H. influenzae*. In one study (Lampe *et al.*, 1976) appropriate antigens were detected in 85–100% of patients with positive cultures and in over half the patients in whom cultures were negative (Table 3). There was one false positive CIE result in 88 patients in whom the aetiology was proven to be due to other bacteria.

Table 3   Bacterial cultures and counterimmunoelectrophoresis of 87 pleural fluid specimens

Bacterial culture	No. of patients	No. with positive CIE		
		S. pneu- moniae	S. aureus	H. in- fluenzae b
S. pneumoniae	19	19	0	0
S. aureus	9	0	8	0
Mixed				
S. aureus and				
S. pneumoniae	3	3	2	0
S. aureus, and				
Pseudomonas sp.	1	0	1	0
S. aureus and				
beta haemolytic				
streptococcus	1	0	1	0
E. coli	3	0	0	1
H. influenzae b	1	0	0	1
Others[a]	5	0	0	0
No growth	45	15	5	3
Totals	87	37	17	5

[a] One each of *Salmonella typhi, Herellea, Pseudomonas, Mima* and *Bacillus sp.*

3. Miscellaneous infections

Group B streptococcal antigens have been detected in urine or serum in a high proportion of patients with group B streptococcal bacteraemia without meningitis (Stechenberg *et al.*, 1970; Edwards *et al.*, 1979; Edwards and Baker, 1979; Kaplan and Feigin, 1979; Naiman and Albritton, 1980; Webb and

Baker, 1980). Several investigators found antigen by CIE in one or more body fluids in essentially all patients with severe group B infections. Pneumococcal antigens have been detected by CIE in 80% of patients with pneumococci cultured from middle ear aspirates (Leinonen, 1980); however, pneumococcal antigens were also detected in 15% of aspirates from which other organisms were cultured.

Several investigators have reported the detection of *Pseudomonas* antigens in sera by CIE in 30–92% of patients with serious *Pseudomonas* diseases (Bartram *et al.*, 1974; Marier and Andriole, 1975; Adams *et al.*, 1976).

Three groups of investigators have reported the detection of *Klebsiella* antigens in serum or urine from patients with *Klebsiella* sepsis. Serum from 8 of 31 patients with *Klebsiella* bacteraemia contained *Klebsiella* capsular antigen by CIE (Pollack, 1976). Parker (1979) reported that *Klebsiella* capsular polysaccharide was detected in 9 of 13 patients with bacteraemia. No cross-reacting antigens were detected in either study in patients with bacteraemia due to organisms other than *Klebsiella* including several enterobacterial species. Simpson and Speller (1977) studied 36 patients for the presence of antigens of *Klebsiella aerogenes* serotype K2. Antigens were detected in serum and urine from 3 patients with bacteraemia and in urine from 21 patients with *K. aerogenes* urinary tract infections. The antigen was not detected in serum or urine from 12 patients with urinary colonization with other Gram-negative bacteria.

CIE has been reported to detect toxins of *Clostridium perfringens* (Naik and Duncan, 1977) and *Clostridium difficile* (Ryan *et al.*, 1980) in the faeces of infected subjects. CIE detected toxin of *Clostridium difficile* which could not be detected by tissue culture.

Regarding specificity, although a large number of cross-reactions have been reported between antisera to various bacteria and broth cultures of other bacteria (Finch and Wilkinson, 1979), cross-reactions in specimens from infected patients have been infrequent (Higashi *et al.*, 1974; Ribner *et al.*, 1975) except for the known cross-reactions between *E. coli* K1 and type B meningococci.

E. Comparison of CIE with other antigen detection methods

Several investigators have compared antigen detection by CIE with latex agglutination, enzyme-linked immunosorbent assays (ELISA) or radioimmunoassays. These will be discussed in detail in later sections of this chapter. Briefly, one radioimmunoassay detected *H. influenzae* polysaccharide 10- to 15-fold better than CIE (O'Reilly *et al.*, 1975). Latex agglutination was more effective than CIE in detecting antigens in patients with bacterial meningitis and group B streptococcal bacteraemia (Severin, 1972; Whittle *et al.*, 1974;

Ward et al., 1978; Edwards et al., 1979; Leinonen, 1980; Webb and Baker, 1980). ELISA was more sensitive than CIE in detecting antigens in spinal fluid from patients with meningitis due to *N. meningitidis*, *S. pneumoniae* and *H. influenzae* (Beuvery et al., 1979).

III. LATEX AGGLUTINATION

A. General aspects

Latex agglutination is an immunoassay system which relies on the tendency of proteins to adsorb to polystyrene. Polystyrene latex particles coated with appropriate antibodies undergo visible agglutination when exposed to the appropriate antigen (Fig. 3). Antigen detection by latex agglutination is simple, very rapid, and inexpensive. The rapid diagnosis of disseminated cryptococcosis by latex agglutination is the first immunological test for microbial antigen to gain widespread acceptance in hospital clinical laboratories.

Immunoglobulin-coated latex spheres were first used to detect rheumatoid factor, an immunoglobulin M which binds to aggregated immunoglobulin G (Singer and Plotz, 1956). Soon after, Singer et al. (1957) demonstrated that particles sensitized with specific rabbit immunoglobulin could detect C-reactive protein. Keele and Webster (1961) similarly detected human growth hormone at 300 ng ml $^{-1}$, and in 1963 Bloomfield et al. detected *Cryptococcus neoformans* polysaccharide in serum and spinal fluid from patients with disseminated cryptococcosis. Since then the technique has been widely applied to the rapid diagnosis of microbial infections by antigen detection.

B. Technical aspects

Polystyrene latex particles with a diameter of 0.81 μm, purchased from various commercial sources, have been used for most published latex particle immunoassays. Immunoglobulins prepared by precipitation with sodium or ammonium sulphate are generally used to sensitize the particles (Bloomfield et al., 1963; Newman et al., 1970; Goodman et al., 1971; Bennett and Bailey, 1971; Severin, 1972; Hechemy et al., 1974; Whittle et al., 1974; McCarthy, 1975; Coonrod and Rylko-Bauer, 1976; Leinonen and Herva, 1977; Bromberger et al., 1980; Scott et al., 1980), but whole antisera have been used successfully by a few investigators (Singer et al., 1957; Salomon and Tew, 1968; Ward et al., 1978). Some antisera are clearly superior to others for latex particle immunoassays, and several antisera should be tested if the first one tested provides inadequate sensitivity (Kumar and Nankervis, 1980).

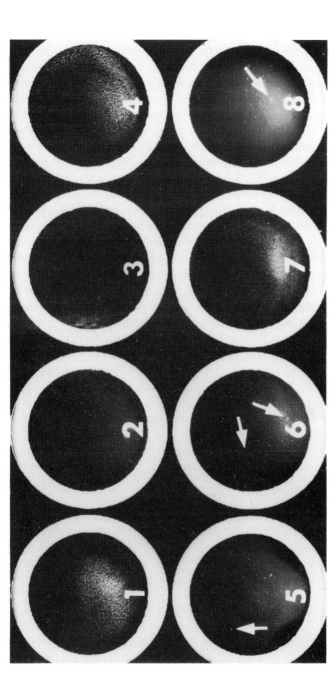

Fig. 3 Latex agglutination for cryptococcal antigen. Wells 1, 2 and 4 contain latex particles coated with anticryptococcal IgG. Wells 5–8 contain latex particles coated with nonimmune IgG. The test specimens in the wells are: (1) and (5) — positive control antigen; (2) and (6) —negative control antigen; (3) —empty; (7) —anti-immunoglobulin G; (4) and (8) — cerebrospinal fluid from a patient with *Cryptococcus neoformans* meningitis. The solitary white spots (*arrows*) are photographic artefacts not visible in the actual test; several attempts to eliminate them were unsuccessful. Wells 1, 4 and 7 represent positive reactions; wells 2, 5, 6 and 8 are negative.

To sensitize the latex particles, they are often diluted to provide a stock suspension which, when diluted 1:100, yields an absorbance at 650 nm of 0.3 (Bloomfield *et al.*, 1963). Investigators using particles supplied by Difco Laboratories often use them without dilution (Severin, 1972; Bromberger *et al.*, 1980). When the concentration of latex particles is too low, agglutination is difficult to see; when the concentration is too high, spontaneous precipitation may occur (Singer and Plotz, 1956). One part latex solution is mixed with an equal volume of optimally diluted whole serum or gamma globulin. Although the optimum dilution must be determined for each antiserum, dilutions of gamma globulin ranging from 1:20 to 1:160, or about 80 to 320 µg ml^{-1}, have been optimal (Bloomfield *et al.*, 1963; Newman *et al.*, 1970; Bennett and Bailey, 1971; Goodman *et al.*, 1971; Severin, 1972; Whittle *et al.*, 1974; Coonrod and Rylko-Bauer, 1976; Leinonen and Herva, 1977; Bromberger *et al.*, 1980). For producing "polyvalent" particles sensitized with multiple globulin preparations with multiple specificities, a modified sensitizing procedure using sedimented latex particles appears superior to the standard procedure (Hechemy *et al.*, 1974). A glycine saline buffer, consisting of 7.3 g glycine and 10 g sodium chloride, adjusted to pH 8.2 with 1.0 N sodium hydroxide, and to 1000 ml with distilled water (Newman *et al.*, 1970), is used by virtually all investigators as the diluent for latex particles and immunoglobulin. The pH must be kept between 8.2 and 9.0: below pH 8.0, spontaneous precipitation of gamma-globulin-coated particles occurs; above pH 10.0, agglutination is inhibited (Singer and Plotz, 1956). Adsorption is essentially complete in two hours (Singer *et al.*, 1963). A borate saline buffer, pH 8.0, has been used with success (Bennett and Bailey, 1971).

The "sensitized" latex particles are then stored at 4°C, usually after further two- to fourfold dilution in 0.1 to 1% bovine serum albumin in glycine-buffered saline containing 0.1–0.2% sodium azide to inhibit microbial growth (Leach and Ruck, 1971; Severin, 1972; Hechemy *et al.*, 1974; Leinonen and Herva, 1977; Bromberger *et al.*, 1980). The bovine serum albumin is added to prevent autoagglutination; Hechemy *et al.* (1974) found defatted bovine serum albumin (Sigma type F) superior to standard bovine albumin for this purpose. It is important that the latex particles should not be exposed to bovine serum albumin or other proteins until they have been fully adsorbed with gamma globulin, since other proteins may prevent adsorption of gamma globulin to polystyrene (Pesce *et al.*, 1977). Attempts to remove unadsorbed globulin from the reaction system by washing the coated particles may result in nonspecific agglutination (Singer and Plotz, 1956). After sensitization the particles remain useful for at least several months. Coonrod and Rylko-Bauer (1976) noted a fourfold drop in sensitivity with several of their sensitized particle preparations between two and four months of storage; however, their storage solution did not contain bovine serum albumin. Others have reported stability of the sensitized particles for at least 3 months (Bloomfield *et al.*, 1963; Leach and Ruck, 1971), 4 months (Whittle *et al.*, 1974), 6 months (Newman *et al.*, 1970; McCarthy, 1975), 12 months (Severin, 1972), and 24 months (Ward *et al.*, 1978).

For the actual assay, 20–50 μl of the test specimen and 10–20 μl of sensitized latex particles are mixed together on a scrupulously cleaned slide. The slide is agitated manually or on a rotary shaker at room temperature. Mixing is usually terminated in two minutes (Kaufman and Blumer, 1968; Newman *et al.*, 1970; Leach and Ruck, 1971; Hechemy *et al.*, 1974; Leinonen and Herva, 1977; Scott *et al.*, 1980) although others have chosen three (Severin, 1972; Whittle *et al.*, 1974; Coonrod and Rylko-Bauer, 1976), five (Bramner *et al.*, 1974), ten (Bennett and Bailey, 1971), and 45 minutes (Ward *et al.*, 1978). Prolonging incubation beyond the established time may lead to false-positive reactions (International Biological Laboratories, Inc., Rockville, MD). No explanation for the longer reaction times was provided. Humidified chambers must be used for the long incubation times to prevent reagent desiccation (Ward *et al.*, 1978). When dilutions of the sample are to be tested, glycine-buffered saline containing bovine serum albumin is the usual diluent.

The reactions are then scored visually as 0 to 4 + as described by Newman *et al.* (1970), preferably with clear glass slides read by indirect lighting against a black background (Coonrod and Rylko-Bauer, 1976). Some investigators accept only 2 + or greater agglutination as positive because of numerous 1 + reactions in control specimens (Bloomfield *et al.*, 1963; Hechemy *et al.*, 1974; Coonrod and Rylko-Bauer, 1976; Scott *et al.*, 1980).

C. Problems with latex particle immunoassays

Fifty to 95% of sera containing rheumatoid factor will agglutinate latex particles coated with rabbit or guinea pig gamma globulins (Bennett and Baily, 1971; Klossner and Willman, 1973; Gordon and Lapa, 1974; Ohya *et al.*, 1974; Rutstein *et al.*, 1978). Rheumatoid factor may be present in the sera of 3% or more of humans who do not have rheumatoid arthritis (Plotz and Singer, 1956) and in spinal fluid from up to 39% of patients with diverse central nervous system disorders (Lund-Olesen, 1969). Therefore, the inclusion of latex particles coated with nonimmune gamma globulin as controls and/or treatment of specimens to eliminate rheumatoid factor is mandatory in latex particle agglutination tests for microbial antigens. When latex particles coated with nonimmune gamma globulin have been included as controls, 3–18% of all sera tested (Leach and Ruck, 1971; Desmyter, 1973; Zalan *et al.*, 1973; Hopkins and Dos, 1974; Ohya *et al.*, 1974; Martin-Sosa and Berron, 1975; Ward *et al.*, 1978) and 2% of cerebrospinal fluids (Newman *et al.*, 1970; Whittle *et al.*, 1974) agglutinated the control particles. Martin-Sosa and

Berron (1975) estimated that approximately 50% of the nonspecific positive serum reactions were due to rheumatoid factor. To evaluate such specimens for antigens, the manufacturer of a commercial kit for detecting cryptococcal antigens (International Biological Laboratories, Inc., Rockville, MD) recommends testing serial dilutions of the test specimen with the nonimmune and immune globulin coated particles; if the titre of the specimen with the immune globulin coated particles is fourfold higher than with the control particles the test should be regarded as positive for cryptococcal antigen. Limited data suggests this recommendation is valid (Prevost and Newell, 1978). Alternatively, rheumatoid factor activity can be eliminated or greatly reduced by treating specimens with 0.0065 molar 2-mercaptoethanol or 0.003 molar dithiothreitol (Burrell et al., 1972; Gordon and Lapa, 1974; Rutstein et al., 1978; Ward et al., 1978). Specimens so treated should be tested within three hours because the rheumatoid factor activity tends to return with time (Gordon and Lapa, 1974). Zalan et al. (1973) eliminated rheumatoid factor by combining heating at 62°C for ten minutes with adsorption with goat or rabbit antihuman IgM, neither treatment alone being satisfactory. Heating spinal fluid at 100°C for 15 min eliminated false-positives in a latex test for H. influenzae meningitis (Newman et al., 1970). Obviously the antigen being detected must be unaffected by these treatments for them to be useful.

Body fluid components destroyed by heating at 56°C for 15–30 min, presumably early complement components, may also cause weak nonspecific agglutination of globulin-coated latex particles (Ewald and Schubart, 1966). Martin-Sosa and Berron (1975) found that about one-third of the nonspecific reactions in a latex agglutination test for hepatitis B could be eliminated by heating at 56°C for 30 min, and such heating is recommended in latex agglutination tests for cryptococcal antigen (Gordon and Vedder, 1966; Kaufman and Blumer, 1968; Goodman et al., 1971; International Biological Laboratories, Inc., Rockville, MD). Several investigators have not, however, found this treatment effective in eliminating false-positive reactions (Hopkins and Das, 1974; Coonrod and Rylko-Bauer, 1976). Specimens tested immediately after collection appear more likely to yield nonspecific agglutination by this mechanism than those tested after 24 hours or more of storage (Ohya et al., 1974; Perkins et al., 1974). Thus, heating at 56°C for 30 min should probably be routinely performed for latex agglutination tests, especially of freshly tested specimens, unless the antigen is destroyed by such treatment.

Bromberger et al. (1980) claimed that crystals and mucus in urine caused strong nonspecific agglutination in a latex agglutination test for group B streptococcal antigen which could be eliminated by centrifugation of the urine prior to testing.

Prozone phenomena in the presence of high rheumatoid factor levels were first noted as a cause of false-negative latex tests for rheumatoid factor (Singer *et al.*, 1957). Subsequently, high antigen concentrations have been shown to cause false negatives because of the prozone effect (Kelle and Webster, 1961; Bloomfield *et al.*, 1963; Newman *et al.*, 1970; Leinonen and Herva, 1977). Nonreactive specimens should therefore be tested at several dilutions before being regarded as lacking antigen.

Day to day interpretation of results is sufficiently variable to require the inclusion of weak positive and negative controls with each day's testing (Coonrod and Rylko-Bauer, 1976). Serum may or may not diminish the sensitivity of latex agglutination (Coonrod and Rylko-Bauer, 1976; Scheifele *et al.*, 1979). Contamination of test samples with *S. aureus* would be expected to yield false-positive results (Hechemy *et al.*, 1974), presumably caused by staphylococcal protein A.

A final problem with latex agglutination is that the limited surface area available for antibody adsorption limits the effectiveness of a single latex agglutination test for detecting multiple antigens. This has been particularly noted in tests for pneumococcal polysaccharides; Leinonen (1980) found latex particles sensitized with pneumococcal Omniserum less capable of detecting the various polysaccharide types than counterimmunoelectrophoresis using the same Omniserum. Since Omniserum is standardized for the pneumococcal quellung test rather than precipitating or agglutinating antibodies, lot-to-lot variability in its ability to detect antigens in latex agglutination might be expected (Coonrod and Rylko-Bauer, 1976). Furthermore, the relatively high concentration of Omniserum globulin necessary to sensitize latex particles appears to increase the problem of nonspecific agglutination (Coonrod and Rylko-Bauer, 1976).

D. Applications and comparative sensitivities of latex agglutination assays

1. *Haemophilus influenzae infections*

Latex agglutination detects *H. influenzae* type b capsular polysaccharide at $0.2-5.0\,\text{ng ml}^{-1}$, depending upon the investigator (Leinonen and Kayhty, 1978; Ward *et al.*, 1978; Scheifele *et al.*, 1979). Serum did not diminish the sensitivity (Ward *et al.*, 1978; Scheifele *et al.*, 1979). When compared to CIE, latex agglutination was consistently 2- to 32-fold more sensitive for detecting *H. influenzae* polysaccharide in prepared solution or in serially diluted antigen-positive spinal fluid (Whittle *et al.*, 1974; Leinonen and Kayhty, 1978; Ward *et al.*, 1978; Scheifele *et al.*, 1979). Latex agglutination was 10-fold less sensitive than a liquid-phase radioimmunoassay for detecting the polysaccharide in prepared solution (Leinonen and Kayhty, 1978).

In five series, 114 of 127 (90%) spinal fluids collected before or soon after initiation of antibiotic therapy for *H. influenzae* meningitis were positive. The range of positive results was 74–100% (Newman *et al.*, 1970; Whittle *et al.*, 1974; Leinonen and Kayhty, 1978; Ward *et al.*, 1978; Thirumoorthi and Dajani, 1979). Latex agglutination (LA) was somewhat more sensitive than CIE in actual clinical use: 25/25 (LA) v. 20/24 (CIE) (Ward *et al.*, 1978); 15/16 (LA) v. 14/16 (CIE) (Whittle *et al.*, 1974). Latex agglutination was slightly less sensitive than radioimmunoassay (RIA): 14/19 (LA) v. 16/19 (RIA). Latex agglutination was also more sensitive than the Gram stain (GS): 15/16 (LA) v. 11/16 (GS) (Whittle *et al.*, 1974); 15/17 (LA) v. 14/17 (GS) (Ward *et al.*, 1978).

Regarding specificity, Newman *et al.* (1970) encountered nonspecific positivity in 2.3% of 558 control spinal fluid specimens. Most of these were retested after heating at 100°C for 15 min and all became negative. True positives were not affected by this treatment. Ward *et al.* (1978) encountered no false-positives in 34 control spinal fluids tested by latex agglutination.

Serum is positive by latex agglutination almost as frequently as spinal fluid in *H. influenzae* meningitis (Ward *et al.*, 1978; Thirumoorthi and Dajani, 1979) and is often positive in *H. influenzae* epiglottitis, cellulitis, and pneumonia. For these nonmeningitic infections, latex agglutination was more sensitive than CIE (Ward *et al.*, 1978). The superiority of latex agglutination over CIE for detecting antigen in serum has been confirmed in a monkey *H. influenzae* infection model (Scheifele *et al.*, 1979). However, serum false-positivity was seen in 11 of 60 human controls tested by latex agglutination and 7 of 58 tested by CIE (Ward *et al.*, 1978). Dithiothreitol treatment eliminated the latex agglutination false-positives; phenol extraction eliminated the false positives by CIE. Antigen may be detected in urine by latex agglutination (29/37) more frequently than by CIE (19/37) in *H. influenzae* infections (Thirumoorthi and Dajani, 1979).

2. *Streptococcus pneumoniae* infections

Latex particles sensitized with pneumococcal Omniserum detect pneumococcal polysaccharides at 12 to 1600 ng ml^{-1}, depending on the serotype (Coonrod and Rylko-Bauer, 1976; Leinonen, 1980). No consistent superiority of latex agglutination or CIE was seen among the many serotypes. For example, latex agglutination detected serotype 1 polysaccharide at 1600 ng ml^{-1}, CIE at 400 ng ml^{-1}; however, for serotype 3, latex agglutination detected 12 ng ml^{-1}, and CIE 50 ng ml^{-1} (Coonrod and Rylko-Bauer, 1976). The type 7 and 14 polysaccharides, which cannot be detected by CIE under standard conditions, were each detected by latex agglutination at 25 ng ml^{-1}. Pooled spinal fluid from pneumococcal meningitis patients was positive at a 1/64 dilution by both methods.

Whittle *et al.* (1974) found spinal fluid pneumococcal antigens in 82% of 87 meningitis patients by latex agglutination and 98% by CIE. Only 67% had positive Gram stains. Some patients had already received antibiotics when the spinal fluid was obtained. In 11 pretreatment spinal fluids, Coonrod and Rylko-Bauer (1976) found antigen in 64% by latex agglutination, 73% by CIE, 82% by one or both procedures, and 82% by Gram stain. As a single procedure, CIE appears somewhat superior to latex agglutination for diagnosing pneumococcal meningitis. In pretherapy specimens, neither procedure offers much, if any, improvement over the Gram stain.

CIE was superior to latex agglutination for detecting antigens in 50 cases of pneumococcal pneumonia: 40% positive (CIE); 22% (LA); 52% (CIE + LA). The superiority of CIE in this study was due, in part, to the relatively high frequency of serogroup 1 infections, which the Omniserum batch used to prepare the latex agglutination test detected poorly (Coonrod and Rylko-Bauer, 1976). CIE was also superior to latex agglutination for detecting pneumococcal antigen in middle ear fluids from which pneumococci were grown: 76% (CIE) v. 63% (LA) v. 88% (CIE + LA) (Leinonen, 1980).

False-positive pneumococcal antigen latex agglutination results occurred in 4 of 23 spinal fluids from patients with *H. influenzae* meningitis and in none of 22 other specimens (Coonrod and Rylko-Bauer, 1976). No attempt was made to retest the specimens after heating or dithiothreitol treatment. The false-positive results were readily detected by the control latex particles.

In summary, latex agglutination has little to offer over the Gram stain for diagnosing pneumococcal meningitis unless therapy has already been given. It is also insufficiently sensitive to be of much value for diagnosing pneumococcal pneumonia.

3. Neisseria meningitidis infections

Latex agglutination detected group A *N. meningitidis* polysaccharide at 10 ng ml^{-1} and group C polysaccharide at 25 ng ml^{-1}; this was, respectively, five and three times better sensitivity than CIE (Leinonen and Kayhty, 1978).

Three reasonably large studies have assessed latex agglutination for detecting meningococcal antigens in group A meningococcal meningitis. In these studies 84% of 192 patients were positive, ranging from 67% to 93% (Severin, 1972; Whittle *et al.*, 1974; Leinonen and Kayhty, 1978). Type-specific antigens were detected in 86% of 21 group C meningitis patients' spinal fluids (Severin, 1972; Leinonen and Kayhty, 1978). Latex agglutination was more sensitive than CIE in one study—25/27 (LA) v. 20/27 (CIE), (Severin, 1972)—and of equivalent sensitivity in another (Whittle *et al.*, 1974) for diagnosing group A meningococcal infections. Leinonen and Kayhty (1978) found latex agglutination to be as sensitive as radioimmunoassay for group A infections: 26/39 (LA) v. 25/39 (RIA). Latex agglutination was also more sensitive than combined Gram stain and culture (GS/C) in an African population with group A meningococcal meningitis: 111/126 (LA) v. 100/126

(GS/C) (Whittle *et al.*, 1974); some of these patients were tested after antibiotics had been started.

4. Group B streptococcal infections

Latex agglutination was 8- to 16-fold more sensitive than CIE for detecting group specific antigens of group B streptococci but 4- to 64-fold less sensitive for detecting type-specific antigens. Of three spinal fluids from patients with group B streptococcal meningitis all were positive in both assays. In children with various types of group B streptococcal infections, antigen was detected in unconcentrated urine in 7/11 (LA) and 1/11 (CIE); in 25-fold concentrated urine in 11/11 (LA) and 8/11 (CIE) and in serum in 2/8 (LA) and 0/8 (CIE) (Bromberger *et al.*, 1980). False-positives were not seen in 114 control specimens. Thirumoorthi and Dajani (1979) were not able to detect group B streptococcal antigens in any of 10 spinal fluids or three urines from patients with group B streptococcal meningitis.

5. Disseminated cryptococcal infections

Cryptococcal antigen can be detected by latex agglutination in the serum and/or spinal fluid of 80–95% of patients with cryptococcal meningitis (Bloomfield *et al.*, 1963; Kaufman and Blumer, 1968; Bennett and Bailey, 1971), including some patients whose cultures and india ink preparations are negative during life but proven by autopsy to have the illness (Goodman *et al.*, 1971; Snow and Dismukes, 1975). Antigen has also been detected in the serum of patients with cutaneous cryptococcosis and in serum or pleural fluid from cryptococcal pneumonia patients (Gordon and Vedder, 1966; Fisher and Armstrong, 1977; Young *et al.*, 1980). False-positive results occur but are recognized by their ability to agglutinate control latex particles coated with nonimmune guinea pig gamma globulin. Other fungal infections do not appear to cross-react in the assay (Kaufman and Blumer, 1968). In a recently reported false-positive cerebrospinal fluid test in a patient with *Klebsiella pneumoniae* prevertebral abscess, the authors did not state whether control particles were tested (MacKinnon *et al.*, 1978).

Recently, an enzyme-linked radiosorbent immunoassay was reported which is capable of detecting cryptococcal polysaccharide at 6.25 ng ml^{-1} as opposed to the 35 ng ml^{-1} possible with latex agglutination. The enzyme immunoassay detected antigen in several patients who were negative by latex agglutination. Only four patients' data were presented to compare the two assays (Scott *et al.*, 1980).

6. Hepatitis B

A latex agglutination test for hepatitis B surface antigen was found comparable in sensitivity to CIE and complement fixation but less sensitive than solid-phase radioimmunoassay. False-positive reactions occurred in 0.4–1.8% of specimens tested (Bramner *et al.*, 1974). Since commercial radioimmunoassays and enzyme immunoassays are available, the latex agglutination test would appear to have little appeal, at least in industrialized countries.

7. Other latex agglutination tests

A very sensitive latex agglutination test for *S. aureus* type B enterotoxin has been described; its clinical utility has not been reported (Salomon and Tew, 1968). A sensitive latex assay for detecting EDTA-extractable *E. coli* antigens has been developed, but again its clinical utility has not been reported (Hechemy *et al.*, 1974).

IV. RADIOIMMUNOASSAY

A. General aspects

Radioimmunoassay, introduced in 1960 by Yalow and Berson, for hormone detection has subsequently been successfully applied to the rapid diagnosis of microbial infections by antigen detection. In standard liquid-phase systems unlabelled and radiolabelled antigens compete for attachment to specific antibodies. The resultant antibody–antigen complexes are then separated from free antibodies and antigens. The amount of radiolabelled antigen in the complexes is then inversely related to the amount of unlabelled antigen in the test sample. Although highly sensitive, the liquid-phase system is time-consuming because of the long incubation times and labour intensive because of the need to separate the antibody–antigen complexes from the free antigens and antibodies. Subsequently, solid-phase radioimmunoassays were developed using antibodies attached to insoluble support structures. The application of radioimmunoassay to diagnosing microbial infections will be discussed in this section.

B. Technical aspects

1. Direct solid phase radioimmunoassay (SPRIA) (Fig. 4a)

(a) Solid-phase antibody coating step
Most solid-phase radioimmunoassays use specific antibodies attached by adsorption to an insoluble support. Acceptable solid-phase supports have included polystyrene or polypropylene tubes (Catt *et al.*, 1970), polyvinyl microtitre plates (Purcell *et al.*, 1976), Sepharose 4B (Poor and Cutler, 1979),

microcrystalline cellulose particles (Thornley *et al.*, 1979) or protein A rich *Staphylococcus aureus* (Shaffer *et al.*, 1979b). Radioimmunoassay studies comparing different solid phase supports are not available, although the studies discussed in the next section on enzyme immunoassays probably apply to radioimmunoassay.

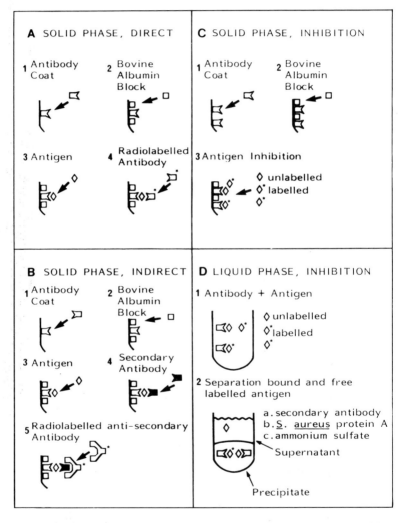

Fig. 4 Radioimmunoassay methods are outlined here and discussed in more detail in the text.

Antisera used in the solid phase coating step should be late, presumably high affinity sera. In our SPRIA for *Legionella pneumophila*, antiserum harvested 16 months after initiation of immunization provided an assay which was 40- to 80-fold more sensitive than an assay established with serum from the same rabbit after only six weeks. Immunization methods and antiserum selection have been reviewed by Overby and Mushawar (1979). Diluted whole antisera, gamma globulins precipitates, and immunoglobulin G fractions have all been used to coat the solid-phase. Although diluted whole antiserum may be adequate (Minta *et al.*, 1973), most investigators use immunoglobulin G fractions. Immunoglobulin M antibodies, although offering a larger number of antigen-binding sites than immunoglobulin G antibodies, have not worked in our assay for staphylococcal antigens or in an assay for *Brucella* antigens (Wilson *et al.*, 1977). The coating antibody concentration should be determined for new radioimmunoassays. Although antigen binding may be greater in tubes coated with concentrated antibody solutions (Foti *et al.*, 1975), sensitivity may be less than when lower antibody concentrations are used (Salmon *et al.*, 1969). In our systems, sensitivity is stable until critically low concentrations of coating antibodies are used (Fig. 5). We have generally chosen $10–20 \, \mu g \, ml^{-1}$.

Catt and Tregear (1967) stated that antibodies should be diluted in slightly alkaline, low ionic strength buffers for tube coating. Rising ionic strength inversely affects antibody attachment to the solid phase (Kotoulas and Moroz, 1971), but pH has limited effects over a range from 6.6–9.6 (Baumann *et al.*, 1969; Askenase and Leonard, 1970). Coating antibodies should not be diluted in protein-containing buffers, which interfere with attachment (Askenase and Leonard, 1970; Koutoulas and Moroz, 1971; Rosenthal *et al.*, 1973).

Coating appears to occur more rapidly at higher temperatures (Foti *et al.*, 1975; Minta *et al.*, 1973; Baumann *et al.*, 1969). Binding increases with time (Catt *et al.*, 1970), but a plateau is reached in one to two hours at frequently used coating concentrations. If appropriate antibody concentrations are used, assay sensitivity and accuracy are not improved by prolonged incubation of the antibody binding step, and a one-hour incubation has worked well in most assays (Foti *et al.*, 1975; Minta *et al.*, 1973). If very low concentrations of antibody must be used, prolonged incubation may be necessary (see discussion under Enzyme Immunoassays).

Following incubation, unadsorbed antibodies are aspirated and the tubes are washed from one to five times, usually with saline or the buffer used in the coating step. Under the usual coating conditions, less than 1% of the coating antibodies bind to the tube (Salmon *et al.*, 1969). Antibodies coated in this manner adhere sufficiently well to the plastics to allow numerous washes during subsequent assay steps (Catt *et al.*, 1970).

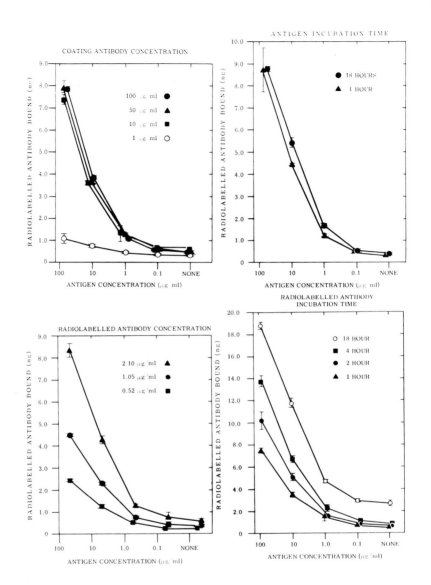

Fig. 5 Direct solid-phase radioimmunoassay conditions. Data obtained with the staphylococcal antigen assay diagrammed in Fig. 4a (Wheat *et al.*, 1978). Sensitivity was similar (1 µg ml^{-1}) in tubes coated with 10–100 µg ml^{-1} of the IgG fraction of rabbit anti-*S. aureus* (*top left*). Sensitivity was only 10 µg ml^{-1} in tubes coated with 1 µg ml^{-1} antibody. Sensitivity was stable at radio-labelled antibody concentrations from 0.52–2.10 µg ml^{-1}, although the curve was shifted upward with higher labelled antibody concentrations (*bottom left*). Sensitivity was not improved by prolonging incubation of antigen in the coated tubes (*top right*). Prolonging the radiolabelled antibody incubation time shifted the curve upward without improving sensitivity, 1 µg ml^{-1} (*bottom right*).

(b)   Protein filler step

In most solid-phase radioimmunoassays, a protein solution is next added to the tubes or plates to block remaining unoccupied binding sites and prevent nonspecific attachment of subsequently added materials (Fig. 4a, step 2) (Askenase and Leonard, 1970; Rosenthal *et al.*, 1973; Minta *et al.*, 1973; Purcell *et al.*, 1976). Bovine serum albumin at 10–50 μg ml $^{-1}$ in the same buffer used in the antibody-coating step has been used most frequently. Optimal incubation conditions have not been reported. Bovine serum albumin at 50 μg ml $^{-1}$, incubated for one hour at 37°C, has worked well in our laboratory. Tubes coated with antibody and bovine serum albumin can be stored at 4°C for at least four to six weeks until use without loss of sensitivity or accuracy (Catt *et al.*, 1970).

(c)   Antigen step

In the third step, samples to be tested for antigen are added to the antibody-coated tubes. Antigens attach specifically to the solid-phase antibodies. If dilutions of antigen standards or test samples are to be assayed, they are usually diluted in the same protein-containing solution used in the blocking step, although in some of our assays we have found protein to be unnecessary. Incubation temperature and duration have varied in reported studies (Prince and Jass, 1974; Askenase and Leonard, 1970). Sensitivity was not improved by prolonged incubation at 37°C in our assays (Fig. 5). The duration of this step should be evaluated for new essays since optimal conditions probably vary.

(d)   Radiolabelled antibody step

After aspirating and washing, antigens adherent to the solid-phase antibodies are detected by specific radiolabelled antibodies in direct, or single antibody sandwich, solid-phase assays. The same immunoglobulin preparation used for tube coating can be used in this step, although antibodies produced in a second animal species can also be used (Overby and Mushawar, 1979). Antibodies should be at least partially purified prior to radiolabelling. Without purification, other serum proteins would also be radiolabelled, resulting in high nonspecific background radioactivity and poor assay sensitivity. Immunoglobulin G antibodies obtained by Sephadex G200 or DEAE chromatography are generally used (Overby and Mushawar, 1979). Some have used monospecific antibodies purified by affinity chromatography or by immunoprecipitation with the specific antigen. Antibodies are isolated from the resolubilized immune complexes by dissociation at low pH followed by separation of the free antibodies and antigens by molecular sieve or ion exchange chromatography (Ling and Overby, 1972; Overby *et al.*, 1973). Studies comparing the sensitivity and specificity of solid-phase radioimmunoassays using such monospecific antibodies to assays using the whole immunoglobulin G fraction of immune sera have not been reported.

Radiolabelling methods have been reviewed by Overby and Mushawar (1979), Felber (1978) and Chervu and Murty (1975). The chloramine T method of Hunter and Greenwood, or a modification, using $Na^{125}I$ has been used most frequently (Hunter, 1971), but other methods may cause less iodination damage (Overby and Mushawar, 1979). We have used the chloramine T method, with the ratio of chloramine T to protein being 20 μg mg^{-1} and of $Na^{125}I$ to protein being 5 mCi mg^{-1}, and the reaction time, 10 min. The reaction is terminated with sodium metabisulphite, 20 μg ml mg^{-1} of protein. After adding an equal volume of 0.04% potassium iodide in 10% bovine serum albumin in the iodination buffer, radiolabelled antibodies are separated from free radioactive iodide by chromatography on disposable columns of Sephadex G25 (Pharmacia Fine Chemicals). Any residual unbound radioactive iodide can be further reduced by dialysis if nonspecific background radioactivity seems too high (Overby and Mushawar, 1979). Using this method, radiolabelled antibodies with specific activities of 0.4 and 2.0 mCi mg^{-1} protein are usually produced. Radiolabelled antibodies may be used for four to eight weeks.

The optimum concentration of radiolabelled antibodies should be determined by testing serial dilutions of antigen with various concentrations of labelled antibodies. Assay sensitivity may be impaired at very low concentrations of radiolabelled antibodies; however, beyond a certain point, increasing the concentrations of labelled antibodies causes both increased binding to antigens and nonspecific background binding without improving assay sensitivity (Fig. 5). We have generally used a concentration of 1–4 μg ml^{-1}.

Little information is available about the optimum incubation conditions for this step. Most have diluted the labelled antibodies in solutions containing 10–100 mg ml^{-1} of protein, usually bovine serum albumin, to reduce nonspecific binding to tubes lacking antigen. Although incubation at 50°C may be better than lower temperatures (Prince and Jass, 1974), most have used 37°C. The duration of incubation should be studied for each assay. We have found one hour at 37°C to be adequate. Prolonging incubation may increase both specific and nonspecific binding without improving sensitivity (Fig. 5).

(e)   Expressing results

Determination of positivity requires testing appropriate specimens from uninfected controls. Specific definitions of positivity depend on the accuracy and reproducibility of the assay in addition to the range of results in controls. Generally, cutoffs separating positive and negative results are chosen which maximize the sensitivity in infected subjects and minimize false-positive results in controls. Cutoffs may be based on standard deviations above the mean of the negative control group, i.e. 2 to 5 SD above the mean, or on a ratio of the mean of the test sample to the mean of the control group, i.e. 2.1 times the mean (Overby et al., 1973). Appropriate negative controls should generally be included each time the assay is run. Using 5 to 10 negative controls for daily determinations, cutoffs based on ratios of the mean have, in our experience, been more reproducible than those based on standard deviations. The number of aliquots to be assayed for each specimen depends on the tube-to-tube variability of the assay. Tube-to-tube variability, expressed as the coefficient of variation — (SD of the mean)/(mean of the tubes tested for a sample) × 100 — should be 10% or less (Catt, 1969). We have generally tested three or four tubes for each specimen with acceptable tube-to-tube variability for 90% of specimens.

2.   Antigen assay in antigen-coated tubes

One method for improving assay specificity is to coat the solid phase with the specific antigen to be detected (Salmon et al., 1969). Antibodies are then attached to the solid-phase antigen rather than directly to the solid phase. After a subsequent filler step, these tubes are then used to detect antigen as described above for the direct assay. Presumably, only specific antibodies attach to the solid phase in this assay method whereas other immunoglobulins would also bind in the direct coating method. Assay sensitivity and accuracy are reported to be improved using tubes coated in this manner (Salmon et al., 1969).

3.   Indirect, or double-antibody sandwich, solid phase radioimmunoassay

(a)   General aspects

The first three steps in indirect assays are similar to those just described for direct assays. Unlabelled antibodies from an animal species different from that from which the tube coating antibodies are derived are used to detect the antigens bound to the solid-phase antibodies, as shown in Fig. 4b. This second antibody is then measured with radiolabelled anti-immunoglobulin G antibodies specific for the animal species which produced the second antibody. Conditions for the first four steps should be similar to those used in direct assays.

(b)   Radiolabelled anti-immunoglobulin step (step 5 in Fig. 4b)

Most investigators have used commercially available immunoglobulin G antibodies to the Fc fragment of the second antibody. Nonspecific background radioactivity is reduced if the labelled antibody is diluted in bovine serum albumin (Rosenthal *et al.*, 1973). Studies establishing optimal conditions for the second antibody and the labelled antibody step have not been reported for indirect assays, so assay conditions should be evaluated thoroughly for new indirect assays. As pointed out in a later section indirect enzyme assays are more sensitive than direct assays, and the same is probably true of radioimmunoassays, although proof is lacking. The advantage of indirect assays is that a single radiolabelled antibody can be used for multiple antigen assays if the same animal species provides the antisera, thus decreasing the expense, risks and inconvenience of radioiodination. A disadvantage is the requirement for antisera from two animal species for each assay.

4. Solid phase inhibition assays

(a)   Direct competition inhibition assays
Several types of solid phase inhibition assays have been described. In the simplest method, unlabelled antigens in the test specimen compete with radiolabelled antigen for the solid phase antibodies (Fig. 4c). The first two steps are similar to those in the direct assay. The coating antibody concentration should be sufficient to bind 60–80% of the labelled antigen (Baumann *et al.*, 1969). A prozone may occur with excessive coating antibody (Ceska, 1970), and so coating conditions must be evaluated carefully.

(b)   Competition step in direct competition assays
The test samples containing the purported antigen and radiolabelled antigen are added to the coated tubes. Alternatively, unlabelled antigens or unknowns may be added to the coated tubes before the labelled antigen, with similar sensitivity (Baumann *et al.*, 1969). Sensitivity may be increased through the use of relatively low concentrations of coating antibodies and labelled antigens (Baumann *et al.*, 1969). At 37°C nearly maximum antigen binding occurs within 5 hours (Ceska *et al.*, 1970). At 4°C incubation for up to 48 hours may be necessary (Ceska *et al.*, 1978; Foti *et al.*, 1975). Sensitivity may be improved by prolonging incubation of unlabelled antigens in coated tubes for 24 hours in sequential inhibition assays (Minta *et al.*, 1973). Once adherent to the solid phase antibodies, unlabelled antigens are not eluted by the labelled antigens (Minta *et al.*, 1973).

(c)   Antigen inhibition competition assays
Another type of solid phase inhibition assay uses antigen-coated tubes. Antigens present in standards and unknowns are detected by inhibition of attachment of specific antibodies to the coated tubes. Specific antibodies attached to the solid phase antigen can be detected by ^{125}I-labelled *S. aureus*

protein A, which attaches to the Fc fragment of immunoglobulin G of many animal species (Avraham *et al.*, 1980) or by ^{125}I-labelled anti-immunoglobulin G (Zollinger and Mandrell, 1977).

5.   Liquid phase inhibition radioimmunoassay

(a)   General aspects
Liquid phase assays have been useful for detecting several microbial antigens. Labelled and unlabelled antigens compete for binding to specific antibodies in a solution (Fig. 4d). After equilibrium has occurred, antigen–antibody complexes are removed from solution by a variety of separation methods. Unlabelled antigens in test samples are quantitated by comparing their inhibition of radiolabelled antigen binding to a standard inhibition curve with known concentrations of unlabelled antigens. Such assays may be more sensitive than solid phase assays (Arends, 1971; Hollinger *et al.*, 1971; Robern *et al.*, 1975) but they are labour intensive and slow.

(b)   Antigen–antibody binding step
The primary antibody concentration should be determined for each assay. A concentration which binds 50% of the labelled antigen should be used (Goldsmith, 1975; Russ *et al.*, 1976). The working dilution of the primary antibody should contain at least 2–5 µg of protein to form sufficient precipitate for the subsequent separation step. Assay sensitivity is improved using labelled antigens of high specific activity (Chervu and Murty, 1975; Goldsmith, 1975), but excess introduction of iodine into some antigens may decrease their affinity for antibodies. The unlabelled and labelled antigens may be added to the specific antibodies sequentially or simultaneously. The sequential method may be more sensitive (Felber, 1978). The antibodies and antigens should be diluted in protein-containing solutions such as bovine serum albumin or normal rabbit serum to minimize nonspecific binding to the glass tubes in which the reaction is conducted (Parker, 1972; Kayhty, 1977). Most have used at least overnight incubation. Incubation should be at 4°C if the incubation time is more than 8 hours (Parker, 1972).

(c)   Separation step
Antibody-bound labelled antigen must be separated from free labelled antigens. Separation methods have been thoroughly reviewed elsewhere (Parker, 1972; Ratcliffe, 1974; Felber, 1978). Precipitation of the antibody–antigen complexes with secondary antibodies specific for the primary antibody or with ammonium or sodium sulphate have been used most frequently. Incubation at 4°C for 16–48 hours is necessary using the secondary antibody method (Parker, 1972). Subsequent washing should also

be done at 4°C to prevent solubilization of the precipitate. Separation techniques based on the ability of protein A-rich *S. aureus* to bind the Fc fragment of immunoglobulin G of many animals have recently been described (Polakova, 1979; Frohman *et al.*, 1979). Antigen–antibody complexes attached to the staphylococci can be easily separated from free antigens by centrifugation. In contrast to the slow secondary antibody separation method, separation can be completed in 10 minutes without loss of sensitivity.

C. Problems

Antigen detection in solid-phase assays may be inhibited by serum factors which are destroyed by heating at 56°C (Robern *et al.*, 1975; Tabbarah *et al.*, 1979; Kohler *et al.*, 1980). These heat-labile inhibitory factors are also inactivated by heparin and, partially, by zymosan (Tabbarah, 1979; Kohler *et al.*, 1980). Presumably, early complement components cause part of this heat-labile inhibition by attaching to the solid phase and preventing antigen attachment; it is postulated that C1q recognizes the solid phase antibodies as immune complexes (Tabbarah *et al.*, 1979). The sensitivity of solid phase radioimmunoassays for *Pseudomonas*, staphylococcal and hepatitis B surface antigens was increased 4- to 16-fold by preheating serum samples at 56°C for 30 min before testing (Tabbarah *et al.*, 1979). Mechanisms for this heat-labile inhibition have not been fully elucidated.

In addition to the heat-labile inhibitory factors, serum factors stable to heating at 56°C for 30 min may inhibit antigen detection (Wheat *et al.*, 1979). These heat-stable inhibitors appear to be antibodies specific for the antigen being assayed. Antigens within immune complexes may be poorly detected in radioimmunoassays (O'Reilly *et al.*, 1976; Wheat *et al.*, 1979; Weiner and Coats-Stephen, 1979). Several methods have been described to dissociate these immune complexes to permit detection of the freed antigens (O'Reilly *et al.*, 1976; Coonrod and Leach, 1978; Weiner and Coats-Stephen, 1979), but thermodissociation is the simplest (Tabbarah *et al.*, 1980). In the thermodissociation method immune complexes are precipitated from the serum with ammonium sulphate. The resuspended complexes are then heated at 90°C; this frees the antigen from the complex and irreversibly denatures the antibody, preventing reassociation of the complex when the temperature is lowered. This thermodissociation method was necessary to detect circulating staphylococcal antigens in the blood of patients with *S. aureus* bacteraemia (Tabbarah *et al.*, 1980). Similar methods which also concentrate clinical samples, permitting detection of antigen at levels below the usual assay sensitivity, have been described (Doskeland and Berdal, 1980).

D. Applications

Published studies using radioimmunoassay for microbial antigen detection are summarized in Table 4. Polyribophosphate could be detected in the serum, in spinal fluid, or in both at concentrations ranging from 1 to 1100 ng ml $^{-1}$ in all of 36 patients with *H. influenza* type b meningitis (O'Reilly *et al.*, 1975). Antigen was detected only after dissociating immune complexes with citric acid pepsin treatment in 12 of 45 samples from the 36 patients. Antigen concentration and duration of antigenaemia correlated with clinical severity.

Group A and C meningococcal polysaccharides can also be detected by radioimmunoassay in the spinal fluid of about 75% of patients with meningococcal meningitis (Kayhty *et al.*, 1977).

A solid-phase assay for *P. aeruginosa* antigens was a sensitive and specific method for rapidly identifying patients with *P. aeruginosa* urinary tract infections (Kohler *et al.*, 1979). At least 10^5 CFUs ml $^{-1}$ of *P. aeruginosa* were required for a positive result. The antigens detected were both associated with the bacterial cells and released into the growth media. Using that same assay, antigen could also be detected in the blood of granulocytopenic rabbits with *P. aeruginosa* bacteraemia (Kohler *et al.*, 1980). Assay sensitivity was improved by heating the serum sample for 30 min at 56°C before testing. Whereas antigen could be detected in four of five rabbits with $> 10^3$ CFUs of *P. aeruginosa* per ml of blood, results were negative in 15 rabbits with lower colony counts. The antigen detected by this assay has not been identified.

Antigens were detected by a direct solid-phase radioimmunoassay in the blood of rabbits with *S. aureus* endocarditis (Wheat *et al.*, 1978). Although serum impaired the *in vitro* sensitivity of this assay (Tabbarah *et al.*, 1979), heat treatment at 56°C for 30 min did not improve the clinical sensitivity. Antigen levels did not correlate with quantitative blood culture results. Staphylococcal antibodies present in human sera were shown to impair antigen detection (Wheat *et al.*, 1979); circulating antigen could be detected in early sera from only 1 of 20 patients with *S. aureus* bacteraemia (Wheat *et al.*, 1979). After thermodissociation of immune complexes, antigen could be detected in early sera from 4 of 26 patients with *S. aureus* bacteraemia (Tabbarah *et al.*, 1980). Three of 5 patients with endocarditis but only 1 of 21 with other staphylococcal infection were antigenaemic. Antigen was not detected in the urine of patients with staphylococcal bacteraemia (Wheat, unpublished observation). The staphylococcal antigen detected in the rabbits and humans appeared in the void of a Sepharose 4B column, was immunologically stable at 100°C for 30 min, was sensitive to pepsin but not to ribonuclease or deoxyribonuclease, and did not form a precipitin line by immunodiffusion or immunoelectrophoresis against staphylococcal antisera (Wheat, unpublished observation).

Table 4 Antigen detection in infections by radioimmunoassay

Antigen	Assay	Detection limit	Infection	Test sample	Special treatment	Clinical sensitivity	False positives	Reference
H. influenzae polyribophosphate	Liquid-phase inhibition	0.5 ng ml^{-1}	Meningitis humans	Serum CSF	Citric acid–pepsin Citric acid–pepsin	34/38 11/12	Not stated	O'Reilly et al. (1975)
H. influenzae capsular polysaccharide	Liquid-phase inhibition	0.5 ng ml^{-1}	Meningitis humans	CSF	No	14/15	0/22	Kayhty et al. (1977)
Group A & C meningococcal capsular polysaccharides	Liquid-phase inhibition	2 ng ml^{-1}	Meningitis humans	CSF	No	GpA 18/23 GpC 2/4	0/22 0/22	Kayhty et al. (1977)
P. aeruginosa antigens	Solid-phase direct	Not stated	Urinary tract, humans	Urine	No	13/17	3/121	Kohler et al. (1979)
P. aeruginosa antigens	Solid-phase direct	Buffer 0.5 µg ml^{-1} Serum 10 µg ml^{-1}	Bacteraemia, granulocyto-penic rabbits	Serum	Heat 56°C×30 min	4/20	0/38	Kohler et al. (1980)
S. aureus antigens	Solid-phase direct	Buffer 0.31 µg ml^{-1}, rabbit serum 1.25 µg ml^{-1}	Endocarditis, rabbits	Serum	No	12/12	0/54 (1978)	Wheat et al.
S. aureus antigens	Solid-phase direct	Buffer 0.31 µg ml^{-1}, human serum 10 µg ml^{-1}	Endocarditis, humans	Serum	Ammonium sulphate pre-cipitation, 90°C×15 min	4/26	0/93	Tabbarah et al. (1980)
L. pneumophila antigens	Solid-phase direct	Not stated	Legionnaires disease, humans	Urine	No	9/9	0/241	Kohler et al. (1981)
Gonococcal antigens	Solid-phase direct	Not stated	Gonorrhoea, humans	Urine 2000 g× 10 min sediment	1. 37°C×30 min 2. Glacial acetic acid pH 5.5 3. Enzymes	41/56	0/27	Thornley et al. (1979)

Antigen/agent	Assay format	Sensitivity	Disease/host	Sample	Pretreatment	Positive	Controls	Reference
C. albicans antigens	Solid-phase direct	100 ng ml^{-1}	Candidiasis mice	Serum	No	19/27	0/15	Poor and Cutler (1979)
Candida mannan	Liquid-phase inhibition	0.3 ng ml^{-1}	Candidiasis, rabbits humans	Serum Serum	Not stated	15/29 2/2	0/73 0/9	Weiner (1979, 1980a)
Aspergillus fumigatus antigens	Solid-phase inhibition	0.5 µg ml^{-1}	Aspergillosis, rabbits humans	Serum	Centrifugation, dialysis distilled water	4/6	Not stated	Shaffer et al. (1979a) Shaffer et al. (1979b)
Aspergillus fumigatus antigens	Liquid-phase inhibition	3.1 ng ml^{-1}	Aspergillosis, rabbits humans	Serum Serum Pleural fluid	Acidification, heat 96°C	40/51 4/7 1/1	1/101 0/79 0/2	Weiner (1979) Weiner (1980a)
Coccidiodes immitis antigens	Liquid-phase inhibition	Not stated	Coccidiodomycosis	Serum	Acidification, heat 96°C	3/5	2/60	Weiner (1980b)
Hepatitis A virus	Solid-phase direct	Not stated	Hepatitis A, humans	Stool	Isopycnic band, zonal separation, preparative electrophoresis	2/?	Not stated	Purcell et al. (1976)
Hepatitis A virus	Solid-phase direct	Not stated	Hepatitis A, humans chimpanzees marmoset	Stool Serum Liver Stool	Isopycnic banding	1/1 4/4 1/1 4/4	Not stated 0/3 0/1 3/295	Hollinger et al. (1977)
Adenovirus	Solid-phase indirect	0.1 ng ml^{-1}	Gastroenteritis, humans	Stool	None	36/36	1/78	Halonen et al. (1980)
Rotavirus	Solid-phase direct	Not stated	Gastroenteritis, humans	Stool	2% stool filtrate	60/60	1/83	Cukor et al. (1978)
Reovirus	Solid-phase direct	Not stated	Gastroenteritis, humans	Stool	2% stool filtrate	12/22	Not stated	Kalica et al. (1977)
Norwalk agent	Solid-phase inhibition	Not stated	Gastroenteritis, humans	Stool	Stool filtrate			Greenberg and Kapikian (1978)

We have developed a sensitive and specific direct solid-phase radioimmunoassay for *Legionella pneumophilia* antigen(s) (Kohler *et al.*, 1981a). When collected within the first several days of the onset of therapy, the antigen is detectable in about 80% of patients (Kohler *et al.*, 1981b). In one patient, antigen remained present for 18 weeks following initiation of therapy; generally, however, the antigen disappears sooner. The antigen is heat stable at 100°C for 30 min, pepsin and trypsin resistant, and has a molecular weight of approximately 10 000.

Gonococcal antigens can be detected in the urinary sediments of patients with gonorrhoea but not in patients with nonspecific urethritis (Thornley *et al.*, 1979). Urines must be heated at 37°C for 30 min and acidified to pH 5.5 with glacial acetic acid to dissolve insoluble materials. Antigens are found in the $2000 \times G$ leucocyte sediment rather than the urine. Sediments must be treated with soy-bean trypsin inhibitor to overcome the inhibitory effect of urinary substances, presumably proteases, and with deoxyribonuclease and ribonuclease to prevent nonspecific binding to the radiolabelled gonococcal antibodies. The radioimmunoassay result correlates directly with the urinary concentration of leucocytes and gonococcal colony-forming units. The antigens have not been characterized.

Radioimmunoassay has also been applied to the diagnosis of fungal infections. Circulating *Candida* antigens were detected in sera from 70% of infected mice whereas blood cultures were positive in only 10% (Poor and Cutler, 1979). These mice had been injected intravenously with $2–4 \times 10^6$ *C. albicans* from 1–5 days before testing. All had extensive candidiasis demonstrated by colony counts between 0.9 and 22.3×10^6 *Candida* per gram of kidney tissue. Using a more sensitive liquid phase inhibition assay capable of detecting 0.3 ng ml^{-1} of *Candida* mannan, antigenaemia was demonstrated in rabbits and in 2 of 2 humans with systemic candidiasis (Weiner and Coats-Stephen, 1979; Weiner, 1980a).

Aspergillus antigen could be detected in a direct competition inhibition solid phase assay using a tyramine conjugated, partially purified alkaline extract of *Aspergillus fumigatus* radioiodinated with Na^{125}I (Shaffer *et al.*, 1979a). Centrifugation of serum specimens to remove protein and dialysis against distilled water at 4°C was necessary to overcome serum inhibitory effects. Antigen was first detected on the third day after intravenous injection of 3×10^7 *A. fumigatus*. Antigenaemia occurred in 4 of 6 rabbits, whereas blood cultures were negative. Despite poor *in vitro* sensitivity, 10–100 μg ml^{-1} antigen could also be detected in humans with aspergillosis using a similar assay (Shaffer *et al.*, 1979b). Deproteinization with perchloric acid and tenfold concentration of samples was necessary before testing. Of the 3 antigenaemic patients, 2 had negative blood cultures despite disseminated aspergillosis at autopsy. False positive results occurred in 2 patients with histoplasmosis, 1 with cryptococcal meningitis, and 1 with leukaemia, thus limiting the usefulness of the assay. The circulating antigen was not characterized.

Using a more sensitive liquid phase inhibition assay antigen was detected in 78% of rabbits with experimental aspergillosis but not in normal rabbits or rabbits with disseminated candidiasis (Weiner and Coats-Stephen, 1979). Antigenaemia peaked during the most fulminant period of the infection, days 2 to 5 after intravenous injection, and decreased thereafter. Maximum sensitivity required fivefold dilution, acidification, and heating of the serum at 96°C. Presumably, in addition to free antigens, antigens released from immune complexes were detected following this treatment. The circulating antigen was not characterized. Using the same assay, antigen could be detected in the serum from 4 of 7 humans with systemic aspergillosis and the pleural fluid of a single patient with aspergillus empyema, but not in controls (Weiner, 1980a). Serum antigen concentrations ranged from 271 to 682 ng ml^{-1}. Blood cultures were negative in four antigenaemic patients despite extensive aspergillosis at autopsy. Circulating antigen has also been detected in patients with coccidiodomycosis; however, false-positive results occurred in a patient with histoplasmosis and another with bacterial sepsis (Weiner, 1980b).

In addition to hepatitis B, which will not be reviewed here, radioimmunoassays have been described for several other viral antigens; these are summarized in Table 4. Hepatitis A virus antigens have been detected in the stools of infected humans (Purcell et al., 1976; Hollinger et al., 1975) and liver and serum of infected marmosets and chimpanzees (Hollinger et al., 1975). Adenovirus (Halonen et al., 1980), rotavirus (Cukor et al., 1978), reovirus (Kalica et al., 1977), Norwalk agent (Greenberg and Kapikian, 1978), Newcastle disease virus (Spira et al., 1976), and Western Equine Encephalomyelitis virus (Levitt et al., 1976) antigen assays have also been described. As antiviral chemotherapies are developed, assays for viral antigens may become valuable clinical tools because of the difficulty and delay in culturing viruses.

Other assays, not summarized in Table 4, have been developed for Brucella antigens (Wilson et al., 1977), E. coli enterotoxin (Greenberg et al., 1977), E. coli and Salmonella lipopolysaccharides (Munford and Hall, 1979), S. aureus enterotoxins (Bukovic and Johnson, 1975; Robern et al., 1975; Johnson et al., 1972), cholera toxin (Ceska et al., 1978), Clostridium botulinum C toxin (Boroff and Shu-Chenn, 1973), Histoplasma capsulatum M antigens (Reiss et al., 1977), leptospiral lipopolysaccharide (Kawaoka et al., 1979), influenza virus (Russ et al., 1976; Polakova et al., 1979), and Herpesvirus hominis (Forghani et al., 1974; Enlander et al., 1976).

V. ENZYME-LINKED IMMUNOASSAY

A. General aspects

Enzyme-linked immunoassay is an immunological method for detecting and measuring antigens or antibodies which is based on the same principles as radioimmunoassay. The key difference is that for enzyme immunoassays the antigen or antibody is conjugated to an enzyme rather than a radioactive isotope. The enzyme is then detected by its ability to convert a colourless substance to a coloured one. Obviously the method requires that, in the enzyme–immunoglobulin conjugate, the enzyme retains its enzymatic activity and the antigen or antibody its immunological activity.

Solid-phase enzyme immunoassays are usually used. Such systems are called enzyme-linked immunosorbent assays (ELISAs). The reaction of antigen and antibody takes place after one or the other has been attached in an earlier step to a solid phase, usually a plastic, by adsorption or covalent bonding. For antigen detection several types of systems have been used. For competitive assays, either direct competition or antigen inhibition methods may be used. In the direct competition competitive assay, which is analogous to the solid phase inhibition assay shown in Fig. 4c, the solid-phase reactant is antibody. The test sample is mixed with a predetermined quantity of antigen–enzyme conjugate, and the mixture is exposed to the solid-phase antibody. If no antigen is present in the test sample, the antigen–enzyme conjugate binds the solid-phase antibody, producing a large colour change in the next step of the procedure. If a large quantity of antigen is present in the test sample, almost none of the antigen–enzyme conjugate binds to the solid-phase antibody. Quantitation of antigen requires construction of a curve relating the amount of antigen–conjugate bound to the solid-phase as a function of antigen concentration in the test sample. This method requires that the antigen in question be available in pure form and that it have reactive groups which allow coupling to an enzyme.

In the antigen-inhibition competitive assay, antigen is bound to the solid phase. The test sample is mixed with a predetermined amount of antibody–enzyme conjugate, then the mixture is exposed to the solid-phase antigen. The amount of enzyme–antibody conjugate which binds to the solid-phase antigen will be inversely related to the amount of antigen in the test sample. This method requires monospecific antibody conjugates or a purified antigen which will adsorb to the solid phase.

The most frequently used enzyme immunoassay for detecting microbial antigens is the sandwich solid-phase system (Figs 6 and 7). Antibody is attached to the solid phase. The test sample is then exposed to the solid-phase antibody, to which the antigen, if present, will bind. The solid-phase

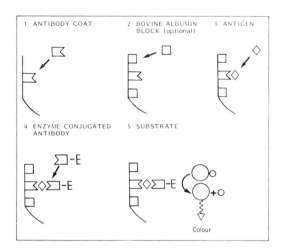

Fig. 6   Schematic representation of the steps in the single-antibody sandwich, or direct, ELISA. In step 1, the antibody, usually purified IgG, binds to the solid-phase, usually by adsorption. In this diagram, the solid phase is the inside wall of a polystyrene tube. After this step (and also after steps 2–4) the solution is aspirated from the tubes and the tubes rinsed. Remaining protein adsorption sites may be blocked with a protein such as bovine serum albumin (step 2). Many investigators have found that inclusion of a detergent in the buffer used for step 4 eliminates the need for a blocking step. In the third step, the test specimen is added to the tubes. Antigen, if present, binds to the solid-phase antibodies. In step 4 of the direct system, anti-antigen IgG which is covalently conjugated with an enzyme (-E), binds to the antigen, completing the sandwich. In step 5 a colourless substrate is added to the tubes. If enzyme–immunoglobulin conjugates remain bound to the tubes from earlier steps, the enzyme will cleave the substrate to yield a coloured breakdown product which can be assayed visually or spectrophotometrically.

antibody–antigen complex is then rinsed free of unbound test sample and exposed again to antibodies reactive against the test antigen. The antibody will react with the antigen held to the solid-phase by the first antibody, forming an antibody–antigen–antibody sandwich on the solid-phase. The solid-phase sandwich is again separated from unreacted test sample by rinsing. The second antibody, if itself conjugated to an enzyme as shown schematically in Fig. 6, can be detected with an appropriate substrate. This is a single-antibody, or direct, sandwich ELISA. Alternatively, the second antibody can itself be detected with an antiimmunoglobulin–enzyme conjugate (Fig. 7). This is a double-antibody, or indirect, sandwich ELISA. In the double-antibody ELISA, the second antibody of the sandwich must be from a different species than the solid-phase antibody; otherwise, the antiimmuno-

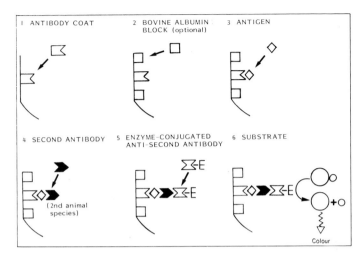

Fig. 7 Double-antibody, or indirect, sandwich ELISA. The first three steps are identical to the single-antibody sandwich ELISA. In step 4 anti-antigen antibody is added to the tubes. The species from which this antibody is obtained must differ from that which is adsorbed to the solid phase; otherwise, the enzyme–anti-antibody conjugate from step 5 would bind to the antibody coating the solid phase. The substrate step is performed as for the single-antibody sandwich ELISA.

globulin conjugate reacts with the solid-phase antibody, producing high background activity.

A liquid-phase enzyme immunoassay, called the homogeneous enzyme immunoassay, takes advantage of the observation that enzymes conjugated to small antigens are unable to function when the antigen is bound to antibody. Such an antigen–enzyme conjugate would therefore remain active enzymatically in the presence of antibodies if a large excess of unconjugated antigen is present in the test sample. If no free antigen is present, the antigen–enzyme conjugate would be inactivated enzymatically by reaction with antibody. This system requires that the antigen be small.

B.   Technical aspects of ELISA

1.   The solid phase
The most popular solid phases are microtitre plates made of polystyrene or polyvinyl chloride. The inside walls of the wells of the plates are used as the solid-phase adsorption surface. Each plate contains 96 sample wells, and a large number of samples can be tested in each plate. Colour development in each well can be measured directly from the plates with special colorimeters,

and an entire plate can be analysed quantitatively in less than five minutes. Plates are also easily read if visual interpretation of colour changes is used. Sipple and Voller (1980) found polystyrene plates more suitable for a double-antibody sandwich assay for *Neisseria meningitidis* envelope antigens, producing fourfold better sensitivity than polyvinyl plates. Wetherall *et al.* (1980) also preferred polystyrene over polyvinyl plates for a single antibody sandwich ELISA for *Haemophilus influenzae* type B polyribophosphate. Yolken (1978) stated that polyvinyl plates were superior, but Araujo and Remington (1980a) found no differences between polystyrene and polyvinyl plates, so the issue is obviously not resolved. The edge wells of microtitre plates, for unknown reasons, produce aberrant results so often that several groups suggest not using them for testing unknowns (Denmark and Chessum, 1978; Yolken, 1978). Yolken (1978) has cautioned against using tissue-culture microtitration plates, which produce nonspecific positive reactions due to a coating on the plastic. Finally, batches of microtitre plates obtained from the same manufacturer may vary in their suitability for use (Araujo and Remington, 1980; Denmark and Chessum, 1978). The causes of this variability are unknown.

If the solution must be aspirated into a rapid sampling device for absorbance measurement, we have observed that separate plastic tubes, rather than microtitre plates, allow easier access to the aspiration tubing used on low volume rapid samplers. Plastic balls (Stiffer-Rosenberg and Fey, 1978; Drow *et al.*, 1979) and discs (Halbert and Anken, 1977) have also been used successfully. Stiffler-Rosenberg and Fey (1978) preferred plastic balls to tubes or plates so that the solid-phase antibody could be exposed to a large volume of food extract in an assay for staphylococcal enterotoxins A, B, and C. The 6-mm diameter antibody-coated balls were tumbled through 20 ml of food extract during the test sample incubation step, theoretically allowing greater sensitivity than could be found with the small volumes and solid-phase surface areas available in microtitre plates. Hendry and Herrmann (1980) found that HCl-treated nylon balls acted as an excellent solid phase for covalent linkage of antibodies to eliminate the problem of antibody desorption during later assay steps. Their assay sensitivity for IgE was improved tenfold when covalently-coupled antibody coated nylon balls rather than conventionally adsorbed polystyrene wells were used. Whether nylon will be superior to polystyrene or polyvinyl chloride remains to be confirmed. A disadvantage with balls and discs is the need for their transfer from tube to tube during the various steps of the procedure, particularly the substrate step.

In summary, polystyrene and polyvinyl chloride microtitre plates and tubes have all been used successfully in ELISAs. Conflicting claims of superiority of one plastic over another may reflect differences in assay procedures or batch variation in plates. Improved solid phases with elimination of batch-to-batch variability, increased but constant surface area, and ease of covalent bonding (e.g. nylon) will hopefully be available in the future.

2. Coating the solid phase with antibody

Most successful solid-phase immunoassays take advantage of the tendency of proteins to adsorb to plastics. Since IgG binds polystyrene as well at pH 9, at which the protein's net charge is negative, as at pH 4, at which the net charge is positive, electrostatic forces appear to be relatively unimportant in the interaction; at both pHs the net surface charge on the polystyrene is negative (Oreskes and Singer, 1961). Van Oss and Singer (1966) theorized that hydrophobic bonding is the most important binding force; they demonstrated slightly decreased binding of IgG to polystyrene latex particles when the reaction occurred in buffers with decreased ionic strength. More recent experiments, however, showed increased binding of IgG as the molarity of the solvent dropped from 4.0 to 0.5 (Tsang et al., 1980). Thus, the exact nature of the adsorptive forces is currently unclear.

Experiments with polystyrene latex spheres suggest that the globulin molecules adsorb to the plastic with their long axes parallel to the sphere surface (Oreskes and Singer, 1961). Random adsorption of this type should, when complete, leave a small proportion of the plastic surface available for additional adsorption. Kinetic studies confirm that a secondary adsorption reaction occurs when the plastic surface has adsorbed the maximum number of molecules in this fashion. The secondary adsorption involves formation of a protein bilayer due to protein–protein adsorptive interactions and/or adsorption of additional IgG molecules to the small patches of remaining plastic surface with the long axis of the molecule perpendicular to the plastic surface (Oreskes and Singer, 1961). After adsorption, the IgG molecules appear to undergo a conformational change, as indicated by an increase in the number of acid-titrable groups (Kochwa et al., 1967).

Anionic, cationic, and nonionic detergents inhibit adsorption of IgG to polystyrene (van Oss and Singer, 1966).

Antisera for coating tubes have been obtained from rabbits, guinea pigs, horses, burros, sheep, and humans. No species superiority, in terms of ability to adsorb to solid phases and function in the immunoassay, have been reported. Generally, laboratory animals have been immunized or infected for at least 6 to 12 weeks before harvesting the antisera to be used for the assay (Clark and Adams, 1977; Araujo and Remington, 1980; Kozaki et al., 1979; Harding et al., 1980). As noted in the radioimmunoassay section of this chapter, we have obtained greater sensitivity with antiserum harvested 16 months into immunization than that harvested at 6 weeks. Investigators using commercially prepared antisera for assays have reported better success with antisera from certain sources than others (Kozaki et al., 1979; Wetherall et al.,

1980). Thus, while one antiserum may fail to yield a satisfactorily sensitive assay, another may perform adequately. Our impression from our own work is that about one-third of rabbits immunized with whole bacterial vaccines will produce very high-titred antisera, and that antisera harvested late (months) during the immunization work better than those harvested earlier.

Successful assays have been devised in which whole antiserum, gamma globulin precipitates, purified IgG fractions, IgG F(ab)$_2$ fragments, and monoclonal IgG were used. The adsorption of protein to plastic is nonspecific; serum proteins other than IgG bind equally well (Pesce et al., 1977). It follows, therefore, that elimination of non-IgG proteins from the adsorption solution should increase the amount of IgG bound to the plastics; this has been verified experimentally (Pesce et al., 1977). The use of monospecific IgG antibodies would additionally increase the number of specific antibodies bound to the solid phase. Thus, particularly when antisera with low levels of antigen-specific IgG must be used, purified IgG should be used to coat tubes. In high-quality hyperimmune sera, however, adequate numbers of antigen-specific antibody molecules will adsorb to the plastic to allow antigen detection (Notermans et al., 1978; Mathieson et al., 1978; Chao et al., 1979). Increasing the number of antibody molecules beyond this adequate "threshold" (e.g. by coating with purified IgG) would not be expected to increase sensitivity significantly (Mathieson et al., 1978). However, if the number of antigen-specific IgG antibodies were only slightly above the "threshold" level for antigen detection, increasing amounts of antigen would quickly saturate the available binding sites. Increasing the number of antigen-specific molecules should therefore increase the working range of the assay to higher antigen concentrations for a given dilution of the test sample.

When whole antisera provide inadequate sensitivity or inadequate working range, acceptably pure gamma globulin may be prepared by precipitation with sodium or ammonium sulphate (Kibrick et al., 1948; Hebert et al., 1973). Immunoglobulin G may be prepared with diethylaminoethyl (DEAE) cellulose either by batch or column procedures (Sober et al., 1956; Baumstark et al., 1968), by precipitation with caprylic acid (Steinbach and Audran, 1969) or by elution of serum or gamma globulin precipitates through G200 Sephadex (Flodin and Killander, 1962). Thus, although in some cases whole antiserum can be used the degree of purification of antibodies needed for tube coating for a given ELISA must be determined by trial and error.

As noted later, the use of F(ab)$_2$ fragments from IgG antibodies decreases the frequency of false-positive reactions due to rheumatoid factor activity (Araujo and Remington, 1980). This observation, if verified by others, may be important if sera are the major specimens being tested. F(ab)$_2$ fragments also appear to increase the working range of the assay.

Araujo et al. (1980) compared hybridoma monoclonal antibodies to purified IgG from a hyperimmune rabbit for tube coating. The purified IgG from the hyperimmune rabbit produced a more sensitive ELISA for detecting *Toxoplasma gondii* antigens *in vitro* and in infected patients than assays prepared with several monoclonal lines. A fairer comparison of monoclonal antibodies with standard IgG preparations awaits development of mono-clonal ELISAs for purified, well-characterized antigens.

When whole antiserum is used to coat polystyrene, immunoglobulin coating of the surface reaches saturation at about a 1/500 dilution of the antiserum; generally, therefore, using more concentrated solutions would be wasteful of the antiserum (Pesce *et al.*, 1977). When either gamma globulin or purified IgG at 25°C are allowed 24 hours to adsorb to polystyrene, adsorption at 1 μg ml^{-1} is as good as or better than at 0.1, 0.5, 2, 10, or 25 μg ml^{-1} (Tsang *et al.*, 1980). For incubation times of an hour or less adsorption of maximal amounts of IgG or gamma globulin can be achieved with 2–10 μg ml^{-1} (Clark and Adams, 1977; Tsang *et al.*, 1980; Wetherall *et al.*, 1980). Pesce *et al.* (1977) found that maximal binding occurs at 25 μg ml^{-1} although the next lower concentration tested was 2.5 μg ml^{-1}. Thus, one's priorities (availability of time v. availability of antibodies) partially determine the concentration selected. Most assays have used 2–20 μg ml^{-1} (Clark and Adams, 1977; Stevens and Tsiantos, 1979; Wetherall *et al.*, 1980; Harding *et al.*, 1980; Richardson *et al.*, 1979; van Knapen *et al.*, 1977; Yolken *et al.*, 1977; Notermann *et al.*, 1978). Higher concentrations have also been used, although it is not clear whether the high concentrations were necessary (Warren *et al.*, 1977; Lehmann and Reiss, 1980; Wolters *et al.*, 1976). If satisfactory results are not achieved with 2–20 μg ml^{-1}, it seems likely that a better antiserum is needed. Higher concentrations may be optimal when F(ab)$_2$ fragments or monoclonal antibodies are used (Araujo and Remington, 1980; Araujo *et al.*, 1980). Large excesses of coating antibodies should probably be avoided, since poorly adsorbed antibody could be eluted during subsequent incubations (Kochwa *et al.*, 1967; Engvall and Perlmann, 1972) and compete with solid-phase antibody for antigen, potentially reducing assay sensitivity (Clark and Adams, 1977).

pHs ranging from 4.1 to 9.0 have little consistent effect on the binding of IgG to polystyrene (van Oss and Singer, 1966; Tsang *et al.*, 1980). In many assays coating is carried out at a pH of 9.6. Yolken (1978) stated that immunoglobulins bind best to polyvinyl plates at pH 9.6; date supporting this contention were not provided. Ionic strength also appears to have minor effects on adsorption. Tsang *et al.* (1980) found that adsorption was slightly better from 0.5 molar NaCl than higher concentrations up to 4.5 molar; at lower NaCl concentrations, adsorption appeared to be erratic. A variety of diluents have been successfully used, most often 0.05 to 1.0 molar carbonate buffer at pH 9.6 to 9.8 (Engvall *et al.*, 1971; Richardson *et al.*, 1979; Yolken *et* al., 1977; Araujo and Remington, 1980; Schetters et al., 1980) or phosphate buffered saline, pH 7.2 to 7.4 (Matthiesen et al., 1978; Kozaki et al., 1979; Harding et al., 1980; van Knapen and Panggabean, 1977; Notermans et al., 1978; Engvall et al., 1971). Other proteins and detergents should be avoided in the tube coat diluents since they inhibit binding of the IgG (van Oss and Singer, 1966).

Raising the incubation temperature to 37°C permits one to decrease the binding time. Tsang et al. (1980) found that, for a 1.0 μg ml^{-1} solution of IgG, maximal binding at 4°C required 24 hours, at 25°C, 2 hours, and at 37°C, 1 hour.

Hendry and Herrmanns (1980) found that covalent linkage of immunoglobulins to the solid phase (nylon balls) increased the binding capacity of the balls for antigen when compared to attachment by adsorption. In addition to increasing the amount of antibody bound to the nylon balls, covalent binding with glutaraldehyde greatly diminished desorption of the immunoglobulin from the balls during a subsequent washing procedure. This technique deserves further study as it might be expected to increase the reproducibility and working range of ELISAs.

3. The filler step

If additional solid-phase adsorption sites remain on the solid phase following the coating of immunoglobulins nonspecific adsorption of antigen or antibody conjugates during later steps of the assay might increase the assay background and decrease the sensitivity. Matthiesen et al. (1978) found that 1% bovine serum albumin, as a second coating agent, or filler, increased the sensitivity of their sandwich ELISA for hepatitis A antigen by lowering the background activity. Drow et al. (1979) found that a filler step with 10% fetal calf serum was necessary to eliminate nonspecific binding in their ELISA for H. influenzae type b polyribophosphate; 10% foetal calf serum was superior to 2% bovine serum albumin. Locarnini et al. (1978) chose 1% bovine serum albumin as their filler, and Schetters et al. (1980) used homologous preimmune rabbit serum.

On the other hand, in the majority of antigen ELISAs reported, the filler step has been omitted (Wolters et al., 1976; van Knapen and Panggabean, 1977; Warren et al., 1977; Yolken et al., 1977a,b; Notermans et al., 1978; Harding et al., 1979; Kozaki et al., 1979; Chao et al., 1979; Araujo and Remington, 1980; Harding et al., 1980; Lehmann and Reiss, 1980; Sipple and Voller, 1980). The authors of these reports did not state whether filler steps were tested, but in most cases their assays functioned well without filler steps. Because the filler step adds time, work, and expense (particularly fetal calf serum), the need for this step should be determined for individual assay systems.

4. The test sample, or antigen, step

Serum contains heat-labile inhibitors of solid-phase immunoassays, presumably components of the complement system (Tabbarah et al., 1979). The proposed mechanisms for this effect were discussed in the radioimmunoassay section of this chapter. Heating the serum at 56°C for 30 min eliminates much of this inhibitory activity and also inactivates intrinsic alkaline phosphatase. In some assay systems heating of serum samples before testing in the ELISA is routinely performed (Drow et al., 1979; Harding et al., 1979, 1980; Segal et al., 1979); this step improved the sensitivity approximately 100-fold in an ELISA for mannan (Harding et al., 1980). In other assay systems, this inhibitory effect is not seen (Drow and Manning, 1980).

Concentrating antigen from test specimens may improve assay sensitivity. Doskeland and Berdal (1980) described simple methods for concentrating serum, spinal fluid, urine, and other fluids; their methods require that the antigen be ethanol precipitable and/or stable at 100°C for 3 min. Commercially available disposable ultrafiltration cells can also be used for concentrating if the molecular weight of the antigen is greater than 15 000 (Amicon Corp., Lexington, MA, USA). A simple method for freeing heat-stable antigens from antigen–antibody complexes and simultaneously destroying the immunoglobulin has been described (Tabbarah et al., 1980).

Respiratory secretions may be liquefied with equal volumes of 2% N-acetyl cysteine (Drow et al., 1979). Antigens have also been successfully detected in 2–10% stool filtrates (Yolken et al., 1977; Locarnini et al., 1978; Merson et al., 1980).

The reaction kinetics of ^{125}I-albumin with solid-phase antialbumin was studied by Pesce et al. (1977). Approximately 10–25% of the antigen which could bind in 24 hours of incubation bound within 3 min. Thereafter, binding occurred more slowly and linearly, so that, for 1.0 μg ml^{-1} of albumin, 50% had bound within 30 min and 90% within 6 hours. For albumin concentrations of 10 and 100 μg ml^{-1}, 50% of that which could bind in 24 hours had bound in 3 hours, and 90% in 17 hours. Although not specifically stated, it appears that the reaction temperature was 4°C. Thus, from this data, it would appear that maximum sensitivity should occur with antigen-step incubation times approaching 24 hours. Mathiesen et al. (1978) and Chao et al. (1979) found 24 hour incubations superior to shorter periods for optimizing sensitivity.

Despite such data most investigators have used much shorter incubation times for the antigen steps. Sipple and Voller (1980) in an assay for N. meningitidis envelope antigen, found 1 hour at 37°C to work as well as 16 hours at 37°C. For other assays, although relatively short incubation periods were used, it was unclear whether longer incubations were studied. These periods and temperatures included 30 min at 43°C (Holbert and Auken, 1977),

45 min at 40°C (Drow *et al.*, 1979), 60 min at 37°C (Yolken *et al.*, 1977), 90 min at 37°C (Notermans *et al.*, 1978; Kozaki *et al.*, 1979); 2 hours at 22–37°C (Wolters *et al.*, 1976; Araujo and Remington, 1980; Merson *et al.*, 1980; Wetherall *et al.*, 1980), 3 hours at 37°C (Harding *et al.*, 1979, 1980; Richardson *et al.*, 1979) and 4 hours at 37°C (van Knapen and Panggabean, 1977).

Thus, 1–4-hour antigen-step incubation periods appear to be adequate for most assay systems, although overnight and 24-hour incubations have improved assay sensitivity in others.

5. First antibody step in the double-antibody (indirect) sandwich assay

Use of the double-antibody sandwich technique requires that antisera from two species of animals be available; otherwise, the anti-immunoglobulin–enzyme conjugate reacts with the solid-phase antibody as well as the second antibody, producing high background activity. Likewise, an extra incubation step is required which increases the work time, and expense. On the other hand, if assays for multiple antigens are to be performed, a single antiglobulin or staphylococcal protein A conjugate can be used for all assays. Furthermore, a multiplication effect, resulting from the reaction of several antiglobulin–enzyme conjugates with each of the second species antibodies might increase the assay sensitivity.

Kozaki *et al.* (1979) reported that the double-antibody sandwich technique is 8–10 times more sensitive for detecting *Clostridium botulinum* type B toxin than the single-antibody sandwich. Yolken and Stopa (1980) compared eight ELISA techniques for detecting cytomegalovirus antigens, including several variations of the double-antibody sandwich technique. The double-antibody sandwich techniques using antiglobulin enzyme – or staphylococcal protein A – rabbit peroxidase–antiperoxidase complex conjugates were fourfold more sensitive than the standard single-antibody sandwich. When a staphylococcal protein A–horseradish peroxidase conjugate was used to detect the second antibody, the sensitivity was the same as with the single-antibody sandwich. Thus, if four- to tenfold improvement in sensitivity is needed, use of the double-antibody sandwich technique may be worth the added time, effort, and expense needed to obtain the extra antiserum and to perform the assay.

Most investigators have used diluted whole antiserum for this step (Chao *et al.*, 1979; Drow *et al.*, 1979, 1980; Kozaki *et al.*, 1979; Drow and Manning, 1980; Yolken and Stopa, 1980). Dilutions from 1:160 to 1:500 were chosen on the basis of serial titrations. Caprylic acid purified IgG at $20 \, \mu g \, ml^{-1}$ (Notermans *et al.*, 1978) and affinity-purified IgG at an "optimal concentration" (Merson *et al.*, 1980) have also been used. No published comparisons of these various preparations are available for review. Affinity purification of antibody used in this step will be desirable if crude antigen mixtures (e.g. organism sonicates) have been used to obtain the antiserum and if cross-reactions with extraneous antigenic determinants in test samples could complicate interpretation of assay results. Otherwise, the use of diluted whole antiserum has been a satisfactory and simple approach.

There are no published comparisons of varied time and temperature for this step. Conditions found satisfactory have included 45 min at 40°C (Drow *et al.*, 1979), 60 min at room temperature (Sipple and Voller, 1980), and 90 min at 37°C (Notermans *et al.*, 1978; Chao *et al.*, 1979; Kozaki *et al.*, 1979).

6.   The enzyme–immunoglobulin conjugate

(a)   General considerations
Essential to the success of ELISA are methods for irreversibly linking an enzyme and an immunoglobulin, with maintenance of function of both. Although many potentially useful coupling reactions are available (Kennedy *et al.*, 1976), one of two basic coupling reactions is generally used.

(b)   Glutaraldehyde
Based on the work of Avrameas (1969, 1970) glutaraldehyde ($OHCC_3H_6CHO$) is frequently used to couple immunoglobulins to enzyme. Although the simplest assumption on the nature of the cross linking reaction is the formation of a Schiff's base [R-C-C-N$=$CH-C_3H_6-CH$=$N-C-R$'$] involving the aldehyde functions of the glutaraldehyde and amino groups of the two proteins, the inability of semicarbazole, urea, or strong acids to reverse the cross-linkage suggests the reaction is more complex. In solution commercial aqueous glutaraldehyde exists predominantly as oligomeric and polymeric α, β-unsaturated aldehydes. Long bridges of linear and cyclic glutaraldehyde polymers should therefore form between coupled proteins (Kennedy *et al.*, 1976). The ε-amino group of lysine appears to be the protein amino group primarily involved in the coupling reaction (Korn *et al.*, 1972). Despite its simplicity in practice, the nature of the glutaraldehyde coupling reaction is probably complex and not yet thoroughly understood.

Following glutaraldehyde-mediated coupling of alkaline phosphatase and IgG, both the enzyme and IgG function less efficiently than when uncon-jugated. At the usual glutaraldehyde and IgG concentrations used (1.0–2.8 µmol glutaraldehyde mg^{-1} protein), the reaction product contains unreacted alkaline phosphatase plus a heterogeneous mixture of high molecular weight IgG polymers bound to variable amounts of alkaline phosphatase. The IgG polymers chromatograph in the void volume of G200 Sephadex (Ford *et al.*, 1978) and are therefore quite large.

Alkaline phosphatase–immunoglobulin G conjugates are usually prepared by the method of Engvall *et al.* (1971) or a slightly modified version. Ratios of purified IgG to alkaline phosphatase (mg:mg) have included 1:3 (Engvall *et al.*, 1971), 2:5 (Voller *et al.*, 1977) and 1:1 (Drow *et al.*, 1979). The ratios of glutaraldehyde to protein (μmol:mg) have ranged from 1:1 (Engvall *et al.*, 1971) to 2.8:1 (Voller *et al.*, 1977). Antibody activity diminishes more at 2.5 μmol glutaraldehyde mg^{-1} protein than at 1.0 μmol mg^{-1}; however, more alkaline phosphatase molecules bind the IgG polymers at 2.5 μmol mg^{-1} than 1.0 μmol mg^{-1}. The net effect is similar activity in assays of conjugates prepared with either ratio (Ford *et al.*, 1978).

In the coupling reaction, IgG in phosphate-buffered saline (PBS), pH 7.4, is added to the precipitated alkaline phosphatase (Sigma type VII), dialysed with PBS, then mixed with glutaraldehyde for two hours at room temperature. The glutaraldehyde is then dialysed out and the conjugate stored at 4°C in a solution such as 1% bovine serum albumin in a pH 8.0 tris(hydroxymethyl)aminomethane buffer containing 0.02% sodium azide (Voller *et al.*, 1977). The conjugates can be separated from unreacted alkaline phosphatase by chromatography on gels which will retard the enzyme (molecular weight approximately 10^5). Whether this improves the assay is not clear.

Horseradish peroxidase may be coupled to immunoglobulins with glutaraldehyde. When IgG, horseradish peroxidase, and glutaraldehyde are mixed the predominant reaction is the formation of large IgG polymers with relatively inefficient binding of horseradish peroxidase to the IgG; this is termed the one-step procedure. Alternatively, the horseradish peroxidase can be mixed with a relatively large amount of glutaraldehyde in the absence of IgG. Because each molecule of horseradish peroxidase has only one site which reacts readily with glutaraldehyde (Avrameas and Ternynck, 1971), each molecule of peroxidase couples with one glutaraldehyde or glutaraldehyde polymer molecule, and then contains a single reactive aldehyde group. The "activated" horseradish peroxidase then reacts with IgG in a subsequent step in glutaraldehyde-free solution, yielding conjugates which contain only one IgG molecule per conjugate. Such conjugates are more active than those prepared with the one-step procedure, at least in their ability to react in haemagglutination and precipitin reactions. Unbound horseradish peroxidase can be eliminated since it does not precipitate in 50% saturated ammonium sulphate, although some loss in the immunoreactivity of the precipitated conjugates may accompany this step (Boorsma and Kalsbeck, 1975). Wolters *et al.* (1976) used the two-step procedure to link horseradish peroxidase to gamma globulin in their assay for hepatitis B surface antigen.

(c)   Schiff base formation
Currently, the most widely used procedure for coupling IgG to horseradish peroxidase in microbiological research is the procedure reported in 1974 by

Nakane and Kawaoi (van Knapen and Panggabean, 1977; Locarnini *et al.*, 1978; Notermans *et al.*, 1978; Chao *et al.*, 1979; Kozacki *et al.*, 1979; Harding *et al.*, 1980). As opposed to glutaraldehyde coupling, the efficiency of binding horseradish peroxidase to IgG is markedly improved with this technique, and IgG–IgG complexes do not form. This procedure utilizes the carbohydrate moiety in the horseradish peroxidase molecule, which is a glycoprotein. Free amino groups in the protein portion of the enzyme are blocked with fluorodinitrobenzene. Aldehyde groups are then created in the carbohydrate moiety with sodium *m*-periodate. When the IgG is subsequently added, the aldehyde groups of the enzyme form Schiff bases with free amino groups of the IgG. The Schiff bases are then stabilized with sodium borohydride. Mathiesen *et al.* (1978) found that conjugates prepared by a slight modification of this technique produced better sensitivity in an ELISA for hepatitis A antigen than conjugates produced with the two-step glutaraldehyde technique.

(d)   Horseradish peroxidase v. alkaline phosphatase
Although many enzymes can function in ELISAs (Sharpe *et al.*, 1976) alkaline phosphatase or horseradish peroxidase is generally used. Horseradish peroxidase is considerably cheaper than alkaline phosphatase (Sigma Chemical Co., St Louis, MO). Theoretically, the large aggregates formed during preparation of alkaline phosphatase conjugates should be more likely to react nonspecifically with rheumatoid factor than the IgG monomers in horseradish peroxidase conjugates. The preparation of alkaline phosphatase conjugates with glutaraldehyde, on the other hand, is considerably simpler than preparation of horseradish peroxidase conjugates by formation of Schiff bases. When the two enzymes have been compared in otherwise identical ELISAs for microbial antigens, the sensitivities have been the same (Lehmann and Reiss, 1980; Yolken and Stopa, 1980).

(e)   Use of the enzyme–immunoglobulin conjugates in the immunoassay
Preparations used for conjugation to enzymes have included ammonium sulphate, sodium sulphate, or caprylic acid gamma globulin precipitates (Wolters *et al.*, 1976; van Knapen and Panggabean, 1977; Yolken *et al.*, 1977a; Warren *et al.*, 1977; Waart *et al.*, 1978; Herrman *et al.*, 1979; Richardson *et al.*, 1979; Stevens and Tsiantos, 1979; Wetherall *et al.*, 1980; Yolken and Stopa, 1980); IgG purified by ion exchange chromatography or batch purification (Drow and Manning, 1977; Locarnini *et al.*, 1978; Mathiesen *et al.*, 1978; Schultz *et al.*, 1979; Kozacki *et al.*, 1979; Lehmann and Reiss, 1980; Harding *et al.*, 1980; Schetters *et al.*, 1980; Drow and Manning, 1980), or monospecific IgG prepared by affinity chromatography (Araujo and Remington, 1980). Which—if any—type of preparation is superior is unknown; published comparisons are lacking.

The major consideration in choosing a conjugate diluent is minimization of nonspecific binding of the conjugate to the solid phase. Most investigators therefore use Tween 20 and/or an animal protein such as fetal calf serum or bovine serum albumin in phosphate-buffered saline, pH approximately 7.4. Hermann *et al.* (1979) compared various combinations of Tween 20 (0.05–0.20%) and bovine serum albumin; a diluent containing 2% bovine serum albumin and 0.15–0.20% Tween 20 minimized nonspecific binding. Diluents with 0.15–0.20% Tween 20 without albumin worked almost as well.

The optimal concentration of conjugate must be determined in titration experiments. Schetters *et al.* (1980), in a direct sandwich assay for type C viral protein antigens, found that sensitivity increased as the conjugate concentration was increased; no plateau was reached even at an IgG concentration of $50 \mu g \ ml^{-1}$. Engvall and Perlmann (1972) obtained similar results. Final IgG concentrations in the working dilution of conjugates have ranged from approximately 0.5 to $20 \mu g \ ml^{-1}$ (Mathiesen *et al.*, 1978; Harding *et al.*, 1979, 1980; Wetherall *et al.*, 1980). Presumably, in most cases, the working dilutions which were selected represented a compromise between maximum sensitivity and economy of reagents.

Published data suggest that optimum incubation time may vary among assays. Using an anti-IgG–enzyme conjugate to detect IgG bound to a solid-phase antigen, Engvall and Perlmann (1972) found conjugate binding to be about 50% complete at 1 hour and 70 to 90% complete at 2 hours; overnight was used as the standard incubation time. Clark and Adams (1977) found 6 hours incubation superior to 4, 3, 2, or 1 hour; Mathiesen *et al.* (1978) found 2 hours as good or better than 1, 5, or 7 hours. Many investigators have used a 1-hour incubation at room temperature or 37°C with satisfactory results (van Knapen and Panggabean, 1977; Yolken *et al.*, 1977a,b; Chao *et al.*, 1979; Araujo and Remington, 1980; Sipple and Voller, 1980; Wetherall *et al.*, 1980). Investigators should determine the optimum time and temperature for each assay system.

7. The substrate step

Horseradish peroxidase catalyses the transfer of hydrogen from a hydrogen donor to a peroxide (Maehly and Chance, 1954). For ELISAs, a hydrogen donor is chosen which develops colour following removal of hydrogen. Orthophenylenediamine (OPDA) is felt by Wolters *et al.* (1976) to be the most suitable chromogen because it produces a very sensitive assay, its colour development is easy to stop, and the coloured reaction product is stable for many hours. Because of its light sensitivity, OPDA solutions require fresh preparation and the trays must be incubated in the dark. Unfortunately, OPDA is mutagenic (Ames *et al.*, 1975; Voogt *et al.*, 1980). Another peroxidase substrate, 5-aminosalicylic acid (5-ASA), is not mutagenic (Voogt et al., 1980) but, as commercially supplied, tends to undergo spontaneous colour change. Furthermore, the reaction of off-the-shelf 5-ASA with horseradish peroxidase is impossible to stop completely. However, these difficulties with 5-ASA may be overcome if the commercially supplied material is recrystallized in the presence of sodium bisulphite and stored in an EDTA phosphate buffer (Ellens and Gielkens, 1980). In most horseradish peroxidase ELISAs for microbial antigens currently performed, the peroxide used is hydrogen peroxide and the hydrogen donor, 5-ASA (van Knapen and Panggabean, 1977; Locarnini et al., 1978; Notermans et al., 1978; Kozaki et al., 1979; Chao et al., 1979; Harding et al., 1979). The reaction is usually terminated after 30–60 min with sodium hydroxide, and the purple-brown colour is measured visually or with a spectrophotometer.

In alkaline phosphatase ELISAs, p-nitrophenyl phosphate (PNPP) is the chromogenic substrate. Phosphate is cleaved from the PNPP to yield the yellow-coloured sodium salt of p-nitrophenol (Bessey et al., 1946). PNPP appears not to be mutagenic (Voogt et al., 1980). The reaction is carried out at pH 9.8 in either cabonate (Engvall et al., 1971) or diethanolamine (Warren et al., 1977) buffer, then terminated with sodium hydroxide in 30–60 min. The yellow colour is then read visually or measured with a spectrophotometer. Major temperature differences between samples at the time of spectrophotometric analysis should be avoided, since the absorbance of alkaline solutions of PNPP at 404 nm increases linearly with increasing temperature (Burtis et al., 1979).

Through the use of alternative substrates which produce fluorescent or luminescent breakdown products, assays with sensitivities better than standard ELISA have been reported. In the presence of horseradish peroxidase isoluminol is oxidized by hydrogen peroxide. Light accompanies this reaction and can be measured in a liquid scintillation counter. Pronovost et al. (1981) reported that their chemiluminescent ELISA is 50 to 100 times more sensitive than a standard ELISA for detecting antibodies to and antigens of Herpes simplex. Similarly, alkaline phosphatase catalyses the hydrolysis of 4-methyl umbelliferyl phosphate to yield a fluorescent product which can be quantitated in a fluorocolorimeter. Rotavirus antigens were detected in stool suspensions about 100 times better with the fluorescent substrate–fluorocolorimeter system than the standard chromogenic–colorimeter system (Yolken and Stopa, 1979a). Further experience with such systems is needed before these encouraging results can be accepted a universally applicable. Improved instruments must also be developed which can permit quantitation of light emission or fluorescence directly from the wells of microtitre trays before laboratory acceptance is likely.

8. Reading assay results

Several investigators have found that visual analysis of ELISA results produces comparable results to reading by spectrophotometers (Harding *et al.*, 1979, 1980; Araujo and Remington, 1980), but others have found two- to tenfold improvement in sensitivity when absorbance measurements are made (Wolters *et al.*, 1976; Clark and Adams, 1977). In many diagnostic assays visual readings provide satisfactory results (Rotazyme[R], Abbott Laboratories, North Chicago, Ill.; van Knapen and Panggabean, 1977; Kozaki *et al.*, 1978; Locarnini *et al.*, 1978; Araujo and Remington, 1980; Lehmann and Reiss, 1980).

For antigen quantitation, spectrophotometric analysis is necessary, and a standard curve with purified antigen must be determined. Spectrophotometers are available which can read all 96 wells of a suitable microtitre plate in less than five minutes (Yolken *et al.*, 1977b) making quantitation almost as rapid as visual inspection (Fig. 8). The working range of typical sandwich

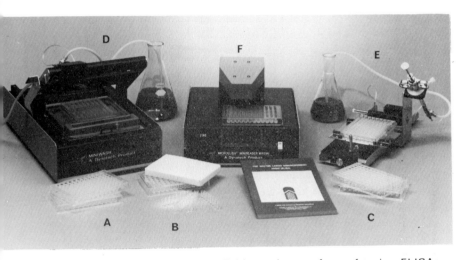

Fig. 8 Examples of commercially available equipment for performing ELISAs. A, B, C are several types of plastic trays, each containing 96 wells. Each well can serve as the solid phase for performing a single assay on a single sample. Instrument D sequentially aspirates and refills each row of the plate to effect multiple rinses of the wells in a short period of time. Instrument E permits addition of a reagent to the wells one row at a time (as would be required in steps 1, 2, 4 and 5 of Fig. 6). Instrument F is a manually operated photometer which measures absorbance values from solutions in the tray wells, one well at a time. Instruments that automatically read, report, and print out the absorbance values for all 96 wells are also available. (Courtesy of J. Eisenmann, Dynatech Laboratories, Inc., Alexandria, Virginia, USA.)

ELISAs is about 10^2 (Maiolini and Masseyeff, 1975; Drow *et al.*, 1979; Schultz *et al.*, 1979; Pepple *et al.*, 1980).

Conversion of spectrophotometer readings to positive versus negative results has been handled in several ways. Generally, the test sample absorbance is divided by the absorbance of suitable negative controls to yield a ratio. Ratios of 2.0 (Wolters *et al.*, 1976; Yolken *et al.*, 1977a; Waart *et al.*, 1978; Beuvery *et al.*, 1979; Chao *et al.*, 1979; Harding *et al.*, 1978, 1980; Merson *et al.*, 1980) or 3.0 (Ellens and deLeeuw, 1977) have been used. Alternatively, positivity may be defined as an absorbance of a test sample exceeding the negative controls by an empirically determined value (Halbert and Anken, 1977) or by two or three standard deviations (Pepple *et al.*, 1980; Sipple and Voller, 1980).

Examples of the type of equipment which may be purchased to improve laboratory efficiency in performing and reading ELISAs is shown in Fig. 8. The total cost for the instruments and materials shown in Fig. 8 was approximately $5900 in 1981. A directory of North American, European and Japanese manufacturers of instruments and reagents for ELISAs and other immunoassays is published in the March, 1981 issue of "Frontiers in Immunoassay" Vol. II, No. 3 (Scientific Newsletters, Inc., P.O. Box 4546, Anaheim, CA 92803, USA).

9. Wash solutions

After each step in the sandwich ELISA the solid phase must be rinsed to eliminate weakly adsorbed nonspecific protein from the step just completed. Although solutions of the detergent Tween 20 increase desorption of the solid-phase IgG (Engvall *et al.*, 1971; Herrmann *et al.*, 1979), most investigators use 0.05% Tween 20 in tap water or buffered saline as the wash solution after each step in the assay (van Knapen and Paggabean, 1977; Warren *et al.*, 1977; Yolken *et al.*, 1977; Mathiesen *et al.*, 1978; Notermans *et al.*, 1978; Chao *et al.*, 1979; Araujo and Remington, 1980; Lehmann and Reiss, 1980). Wolters *et al.* (1976) used a Tris buffer and Locarnini *et al.* (1978) used saline, neither containing Tween 20; Richardson *et al.* (1979) washed with buffered saline containing both Tween 20 and 5% chicken plasma. Whether Tween 20 actually improves assay sensitivity and reproducibility has not been rigorously demonstrated in published reports.

10. Competitive ELISAs

In the antigen inhibition competitive ELISA, the antigen is adsorbed to the solid phase. Antigen in the test sample is then measured by its ability to inhibit binding of an antibody–enzyme conjugate to the solid-phase antigen. Yolken and Stopa (1980) compared an antigen inhibition competitive ELISA with single- and double-antibody sandwich ELISAs for detecting cytomegalovirus antigens. The sensitivity with the antigen inhibition ELISA was 64-fold less than with the double-antibody sandwich ELISAs and 16-fold less than with the single-antibody sandwich ELISA.

In direct competition ELISAs, antibody is adsorbed to the solid phase. The presence of antigen in the test sample is determined by its ability to inhibit the binding of an antigen–enzyme conjugate to the solid-phase antibody. Belanger et al. (1973) compared direct competition versus double-antibody sandwich ELISAs for detecting rat alpha-fetoprotein and found the assays to have comparable sensitivities. Rissing et al. (1980) compared direct competition and antigen inhibition ELISAs using rabbit IgG as the test antigen. The assay sensitivities were similar, but the slope of the inhibition curve was steeper and the range of colour greater with the direct competition assay. For the direct competition system a purified antigen must be available and it must be capable of conjugation to a protein.

Polin and Kennett (1980) successfully used an antigen inhibition ELISA to detect type III group B streptococcal polysaccharide to as low as 10 µg ml^{-1} and used it to detect the polysaccharide in cerebrospinal fluid from infected infants. The solid-phase antigen consisted of whole bacteria; monoclonal antibodies in the conjugate provided the assay with specificity. Segal et al. (1979) detected Candida albicans mannan in patients with systemic Candida infections using an antigen inhibition system, and Stiffler-Rosenberg and Fey (1978) detected as little as 0.1 ng ml^{-1} of staphylococcal enterotoxin using a direct competition ELISA. Thus, the potential utility of competitive ELISAs has been demonstrated although few have chosen them for detecting microbial antigens. Whether competitive ELISAs are uniformly less sensitive than sandwich assays, as found by Yolken and Stopa, awaits confirmation by others.

11. Storing ELISA components

Few reports have rigorously defined the useful storage period of antibody-coated solid phases. Using disks coated with affinity-purified, covalently bonded horse antihepatitis B surface antigen, Halbert and Anken (1977) demonstrated continued usefulness after 13 months storage if lyophilized and stored dry at either refrigerator or room temperature. Clark and Adams (1977) found coated polystyrene microtitre plates to be useful for "several weeks" when stored at −18°C and Harding et al. (1980) claimed that coated polyvinyl plates could be stored in a moist chamber at 4°C for at least four weeks without loss of activity. Drow et al. (1979) stored coated polystyrene balls, after drying, in capped tubes at 4°C; full activity of the balls persisted for more than one month.

Antibody–enzyme conjugates are stable in solutions containing sodium azide at 4°C for at least 3–4 months (Arameas, 1969; Nakane and Pierce, 1967;

Engvall and Perlmann, 1972), and Engvall *et al.* (1971) used one conjugate for over one year. Lyophilized conjugates are stable for "indefinite" (presumably very long) periods (Nakane and Pierce, 1967). This is in contrast to ^{125}I tagged antibodies or antigens, which lose half their radioactivity every 60 days.

C. Problems with ELISAs

Rheumatoid factor (or rheumatoid-factor-like activity) may cause false-positive results in sandwich ELISAs (Wolters *et al.*, 1977; Waart *et al.*, 1978; Yolken and Stopa, 1979b; Araujo and Remington, 1980). Rheumatoid factor is IgM which binds IgG, particularly aggregated IgG. Solid-phase IgG is apparently recognized as "aggregated" by rheumatoid factor, and IgG–enzyme conjugates, particularly those prepared by one-step glutaraldehyde treatment, consist of large IgG polymers. Thus, rheumatoid factor can bridge the solid-phase and conjugated IgGs, producing false positivity in ELISAs. Araujo and Remington (1980) eliminated this problem by using only the $F(ab)_2$ portion of the IgG molecules, prepared by pepsin digestion, for coating the solid-phase. This eliminates the Fc, or rheumatoid-factor-binding portion, of the IgG molecule. Other methods for eliminating or diminishing false positivity presumably due to rheumatoid factor or similar activity include treatment with 2-mercaptoethanol (Yolken and Stopa, 1979b; Araujo and Remington, 1980), *N*-acetylcysteine (Yolken and Stopa, 1979b), heating at $100°C$ for 3 min (Doskeland and Berdal, 1980), or absorption with IgG-coated latex particles (Araujo and Remington, 1980), or whole serum or globulin from various animal species (Halbert and Auken, 1977; Yolken and Stopa, 1979b; Pepple *et al.*, 1980). Specific inhibition of positivity as demonstrated after premixing the test specimen with antigen-specific and with nonimmune sera (Wolters *et al.*, 1977; Yolken *et al.*, 1977; Waart *et al.*, 1978; Kozaki *et al.*, 1979; Merson *et al.*, 1980; Wetherall *et al.*, 1980) or by comparing the effect of antigen-specific immune versus nonimmune serum added to assay wells between the antigen and conjugate steps (Kacaki *et al.*, 1977; Locarnini *et al.*, 1978; Mathiesen *et al.*, 1978; Chao *et al.*, 1979) have both been used successfully to distinguish true from false positives. It is possible that factors in addition to rheumatoid factor may be eliminated by these procedures as causes of false positivity.

Another potential cause for false positivity is the existence in some test materials, particularly faeces, of numerous antigenic determinants expected to give rise to "natural" antibodies in animals whose sera may be used as antisera (Mathiesen *et al.*, 1978; Merson *et al.*, 1980). This problem may be overcome by using serum obtained prior to immunization from the same animal from which the hyperimmune serum is obtained; the preimmune serum should lock detection of nonspecific antigens but not the test antigen (Mathiesen *et l.*, 1978). Alternatively, affinity-purified or hybridoma-produced monos-ecific antibodies can be used.

Contamination of specimens with protein-A-containing staphylococci is nother potential source for false-positive reactions (Wetherall *et al.*, 1980). uch specimens should become negative when absorbed with nonspecific IgG.

Other problems, such as batch-to-batch variation in adsorption properties f solid phases and inhibitory effects of serum, have already been discussed nd will not be dealt with in further detail.

). Comparison of ELISA with other antigen-detection methods

LISA is 8 to 250 times more sensitive than counterimmunoelectrophoresis or detecting various purified microbial antigens in prepared solutions Beuvery *et al.*, 1979; Harding *et al.*, 1979, 1980; Pepple *et al.*, 1980; Wetherall *t al.*, 1980). ELISA is also more sensitive than CIE for detecting antigens in arious body fluids from infected animals and humans (Wolters *et al.*, 1976; Beuvery *et al.*, 1979; Drow *et al.*, 1979; Harding *et al.*, 1979; Richardson *et al.*, 979; Pepple *et al.*, 1980). CIE is faster than ELISA, involves less labour and ss expensive equipment, and difficulty with rheumatoid factor has not been eported, so it may be preferred if its sensitivity is adequate for the task at and. In most instances, however, for rapid diagnosis by antigen detection, he improved sensitivity of ELISA makes it the preferred procedure.

Latex agglutination is much simpler and cheaper than ELISA but is less ensitive (Pepple *et al.*, 1980). Rheumatoid factor produces false agglutination n latex agglutination as well as ELISA. Again, ELISA is preferable to latex gglutination when high sensitivity is needed. ELISA may be similarly ompared to haemagglutination inhibition procedures (Wolters *et al.*, 1976; chultz *et al.*, 1979).

ELISA is similar in sensitivity to solid-phase radioimmunoassay as etermined by comparing systems which use different immunological reagents o detect hepatitis B surface antigen (Wolters *et al.*, 1976, 1977; Halbert and uken, 1977; Kacaki *et al.*, 1978); in these studies, the sensitivities were similar ven if visual results were used for interpreting the ELISA. The two techniques ave also been found to have similar sensitivities for detecting *E. coli* nterotoxin (Yolken *et al.*, 1977a), hepatitis A virus (Locarnini *et al.*, 1978; Mathiesen *et al.*, 1978), and rotavirus (Yolken *et al.*, 1977b); in these studies, he same immunological reagents were used to perform the assays.

One ELISA for detecting hepatitis B surface antigen produced many more alse-positive results on screening than the solid-phase radioimmunoassay, ecessitating confirmatory testing on 2.2% of all specimens tested by ELISA; Kacaki *et al.*, 1978). Sixty-one per cent of all specimens called positive by

ELISA but only 3% of those called positive by RIA were falsely positive. The assays differed significantly in that monospecific antibody was used in the radioimmunoassay whereas polyspecific immunoglobulin was used in the ELISA. In another ELISA for hepatitis B surface antigen in which monospecific antibodies were used, the false positivity rate was only slightly higher with the ELISA than the solid-phase radioimmunoassay (Halbert and Auken, 1977). Thus, the two assay systems appear to have comparable sensitivities and specificities.

E. Applications of ELISA

At the time of publication we are aware of only two microbial antigens for which commercially available kits are available, hepatitis B surface antigen and rotavirus. As noted earlier, the ELISA for diagnosing hepatitis B is as sensitive as solid-phase radioimmunoassay; either assay system is optimal among currently available methods for diagnosing hepatitis B. Rotazyme (Abbott Laboratories, North Chicago, ILL.) is the only practical commercially available method for diagnosing rotavirus infections and is at least as sensitive as immune electronmicroscopy (Yolken *et al.*, 1977b). At 1981 prices, the cost for the kit itself contributes about $3.10 per patient to the cost of the test, assuming about 8 patients are tested each day the assay is run.

A kit for detecting amoebic antigens in faeces has been developed (IMMUNOZYME *Entamoeba histolytica* Antigens Reagent Set, Millipore Corp., Bedford, MA). The assay was positive on 159 of 163 stool samples from patients with microscopy evidence of amoebiasis. Multiple stool samples were needed to detect many of the positive specimens by microscopy; the ELISA was much more efficient. However, 410 ELISA-positive stool specimens of the 1177 tested were microscopy negative; whether these were true or false positives could not be stated. Thus, the chief value of the test is that patients with ELISA-negative samples can be assumed to be microscopy negative, eliminating the need for further testing in these patients. This should be particularly valuable in areas where amoebiasis is infrequent. However, interpretation of positive ELISA results is impossible until the meaning of the ELISA-positive microscopy-negative specimens is delineated (data from D. M. Root, Millipore Corporation). The test will presumably be marketed in the near future.

ELISA systems have been tested in other human infections, and many should theoretically be convertible to commercial production. Toxoplasmosis antigens were detected in the serum of 14 of 22 patients with acute toxoplasmosis but not in serum of 28 normal or 55 chronically infected humans. Antigens were also present in 2 of 2 amniotic fluids and 4 of 6 spinal fluids from cases of congenital toxoplasmosis (Araujo and Remington, 1980).

In three studies ELISA was positive in 95% of 22 spinal fluids from patients with *H. influenzae* meningitis. No false positives were seen in 136 control spinal fluids (Beuvery *et al.*, 1979; Drow *et al.*, 1979; Pepple *et al.*, 1979). Urine and serum specimens were also often positive (Drow *et al.*, 1979; Pepple *et al.*, 1980). Specific antigens were detected by ELISA in spinal fluid from all of 10 patients with pneumococcal meningitis and from 7 of 8 with meningococcal meningitis; all of 86 control specimens were negative (Beuvery *et al.*, 1979). Polin and Kennett (1980) detected specific antigens by ELISA in all of 11 spinal fluids from patients with group B streptococcal meningitis and in none of 10 sterile fluids. Thus, ELISA appears very sensitive for diagnosing the common types of bacterial meningitis. However, larger numbers of specimens from patients and controls must be tested and compared with conventional techniques such as the Gram stain before the true sensitivity, specificity, and need for these assays is known.

ELISA detected hepatitis A virus in stools from 18 of 20 patients with hepatitis A virus by immune electronmicroscopy and in none of 31 with other types of hepatitis or 13 with other illnesses. A blocking test was required to eliminate many false positive results (Locarnini *et al.*, 1978).

Of 29 pharyngeal secretions culture-positive for respiratory syncytial virus, 79% were ELISA-positive. A positive result was obtained in 1 of 36 specimens which did not grow the virus (Chao *et al.*, 1979). Sarkkinen *et al.* (1981) detected adenovirus antigens in all of 11 nasopharyngeal specimens from immunofluorescence-positive specimens and in none of 83 immuno-fluorescence-negative specimens. ELISA thus shows great promise for improving the rapid diagnosis of viral respiratory infections and will assume particular importance if safe and effective antiviral drugs are developed.

In diarrhoeal diseases the effectiveness of ELISA for detecting rotavirus antigens has been discussed. In toxigenic *E. coli* diarrhoea the labile enterotoxin was detected in 26 of 28 stool specimens from patients with moderate to severe symptoms and in whom the presence of toxin-producing *E. coli* was confirmed by standard methods; 5 of 21 other specimens were positive, although toxigenic *E. coli* could not be demonstrated (Merson *et al.*, 1980). Further studies of sensitivity and specificity are needed, but the assay appears promising.

ELISAs for detecting *Candida* antigens (Warren *et al.*, 1977; Segal *et al.*, 1979; Harding *et al.*, 1980), *Aspergillus* antigens (Richardson *et al.*, 1979), and staphylococcal enterotoxins have been described but have not yet been tested in adequate numbers of well-documented human infections to assess their potential.

REFERENCES

Adams, M. B., Aguilar-Torres, F. G. and Rytel, M. W. (1976). *Surg. Forum* **27**, 3–5.

Ames, B. N., Kammen, H. O. and Yamasaki, E. (1975). *Proc. Nat. Acad. Sci. USA* **72**, 2423–2427.

Anhalt, J. P., Kenny, G. E. and Rytel, M. W. (1978). *Cumitech* **8**, pp. 1–11. Cumulative Techniques and Procedures in Clinical Microbiology. American Society for Microbiology.

Araujo, F. G. and Remington, J. S. (1980). *J. Infect. Dis.* **141**, 144–150.

Araujo, F. G., Handman, E. and Remington, J. S. (1980). *Infect. Immun.* **30**, 12–16.

Arends, J. (1971). *Acta Endocrin.* **68**, 425–430.

Askenase, P. W. and Leonard, E. J. (1970). *Immunochem.* **7**, 29–41.

Avraham, H., Spira, D. T., Gorsky, Y. and Sulitzeanu, D. (1980). *J. Immunological Methods* **32**, 151–155.

Avrameas, S. (1969). *Immunochem.* **6**, 43–52.

Avrameas, S. (1970). *Intern. Rev. Cytol.* **27**, 349–385.

Avrameas, S. and Ternynk, T. (1969). *Immunochem.* **6**, 53–66.

Bartram, C. E., Crowder, J. G., Beeler, B. and White, A. (1974). *J. Lab. Clin. Med.* **83**, 591–598.

Baumann, J. B., Girard, J. and Vest, M. (1969). *Immunochem.* **6**, 699–713.

Baumstark, J., Laffen, R. and Bardawil, W. (1964). *Arch. Biochem. Biophys.* **108**, 514–522.

Belanger, L., Sylvestre, C. and Dufour, D. (1972). *Clin. Chim. Acta* **48**, 15–18.

Bennett, J. E. and Bailey, J. W. (1971). *Amer. J. Clin. Pathol.* **56**, 360–365.

Bessey, O. A., Lowry, O. H. and Brock, M. J. (1946). *J. Biol. Chem.* **164**, 321–329.

Beuvery, E. C., van Rossum, F., Lauwers, S. and Coignau, H. (1979). *Lancet* **1**, 208.

Bloomfield, N., Gordon, M. A. and Dumont, F. E. (1963). *Proc. Soc. Exp. Biol. Med.* **114**, 64–67.

Boorsma, D. M. and Kalsbeek, G. L. (1975). *J. Histochem. Cytochem.* **23**, 200–207.

Boroff, D. A. and Shu-Chenn, G. (1973). *Appl. Microbiol.* **25**, 545–549.

Bramner, K. W., Leach, J. M. and Butt, W. D. (1975). *Develop. Biol. Stand.* **30**, 58–67.

Bromberger, P. I., Chandler, B., Gezon, H. and Haddow, J. E. (1980). *J. Pediatr.* **96**, 104–106.

Bukovic, J. A. and Johnson, H. M. (1975). *Appl. Microbiol.* **30**, 700–701.

Burrell, C. J., Dickson, J. D., Gerber, H., McCormick, J. N. and Marmion, B. P. (1972). *Br. Med. J.* **4**, 23–24.

Burtis, C. A., Seibert, L. E., Baird, M. A. and Sampson, E. J. (1977). *Clin. Chem.* **23**, 1541–1547.

Catt, K. J. (1970). *Acta Endocr.* **63**, 222–246.

Catt, K. and Treagear, G. W. (1967). *Science* **158**, 1570–1572.

Catt, K. J., Tregear, G. W., Burger, H. G. and Skermer, C. (1970). *Clin. Chim. Acta* **27**, 267–279.

Ceska, M., Grossmuller, F. and Lundkvist, U. (1970). *Acta Endocr.* **64**, 111–125.

Ceska, M., Effenberger, F. and Grossmuller, F. (1978). *J. Clin. Microbiol.* **7**, 209–213.

Chao, R. K., Fishaut, M., Schwartzman, J. D. and McIntosh, K. (1979). *J. Infect. Dis.* **139**, 483–486.

Chervu, L. R. and Murty, D. R. K. (1975). *Sem. Nucl. Med.* **5**, 157–172.

Chessum, B. S. and Denmark, J. R. (1978). *Lancet* **1**, 161.

Clark, M. F. and Adams, A. N. (1977). *J. Gen. Virol.* **34**, 475–483.

Colding, H. and Lind, I. (1977). *J. Clin. Microbiol.* **5**, 405–409.
Congeni, B. L. and Nankervis, G. A. (1978). *Amer. J. Dis. Child.* **132**, 684.
Coonrod, J. D. and Drennan, D. P. (1976). *Ann. Intern. Med.* **84**, 254–260.
Coonrod, J. D. and Leach, R. P. (1978). *J. Clin. Microbiol.* **8**, 257–259.
Coonrod, J. D. and Rylko-Bauer, B. (1976). *J. Clin. Microbiol.* **4**, 168–174.
Coonrod, J. D. and Rytel, M. W. (1972). *Lancet* **1**, 1154–1159.
Cruickshank, R. (1938). *J. Path. Bact.* **46**, 67–75.
Cukor, G., Berry, M. K. and Blacklow, N. R. (1978). *J. Infect. Dis.* **138**, 906–910.
Denis, F., Samb, A. and Chrion, U. P. (1977). *J.A.M.A.* **238**, 1248–1249.
Denmark, J. R. and Chessum, B. S. (1978). *Med. Lab. Sci.* **35**, 227–232.
Desmyter, J. (1973). *Vox Sang.* **24**, 88–94.
Dochez, A. R. and Avery, O. T. (1917). *J. Exp. Med.* **26**, 447–493.
Donaldson, P. and Pennington, K. (1965). *J. Immunol.* **94**, 710–714.
Doskeland, S. O. and Berdal, B. P. (1980). *J. Clin. Microbiol.* **11**, 380–384.
Drow, D. L. and Manning, D. D. (1980). *J. Clin. Microbiol.* **11**, 641–645.
Drow, D. L., Maki, D. G. and Manning, D. D. (1979). *J. Clin. Microbiol.* **10**, 442–450.
Edwards, M. S. and Baker, C. J. (1979). *J. Pediatr.* **94**, 286–288.
Edwards, M. S., Kasper, D. L. and Baker, C. J. (1979). *J. Pediatr.* **95**, 202–205.
Edwards, E. A., Muchl, P. M. and Peckinpaugh, R. D. (1972). *J. Lab. Clin. Med.* **80**, 449–454.
Ellens, D. J. and de Leeuw, P. W. (1977). *J. Clin. Microbiol.* **6**, 530–532.
Ellens, D. J. and Gielkens, L. J. (1980). *J. Immunol. Meth.* **37**, 325–332.
El-Refaie, M. and Dulake, C. (1975). *J. Clin. Path.* **28**, 801–806.
Ende, J. V. D., Kloppers, L. L., Hyland, J. and Lennon, M. E. (1977). *South Afr. Med. J.* **51**, 800–802.
Engvall, E., Jonsson, K. and Perlmann, P. (1971). *Biochim. Biophys. Acta* **251**, 427–434.
Engvall, E. and Perlmann, P. (1972). *J. Immunochem.* **109**, 129–135.
Enlander, D., Dos Remedios, L. V., Weber, P. M. and Drew, L. (1976). *J. Immunol. Methods* **10**, 357–362.
Ewald, R. W. and Schubart, A. F. (1966). *J. Immunol.* **97**, 100–105.
Feigen, R. D., Stechenberg, B. W., Chang, M. J., Dunkle, L. M., Wong, M. L., Palkes, H., Dodge, P. R. and Davis, H. (1976a). *J. Pediat.* **88**, 542–548.
Feigin, R. D., Wong, M., Shackelford, P. G., Stechenberg, B. W., Dunkle, L. M. and Kaplan, S. (1976b). *J. Pediat.* **89**, 773–775.
Felber, J. P. (1978). *Adv. Clin. Chem.* **20**, 130–179.
Feldman, W. E. (1977). *Med. Intelligence* **296**, 433–435.
Finch, C. A. and Wilkinson, H. W. (1979). *J. Clin. Microbiol.* **10**, 519–524.
Fisher, B. D. and Armstrong, D. (1977). *N. Engl. J. Med.* **297**, 1440–1441.
Flodin, P. and Killander, J. (1962). *Biochim. Biophys. Acta* **63**, 403–410.
Ford, D. J., Radin, R. and Pesce, A. J. (1978). *Immunochem.* **15**, 237–243.
Forghani, B., Schmidt, N. J. and Lennette, E. H. (1974). *Appl. Microbiol.* **28**, 661–667.
Fossieck, B., Craig, R. and Patterson, P. Y. (1973). *J. Infect. Dis.* **127**, 106–109.
Foti, A. G., Herschman, H. and Cooper, J. F. (1975). *Cancer Res.* **35**, 2446–2452.
Frohman, M. A., Frohman, L. A., Goldman, M. B. and Goldman, J. N. (1979). *J. Lab. Clin. Med.* **93**, 614–621.
Goldsmith, S. J. (1975). *Sem. Nucl. Med.* **5**, 125–152.
Goodman, J. S., Kaufman, L. and Koenig, M. G. (1971). *N. Engl. J. Med.* **285**, 434–436.

Gordon, M. A. and Lapa, E. W. (1974). *Amer. J. Clin. Pathol.* **61**, 488–494.
Gordon, M. A. and Vedder, D. K. (1966). *J.A.M.A.* **197**, 961–967.
Granoff, D. M., Cogen, B., Baker, R. and Ogra, P. (1977). *Amer. J. Dis. Child.* **131**, 1357–1362.
Greenberg, H. B. and Kapikian, A. Z. (1978). *J. Amer. Vet. Med. Assoc.* **173**, 620–623.
Greenberg, H. B., Sack, D. A., Rodriguez, W., Sack, R. B., Wyatt, R. G., Kalica, A. R., Horswood, R. L., Chanock, R. M. and Kapikian, A. Z. (1977). *Infect. Immun.* **17**, 541–545.
Greenwood, B. M., Whittle, H. E. and Dominic-Rajkovic, O. (1971). *Lancet* **2**, 519–521.
Halbert, S. P. and Anken, M. (1977). *J. Infect. Dis.* **136**, S318–S323.
Halonen, P., Sarrkkinen, H., Arstila, P., Hjertsson, D. and Torfason, E. (1980). *J. Clin. Microbiol.* **11**, 614–617.
Harding, S. A., Scheld, W. M., McGowan, M. D. and Sande, M. A. (1979). *J. Clin. Microbiol.* **10**, 339–342.
Harding, S. A., Brody, J. P. and Normansell, D. E. (1980). *J. Lab. Clin. Med.* **95**, 959–966.
Hebert, G. A., Pelham, P. L. and Pittman, B. (1973). *Appl. Microbiol.* **25**, 26–36.
Hechemy, K., Stevens, R. W. and Gaafar, H. A. (1974). *Appl. Microbiol.* **28**, 306–311.
Hendry, R. M. and Herrmann, J. E. (1980). *J. Immunol. Meth.* **35**, 285–296.
Herrmann, J. E. and Collins, M. F. (1976). *J. Immunol. Meth.* **10**, 363–366.
Herrmann, J. E., Hendry, R. M. and Collins, M. F. (1979). *J. Clin. Microbiol.* **10**, 210–217.
Higashi, G. I., Sippel, J. E., Girgis, N. E. and Hassan, A. (1974). *Scand. J. Infect. Dis.* **6**, 233–235.
Hill, H. R. (1981). *In* "Second Aspen Conference on Clinical Relevance of Microbiology" (H. Summers, ed.) College of American Pathologists. Chicago.
Hoffman, T. A. and Edwards, E. A. (1972). *J. Infect. Dis.* **126**, 636–644.
Hollinger, F. B., Vorndam, V. and Dreesman, G. R. (1971). *J. Immunol.* **107**, 1099–1111.
Hollinger, F. B., Bradley, D. W. and Maynard, J. E. (1975). *J. Immunol.* **115**, 1464–1466.
Holmgren, J. and Svennerholm, A. M. (1973). *Infect. Immun.* **7**, 759–763.
Hopkins, R. and Das, P. C. (1974). *J. Clin. Pathol.* **27**, 40–44.
Hunter, W. M. (1971). *In* "Radioimmunoassay Methods", (K. E. Kirkham, W. M. Hunter, ed.) p. 3, Churchill Livingstone, Edinburgh.
Ingram, D. L., Anderson, P. and Smith, D. H. (1972). *J. Pediat.* **81**, 1156–1159.
Jackson, L. J., Sottile, M. I. and Aguilar-Torres, J. (1978). *Amer. J. Med.* **64**, 629–633.
Johnson, H. M., Bukovic, J. A. and Kauffman, P. E. (1972). *Infect. Immun.* **5**, 645–647.
Johnson, H. M., Bukovic, J. A., Kauffman, P. E. and Peeler, J. T. (1971). *Appl. Microbiol.* **22**, 837–841.
Kacaki, J., Wolters, G., Kuijpers, W. L. and Schuurs, A. (1977). *J. Clin. Pathol.* **30**, 894–898.
Kacaki, J., Wolters, G., Kuijpers, L. and Stulemeyer, S. (1978). *Vox Sang.* **35**, 65–74.
Kalica, A. R., Purcell, R. H. and Sereno, M. M. (1977). *J. Immunol.* **118**, 1275–1279.
Kaplan, S. L. and Feigin, R. D. (1979). *In* "Rapid Diagnosis in Infectious Diseases" (Rytel, M. W., ed.) pp. 105–112. CRC Press, Boca Raton, FL.
Kaufman, L. and Blumer, S. (1968). *Appl. Microbiol.* **16**, 1907–1912.
Kawaoka, Y., Naiki, M. and Yanagawa, R. (1979). *J. Clin. Microbiol.* **10**, 313–326.
Kayhty, H., Makela, P. H. and Ruoslahti, E. (1977). *J. Clin. Path.* **30**, 831–833.

Keele, D. K. and Webster, J. (1961). *Proc. Soc. Exp. Biol. Med.* **106**, 168–170.
Kennedy, J. H., Kricka, L. J. and Wilding, P. (1976). *Clin. Chim. Acta* **70**, 1–31.
Kibrick, A. C. and Blonstein, M. (1948). *J. Biol. Chem.* **176**, 983–987.
Klossner, J. L. and Willman, K. (1973). *Lancet* **1**, 322–323.
Kochwa, S., Brownell, M., Rosenfield, R. E. and Wasserman, L. R. (1976). *J. Immunol.* **99**, 981–986.
Kohler, R. B., Wheat, L. J. and White, A. (1979). *J. Clin. Microbiol.* **9**, 253–258.
Kohler, R. B., Wheat, L. J. and White, A. (1980). *J. Clin. Microbiol.* **12**, 39–43.
Kohler, R. B., Zimmerman, S. E., Wilson, E., Allen, S. D., Edelstein, P. H., Wheat, L. J. and White, A. (1981a). *Ann. Intern. Med.* **94**, 601–605.
Kohler, R. B., Winn, W. E., Wheat, L. J. and Girod, J. C. (1981b). 3rd International Symposium on Rapid Methods and Automation in Microbiology, Washington, D.C., May 26–30.
Korn, A. H., Feairheller, S. H. and Filachione, E. M. (1972). *J. Mol. Biol.* **65**, 525–529.
Kotoulas, A. O. and Moroz, L. A. (1971). *J. Immunol.* **106**, 1630–1640.
Kozaki, S., Dufrenne, J., Hagenaars, A. M. and Notermans, S. (1979). *Jap. J. Med. Sci. Biol.* **32**, 199–205.
Kumar, A. and Nankervis, G. A. (1980). *J. Pediatr.* **96**, 786.
Lampe, R., Major, M., Chottipitayasunondh, T. and Sunakorn, P. (1976). *J. Pediat.* **88**, 557–560.
Leach, R. P. and Coonrod, J. D. (1977). *Amer. Rev. Resp. Dis.* **116**, 847–851.
Leach, J. M. and Ruck, B. J. (1971). *Br. Med. J.* **4**, 597–598.
Lehmann, P. F. and Reiss, E. (1980). *Mycopathol.* **70**, 83–88.
Leinonen, M. K. (1980). *J. Clin. Microbiol.* **11**, 135–140.
Leinonen, M. and Herva, E. (1977). *Scand. J. Infect. Dis.* **9**, 187–191.
Leinonen, M. and Kayhty, H. (1978). *J. Clin. Pathol.* **31**, 1172–1176.
Levitt, N. H., Miller, H. V. and Eddy, G. A. (1976). *J. Clin. Microbiol.* **4**, 382–383.
Ling, C. M. and Overby, L. R. (1972). *J. Immunol.* **109**, 834–841.
Locarnini, S. A., Garland, S. M., Lehmann, N. I., Pringle, R. C. and Gust, I. D. (1978). *J. Clin. Microbiol.* **8**, 277–282.
Lund-Olesen, K. (1969). *Dan. Med. Bull.* **16**, 46–47.
McCarthy, D. H. (1975). *J. Gen. Microbiol.* **89**, 384–386.
McCracken, G. H., Jr, Sarff, L. D., Glode, M. P. and Mize, S. G. (1974). *Lancet* **2**, 246–250.
MacKinnon, S., Kane, J. G. and Parker, R. H. (1978). *J.A.M.A.* **240**, 1982–1983.
Maehly, A. C. and Chance, B. (1954). *In* "Methods of Biochemical Analysis" (G. Glick, ed.) Vol. I, pp. 357–423. Interscience Publishers, Inc., New York, N.Y.
Maiolini, R. and Masseyeff, R. (1975). *J. Immunol. Meth.* **8**, 223–234.
Marier, R. and Andriole, V. T. (1975). *Clin. Res.* **23**, 308A.
Martin-Sosa, S. and Berron, R. (1975). *Develop. Biol. Stand.* **30**, 68–72.
Mathiesen, L. R., Feinstone, S. M., Wong, D. C., Skinhoej, P. and Purcell, R. H. (1978). *J. Clin. Microbiol.* **7**, 184–193.
Merson, M. H., Yolken, R. H., Sack, R. B., Froehlich, J. L., Greenberg, H. B., Huq, I. and Black, R. W. (1980). *Infect. Immun.* **29**, 108–113.
Michaels, R. H. and Poziviak, C. S. (1976). *J. Pediat.* **88**, 72–74.
Minta, J. O., Goodkofsky, I. and Lepow, I. H. (1973). *Immunochem.* **10**, 341–350.
Munford, R. S. and Hall, C. I. (1979). *Infect. Immun.* **26**, 42–48.
Naik, H. S. and Duncan, C. L. (1978). *J. Clin. Microbiol.* **7**, 337–340.
Naiman, H. L. and Albritton, W. L. (1980). *J. Infect. Dis.* **142**, 524–531.
Nakane, P. K. and Kawaoi, A. (1974). *J. Histochem. Cytochem.* **22**, 1084–1091.

Nakane, P. K. and Pierce, G. B. (1967). *J. Cell Biol.* **33**, 307–318.
Neill, J. M., Sugg, J. Y. and McCauley, D. W. (1951). *Proc. Soc. Exp. Biol. Med.* **77**, 775–783.
Newman, R. B., Stevens, R. W. and Gaafar, H. A. (1970). *J. Lab. Clin. Med.* **76**, 107–113.
Notermans, S., Dufrenne, J. and van Schothorst, M. (1978). *Jap. J. Med. Sci. Biol.* **31**, 81–85.
Ohya, T., Ohya, F. and Tomimura, K. (1974). *Nagoya J. Med. Sci.* **37**, 29–32.
O'Reilly, R. J., Anderson, P., Ingram, D. L., Peter, G. and Smith, D. H. (1975). *J. Clin. Invest.* **56**, 1012–1022.
Oreskes, I. and Singer, J. M. (1961). *J. Immunol.* **86**, 338–344.
Overby, L. R. and Mushahwar, I. K. (1979). *In* "Rapid Diagnosis in Infectious Disease" (M. W. Rytel, ed.) pp. 40–68. CRC Press, Boca Raton, FL.
Overby, L. R., Miller, J. P., Smith, I. D., Decker, R. H. and Ling, C. M. (1973). *Vox Sang. Suppl.* **24**, 102–113.
Parker, C. W. (1972). *In* "Progress in Clinical Pathology" (M. Stefanini, ed.) Vol. IV, pp. 103–141. Grune and Stratton, New York and London.
Parker, R. H. (1979). *In* "Rapid Diagnosis in Infectious Diseases" (M. W. Rytel, ed.) pp. 1250–1300. CRC Press, Boca Raton, FL.
Pepple, J., Moxon, E. R. and Yolken, R. H. (1980). *J. Pediatr.* **97**, 233–237.
Perlino, C. A. and Shulman, J. A. (1976). *J. Lab. Clin. Med.* **87**, 496–501.
Pesce, A. J., Ford, D. J., Gaizutis, M. and Pollak, V. E. (1977). *Biochim. Biophys. Acta* **492**, 399–407.
Polakova, K., Sintovicona, M., Chorvath, B., Russ, G., Style, B. and Sourek, J. (1979). *Acta Virol.* **23**, 107–112.
Polin, R. A. and Kennett, R. (1980). *J. Pediatr.* **97**, 540–544.
Pollack, M. (1976). *Infect. Immun.* **13**, 1543–1548.
Poor, A. H. and Cutler, J. E. (1979). *J. Clin. Microbiol.* **9**, 362–368.
Prevost, E. and Newell, R. (1978). *J. Clin. Microbiol.* **8**, 529–533.
Prince, A. M. and Jass, D. (1974). *Vox Sang.* **26**, 209–221.
Pronovast, A. D., Baumgarten, A. and Hsiung, G. D. (1981). *J. Clin. Microbiol.* **13**, 97–101.
Purcell, R. H., Wong, D. C., Moritsugu, Y., Dienstag, J. L., Routenberg, J. A. and Bogg, J. D. (1976). *J. Immunol.* **116**, 349–356.
Ratcliffe, J. G. (1974). *Br. Med. Bull.* **30**, 32–37.
Ribner, R., Keusch, G. T. and Robbins, J. B. (1975). *Ann. Intern. Med.* **83**, 370–371.
Richardson, M. D., White, L. O. and Warren, R. C. (1979). *Mycopathol.* **67**, 83–88.
Rissing, J. P., Buxton, T. B., Talledo, R. A. and Sprinkle, T. J. (1980). *Infect. Immun.* **27**, 405–410.
Robern, H., Dighton, M. and Dickie, N. (1975). *Appl. Microbiol.* **30**, 525–529.
Robbins, J. B., McCracken, G. H., Gotschidh, E. C., Orskow, F. and Hanson, L. A. (1974). *N. Engl. J. Med.* **290**, 1216–1220.
Rosenthal, J. D., Hayashi, K. and Notkins, A. L. (1973). *Appl. Microbiol.* **25**, 567–573.
Russ, G., Styk, B. and Varechova, E. (1976). *Acta Virol.* **20**, 460–465.
Rutstein, J. E., Holahan, J. R., Lyons, R. M. and Pope, R. M. (1978). *J. Lab. Clin. Med.* **92**, 529–535.
Ryan, R. W., Kwasnik, I. and Tilton, R. C. (1980). *J. Clin. Microbiol.* **12**, 776–779.
Rytel, M. W. (1979). *In* "Rapid Diagnosis in Infectious Diseases" (Rytel, M. W., ed.) pp. 91–103. CRC Press, Boca Raton, FL.
Salmon, S. E., Mackey, G. and Fudenberg, H. H. (1969). *J. Immunol.* **103**, 129–137.

Salomon, L. L. and Tew, R. W. (1963). *Proc. Soc. Exp. Biol. Med.* **129**, 539–542.
Sarkkinen, H. K., Halonen, P. E., Arstila, P. P. and Salmi, A. A. (1981). *J. Clin. Microbiol.* **13**, 258–265.
Scharpe, S. L., Cooreman, W. M., Blomme, W. J. and Laekeman, G. M. (1976). *Clin. Chem.* **22**, 733–738.
Scheifele, D. W., Daum, R. S., Syriopoulou, V. P., Siber, G. R. and Smith, A. L. (1979). *Infect. Immun.* **23**, 827–831.
Schetters, H., Hehlmann, R., Erfle, V. and Ramanarayaban, M. (1980). *Infect. Immun.* **29**, 972–980.
Schultz, W. W., Phipps, T. J. and Pollack, M. (1979). *J. Clin. Microbiol.* **9**, 705–708.
Scott, E. N., Muchmore, H. G. and Felton, F. G. (1980). *Amer. J. Clin. Pathol.* **73**, 1–6.
Segal, E., Berg, R. A., Pizzo, P. A. and Bennett, J. E. (1979). *J. Clin. Microbiol.* **10**, 116–118.
Severin, W. P. J. (1972). *J. Clin. Path.* **25**, 1079–1082.
Shaffer, P. J., Medoff, G. and Kobayashi, G. S. (1979a). *J. Infect. Dis.* **139**, 313–319.
Shaffer, P. J., Kobayashi, G. S. and Medoff, G. (1979b). *Amer. J. Med.* **67**, 627–630.
Simpson, R. A. and Speller, D. C. E. (1977). *Lancet* **1**, 1206–1207.
Singer, J. M. and Plotz, C. M. (1956). *Amer. J. Med.* **21**, 888–892.
Singer, J. M., Plotz, C. M., Pader, E. and Elster, S. K. (1956). *Amer. J. Clin. Pathol.* **28**, 611–617.
Singer, J. M., Altmann, G., Goldenberg, A. and Plotz, C. M. (1960). *Arth. Rheumatism* **3**, 515–521.
Singer, J. M., Oreskes, I., Hutterer, F. and Ernst, J. (1963). *Ann. Rheum. Dis.* **22**, 424–428.
Sippel, J. E. and Voller, A. (1980). *Trans. Royal Soc. Trop. Med. Hyg.* **74**, 644–648.
Snow, R. M. and Dismukes, W. E. (1975). *Arch. Intern. Med.* **135**, 1155–1157.
Sober, H. A., Gutter, F. J., Wyckoff, M. M. and Peterson, E. A. (1956). *Amer. Chem. Soc. J.* **78**, 756–763.
Spencer, R. C. and Savage, M. A. (1975). *J. Clin. Path.* **29**, 187–190.
Spira, G., Silvian, I. and Zakay-Rones, Z. (1976). *J. Immunol.* **116**, 1098–1092.
Stechenberg, B. W., Schreiner, R. L., Grass, S. M. and Shackelford, P. G. (1979). *Pediatrics* **64**, 632–634.
Steinbuch, M. and Audran, R. (1969). *Arch. Biochem. Biophys.* **134**, 279–284.
Stevens, W. A. and Tsiantos, J. (1979). *Microbios Lett.* **10**, 29–32.
Stiffler-Rosenberg, G. and Fey, H. (1978). *J. Clin. Microbiol.* **8**, 473–479.
Tabbarah, Z. A., Kohler, R. B., Wheat, L. J., Griep, J. S. and White, A. (1979). *J. Infect. Dis.* **140**, 822–825.
Tabbarah, Z. A., Wheat, L. J., Kohler, R. B. and White, A. (1980). *J. Clin. Microbiol.* **11**, 703–709.
Thirumoorthi, M. C. and Dajani, A. S. (1979). *J. Clin. Microbiol.* **9**, 28–32.
Thornley, M. J., Wilson, D. V., De Hormaeche, R. D., Oates, J. K. and Coombs, R. R. A. (1979). *J. Medical Microbiol.* **12**, 161–175.
Tilton, R. C. (1978). "CRC Critical Reviews in Clinical Laboratory Sciences" pp. 347–365. CRC Press, Cleveland, OH.
Trollfors, B., Berntsson, E., Elgefors, B. and Kaijser, B. (1979). *Scand. J. Infect. Dis.* **11**, 31–34.
Tsang, V., Wilson, B. and Maddison, S. (1980). *Clin. Chem.* **26**, 1255–1260.
Tuazon, C. U. and Sheagren, J. M. (1976). *Ann. Intern. Med.* **84**, 543–546.
Tugwell, P. and Greenwood, B. M. (1975). *J. Clin. Pathol.* **28**, 118–123.
Van Knapen, F. and Panggabean, S. O. (1977). *J. Clin. Microbiol.* **6**, 545–547.

388 R. B. Kohler, L. J. Wheat and A. White

van Oss, C. J. and Singer, J. M. (1966). *J. Reticuloendothelial Soc.* **3**, 29–40.
Vincent, M. H. and Bellot, M. (1909). *Bulletin De L'Academie de Medicine S. Serie* **61–62**, 326–332.
Voller, A., Bartlett, A., Bidwell, D. E., Clark, M. F. and Adams, A. N. (1976). *J. Gen. Virol.* **33**, 165–167.
Voller, A. and Bidwell, D. E. (1980). *Clin. Immunol. Newsl.* **1**, 5–7.
Voller, A., Bidwell, D. E. and Bartlett, A. (1976). *Bull. WHO* **53**, 55–65.
Voogt, C. E., Van Der Stel, J. J. and Jacobs, J. J. J. S. S. (1980). *J. Immunolog. Meth.* **36**, 55–61.
Waart, M., Snelting, A., Cichy, J., Wolter, G. and Schuurs, A. (1978). *J. Med. Virol.* **3**, 43–49.
Ward, J. I., Siber, G. R., Schieifele, D. W. and Smith, D. H. (1978). *J. Pediatr.* **93**, 37–42.
Warren, R. C., Bartlett, A., Bidwell, D. E., Richardson, M. D., Voller, A. and White, L. O. (1977). *Br. Med. J.* **1**, 1183–1185.
Webb, B. J. and Baker, C. J. (1980). *J. Clin. Micro.* **12**, 442–444.
Weiner, M. H. and Coats-Stephen, M. (1979). *J. Lab. Clin. Med.* **93**, 111–119.
Weiner, M. H. (1980a). *Clin. Res.* **28**, 5, 832A. (abstract).
Weiner, M. H. (1980b). *Ann. Intern. Med.* **92**, 793–796.
Wetherall, B. L., Hallsworth, P. G. and McDonald, P. J. (1980). *J. Clin. Microbiol.* **11**, 573–580.
Wheat, L. J., Kohler, R. B. and White, A. (1978). *J. Infect. Dis.* **138**, 174–180.
Wheat, L. J., R. Kohler and White, A. (1979). *J. Infect. Dis.* **140**, 25–30.
Whittle, H. C., Tugwell, P., Egler, L. J. and Greenwood, B. M. (1974). *Lancet* **2**, 619–621.
Whittle, H. C., Greenwood, B. M., Davidson, N. M. and Tompkins, A. (1975). *Amer. J. Med.* **58**, 823–828.
Wiernik, A., Jarstrand, C. and Tunevall, G. (1978). *Scand. J. Infect. Dis.* **10**, 173–176.
Wilson, D. V., Thornley, M. J. and Coombs, R. R. A. (1977). *J. Med. Microbiol.* **10**, 281–292.
Wisdom, G. B. (1976). *Clin. Chem.* **22**, 1243–1255.
Wolters, G., Kuijpers, L., Kacaki, J. and Schuurs, A. (1976). *J. Clin. Pathol.* **29**, 873–879.
Wolters, G., Kuijpers, L., Kacaki, J. and Schuurs, A. (1977). *J. Infect. Dis.* **136**, S311–S317.
Yalow, R. S. (1978). *Science* **200**, 1236–1245.
Yolken, R. H. (1978). *Hosp. Prac.* **13**, 121–127.
Yolken, R. H. and Stopa, P. J. (1979a). *J. Clin. Microbiol.* **10**, 317–321.
Yolken, R. H. and Stopa, P. J. (1979b). *J. Clin. Microbiol.* **10**, 703–707.
Yolken, R. H. and Stopa, P. J. (1980). *J. Clin. Microbiol.* **11**, 546–551.
Yolken, R. H., Greenberg, H. B., Merson, M. H., Sack, R. B. and Kapikian, A. Z. (1977b). *J. Clin. Microbiol.* **6**, 439–444.
Yolken, R. S., Wha Kim, H., Clem, T., Wyatt, R. G., Chanock, R. M., Kalica, A. R. and Kapikian, A. Z. (1977b). *Lancet* **2**, 263–266.
Young, E. J., Hirsh, D. D., Fainstein, V. and Williams, T. W. (1980). *Amer. Rev. Resp. Dis.* **121**, 743–747.
Zollinger, W. D. and Mandrell, R. E. (1977). *Infect. Immun.* **18**, 424–433.

10 Perspectives on the development of a new vaccine against *Pseudomonas aeruginosa* infection

J. YUZURU HOMMA

I. INTRODUCTION

Pseudomonas aeruginosa is widely distributed in the environment but rarely causes infection in normal hosts. However, in patients with underlying diseases, severe thermal injury and organ transplants, it is one of the most frequently isolated pathogens, giving rise to a wide variety of diseases, such as acute overwhelming septicaemia and chronic suppurative infections, as well as superficial harmless colonization (Young and Armstrong, 1972). Thus *P. aeruginosa* infection is intimately related to the defence mechanisms which protect the host. Remarkable progress has been made in research on the parasite, and it has been found that there is great diversity in virulence among the various strains of *P. aeruginosa*. Several metabolites related to the virulence of the bacterium have been identified and characterized. Some of the effects of strains producing toxic metabolites on the host with infection due to the bacterium have also been clarified.

As for the host defence mechanisms against *P. aeruginosa* infection, Aduan and Reynolds (1979) have published a detailed review on the cell-mediated responses to *Pseudomonas* infection, and Høiby (1979) in the same monograph has written on humoral response to the infection.

Using immunologically deficient mice and inbred mice, Nomoto (1977) and Maejima (1977) confirmed that cell-mediated immunity plays only a minor role in *Pseudomonas* infections. The host resistance against *P. aeruginosa* appears to depend mainly on humoral immune phagocytic action.

389

What kinds of specific antibodies then are needed for effective prophylaxis of *P. aeruginosa* infection? The exotoxin alone of *Corynebacterium diphtheriae* is responsible for diphtheria, and so toxoid and antiserum are used for prophylaxis and treatment of diphtheria. In *P. aeruginosa* infection, the bacterium multiplies at the site of infection. Overwhelming septicaemia and the elaboration of toxic metabolites such as exotoxin, protease and elastase, etc. may then take place during the course of infection, and their harmful activities have been demonstrated both *in vitro* and in experimental animals. Accordingly, to prevent pseudomonal infection, the growth of *P. aeruginosa* should be suppressed by enhancing the ingestion and killing of bacteria by polymorphonuclear leucocytes by virtue of complements and specific antibodies against outer membrane constituents of *P. aeruginosa*. At the same time the toxic effects of the metabolites should be countered by neutralizing antibodies.

Consequently, it is first necessary to identify virulence factors from the various kinds of metabolites. Then the effect of antibodies against the metabolites presumed to be the virulence factors must be evaluated in the course of *Pseudomonas* infection.

This chapter will review many animal experiments which indicate that one or more virulence factors are important in *Pseudomonas* infection, thus requiring immunization with a set of antigens for complete protection against invasion by *P. aeruginosa*.

II. VIRULENCE-ASSOCIATED FACTORS

The pathogenicity of opportunistic pathogens is not easily determined. In pathogenicity the role of a substance produced by an opportunistic pathogen depends on its toxicity and the quantity produced. It must also be taken into consideration whether the substance is actually produced in the host and, if produced, whether its toxic activity can actually be demonstrated in the host or disappears easily, for instance, by neutralization, inhibition or destruction with host plasma or enzymes. Therefore animal experiments are essential for determining the pathogenic action of a toxic substance which is presumed to be a virulence factor. If the substance is antigenic, one method for identifying its pathogenicity is to perform protective animal experiments. Animals immunized with the substance are challenged with the viable pathogen to observe whether they can withstand the infection. However, a pathogenic micro-organism may produce many metabolites, so even when immunization with the substance alone is ineffective in protecting against infection, the experiment should be repeated, immunizing the animals with the substance being tested with other metabolites and/or somatic antigens.

Enzyme inhibitors as well as other substances neutralizing toxic effects of metabolites can also facilitate the analysis of microbial virulence, where this may depend on combined and synergistic activities of metabolites.

Genetic research selecting mutants, such as strains deficient in producing the specified substance presumed to be related to virulence, will provide an important and promising approach to clarify the pathogenic roles of the substance. Mutants producing serologically identical but non-toxic proteins similar to a toxin will also facilitate the development of a new and effective vaccine.

A. Exotoxin*

The importance of exotoxin in the pathogenesis of *P. aeruginosa* infections is becoming increasingly recognized. Although exotoxin of *P. aeruginosa* possesses a potential toxicity as great as that of *Corynbacterium diphtheriae*, there are few reports on patients with *P. aeruginosa* infection indicating such severe symptoms as those encountered in cases of diphtheria.

The exotoxin inhibits cellular protein synthesis by catalyzing the transfer of the adenosine 5'-diphosphate ribose (ADPR) portion of nicotinamide adenine dinucleotide (NAD) to mammalian elongation factor 2 (EF-2) (Iglewski and Kabat, 1975; Iglewski *et al.*, 1977). Thus exotoxin produced by *P. aeruginosa* shows potent toxicity with a mechanism of action similar to that of diphtheria toxin.

The histopathology and serum enzyme levels of mice inoculated intravenously with *P. aeruginosa* exotoxin were studied by Pavlovskis *et al.* (1976). The toxin exerted a marked effect on the liver but elicited no demonstrable microscopic changes in other organs. The microscopic lesions caused in the liver by a single injection of two 50% lethal doses (LD_{50}) of toxin (2.3 µg) were characterized by necrosis, cellular swelling, and fatty change within 4–8 hours and near total hepatocellular necrosis at 48 hours. Hepatonecrosis was accompanied by a parallel rise in serum levels of aspartic and alanine aminotransferases and alkaline phosphatase.

Data reported by Saelinger *et al.* (1977) suggest that *Pseudomonas* exotoxin produced by bacteria multiplying at the burn site enters the circulatory system and is disseminated to liver and other organs where it acts by depletion of EF-2, resulting in a reduction in protein synthesis. Similarly Pavlovskis *et al.* (1978) reported that one of the primary effects of *P. aeruginosa* exotoxin during experimental infection was the inactivation of EF-2 in various mouse organs. Whereas EF-2 activity was reduced in all organs examined from PA103-infected animals, the largest decrease was observed in the liver, where the active EF-2 levels were reduced by 70–90%.

* In this chapter exotoxin A is referred to simply as exotoxin.

As mentioned below (Section II B), two distinct proteases produced by *P. aeruginosa*, alkaline protease and elastase, are responsible for some of the gross corneal damage seen in *Pseudomonas* keratitis (Kreger and Griffin, 1974; Kawaharajo and Homma, 1975c). However, Ohman *et al.* (1980) presented data indicating that in experimental infections of mouse cornea, the exotoxin of *P. aeruginosa* contributes to the organism's pathogenicity. After traumatization, the cornea was infected with wild-type parental toxin-producing strains and two toxin-deficient mutants (Tox⁻). The infections produced by both toxin-mutants were less severe than infections produced by their parental strains. Addition of subdamaging doses of exotoxin to eyes infected with the Tox⁻ mutant significantly increased its virulence.

Pollack *et al.* (1976, 1977) and Takeshi and Homma (1978) found neutralizing antibody against *Pseudomonas* exotoxin in human serum. The formation of antibody was more pronounced in patients with severe infections due to *P. aeruginosa*. The same authors and Sanai *et al.* (1978) also reported that most *Pseudomonas* strains isolated from patients produced exotoxin. Bjorn *et al.* (1977) investigated the production of exotoxin within *Pseudomonas* species as well as in laboratory strains and clinical isolates of *P. aeruginosa* by assaying the enzyme activity (ADP-ribosyl-transferase). Exotoxin production was detected in approximately 90% of the 111 isolates of *P. aeruginosa*. In contrast none of the other species of *Pseudomonas* examined produced exotoxin. Homma *et al.* (1975a), Cho *et al.* (1978), Homma (1978), and Takeshi and Homma (1978) found high titres of exotoxin, protease and elastase in the sera of patients with panbronchiolitis, cystic fibrosis pulmonary infections, and bovine mastitis due to *P. aeruginosa*. Klinger *et al.* (1978) also reported that the proteases and exotoxin of *P. aeruginosa* are produced in cystic fibrosis pulmonary infections due to *P. aeruginosa*. These results suggest that these exoenzymes and exotoxin may serve as significant virulence factors in chronic *Pseudomonas* infection.

Pollack and Young (1979) suggest from their data that antibodies to *Pseudomonas* toxin and lipopolysaccharide are present at an early stage in the serum of most patients with *P. aeruginosa* septicemia, increase with survival, and are protective, suggesting that antibodies passively provided or actively engendered to both exotoxin and lipopolysaccharide may have therapeutic or prophylactic potential. Accordingly, it should be questioned whether any pathogenic role is played by exotoxin in chronic respiratory infections due to *P. aeruginosa* in man. It would also be important to know the clinical effects of exotoxin formation in hosts infected by *P. aeruginosa*, who either have generalized immune insufficiency (e.g. neonates) or who have no neutralizing antibody to exotoxin.

It is not clear why *P. aeruginosa* generally causes only mild infections, unlike *Corynebacterium diphtheriae*, despite the fact that both these bacilli produce the same kind of exotoxin. Data reported by Shinozaki *et al.* (1981) seem to offer some explanation. They measured antibodies against OEP (section IV A), exotoxin, protease and elastase (section II B) by passive hemagglutination (PHA) tests in 256 specimens of sera from normal healthy children and adults, and cord blood. Antibody against exotoxin was detected in cord blood samples. The mean level of antibody titres dropped during the first year of age, then rose and reached a plateau at the age of 2–5 years. Mean antibody titres of OEP by age groups were similar to that of exotoxin. Antibodies to protease and elastase were not detectable initially, but the level rose during the second year of age and reached a plateau during childhood. Antibody to exotoxin and OEP was found in sera of age groups 11 to 30 years, while the rate of acquisition of antibodies to protease and elastase was low. The antibody to exotoxin in the age group 1–4 years is mostly of the IgM type. It is suggested that *Pseudomonas* infections or, more importantly, colonization may be common in infants and young children.

Cross *et al.* (1980) measured antibody to *P. aeruginosa* exotoxin by solid-phase radioimmunoassay. Mean ($\pm$SEM) peak levels of IgG in 24 normal soldiers were $2.6 \pm 0.5\,\mu g\,ml^{-1}$, while mean peak levels in 12 patients colonized with and 13 patients infected in sites other than the blood with exotoxin-producing strains of *P. aeruginosa* were 16.7 ± 7.0 and $17.1 \pm 4.4\,\mu g\,ml^{-1}$, respectively. Levels of IgG were determined in 52 patients with *Pseudomonas* bacteraemia. Those surviving and those dying of bacteraemia due to exotoxin-producing strains had mean peak levels of 25.8 ± 5.5 and $4.6 \pm 2.0\,\mu g\,ml^{-1}$, respectively. The antitoxin response in sera obtained sequentially from bacteraemic patients began shortly after the onset of bacteraemia and decreased gradually, but could be recalled promptly upon reinfection with *P. aeruginosa*. Death from *Pseudomonas* bacteraemia was associated with infection by an exotoxin-producing strain, the presence of underlying disease, the presence of hypotension, and an antitoxin level of $<2\,\mu g\,ml^{-1}$.

The 50% prevalence of detectable antitoxin in the normal persons studied by Cross *et al.* suggests that many people are transiently colonized with *P. aeruginosa* and form antibody to exotoxin. They were able to detect significant quantitative differences in mean antibody levels between bacteraemic patients who survived and those who died as a result of *Pseudomonas* bacteraemia.

B. Protease and elastase

Liu (1966) reported that when protease fractions from *P. aeruginosa* were inoculated intraperitoneally and intravenously in mice, peritoneal and pulmonary haemorrhage was observed. According to Meinke *et al.* (1970), partially purified protease exhibiting elastase activity, when injected intra-peritoneally, resulted in serosal haemorrhage and necrosis of the gastro-intestinal tract, while intranasal and intravenous injections caused pulmonary haemorrhage. Fisher and Aller (1958) and Kreger and Grffin (1974) reported that perforation in the cornea was observed when a crude preparation of protease was inoculated intracorneally into rabbits.

Using crystallized protease and elastase prepared by Morihara (1963, 1964) and Morihara *et al.* (1965), Kawaharajo *et al.* (1974, 1975a,b) examined the effect of each of the enzymes on the internal organs, skin and cornea of experimental animals. They confirmed that a relatively small amount of protease and elastase could cause haemorrhage, ulcerating lesions in the skin of rabbits, and haemorrhage in subcutaneous tissue. The gross and histo-pathological findings observed in experimental animals were apparently quite similar to those seen in human cases of eczema gangraenosum.

Although the development of this kind of haemorrhage on rabbit skin required 50 μg crystalline protease or elastase, 2–5 μg of the enzyme was sufficient to develop histopathological changes. Neutrophil infiltration was seen both in degenerating epidermis and in the muscular layer. Haemorrhagic lesions were scattered in all layers of the dermis.

When crystalline protease and elastase were inoculated intraperitoneally, intravenously, intrapleurally, or intranasally in mice, pulmonary haemor-rhages were observed in most cases. Severe multiple haemorrhages due to destruction of elastic fibres of arteries were found in the lungs without any cellular infiltration. In addition, haemorrhages were seen in parts of the parietal bone, pleura, diaphragm, peritoneum, and serosa of the gastro-intestinal tract. The minimal lethal dose (MLD) values in a 24-hour period according to different routes of inoculation were 60 to 300 μg per mouse.

Using the De test with ligated intestine, Okada *et al.* (1976) found that protease and elastase caused swelling of the intestine on the following day. The test was positive with protease- and elastase-producing strains but negative with non-producing strains. Histology showed severe atrophy of the villi and haemorrhage. Protease caused bleeding from capillaries in the submucosa and atrophy of Auerbach's plexus. Elastase produced severe atrophy of the villi and Auerbach's plexus. Bleeding was less severe for elastase than protease. These observations indicate that protease and elastase play an important role in enteritis due to *P. aeruginosa*. Protease and elastase seem to be related to melaena, bleeding in the skin and mucous membranes and pneumonia in terminal infections due to *P. aeruginosa* in man.

Angiitis due to *P. aeruginosa* is characterized by destruction of the lamina elastica, haemorrhage, and bacterial invasion through the vessel wall, but characteristically does not produce any inflammatory reaction.

Corneal ulcers are often noted in ocular infection with *P. aeruginosa*. To study the pathogenicity of *P. aeruginosa* to corneal tissue, corneal damage was experimentally induced with protease and elastase in mice (Tanaka *et al.*, 1972; Kawaharajo *et al.*, 1974, 1975c; Kreger and Griffin, 1974; Gray and Kreger, 1975). The mouse cornea was experimentally incised, protease and elastase were dropped on it once, and the lesion followed. Opacity was produced in the wounded area of the cornea by 0.8–2 μg of the enzymes, and opacity and ulcers were produced in the cornea by 4–50 μg. Protease and elastase caused very similar histopathological changes in the cornea of mice. The extent of such changes depends upon the dose. Kawaharajo and Homma (1975c) demonstrated differences in virulence between those *Pseudomonas* strains that produce protease and elastase in corneal infections of mice and those that do not. A drop of suspension of viable *P. aeruginosa* strain IF03455 (10^5 ml $^{-1}$) which produced protease and elastase was enough to cause corneal ulcer, but not even an abscess was formed after inoculation of strains which produced neither protease nor elastase in suspensions up to 10^9 ml $^{-1}$. The difference in virulence between enzyme-producing and non-enzyme-producing strains of *P. aeruginosa* was definite in corneal infection. Kawaharajo and Homma (1975c) found that NC5, a strain producing neither protease nor elastase, did not produce even an abscess in the experimental model of corneal ulcer, but the addition of a minute quantity of protease dropped in the eye resulted in ulcer formation. The quantity of protease alone in the inoculation of NC5 was so small that it did not cause corneal ulcer. The most frequent isolate from corneal ulcers in man is *P. aeruginosa*. Judging from these experimental results in mice, these strains possibly produce protease and elastase.

However, as all the strains used in these experiments were exotoxin-producing strains, possible participation of exotoxin on corneal ulcer together with the two enzymes must also be taken into consideration. This will be discussed below.

Okada *et al.* (1980) inoculated *P. aeruginosa* subcutaneously into mice at the sites of burn wounds produced by flames according to the method Holder and Jogan (1971) and Stieritz and Holder (1975). Protease- and elastase-producing strains proved to be highly virulent compared with strains not producing the two enzymes.

Holder and Haidaris (1979) inoculated bacteria subcutaneously at sites of burn wounds. Death did not occur in mice given as much as 1000 bacteria of strain PA103, which produces exotoxin but not protease or elastase, while none survived when mice were given a minute amount of protease together with the same bacterial inoculation. This dose of protease alone was not lethal. The aggressin-like effect of protease was not found when *E. coli* or *Klebsiella* was used in the same experimental model. The protease did not have to be pseudomonal in origin: thermolysin showed the same effect. These experiments using the mouse burn model that resembles human burn wound sepsis show that protease producers are more virulent than protease-deficient strains.

Pavlovskis and Wretlind (1979) obtained evidence indicating that in the experimental mouse burn model (Holder's procedure) protease enhanced the virulence of *P. aeruginosa*. They used a protease-producing strain and two of its protease-deficient mutant strains. The LD_{50} for mice infected with the protease-producing strain was at least 1 log lower than the LD_{50} of the protease-deficient mutants. The addition of purified protease to the infecting inoculum of protease-deficient strains reduced to LD_{50}. Although the generation time *in vitro* was the same for all three bacterial strains used, there were consistently fewer viable bacteria in the blood of mice infected with protease-deficient strains than in the blood of those infected with the protease-producing strain. When a protease-deficient strain was mixed with a protease-producing wild-type strain, the number of protease-producing *Pseudomonas* found in the blood remained constant, whereas the number of protease-deficient organisms increased, suggesting that protease contributed to the invasiveness of the organisms. These experiments clearly indicate that proteases may be important in overcoming the host defence mechanism and act as an aggressin to enhance invasion of bacteria.

Complement is known to act in inflammation as chemotactic phagocytic and bactericidal factors. According to Schultz and Miller (1974), elastase has a destructive action on complement. All but two (C_4 and C_7) of nine components of complement are destroyed by elastase of *P. aeruginosa* inhibiting the movement of polymorphonuclear leucocytes to the site of inflammation and lowering their phagocytic activity. Inflammatory response is further depressed because lysosomal enzymes are not released.

Human plasma α_1-proteinase inhibitor is the body's principal modulator of serine proteases. The elastase of *P. aeruginosa*, which is not inhibited, has been found by Morihara *et al.* (1979) to inactivate this important inhibitor markedly. Thus serine proteases in tissues are probably activated and inflammatory reaction enhanced.

Protease and elastase may be produced in abundance at the site of infection. *P. aeruginosa* proliferates locally at the site of invasion and, by overcoming host resistance, enters the organs, tissues and blood, leading to death of the host.

Because humoral antibody and phagocytosis play major roles in the host defence mechanisms against *P. aeruginosa*, these features of elastase and protease are thought to be intimately related to the pathogenicity of this micro-organism.

C. Cytotoxins

1. Leucocidin

Leucocidin, a toxin described by Scharmann (1976a,b), was formed by close to 4% of 110 strains of *P. aeruginosa* isolated from man and animals. Leucocidin is incorporated into the cellular structure of bacteria and is not released into culture medium after synthesis. Leucocidin incorporated into the cellular structure shows only mild or no specific activity, and is considered to represent the "precursor" of leucocidin. It elutes from the cellular structure after activation by endogenous protease during autolysis, as shown for *Botulinus* toxin by Sakaguchi and Oishi (1976).

Leucocidin purified by Scharmann is a protein with a molecular weight of 27 500, heat labile, and activated by trypsin but not by pronase. Immunization of rabbits by this toxin resulted in formation of neutralizing antibody. The toxin destroys granulocytes of animals and man and human lymphocytes. One microgram of leucocidin destroys as many as 300 000 leucocytes, suggesting an important role in the pathogenicity of *P. aeruginosa*. Leucocidin acts neither on red cells nor on platelets (Scharmann and Porstendorfeer, 1976).

Leucocidin is adsorbed by human granulocytes, the process being accelerated by calcium ions. It is not active at 4°C. Phase contrast microscopy at 37°C reveals that leucocidin causes spheric transformation of granulocytes, process formation on the cell membrane, an increase in cell size, vacuolation in the cytoplasm, and elution of cellular contents within 2–3 min. Similar changes occur in cell lines in culture after addition of leucocidin.

Lutz (1979) isolated this cytotoxin by the improved method described by Scharmann (1976b). The molecular weight of the toxin was estimated by sodium sulphate gel electrophoresis (25 100) and by gel chromatography (22 300–22 800), which was slightly less than the leucocidin isolated by Scharmann (1976b). The protein contains neither carbohydrate nor lipids. In a slide adhesion test with human granulocytes ED_{100} of cell swelling was 9 µg ml^{-1}. The ED_{50} for growth inhibition of chick embryo fibroblasts was 11 µg ml^{-1}. At 44 µg ml^{-1} the toxin liberated half of the haemoglobin in rabbit red cells, but did not haemolyse erythrocytes of sheep, horse and cow. The LD_{50} in mice was 25 ng g^{-1} body weight. In postmortem histological examination of mice, fatty liver necrosis was observed.

This toxin seems to be different from exotoxin A. Staphylococcal leucocidin is toxic only to polymorphonuclear leucocytes (PMN) and macrophages of rabbit, man and mice, whereas the toxin from *P. aeruginosa* is toxic to all cells isolated from parenchyma, their cell lines in cultures and tumour cells except for thrombocytes (Scharmann, 1976b; Frimmer *et al.*, 1976b). The cytopatho-

genic effect was similar in all tests. The toxin causes cardiovascular failure in
mice and rats (Frimmer et al., 1976a).

2. Polymorphonuclear leucocyte (PMN) inhibitor

Nishida et al. (1975) demonstrated a close relationship between the virulence
for mice and the susceptibility of clinical isolates of P. aeruginosa to
phagocytosis and killing by PMN. Furthermore, they found that virulent
strains of P. aeruginosa produce an extracellular substance (PMN inhibitor)
which inhibited phagocytosis and killing by PMN. Nonoyama et al. (1979a,b)
subsequently reported that on purification, PMN inhibitor eluted in a
different fraction from both protease and elastase following DEAE-cellulose
chromatography. According to Nonoyama et al., PMN inhibitor appears to
be a protein with a molecular weight of approximately 65 000 which is
inactivated both by heating and by exposure to proteolytic enzymes. PMN
inhibitor does not inhibit PMN intracellular activity or extracellular release of
lysosomal enzymes but does inhibit Nitro Blue Tetrazolium reduction. PMN
inhibitor has a cytotoxic effect on PMN and inhibits the uptake of [^{14}C]-
tyrosine intact PMN, although it does not inhibit the uptake of either [^{14}C]-
uridine or [^{14}C]-thymine. It has no inhibitory effect on protein synthesis in cell
extracts. The authors mention that further studies are needed to clarify
whether PMN inhibitor is the same substance as exotoxin or leucocidin. PMN
inhibitor seems to be distinct from exotoxin and leucocidin: exotoxin does not
affect the ingestion or killing of bacteria by PMN, and leucocidin has a
molecular weight of 27 000.

Kamimura et al. (1980) found that PMN-resistant strains of P. aeruginosa
had the ability to interfere with phagocytosis of Escherichia coli, whereas
PMN-sensitive strains of P. aeruginosa did not. When mice were infected with
an ordinary nonpathogenic strain of E. coli, the addition of a PMN-resistant
strain of P. aeruginosa resulted in a mortality considerably higher than that
obtained with P. aeruginosa alone, whereas addition of a PMN-sensitive
strain of P. aeruginosa resulted in a mortality no different from that observed
with P. aeruginosa alone. This increased mortality in mixed infection with E.
coli and PMN-resistant P. aeruginosa probably resulted from the facilitation
of tissue invasion by both bacteria from the inoculum site.

3. Mucoid substance

In patients with cystic fibrosis repeated respiratory infections due to P.
aeruginosa causes worsening of the disease (Reynolds et al., 1975, 1976;
Høiby, 1977). Mucoid strains constitute only 0.5–1.7% of P. aeruginosa strains
isolated from ordinary patients but account for 70% of the strains isolated
from patients with cystic fibrosis complicated by respiratory infections (Zierdt
and Williams, 1975).

Sensakovic and Bartell (1974) isolated and purified this mucoid material and found it to differ both chemically and serologically from cell wall lipopolysaccharides. This substance inhibits the phagocytic activities of leucocytes (Schwartzmann and Boring, 1971), possibly due to mechanical inhibitory action on the surface of leucocytes as opposed to any direct injurious effect on leucocytes. The mucous substance inhibits phagocytosis of the homologous strain, washed clear of slime, more severely than that of its heterologous strains. The inhibitory effect of the mucoid material is lost by the additon of antimucoid serum, which is also protective against infections with mucoid *P. aeruginosa* (Mates and Zand, 1973).

In additon, the mucoid substance is known to have leucopenic and lethal actions. Both of these actions are lost after removal of lipids by treatment with acetic acid. The result of animal experiment suggests that leucopenia is ascribable to the deposition in the liver from the bloodstream of leucocytes covered with the mucoid surface material. To discover whether such a mechanism occurs *in vivo*, Dimitracopoulos *et al.* (1974) utilized the phenomenon whereby a minute quantity of mucoid material inhibits indirect haemagglutination reaction due to purified mucoid. This reaction was sensitive enough to detect 1 μg ml^{-1} of mucoid. Experimentally, mucoid in plasma and ascites was determined in mice infected with viable *P. aeruginosa*. The degree of inhibition of indirect haemagglutination increased with time following inoculation of viable bacteria. Such inhibition was not seen in mice inoculated with dead bacteria.

Study of mucoid would be valuable for elucidation of the nature of cystic fibrosis of the pancreas.

Glycolipoproteins were isolated by Dimitracopoulos and Bartell (1980) from the slime of each strain. They appeared to be similar chemically when analysed for gross composition. The toxicity of the isolated glycolipoprotein varied insignificantly, except in one strain. Viable cells of each strain and their respective glycolipoproteins caused leucopenia, which occurs in the course of lethal infection. The antisera to the glycolipoproteins protected mice in every case against infection by homologous strains. In some cases, various degrees of cross-protection were observed.

III. VIRULENCE

One basis for the virulence of *P. aeruginosa* has been attributed to its resistance to the bactericidal effects of normal serum (Young and Armstrong, 1972). Most strains are serum-resistant. *Pseudomonas* strains, however, differ in their resistance or sensitivity to phagocytosis or killing by PMN. The resistant strains were found to be virulent as determined by the lethal dose values for mouse infection (Nishida *et al.*, 1975, 1979a). As the circulating neutrophil and monocyte population and the fixed cells of the reticulo-endothelial system are important in host defence in the case of *Pseudomonas* infections, these properties of *P. aeruginosa* will be considered as important virulence factors. The virulence of a given strain of *P. aeruginosa* differs significantly, depending on the challenge routes, modes of infection and species of experimental animals used.

As mentioned earlier, the difference in virulence between protease- and elastase-producing strains and non-producing strains of *P. aeruginosa* has been proved in animal models, e.g. in corneal ulcer in mice, burn in mice and ligated intestine in rabbits and pneumonia in mink (Shimizu *et al.*, 1976). However, it is unlikely that protease by itself is responsible for the lethality of the organism. Kawaharajo and Homma (1975c), Holder and Haidaris (1979), and Pavlovskis and Wretlind (1979) have suggested that protease or elastase may act as aggressins, overcoming the host's initial defence mechanisms.

Elastase- and protease-producing strains M2, PF2243, IFO3455 and No. 5 are highly virulent when inoculated subcutaneously in the mouse burn model: fewer than 10 live bacteria used in this way can kill mice, while it requires more than 10^6 of the same bacteria to kill mice by intraperitoneal challenge. The LD_{50} of these strains given intraperitoneally is about the same as the LD_{50} of strains PA103, N10 and NC5, which do not produce protease or elastase (Kawaharajo and Homma, 1977). Thus infection by the intraperitoneal route seems to negate any advantage the protease-producing strains might have.

In the case of experimental haemorrhagic pneumonia in mink, the LD_{50} of strain No. 5 is fewer than 100 live bacteria by intranasal injection but more than 10^6 by' subcutaneous injection.

Further evidence for the role of protease and elastase as virulence factors comes from a study in which mink were immunized against *Pseudomonas* infection using a common antigen (designated as OEP) of *P. aeruginosa* with and without protease and elastase toxoids (Homma *et al.*, 1978). Immuniz-ation with OEP plus toxoids provided significantly greater protection than when OEP alone was used. It was also observed that mice immunized with toxoids of elastase and protease showed increased resistance to experimental *P. aeruginosa* infections such as corneal ulcers and burn wounds, suggesting that the exoenzymes contribute to the pathogeneses of the organism (Sections IVB2 and IVC3).

Ohman *et al.* (1980) reported that exotoxin plays at least two roles in corneal infections: inhibition of the host's bacterial clearance mechanism and destruction of corneal tissue. It is clear that several pathogenic factors are involved in corneal infections due to *P. aeruginosa*.

Using the mouse burn model devised by Holder and Jogan (1971) and Stieritz and Holder (1975), direct and indirect evidence has been presented by

Saelinger *et al.* (1977), Stiertz and Holder (1978) and Pavlovskis *et al.* (1976, 1978) that exotoxin is a prime – but not necessarily the only – virulence factor for this organism.

Antibody levels of elastase, protease and exotoxin were found to rise in serum of patients and animals suffering from *P. aeruginosa* infections (Takeshi and Homma, 1978; Cho *et al.*, 1978).

Cytotoxins purified by Scharmann *et al.* (1976a,b) and Lutz (1979) are one of the toxic substances produced by *P. aeruginosa*. However, they were produced by less than 4% of 110 clinical isolates. Both cytotoxins and PMN inhibitor may sometimes play important roles in the pathogenicity of *P. aeruginosa*, significantly reducing the phagocytic and killing activities of PMN at the site of infection.

The mechanism which normally keeps Gram-negative bacilli from the oropharyngeal flora of healthy individuals may become impaired in stress. This colonization is associated with the adherence of the colonizing species to the epithelium. Mediators of adherence that have been studied include surface appendages such as pili or chemical structures of lipopolysaccharide of endotoxin. In *P. aeruginosa* infection, it has been suggested by Sadoff (1974) that pili may mediate bacterial attachment to epithelial cells, as has been shown with *Escherichia coli*. Woods *et al.* (1980) indicated that adherence of *P. aeruginosa* to the upper respiratory epithelium of seriously ill patients *in vitro* could be correlated with the subsequent colonization of the respiratory tract by this opportunistic pathogen. The role of pili in the attachment of *P. aeruginosa* to epithelial cells was studied in an *in vitro* system employing human buccal epithelial cells and *P. aeruginosa* pretreated chemically and serologically. The findings seem to indicate that pili mediate the adherence of *P. aeruginosa* organisms to human buccal epithelial cells. Colonization of epithelial cells is often a critical event in the pathogenesis of *Pseudomonas* infections in the immuno-compromised host.

Recently Moulton *et al.* (1980) demonstrated that motility and/or chemotactic ability were associated with the virulence of *P. aeruginosa* strains. Highly chemotactic and/or motile strains had lower LD_{50}s when tested in a burned mouse model, and motility-deficient mutants were found to be less virulent than their wild type parents in burned rat model (McManus *et al.*, 1980).

IV.   IMMUNOLOGICAL APPROACH TO THE PROPHYLAXIS OF *P. AERUGINOSA* INFECTION

Pennington (1979) has published a review, *Immunotherapy of* P. aeruginosa *Infection*, in which the present status of *P. aeruginosa* vaccines is described in detail. In a review entitled *Immunologic Approaches to the Prophylaxis and Treatment of* P. aeruginosa *Infection*, Young and Pollack (1979) have summarized the results of immunization with *P. aeruginosa* vaccines.

The *P. aeruginosa* vaccines widely used at present for human trials consist mainly of lipopolysaccharides (O antigens). From the observation that animals immunized with lipopolysaccharide can only be protected from exposure to live bacteria with the serologically homologous O antigen, the vaccine must be mixed with as many as lipopolysaccharides as possible if it is to be effective in preventing and treating infections due to *P. aeruginosa* with its numerous serovars.

The serological diversity of the O antigens leads to a variety of serovars. Summarizing the results so far obtained on agglutination reactions (Kodama and Ishimoto, 1976; Yabuuchi *et al.*, 1976; Hirao *et al.*, 1977; Homma *et al.*, 1977; Kono and Sei, 1977; Shionoya *et al.*, 1977; Terada *et al.*, 1977), the Serotyping Committee of the Japan *Pseudomonas aeruginosa* Society (Homma, 1976; Homma *et al.*, 1979) delineated the classification schema based on the major O group antigens of *P. aeruginosa* shown in Table 1. Correspondence of the major O antigens of the 7 schemata used widely throughout the world is shown in Table 1.

As mentioned above, to be effective lipopolysaccharide vaccines must include as wide a variety of O antigens as possible. The most serious problem in utilizing such a vaccine has been adverse side effects. Local as well as systemic symptons, such as chills, fever, headache and malaise, can occur. The inoculation dose of the vaccine is usually restricted by these side-effects, which makes it difficult to elevate antibody titres against all the O antigens included in the vaccine. Moreover, the most widely available lipopolysaccharide vaccines appear to elicit IgM responses preferentially although it appears that IgG-type antibodies are more protective against *Pseudomonas* infection than short-lived IgM antibodies (Bjornson and Michael, 1972).

The relatively high incidence of side-effects from lipopolysaccharide vaccines has prompted a search for less toxic immunizing substances. Pier *et al.* (1978a,b, 1981) isolated a high-molecular-weight alkali-labile polysaccharide (PS) from the slime of *Pseudomonas aeruginosa* immunotype 1 of Fisher *et al.* (1969). An antigen immunologically indistinguishable from PS was also obtained from LPS. PS is non-pyrogenic in rabbits and non-toxic in mice at high doses. The material protects mice from challenge with live, homologous organisms. The chemical nature of PS seems to resemble that of the "O" side chain of LPS but differs in molecular size and chemical composition. Pier *et al.* (1980) immunized volunteers with PS, eliciting minor reactions in one half of them. Further studies are in progress.

Other vaccines, such as ribosomal vaccine (Lieberman, 1978) and flagella vaccine (Montie *et al.*, personal communication) are being developed.

Table 1   Correspondence of O antigen group of *Pseudomonas aeruginosa* of various serotyping systems

O antigen group	Homma	Lanyi	Habs	Liu	Verder Evans	Fisher	Meitert
A	1	1	3	3	VI	—	5
	2			2			2
B	7	3	2	5	I	3	6
	13		5	16H	X	7	16
	16			16L			
				7	7		
C	3	5	8	8	VIII	6	3
D	4	10	9	9	IX	—	14
E	5	7	11	11	III	2	15
F	6	11	4	4	—	—	8
G	8	4	6	6	II	1	1
							4
H	9	2	10	10	—	5	11
I	10	6	1	1	IV	4	13
J	11	12	—	15	—	—	—
				13			
K	12	—	—	14	V	—	—
L	14	13	12	12	VII	—	7
M	15	9					
	17		—	—	—	—	—
	—	8	—	—	—	—	—

From Homma (1976) and Homma *et al.* (1979) (reproduced with permission of the publisher).

Interest has also been directed toward the development of a vaccine containing an antigen common to all strains of *P. aeruginosa*, taking into consideration various virulence factors. It is believed that such a vaccine would offer wider protection and be less toxic than those presently available.

A. Protein common antigen

Homma (1971) isolated a protein moiety which is normally complexed with LPS in the cell wall of *P. aeruginosa*. This cell wall protein, originally labelled cell wall protein A, has now become known as original endotoxin protein (OEP).

OEP vaccine is prepared from an autolysate of *P. aeruginosa* N10, belonging to serotype 5 of Homma's serotype schema. Purified OEP consists of 77% protein, 4.5% total sugars, 8.8% lipid, 4.5% hexosamine and 1.2% phosphorus. The antigen has been proved to possess a common protective property against *P. aeruginosa* infections regardless of serotype and also to possess an antigen common to all the serotype strains of *P. aeruginosa* (Homma, 1971, 1975; Homma and Abe, 1972; Homma *et al.*, 1976; Abe *et al.*, 1975, 1977; Shimizu *et al.*, 1976).

When OEP was subjected to protease digestion, the protein content of the protease-treated OEP was reduced to 17% without change in lipid or sugar composition. The protease-treated OEP no longer possessed a serologically common antigen and was also found to have lost the common protecti've property against infections due to all the serotypes of *P. aeruginosa* (Abe *et al.*, 1977; Tanamoto *et al.*, 1978).

Hirao and Homma (1978a) proved that purified IgG antibodies cross-reacting with the OEP of *P. aeruginosa* (derived from *Vibrio cholerae* immune rabbit sera by OEP-coupled affinity chromatography) protected mice against *P. aeruginosa* infection when compared with the control group, which was injected with 100 µg of normal IgG not containing OEP antibody. The purified antibodies (2.5 µg per mouse) protected animals challenged with approximately 10 000 times the LD_{50} of *P. aeruginosa* for the control group. The common antigen (OEP) of *P. aeruginosa* proved also to be a common antigen of *V. cholerae* both serologically and in possessing infection protective properties. As there is no chemical or serological similarity between *P. aeruginosa* and *V. cholerae* LPS, any cross-reactivity between the two species is likely to be related to the protein moiety of OEP.

Yamamoto *et al.* (1979) reported that immunization with OEP of *P. aeruginosa* produced a high level of protection in mice against *V. cholerae* infection. In immune mouse serum the average OEP–PHA titre was 1600. However, neither vibriocidal nor agglutinin titre against *V. cholerae* was seen in the serum of mice immunized with OEP. Mice were also protected against challenge with *V. cholerae* by the passive administration of anti-OEP rabbit serum.

Haranaka *et al.* (1975) studied the effect of immunosuppressive therapy on fatal *Pseudomonas* infection in mice. Groups of mice were treated with 100 mg kg^{-1} of cyclophosphamide, azathioprine, or cortisone acetate 1 day prior to infection. The differential effect of these drugs on T and B cell lymphocyte populations was examined by the anti-θ cytotoxicity test. The main effect of cortisone and azathioprine was a reduction of T lymphocytes. Cyclophosphamide reduced mainly B cells. In drug-treated animals the LD_{50} of *Pseudomonas* given intraperitoneally was reduced from 2.9×10^3 in controls to 1.2×10^2 organisms ml $^{-1}$. Passive transfer of an anti-OEP antibody $F(ab')_2$ just after the infective challenge gave complete protection to normal and immunosuppressed mice challenged with 200 times the LD_{50} of *Pseudomonas*.

It has been proved that the protein moiety of OEP is responsible for the activity of a serologically common as well as protective antigen in *P.*

aeruginosa and *Vibrio cholerae* (Hirao and Homma, 1978b; Yamamoto *et al.*, 1979) and that it is also responsible for IgE antibody response (Cho *et al.*, 1978). In contrast, antitumour (Hoshi *et al.*, 1973a,b) and interferon-inducing (Kojima *et al.*, 1971) activities, adjuvanticity (Sasaki *et al.*, 1975) and nonspecific protective properties (Fukui *et al.*, 1971) reside in the lipopolysaccharide moiety of the OEP. Tanamoto *et al.* (1978, 1979) and Cho *et al.* (1979) investigated the relationship between the chemical structures of lipopolysaccharides and their derivatives on antitumour and interferon-inducing activities and adjuvanticity. It was shown that, for the inhibition of ascites tumour development, lipid A alone is not sufficient and a saccharide such as 3-deoxymanno-octulonic acid is necessary to link the structure of the lipid A portion. In contrast, the incomplete lipid A with amide-linked fatty acid alone is sufficient to induce interferon. The lipid A portion with an adequate amount of ester-linked fatty acids as well as amide-linked fatty acid is essential to demonstrate adjuvanticity. Thus it seems that adjuvanticity, antitumour and interferon-inducing activities of the lipopolysaccharide can be dissociated according to the chemical structures of lipid A and its derivatives.

In an investigation of immunological cross-reactivity between *P. aeruginosa* and 36 other bacterial species, Høiby (1976) reported that 30 species, representing a wide range of Gram-negative and two Gram-positive microorganisms, showed cross-reactions with an antigen represented by a certain precipitate of the crossed immunoelectrophoretic reference system for *P. aeruginosa*. This antigen (designated CA) was obtained in pure form by a combination of salting-out with 18% (w/v) sodium sulphate and gel filtration on Sephadex G-200 (Sompolinsky *et al.*, 1980). The common antigen was shown to be a protein composed of polypeptide subunits of molecular weight of about 62 000. The molecular weight of CA was estimated as 665 000–900 000, depending on the analytical methods used. The isoelectric point was to be pH 4.4. During *P. aeruginosa* infections the peak level antibody response included increased CA antibodies in patients (Høiby *et al.*, 1980).

It would be of interest to clarify the serological relationship between OEP and CA. It may also be important to determine whether CA contains a fraction of the cytoplasmic membrane of *P. aeruginosa*, as Yamamoto and Homma (1978) have found a serologically common antigen among L-forms of *P. aeruginosa* irrespective of their serovars. This common antigen of L-forms of *P. aeruginosa* was also found to cross-react partially with an L-form of *Streptococcus pyogenes*.

It is also important from a practical viewpoint to investigate whether CA is a common protective antigen of *P. aeruginosa* regardless of serovar.

B. Toxoids of exotoxin, protease and elastase

1. *Exotoxin toxoid*

Abe *et al.* (1978) reported that the toxic activity of exotoxin, dialysed against 1% formalin solutions containing 0.2 M L-lysine at 37°C, was completely neutralized on the first day after dialysis. Addition of L-lysine to the formalin solution was essential for this rapid decrease in toxicity. ADP-ribosylation activity as well as lethality and guinea pig skin necrotizing activity (Takeshi *et al.*, 1977) were found to be completely neutralized.

To estimate immunogenicity of exotoxin toxoid, Abe *et al.* (1978) injected mice twice (1 week apart) in the footpad with 5 μg of the preparation in Freund's incomplete adjuvant. One week after the second injection, the mice were injected twice intraperitoneally with 10 μg of the preparation without adjuvant with an interval of 4 weeks. One ml of the combined antiserum after the 4th injection was found to neutralize 6400 MRD (minimum reacting dose of the skin) and 2100 LD_{50}. ADP-ribosylation activity of rat liver EF-2 of the native exotoxin also proved to be neutralized by the antiserum.

Mice immunized with the exotoxin toxoid in the same manner as above were injected intraperitoneally with 100 μg of the purified exotoxin, 1 μg of which corresponds to a dose of 13 LD_{50} against mice, and observed for 7 days. They showed no toxic symptoms. One ml of the anti-exotoxin rabbit serum was found sufficient to neutralize 20 000 MRD and 8230 LD_{50}. ADP-ribosylation activity of rat liver EF-2 of the exotoxin was neutralized by the anti-exotoxin rabbit serum. From these results it is apparent that exotoxin toxoid was prepared successfully using formalin and L-lysine.

The finding of Abe *et al.* (1978) that exotoxin toxoid can be prepared by using formalin and L-lysine has been confirmed by Pavlovskis *et al.* (personal communication). They used similar preparations to evaluate its immuno-prophylactic potential in a burned mouse *P. aeruginosa* infection model (Holder and Jogan, 1971) which closely resembled human burn sepsis. Results indicate that, in the amounts used, the toxoid had no demonstrable toxicity for the mouse and that it may be useful in prophylaxis of *Pseudomonas* infections.

According to Pavlovskis *et al.*, the formalin and L-lysine treated toxoid showed marked reduction in lethality and in guinea pig skin necrotizing activity, and at least a 200-fold decrease in L-cell cytotoxicity. No tissue damage was detectable by light microscopy, nor was altered S-GOT and S-GPT enzyme activity observed in mice injected with the toxoid. Immunization of mice with 3 or 4 doses (10 μg each) of toxoid and the synthetic adjuvant, *N*-acetylmuramyl-L-alanyl-D-isoglutamine (50 μg), induced high levels of anti-exotoxin antibodies as measured by passive haemagglutination assay and enzyme-linked immunosorbent assay. Immunization with toxoid alone did not induce high levels of circulating antitoxin. A significant increase in survival time and survival rate ($P < 0.01$) was seen in immunized burned and infected mice (50–85%) as compared with control mice immunized with formalinized bovine serum albumin (6–20%). Virtually 100% survival was obtained when preinfection immunization was combined with single dose gentamicin treatment within 24 hours of infection. Immunization with glutaraldehyde-treated exotoxin increased survival time but did not increase survival rate, and the results generally were not as satisfactory as those obtained using formalinized exotoxin.

Cryz et al. (1981a) have also studied the effects of formalin on the structure-activity, antigenicity and immunogenicity of exotoxin. They reported that formalin treatment altered the toxicity, antigenicity and structure of exotoxin in a time-dependent manner but had no adverse effect on enzymatic activity. The addition of L-lysine to formalin–toxin mixtures not only resulted in an increase in the rate and extent to which the above parameters were affected but also completely destroyed enzymatic activity. On dialysis and storage, formalin-derived toxoid was found to undergo partial toxic reversion, whereas a formalin–lysine toxoid did not.

Although there are several discrepancies in the data presented by these laboratories, it can be said that active immunization with formalin–lysine-treated exotoxin and adjuvant induced, in varying degrees, protective immunity against infections in mice and may be of potential use in prophylaxis of P. aeruginosa infections in burned mice.

The protective effect of intravenously administered rabbit anti-exotoxin serum was studied by Pavlovskis et al. (1977) in lethal P. aeruginosa burn infections in mice. Survival after infection with 2 median lethal doses of a toxigenic, low-protease-producing strain (PA103) was enhanced in antitoxin-treated mice compared with controls that had received anti-bovine serum albumin serum ($P = 0.0004$). In contrast, anti-exotoxin had no protective effect in mice challenged with a nontoxigenic strain. After infection with toxigenic organisms there were fewer viable bacteria in blood and liver of mice given antitoxin than in those of controls treated with anti-bovine serum albumin, while there were no significant differences between the two groups after challenge with nontoxigenic organisms. This suggests that P. aeruginosa exotoxin contributes to lethality in the burn infection model, and that its effect is diminished by passive immunization with antitoxin. This may be due to the finding reported by Pavlovskis et al. (1978) that treatment of mice with antitoxin before infection with strain PA103 prevented inactivation of EF-2.

Cryz et al. (1981b,c) have isolated a mutant of P. aeruginosa strain PAO-1, which produces a nontoxic protein immunologically indistinguishable from native toxin. Such studies are important not only for a better understanding of the immunochemistry and structure-function of the toxin molecule, but also for the potential use of the protein as a vaccine.

2. Toxoids of protease and elastase

Homma *et al.* (1978) prepared toxoids of protease and elastase in the following manner. Crystalline protease from *P. aeruginosa* IFO3080 (1 mg ml^{-1}) in 0.1 M phosphate buffer (pH 7) was almost stable in the presence of 8% formalin for 4 days at room temperature. Addition of 0.2 M L-lysine to the reaction mixture resulted in marked decrease of enzymic activity, while addition of L-alanine or acetamide affected it only slightly. Other amino acids such as L-arginine, L-leucine, L-tyrosine, and L-glutamic acid were also ineffective. The effect of pH on the inactivation was about the same within the range 6 to 9.

Accordingly, the protease toxoid was prepared using 8% formalin and 0.2 M L-lysine (pH 7). The mixture was kept at room temperature for 2 days and then passed through a Sephadex G-50 column using distilled water as effluent. The protein fraction corresponding to molecular weight 50 000–60 000 was collected and lyophilized. The amino acid composition of protease toxoid, except for lysine and tyrosine, is very similar to that of the protease used as the starting material. The inconsistency concerning lysine and tyrosine would seem to indicate that lysine used for formalin-treatment of protease was incorporated in the protease toxoid molecule and that all the tyrosine residues of protease were modified by the treatment.

Crystalline elastase derived from *P. aeruginosa* IFO3455 was used for preparing its toxoid. The reaction mixture containing elastase (2 mg ml^{-1}), 4% formalin, and 0.2 M borate buffer (pH 9) was kept overnight at about 4°C. The enzymatic activity was lost almost completely. The mixture was passed through a Sephadex G-50 column (effluent, distilled water) and the protein fraction corresponding to molecular weight 25 000–50 000 was collected and lyophilized. The amino acid composition of elastase toxoid is very similar to that of elastase, except for tyrosine; this is to be expected because of treatment with formalin.

In the serum of rabbits immunized with the protease toxoid or elastase toxoid with Freund's incomplete adjuvant, high antibody levels were found by passive haemagglutination tests using protease- or elastase-sensitized sheep blood cells. At the same time it was proved that these sera also possessed high enzyme-neutralizing activities when mixed with native protease or elastase.

The effectiveness of immunizing mice with protease or elastase toxoid on corneal ulceration due to either protease or elastase was investigated by Hirao and Homma (1978b). Mice immunized with either toxoid were protected from corneal ulcers induced by the homologous but not the heterologous enzyme.

As mentioned in Section II B, Pavlovskis and Wretlind (1979) suggested that protease contributed to the invasiveness of *P. aeruginosa*. In the same paper, they also reported that the survival of mice infected with protease-producing *Pseudomonas* was enhanced by anti-protease serum. Anti-protease serum had no effect in mice infected with protease-deficient mutants.

Phosphoramidon (N-α-rhamnopyranosyloxy-(hydroxyphosphinil)-L-leu cyl-L-tryprophan) from a culture filtrate of *Streptomyces tanashiensis* was found by Suda *et al.* (1973) to be a powerful inhibitor of thermolysin. Further work (Komiyama *et al.*, 1975) indicated that the inhibitor was also highly effective against other neutral metallo proteases from *B. subtilis* and *Streptomyces griseus* K-1. From these results, Morihara and Tsuzuki (1978) proved that phosphoramidon was also a powerful inhibitor of elastases obtained from various *P. aeruginosa* strains. This was consistent with their previous assumption that the elastases produced in different broths of *P. aeruginosa* were identical regardless of strain. The same was true of the proteases (Morihara and Tsuzuki, 1977). These findings suggested that phosphoramidon could be used to neutralize elastase in *Pseudomonas* infections.

The therapeutic effect of phosphoramidon on corneal ulceration due to either *Pseudomonas* elastase or protease was investigated by Kawaharajo and Homma (unpublished data). A suspension of elastase or protease was dropped once onto the incised corneas of mice. The mice were then given phosphoramidon solution either by injection or by eyedrop. Phosphoramidon effectively protected cornea from ulceration caused by elastase but not by protease, although it was ineffective when administered by injection.

Holder and Haidaris (1979) and Holder (1980) presented data indicating that treating burned, *P. aeruginosa* infected mice with a protease inhibitor, α_2-macroglobulin, enhanced survival, but treatment with phosphoramidon did not. Alpha$_2$-macroglobulin treatment causes reduction in bacterial counts in the skin and liver of infected mice 30 hours post burn and infection, and also protects liver EF-2 activity, as compared to controls.

Aoyagi and Umezawa (1975) and Aoyagi *et al.* (1977) have attempted to put enzyme inhibitors derived from various micro-organisms to therapeutic use against various diseases. It seems reasonable to test these enzyme inhibitors, together with α_2-macroglobulin, as alternative therapy, used either alone or in combination with immunization and antibiotics.

Based on experimental results indicating that the pathogenic activities of the virulence factors exotoxin, protease and elastase are neutralized by their homologous antiserum, any consideration of an effective new vaccine must include the three toxoids of exotoxin, protease and elastase.

C. A new multi-component vaccine

1. Background and development

P. aeruginosa produces toxic extracellular substances such as exotoxin, protease and elastase, as well as leucocidin and PMN inhibitor, at the site of infection.

As mentioned above, Young *et al.* (1972) demonstrated *in vivo* that the presence of polymorphonuclear leucocytes (PMNs) is critical to *Pseudomonas* killing but optimal phagocytosis occurs only in the presence of *Pseudomonas*-specific opsonizing antibody and complement. For this reason, increasing antibody titres against *Pseudomonas* somatic surface antigen in the host may be effective in decreasing the incidence and mortality of *Pseudomonas* infection. It appears that IgG-type antibodies are more protective than IgM against *Pseudomonas*.

Lipopolysaccharide appears to elicit IgM response preferentially, while OEP elicits both IgG and IgM. Haranaka *et al.* (1975, 1977) reported that isologous, complement non-binding $F(ab')_2$ against OEP was highly protective against infections in mice compromised by immunosuppressants or ^{60}Co irradiation. They also showed that the phagocytic activity of murine splenic macrophages clearly increased upon addition of specific antibodies against OEP. Addition of antibiotics increased intracellular bactericidal action as well as phagocytic activity.

Okada *et al.* (1980), using the Holder mouse burn model, demonstrated that somatic antigen is essential to the effectiveness of the combined vaccine consisting of OEP and toxoids. As there are more than 13 serogroups of *P. aeruginosa* (Homma, 1976) a common protective somatic antigen such as OEP is necessary as an essential component of the multi-component vaccine. To increase the effectiveness of the vaccine, toxoids of the virulent factors exotoxin, protease and elastase are added to the somatic antigen OEP.

Homma *et al.* (1978) prepared a multi-component vaccine consisting of OEP plus toxoids of protease and elastase, which has been used in experimental animal infections with adjuvant of potash alum or Freund's incomplete adjuvant.

2. Trials in corneal ulcers of animals

The therapeutic effects of vaccination with various vaccines consisting of one, two or three components (protease toxoid, elastase toxoid and/or the common antigen (OEP) of *P. aeruginosa*) were examined by Hirao and Homma (1978b) on mouse corneal ulcers produced by live cultures of *P. aeruginosa*. For the same purpose, administration of a single or combined rabbit immune serum against protease toxoid, elastase toxoid and OEP was conducted. As a result, vaccination with the three-component mixed vaccine or administration of combined rabbit immune serum was found to be most effective in the prevention as well as treatment of corneal ulcers in mice.

To investigate therapy of corneal ulcers caused by *Pseudomonas* infection, Kawaharajo and Homma (1976) examined the synergistic effects of immune γ-globulin fraction containing antibodies against OEP, protease and elastase of *Pseudomonas* on the activity of the antibiotic, dibekacin (DKB), in cornea of mice. The median effective dose (ED_{50}) of DKB alone injected intramuscularly against corneal ulcers caused by strain IFO3455 of *P. aeruginosa* in experimentally incised mice was 620 μg per mouse. When the γ-globulin fraction was given subcutaneously to each mouse prior to infection, central corneal opacity rather than severe ulceration was observed. The immune γ-globulin fraction was far more effective in protecting the cornea from infection than the control calf serum. The ED_{50} values of DKB combined with immune γ-globulin was significantly different from those of DKB and control serum. There was no statistical difference between the ED_{50} values of DKB combined with the calf serum and DKB alone.

Tanaka *et al.* (1978) investigated immunotherapy for experimental *Pseudomonas* keratitis using albino rabbits. Active immunization with OEP, protease toxoid and elastase toxoid was found to be effective in preventing keratitis of corneas incised and infected with *P. aeruginosa* strain IFO3455. Intrastromal injection of the immune serum containing antibodies against OEP, protease toxoid and elastase toxoid showed a significant therapeutic effect on cornea ulcers in rabbits. Ueda *et al.* (1980) also reported that immunization of horses with the three-component mixed vaccine was effective in preventing corneal ulceration due to *P. aeruginosa* IFO3455. Intrastromal injection of the immune serum containing antibodies against OEP and the two toxoids was also effective. Oishi *et al.* (1977) examined therapeutic effects of antibiotics combined with γ-globulin containing OEP and toxoids of protease and elastase and antibiotic on endophthalmitis induced experimentally by *P. aeruginosa* in rabbits and clearly recognized the synergistic effect of DKB and the γ-globulin.

3. Trials on haemorrhagic pneumonia in mink

Because mink, especially as kittens, are known to be very susceptible to *P. aeruginosa* infection, the prophylactic effect of immunization with OEP, protease toxoid and elastase toxoid was examined on experimental as well as enzootic mink haemorrhagic pneumonia due to *P. aeruginosa*.

Enzootic of haemorrhagic pneumonia in mink due to *P. aeruginosa* has been shown to occur world-wide, causing much financial loss (Knox, 1953). Formalinized autologous vaccine was found to be effective in preventing the spread of infection and in protecting against subsequent challenge (Farrel *et al.*, 1958; Mansi *et al.*, 1965; Haagsma and Pereboom, 1965; Nordstoga, 1968; Karlson *et al.*, 1971; Takashima *et al.*, 1975).

(a) Effectiveness of immunization with single- and multi-component vaccines against experimental haemorrhagic pneumonia due to P. aeruginosa *in mink*
Experiments performed by Homma *et al.* (1978) involved a total of 100 female Sapphire mink, 3.5 months old and reared in separate cages.

P. aeruginosa strain No. 5, serotype 8 (according to Homma's schema,

1974, 1976) was used for challenge. This strain produces protease, elastase and exotoxin. The strain was cultured on nutrient agar medium at 37°C for 18 hours and suspended in a nutrient broth. Serial 10-fold dilutions were prepared from this bacterial suspension. A small vinyl tube (1.5 mm) was inserted into the nostril of the mink and 0.5 ml of the inoculum in a syringe was injected into the nasal cavity. Just before inoculation, all the mink were anaesthetized with ether.

Mink were immunized three times in one month with either the single-component or the multi-component vaccine. There was no significant difference between the OEP-passive haemagglutination titres of the sera from mink immunized with OEP alone (group A) and those immunized with the multi-component vaccine (group E). On the 12th day after the last immunization, challenge exposure with $P.$ $aeruginosa$ strain No. 5 (serotype 8 according to Homma's schema, Homma, 1974, 1976) was effected by administration of an inoculum containing serial dilutions from 10^3 to 10^{10} live bacteria into the nostril of each mink. The results are shown in Table 2.

There was no significant difference in the survival of the nonimmunized control group G and control group F, which was immunized with potash alum alone. With the OEP-vaccinated group A and group E immunized with the multi-component vaccine, the LD_{50} values differed clearly from those of the control groups G and F. The multi-component vaccine was much more effective than the single-component OEP vaccine.

The effectiveness of the multi-component vaccine has been investigated by Takeuchi et al. (1979, unpublished data). Mink vaccinated twice at an interval of two weeks with three different doses (50, 100, 200 µg) of each component, OEP, protease toxoid and elastase toxoid, were found to have about the same antibody levels of OEP, protease and elastase and to be given sufficient immunity to resist intranasal infection with $P.$ $aeruginosa$. A similar experiment conducted with the multi-component vaccine showed that this was significantly more effective than the OEP alone.

Pathological findings were as follows. Macroscopically, there was acute haemorrhagic pneumonia (lobar distribution) in dead mink from each experimental group. Microscopically, the lungs showed acute haemorrhagic fibrino-purulent and necrotic pneumonia. The most typical lesions of the disease were vascular changes in the lungs characterized by massive bacterial invasion of arterial and venous walls and a lack of perivascular cuffing. These changes were identical to the "$Pseudomonas$ vasculitis" described in previous reports (Trautwein et al., 1962; Teplits, 1965; Nordstoga, 1968). $Pseudomonas$ vasculitis would appear to be pathognomonic of fulminant infection due to $P.$ $aeruginosa$. In contrast, in surviving mink, although perivascular cuffing in the small arteries and veins was noted, there were no bacteria.

Teplits (1965) suggests that the $Pseudomonas$ septic lesions in the viscera of

Table 2 Immunization effects of the single- and the multi-component vaccine on protection of mink against challenge by *Pseudomonas aeruginosa* strain No. 5 into nostril

Vaccinated group	Challenge inoculum	No. of mink		LD_{50}
		Challenge-exposed	Survivors	
A (OEP)	1.5×10^6	5	2	
	1.5×10^7	5	3	
	1.5×10^8	5	0	$\leq 7.5 \times 10^6$
	1.5×10^9	5	0	
	1.5×10^{10}	5	0	
E (Multi-component vaccine)	1.5×10^6	5	4	
	1.5×10^7	5	4	
	1.5×10^8	5	3	$\leq 1.9 \times 10^8$
	1.5×10^9	5	1	
	1.5×10^{10}	5	0	
F (K-alum)	1.5×10^3	5	4	
	1.5×10^4	5	1	
	1.5×10^5	5	1	$\leq 1.2 \times 10^4$
	1.5×10^6	5	1	
	1.5×10^7	5	0	
G (Non-immunized)	1.5×10^3	5	1	
	1.5×10^4	5	2	
	1.5×10^5	5	2	$\leq 7.5 \times 10^3$
	1.5×10^6	5	1	
	1.5×10^7	5	0	

From Homma *et al.* (1978) (reproduced with permission of the publisher).

rats and skin of rabbits are initiated at the capillary level, that the dense transmural arterial or venous bacillary infiltration characteristics of *Pseudomonas* vasculitis is the consequence of perivascular (centripetal) rather than direct haematogenous invasion, and that the characteristic haemorrhagic necrosis of the lesions is generally attributable to diffuse bacterial tissue invasion, rather than to the vasculitis *per se*.

Homma *et al.* (1978) speculated that *P. aeruginosa*, which was inhaled in fine droplets and deposited along the bronchial or bronchiolar mucosa and possibly even in the alveoli, produced slight catarrhal bronchitis or bronchiolotis. Then, after the breakdown of the surface barrier, the bacteria spread rapidly by both endobronchial and peribronchial routes as well as through connective tissues and blood vessels. Focal desquamative alveolitis was often found in the peribronchial areas. Intramural emigration or partial accumulation of polymorphonuclear leucocytes, sometimes with transmural bacillary penetration, was observed in the walls of the blood vessels. In particular, *P. aeruginosa* strain No. 5 (Homma's serotype 8), producing protease, elastase and exotoxin, used in these experiments, showed high virulence in mink (Shimizu *et al.*, 1974). The protease and elastase from *P. aeruginosa* were capable of inducing haemorrhages in various organs. Thus it seems that *P. aeruginosa* invades the walls of the blood vessels and causes the ensuing vascular injury by direct toxic action resulting in haemorrhagic necrosis of surrounding tissue. In mink, interlobular septa are minor, and confluence of the focal fibrinous pneumonia can result in a lobar distribution. *Pseudomonas* vasculitis in the lungs occasionally causes metastatic septic lesions in other visceral organs, e.g. the regional lymph nodes, liver and kidneys.

In surviving mink, the most characteristic lesions of the lungs were focal desquamative alveolitis and perivascular cuffing. In these vascular lesions, there were usually no bacteria, but sometimes a few phagocytic macrophages were seen.

(b)   Effect of the multi-component vaccine on protection against enzootic of haemorrhagic pneumonia due to P. aeruginosa *in mink*
(i) Vaccination with a single component vaccine (OEP alone) was performed for the first time on an enzootic of pneumonia due to *P. aeruginosa* in mink which occurred in 1974. This was partially effective in preventing the spread of infection (Takashima *et al.*, 1975).

The multi-component vaccine was used for the first time for preventive and therapeutic purposes against an outbreak of haemorrhagic pneumonia in mink in 1975.

From September 5 to October 24, 1975, an enzootic of haemorrhagic pneumonia due to *P. aeruginosa* broke out on three adjoining farms (A, B and C) located in Hokkaido, Japan, each raising about 2000 to 3000 mink. A large number of mink succumbed to the infection on farms A and B, but on farm C only a few died. Half of the mink on farm C had been vaccinated prior to the onset of the enzootic. *P. aeruginosa*, serotype 3 (according to Homma's schema, 1971, 1974), was isolated in abundance from lung, liver, kidney and blood of dead mink. This strain was found to produce protease, elastase and exotoxin.

Some examples of the effects of the vaccine containing OEP alone and that containing OEP plus toxoids, taken from the report of Honda *et al.* (1977), are as follows. The effects of the vaccines were compared in male and female kittens and adult mink in each shed, since the lethality rate in unvaccinated mink is higher in male kittens than in adults (Knox, 1953; Mansi *et al.*, 1965 and Takashima *et al.*, 1975). In shed 4 of farm A, the first death occurred 6 days after the first vaccination. The death rate of mink vaccinated with OEP was lower than that of unvaccinated mink (Fig. 1). The difference in the number of deaths between vaccinated and unvaccinated mink was significant ($P < 0.001$, χ^2 test).

In sheds 5 and 6 of farm A, enzootic occurred and many mink died before vaccination. Of the dead mink, 65.3% (shed 5) and 71.0% (shed 6) died before the first vaccination and in the 8 days after the first vaccination.

In shed 5, the first death occurred 12 days before the first vaccination. The death rate of mink vaccinated with OEP and those not vaccinated was high (49.4% and 46.9%), and the difference between the two was not significant. Vaccination with OEP plus toxoids reduced the death rate by half (23.1%). The difference between OEP plus toxoids and the control was significant ($P < 0.01$).

In shed 6, the first death occurred on September 14, 3 days before the first vaccination. The death rate of male kittens in decreasing order was as follows: unvaccinated mink, those vaccinated with OEP alone, and those vaccinated with OEP plus toxoids (Fig. 1). Although the death rate of mink vaccinated with OEP plus toxoids reached 30.7%, the vaccination was found to be effective compared with the controls ($P < 0.001$). The death rate of kittens vaccinated with OEP alone was 48.4% — lower than the rate of unvaccinated kittens (65.0%) but too high to determine the effectiveness of OEP.

On farm B, the first death occurred on September 20, only 3 days after the first vaccination. The death rate of male kittens vaccinated with OEP plus toxoids was lower than that of unvaccinated mink. The difference in death rate between mink vaccinated with OEP plus toxoids (1.8%) and unvaccinated control (36.9%) mink was significant ($P < 0.001$). With OEP alone, the death rate was 5.1%, thus proving its effectiveness ($P < 0.001$). OEP plus toxoids completely protected female mink from death. OEP alone was considered effective ($P \fallingdotseq 0.05$).

OEP plus toxoids was effective in all sheds and farms. OEP alone was ineffective in sheds 5 and 6 of farm A, where enzootic began prior to the vaccination; however, it was effective on farm B, and in sheds 1, 4 and 7 of farm A, where infection occurred later than in sheds 5 and 6.

On farm C, enzootic did not occur. Only two mink (one unvaccinated and one vaccinated) died. Whether the low number of deaths was due to the fact that mink were vaccinated with OEP was not clear.

The data presented here show that OEP plus toxoids had a marked protective effect on haemorrhagic pneumonia in mink. Further, OEP plus toxoids was found to be more effective than OEP alone. These results are in accord with those obtained in experimental infection in mink.

(ii) The effectiveness of the multi-component vaccine was again confirmed during three separate enzootics of haemorrhagic pneumonia which occurred in the northeastern area of Hokkaido in 1977. This time much larger numbers

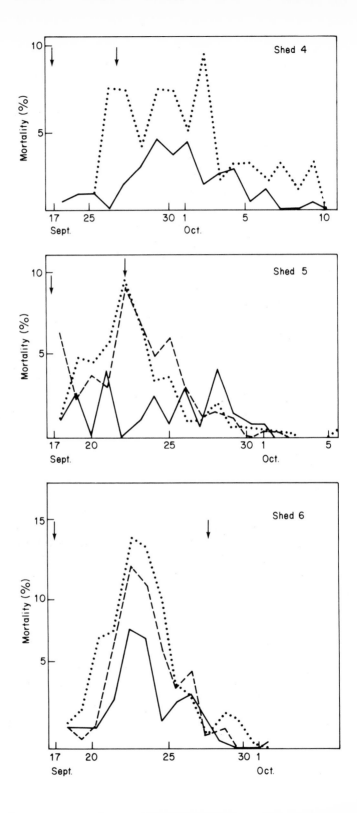

of mink were vaccinated. Some of the cases on farm A are taken from the report of Aoi *et al.* (1979) and mentioned below.

Mink, mostly Sapphire, Dark and Pastel, were raised in long, connected wire cages. Haemorrhagic pneumonia occurred on August 1, 1977 and lasted 35 days. In all, 879 of 7452 mink (11.8%) were lost. The vaccinations were performed on the 21st (Aug. 21) and 22nd (Aug. 22) day after the onset of the infection. Mink were vaccinated once with 200 μg each of OEP, protease and elastase toxoids. The isolates were identified, without exception, as serotype 8, which produces protease, elastase and exotoxin.

In all the sheds with large numbers of deaths, the effectiveness of the multi-component vaccine was confirmed. As examples, the results of shed 1 (male and female kittens), shed 2 (male kittens) and shed 8 (male kittens) are shown in Fig. 2. One dose of the vaccine was sufficient to stop the enzootic. The difference in the number of deaths between vaccinated and unvaccinated mink was significant ($P < 0.001$–$P < 0.05$, χ^2-test).

The period required to reveal the effectiveness of the vaccine was determined in each shed. The mortality rates before and after vaccination were calculated from the number of deaths cumulated daily. The statistical significance of the mortality rate between vaccinated and unvaccinated mink was calculated. On farm A, the enzootic occurred 1 to 13 days before vaccination in sheds 1, 2, 7, 8 and 13. The effect of the vaccine was revealed in male kittens of sheds 1 and 2 within 1 or 2 days. In female kittens of shed 1 and in male kittens of shed 13, the effect of the vaccine was recognized on post-vaccination day 4. The effect of the vaccine appeared 5 days after vaccination in female kittens of shed 2. In the above groups, prior to vaccination there were no significant differences in the mortality rates between those scheduled to be vaccinated and those not.

It is worthy of note, therefore, that the effect of the vaccination was revealed in these sheds within 1–5 days. In male kittens of shed 8, where enzootic broke out 4 days before vaccination, the mortality rate was significantly higher ($P < 0.005$, χ^2-test) in the mink which were to be vaccinated. Seven days after vaccination the mortality rate reversed and became significantly higher ($P < 0.05$, χ^2-test) in the unvaccinated mink. This reversal in mortality rate is of particular interest.

Fig. 1   Death rates of kittens in sheds 4 (♀), 5 (♂) and 6 (♂) of farm A and farm B. ———vaccinated with OEP and toxoids; – – – vaccinated with OEP; .... vaccinated; ↓ date of vaccination.
Note   Mortality indicated as the ratios of the number of deaths to the total number of mink vaccinated. From Honda *et al.* (1977) (reproduced with permission of the publisher).

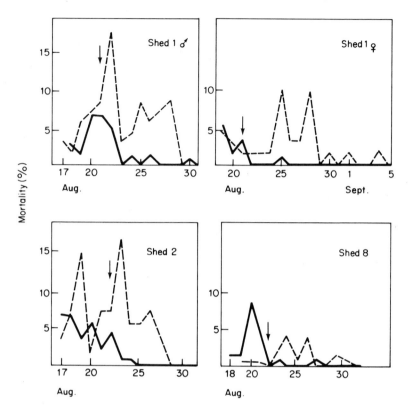

Fig. 2 Death rates of kittens in sheds 1 (♂♀), 2 (♂) and 8 (♂) of farm A. ↓ date of
vaccination; ——— vaccinated with multi-component vaccine; – – – unvaccinated. See note to Fig. 1. From Aoi *et al.* (1979) (reproduced with permission
of the publisher).

*(c)   Comparison of the effects of the multi-component vaccine with those of
formalin-killed cell vaccine on protection against enzootic of haemorrhagic
pneumonia due to* P. aeruginosa *in mink*
The effectiveness of the multi-component vaccine was compared with that of
formalin-killed cell vaccine during an enzootic of haemorrhagic pneumonia in
1979 by vaccination of mink with the two kinds of vaccines. From September
17 to October 10, enzootic haemorrhagic pneumonia broke out on farm A
located in the western area of Hokkaido. In all, 686 of 3838 mink died (17.9%).
The vaccination was performed for the first time on the 3rd day after the onset
of the enzootic.
Sapphire mink were divided into two groups: group A (1956 mink) was

vaccinated with the multi-component vaccine, and a control group B (1879 mink) with formalin-killed cell vaccine. A total of 106 (5.4%) mink were lost in group A and 580 (30.9%) in group B. Each group contained approximately 60% male and 40% female kittens. The isolates were identified as *P. aeruginosa* serotype 8.

The effects of the two vaccines on protection against haemorrhagic pneumonia in mink in each group are shown in Fig. 3. One hundred μg of the multi-component vaccine or 10^9 cells of formalin-killed vaccine was administered to two groups, A and B. The mortality rates in group A vaccinated with the multi-component vaccine and group B vaccinated with the formalin-killed vaccine are shown in Fig. 3. The difference in number of deaths between the two groups was significant. The mortality rate of control group B increased even after vaccination with formalin-killed cells, and 100 μg of the multi-component vaccine was administered to the group B mink only. A dramatic decrease in mortality rate was observed 6 days after this second vaccination (Fig. 3).

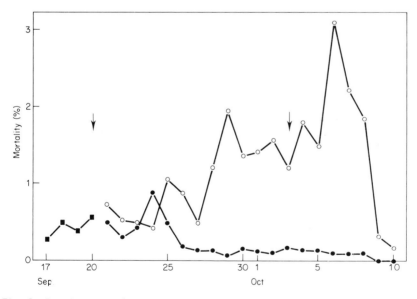

Fig. 3 Death rates of groups A and B. •———• multi component; ○———○ formalin-killed cells; ↓ 100 μg of the multi-component vaccine (group A) or 10^9 cells of formalin-killed cell vaccine (group B) was administered to two groups of mink. ↓ An additional vaccination of 100 μg of the multi-component vaccine was administered to group B only.
See note to Fig. 1. From Abe *et al.* (1981) (reproduced with permission of the publisher).

Table 3 The period required for revealing the effectiveness of the vaccine (Farm A)

Days before vaccination	Sheds in farm A						
	1		2		7	8	13
	M[a]	F[b]	M	F	F	M	M
−13~−5	ND		—[c]	ND			ND
−13~−4	ND		—	P<0.05		ND	—
−13~−3		—	—	—		ND	—
−13~−2		—	—	—		(P<0.01)[a]	—
−13~−1		—	—	—	ND	(P<0.01)	—
−13~0		—	—	—	ND	(P<0.005)	—

Days after vaccination

Days after vaccination							
1	$P<0.025^e$	ND	—	ND	ND	ND	—
1~2	$P<0.005$	ND	$P<0.01$	—	ND	—	—
1~3	$P<0.001$	ND	$P<0.01$	—	ND	—	—
1~4	$P<0.001$	$P<0.01$	$P<0.01$	—	ND	—	$P<0.05$
1~5	$P<0.001$	$P<0.005$	$P<0.01$	$P<0.02$	$P<0.05$	—	$P<0.05$
1~6	$P<0.001$	$P<0.001$	$P<0.001$	$P<0.02$	$P<0.05$	—	$P<0.05$
1~7	$P<0.001$	$P<0.001$	$P<0.001$	$P<0.02$		$P<0.05$	$P<0.05$
1~8	$P<0.001$	$P<0.001$	$P<0.001$	$P<0.02$		$P<0.05$	$P<0.05$
1~9	$P<0.001$	$P<0.001$	$P<0.001$				$P<0.05$
1~10		$P<0.001$	$P<0.001$				$P<0.05$
1~11		$P<0.001$	$P<0.001$				$P<0.05$
1~12		$P<0.001$	$P<0.001$				
1~13		$P<0.001$					
1~14		$P<0.001$					

[a] Male kittens.

[b] Female kittens.

[c] The mortality rate between the mink scheduled to be vaccinated was not significant ($P>0.05$, χ^2-test), before vaccination; the mortality rate between the vaccinated and non-vaccinated mink was not significant ($P>0.05$, χ^2-test), after vaccination.

[d] The parentheses indicate that the mortality rate in the mink scheduled to be vaccinated was higher than that of non-vaccinated mink.

[e] The mortality rate in the vaccinated mink was lower than that of non-vaccinated mink, in the cited statistical significance.

ND: not determined.

—: not significant.

Aoi et al. (1979) (reproduced with permission of the publisher).

From this report it can be concluded that one administration with 100 µg each of OEP and toxoids of protease and elastase sufficed to prevent epidemic of haemorrhagic pneumonia in mink due to *P. aeruginosa*, while a vaccination with formalin-killed cells of strain N10 (serotype 5) was much less effective in preventing the epidemic. The difference in mortality rate between groups A and B was significant ($P < 0.001$, χ^2-test).

It is generally recognized that formalin-killed cells are effective for preventing enzootic, if the serotype of the causative bacteria is the same as that of the bacteria from which the vaccine was prepared. As mentioned above, the common antigen (OEP) alone was effective for preventing enzootic, but it was far less effective compared to the multi-component vaccine comprised of OEP plus toxoids (Abe *et al.*, 1981).

4. Human trials

To prevent septic deaths from *P. aeruginosa*, Sasaki *et al.* (1980) vaccinated severe burn patients with the multi-component vaccine plus exotoxin toxoid. Fluid resuscitation was performed according to Baxter's formula. Cerium nitrate–silver sulphadiazine or silver sulphadiazine was applied to burn wound, and skin grafting was performed 2 weeks after admission.

Vaccinated patients consisted of 21 cases with a burnt surface area of 20–95% (mean 50.7%) and unvaccinated patients, 25 cases with a burnt surface area of 12–100% (mean 51.7%). Only 1 of 7 deaths among the vaccinated cases was a septic death due to *P. aeruginosa*, while 8 of 12 deaths among the unvaccinated patients were septic deaths, including 7 cases of septicaemia due to *P. aeruginosa*. There was no significant difference in wound bacterial cultures between the two groups.

Tachibana *et al.* (1980) and Inatomi *et al.* (1980) administered OEP and protease, elastase and exotoxin toxoids prior to *Pseudomonas* infection to 12 patients with chronic panbronchiolitis. Eight patients have not yet shown any evidence of *P. aeruginosa* superinfection 1 to $3\frac{1}{2}$ years after the start of vaccination. Four patients became colonized with *P. aeruginosa* shortly after the start of the vaccination, but their symptoms did not become worse. Maintenance doses consisting of 50 µg of each component were given intramuscularly at intervals of 3 or 4 weeks. Except for local pain and induration at the site of injection, no severe side-effects were observed.

Although the number of human clinical cases is still too small to judge the effectiveness of the multi-component vaccine, vaccination with OEP and toxoids prior to *Pseudomonas* infection seems worth trying in patients with chronic diffuse panbroncholitis for the prevention of *P. aeruginosa* colonization. Pennington (1979) and Fick and Reynolds (1980) have also considered that early immunization to elicit a primary response before the first *Pseudomonas* respiratory infection has occurred may be truly prophylactic.

Table 4 Results of treatment with anti-*Pseudomonas aeruginosa* γ-globulin (61 cases)

Diagnosis	No. of cases	Markedly effective (1)	Effective (2)	Slightly effective (3)	Ineffective	Unknown	Efficacy rate (%) (1)–(2)	(1)–(2)–(3)
Septicaemia	17		5	1	3	8	29	35
Suspected septicaemia	11	1	2	3	4	1	27	55
Pneumonia	10	1	2	1	4	2	30	40
Pulmonary suppuration	3		2		1		2/3	2/3
Respiratory tract infection	3	1		2			1/3	3/3
Bronchitis	7			1	6		—	1/7
Suspected bronchiectasia	1				1		—	—
Osteomyelitis of the sternum	1					1	—	—
Urinary tract infection	4			1	1	2	—	1/4
Skin infection	2		1		1		1/2	1/2
Corneal abscess	1					1	—	—
Otitis media	1			1	1		—	1/1
Total	61	3	12	10	21	15	25	41

Mashimo *et al.* (1980) (reproduced with permission of the publisher).

To evaluate the effects of anti-*Pseudomonas* γ-globulin clinical investigations were conducted under the auspices of a subcommittee organized by the Japan *Pseudomonas aeruginosa* Society. Machimo *et al.* (1980) prepared human γ-globulin containing antibodies against OEP, protease, elastase and exotoxin from the serum of normal healthy persons whose antibody titres were relatively high. The subcommittee set up a protocol to evaluate the effectiveness of the γ-globulin. Sixty-one cases (32 children and 29 adults) meeting the therapeutic conditions described in the protocol were subjected to clinical evaluations carried out by the subcommittee. Administration of the γ-globulin was conducted on the 61 patients who were found refractory to chemotherapy for at least 3 days of antibiotic treatments.

The γ-globulin was administered at dose levels of 53–652 mg kg^{-1}, 1–3 times per day according to the patient's symptoms and severity of infection. Most patients received a single administration of 100–200 mg kg^{-1}. Results of the treatment with anti-*Pseudomonas* γ-globulin on the 61 cases are shown in Table 3.

In 14 patients with underlying diseases such as leukaemia and malignant tumours, who were presumed to be immunodeficient, efficacy rate was 21%; in 17 patients with general underlying diseases it was 32%. In the 32 children, the γ-globulin was determined as "markedly effective" in 2 cases and "effective" in 5 cases. In the 29 adults, the γ-globulin was "markedly effective" in 1 case and "effective" in 7 cases.

As for side-effects observed during therapy, one patient complained of epigastric and abdominal pain when injected intravenously, but these symptoms disappeared spontaneously upon change to intravenous infusion.

The subcommittee concluded that, according to the study protocol, the γ-globulin showed an efficacy rate of 25% in patients with various underlying diseases.

V. FUTURE PROSPECTS

Antibiotics effective in the treatment of infections due to *P. aeruginosa* have been introduced in recent years. They are valuable for acute infections but usually ineffective against subacute and chronic infections.

Normal immune function is required for chemotherapy to exhibit satisfactory therapeutic effects. Since infections due to *P. aeruginosa* generally occur in individuals with depressed immunity due to physiological immaturity, certain underlying diseases and medical care, immune function must be fully activated for chemotherapy to achieve its purpose. In this regard, serum therapy consisting of anti-*Pseudomonas* γ-globulin containing antibodies of OEP, protease, elastase and exotoxin and leucocyte transfusion is recommended. The vaccine may be given after administration of the *Pseudomonas* immune γ-globulin in such clinical cases as severe burns.

From the above data it is quite possible that antibodies against OEP, protease, elastase and exotoxin are necessary for protection of the host from pseudomonal infections. Many investigators have demonstrated the satisfactory therapeutic effects of the multi-component vaccine or its antisera in experiments on corneal ulcer or burn in mice. Moreover, this vaccine showed definite preventive and therapeutic effects on spontaneous enzootic haemorrhagic pneumonia due to *P. aeruginosa* in mink.

Pseudomonas infections complicating cystic fibrosis patients are generally localized in the lungs. Disseminated infection does not occur, probably because of antibodies produced during the chronic course of the infection. Cho *et al.* (1978) examined antibody titres against OEP, protease, elastase and exotoxin in sera from 30 patients with cystic fibrosis and found high antibody titres in a number of sera, although these differed greatly from serum to serum. Cure of chronic infections caused by *P. aeruginosa* cannot be expected as long as the underlying disease remains uncured, and considerable amounts of protease, elastase, exotoxin and leucocidin would be produced by *P. aeruginosa* at sites of inflammation in the respiratory tract. To be free from the toxic effects of these bacterial products, patients must have ample neutralizing antibodies.

Determination of the antibody level to each of these substances is necessary for proper treatment in clinical cases. Passive haemagglutination tests (Tomiyama *et al.*, 1973; Homma *et al.*, 1975) and enzyme-linked immunosorbent assays (ELISA) (Schultz *et al.*, 1979; Ueda *et al.*, 1982) have been developed for the detection of antibodies to OEP, protease, elastase and exotoxin.

When antibodies to bacterial somatic antigen (OEP), protease, elastase and exotoxin are difficult to detect in patients susceptible to or suffering from pseudomonal infections, both active and passive immunization are recommended to prevent the development of disturbances resulting from infection.

Pavlovskis *et al.* (1977), using the mouse burn model, suggested that *P. aeruginosa* exotoxin contributes to lethality in the burn model used, and this effect is diminished by passive immunization with antitoxin. Hann *et al.* (1976) reported that all strains of *P. aeruginosa* recovered from sputum specimens of patients with cystic fibrosis were found to be coated with antibodies to IgA, IgG, and IgM and with C_3. They also found these humoral factors to be present in sputum. These data indicate that toxic effects of exotoxin, protease and elastase are neutralized in sputum when patients are immunized with these antigens. Pollack and Young (1979) investigated serum antibody responses to exotoxin and type-specific lipopolysaccharide characterized in 52 patients with *P. aeruginosa* bacteraemia and evaluated their comparative protective activities by relating the titres of each at the onset of bacteraemia to subsequent outcome. The data indicate that antitoxin and anti-lipopolysaccharide titres are present early in the serum of most patients with *P. aeruginosa* septicaemia, increase with survival, and are protective, suggesting that antibodies passively provided or actively engendered to both exotoxin and lipopolysaccharide may have therapeutic or prophylactic potential.

As a result of these findings, exotoxin toxoid was added to the multi-component vaccine for administration to human clinical cases. The multi-component vaccine plus exotoxin toxoid has just begun to be used in human clinical cases on chronic panbronchiolitis and burn infections due to the bacillus. Patients immunized with the multi-component vaccine plus exotoxin toxoid are protected from infection because OEP antibody seems to inhibit invasion and proliferation of *P. aeruginosa* and at the same time because antibodies against protease, elastase and exotoxin neutralize the toxic effects of the two enzymes and exotoxin. It is hoped that the vaccine will induce in the patients such "carrier" states as seen in the case of *Vibrio cholerae, Salmonella typhi* and *Corynebacterium diphtheriae*, in which patients do not suffer from the harmful and toxic effects of infection.

In results obtained so far, vaccination with the multi-component vaccine plus exotoxin toxoid significantly reduced the mortality of sepsis due to the bacillus in burn patients (Sasaki *et al.*, 1980). Surprisingly, most patients with chronic panbronchiolitis have not even yet been infected with *P. aeruginosa* more than 3 years after the vaccination. Some of those who did become infected with the bacillus showed no increase in the severity of their symptoms (Tachibana *et al.*, 1980; Inatomi *et al.*, 1980).

The number of human clinical cases which have received vaccination is still too small to judge the effectiveness of the multi-component vaccine plus exotoxin toxoid, so further investigations on the application of the vaccine for various kinds of human clinical infections due to *P. aeruginosa* are needed.

For certain immunocompromised patients, active immunization will sometimes not be effective. Granulocyte transfusion and passive immunization using *Pseudomonas* immune γ-globulin containing high titres of OEP, protease, elastase and exotoxin appear to be a promising approach to prophylaxis and therapy against *Pseudomonas aeruginosa* infection.

ACKNOWLEDGEMENTS

The author wishes to thank Dr Iwao Kato, Professor, Department of Bacterial Infection, Institute of Medical Science, University of Tokyo, Dr Kazuyuki Morihara, Shionogi Research Laboratory, and C. Midori Hamagami for assistance in the preparation of the manuscript.

REFERENCES

Abe, C., Shionoya, H., Hirao, Y., Okada, K. and Homma, J. Y. (1975). *Jpn J. Exp. Med.* **45**, 355–359.

Abe, C., Tanamoto, K. and Homma, J. Y. (1977). *Jpn J. Exp. Med.* **47**, 393–402.

Abe, C., Takeshi, K. and Homma, J. Y. (1978). *Jpn J. Exp. Med.* **48**, 183–186.

Abe, C., Homma, J. Y., Noda, H., Yanagawa, R., Morihara, K., Tsuzuki, H. and Takeuchi, S. (1981). *Zbl. Bakt. Hyg., I. Abt. Orig.* **A249**, 413–417.

Aduan, R. P. and Reynolds, H. Y. (1979). *In "Pseudomonas aeruginosa"* (R. G. Doggett, ed.) pp. 135–152. Academic Press, London and New York.

Aoi, Y., Noda, H., Yanagawa, R., Homma, J. Y., Abe, C., Morihara, K., Ghoda, A., Takeuchi, S. and Ishihara, T. (1979). *Jpn J. Exp. Med.* **49**, 199–207.

Aoyagi, T. and Umezawa, H. (1975). *In* "Proteases and Biological control" (E. Reich, D. B. Rifkin and E. Shaw, ed.). Cold Spring Harbor Conference on Cell Proliferation Vol. 2, 429–454.

Aoyagi, T., Ishizuka, M., Takeuchi, T. and Umezawa, H. (1977). *Jpn J. Antibiotics* **30** Suppl., 121–132.

Bjornson, A. B. and Michael, J. G. (1972). *Infect. Immun.* **5**, 775.

Bjorn, M. J., Vasil, M. L., Sadoff, J. C. and Iglewski, B. H. (1977). *Infect. Immun.* **16**, 362–366.

Callahan, L. T., III (1976). *Infect. Immun.* **14**, 55–61.

Cho, Y. J., Oh, Y. H., Abe, C., Homma, J. Y., Usui, M. and Matsuhashi, T. (1978). *Jpn J. Exp. Med.* **48**, 491–496.

Cho, Y., Tanamoto, K., Oh, Y. and Homma, J. Y. (1979). *FEBS Letters* **105**, 120–122.

Cross, A. C., Sadoff, C., Iglewski, B. H. and Sokol, P. A. (1980). *J. Inf. Dis.* **142**, 538–546.

Cryz, S. J., Jr, Friedman, R. L. and Iglewski, B. H. (1980). *Proc. Nat. Acad. Sci. U.S.A.* **77**, 7199–7203.

Cryz, S. J., Jr, Friedman, R. L., Pavlovskis, O. R. and Iglewski, B. H. (1980b). *Infect. Immun.* **32**, 759–768.

Cryz, S. J., Jr and Iglewski, B. H. (1981b). *Rev. Infect. Dis.* in press.

Cryz, S. J., Jr, Pavlovskis, O. R. and Iglewski, B. H. (1981c). *In* "Seminars in Infectious Diseases" (J. Robbins, ed.). Brian C. Decker Publishers, New York (in press).

Dimitracopoulos, G., Sensakovic, J. W. and Bartell, P. F. (1974). *Infect. Immun.* **10**, 152–156.

Dimitracopoulos, G. and Bartell, P. F. (1980). *Infect. Immun.* **30**, 402–408.

Farrel, R. K., Leader, R. W. and Gorham, J. R. (1958). *Cornell Vet.* **48**, 378–384.

Fich, R., Jr and Reynolds, H. Y. (1980). *In* "Perspective in Cystic Fibrosis (8th International Congress on CF) (J. M. Sturgess, ed.) pp. 335–345. Toronto, Canada.

Ficher, E., Jr and Aller, J. G. (1958). *Am. J. Ophthalmol.* **46**, 249–254.

Fisher, M. W., Devlin, H. B. and Gnabasik, F. J. (1969). *J. Bacteriol.* **98**, 835–836.

Fisher, M. W. (1974). *J. Infect. Dis.* **130**, 149–151.

Frimmer, M., Neuhof, H., Scharmann, W. and Schischke, B. (1976a). *Arch. Exp. Path. Pharmak.* **294**, 85.

Frimmer, M., Homann, J., Petzinger, E., Rufeger, U. and Scharmann, W. (1976b). *Arch. Exp. Path. Pharmak.* **295**, 63.

Fukui, G. M., Homma, J. Y. and Abe, C. (1971). *Jpn J. Exp. Med.* **41**, 489–492.

Gray, L. D. and Kreger, A. S. (1975). *Infect. Immun.* **12**, 419–432.

Gray, L. and Kreger, A. (1979). *Infect. Immun.* **23**, 150–159.

Haagsma, J. and Pereboom, W. J. (1965). *Tijdschr. Diregeneesk.* **90**, 1093–1100.

Hann, S. and Holsclaw, O. S. (1976). *Infect. Immun.* **14**, 114–117.

Haranaka, K., Sugane, K. and Mashimo, K. (1975). *Jpn J. Exp. Med.* **45**, 207–213.

428   J. Yuzuru Homma

Haranaka, K., Matsuo, M. and Mashimo, K. (1977). *Jpn J. Exp. Med.* **47**, 35–40.
Hirao, Y., Homma, J. Y. and Zierdt, C. H. (1977). *Jpn J. Exp. Med.* **47**, 249–254.
Hirao, Y. and Homma, J. Y. (1978a). *Infect. Immun.* **19**, 373–377.
Hirao, Y. and Homma, J. Y. (1978b). *Jpn J. Exp. Med.* **48**, 41–51.
Høiby, N. (1976). *Acta Path. Microbiol. Scand. Sect. C. Suppl.* **262**, 3–96.
Høiby, N. (1977). *Acta Path. Microbiol. Scand. Sect. C. Suppl.* **262**, 1–96.
Høiby, N. (1979). In *"Pseudomonas aeruginosa"* (R. G. Doggett, ed.) pp. 157–185. Academic Press, London and New York.
Høiby, N., Hertz, J. B. and Sompolinsky, D. (1980). *Acta Path. Microbiol. Scand. Sect. C* **88**, 149–154.
Holder, I. A. and Jogan, M. (1971). *J. Trauma* 11, 1041–1046.
Holder, I. A. and Haidaris, C. G. (1979). *Can. J. Microbiol.* **25**, 593–599.
Holder, I. A. (1979). Symposium on *Pseudomonas aeruginosa* Walter Reed Army Institute, Washington D.C.
Homma, J. Y. (1971). *Jpn J. Exp. Med.* **41**, 387–400.
Homma, J. Y. and Abe, C. (1972). *Jpn J. Exp. Med.* **42**, 23–34.
Homma, J. Y. (1974). *Jpn J. Exp. Med.* **44**, 1–12.
Homma, J. Y. (1975). In *"Microbial Drug Resistance"* (S. Mitsuhashi and H. Hashimoto, ed.) pp. 267–279. University of Tokyo Press, Tokyo.
Homma, J. Y., Tomiyama, T., Sano, H., Hirao, Y. and Saku, K. (1975). *Jpn J. Exp. Med.* **45**, 361–365.
Homma, J. Y. (1976). *Jpn J. Exp. Med.* **46**, 329–336.
Homma, J. Y., Abe, C., Okada, K., Tanamoto, K. and Hirao, Y. (1976). In *"Animal, Plant, and Microbial Toxins"* (A. Ohsaka, K. Hayashi and Y. Sawai, ed.) Vol. 1, pp. 499–508. Plenum Publishing Co., New York.
Homma, J. Y., Hirao, Y., Saku, K., Terada, Y. and Sugiyama, J. (1977). *Jpn J. Exp. Med.* **47**, 195–201.
Homma, J. Y. (1978). *Asian Med. J.* **21**, 573–589.
Homma, J. Y., Abe, C., Tanamoto, K., Hirao, Y., Morihara, K., Tsuzuki, H., Yanagawa, R., Honda, E., Aoi, Y., Fujimoto, Y., Goryo, M., Imazeki, N., Noda, H., Ghoda, A., Takeuchi, S. and Ishihara, T. (1978). *Jpn J. Exp. Med.* **48**, 111–133.
Homma, J. Y., Ghoda, A., Goto, S., Jo, K., Kato, I., Kodama, H., Kosakai, N., Kono, M., Shionoya, H., Terada, Y., Tomiyama, T. and Yabuuchi, E. (1979). *Jpn J. Exp. Med.* **49**, 89–94.
Honda, E., Homma, J. Y., Abe, C., Tanamoto, K., Noda, H. and Yanagawa, R. (1977). *Zbl. Bakt. Hyg. I. Abt. Orig. A.* **237**, 297–309.
Hoshi, A., Kanzawa, F., Kuretani, K., Homma, J. Y. and Abe, C. (1973a). *Gann* **63**, 503–504.
Hoshi, A., Kanzawa, F., Kuretani, K., Homma, J. Y. and Abe, C. (1973b). *Gann* **64**, 523–525.
Iglewski, B. G. and Kabat, D. (1975). *Proc. Natl Acad. Sci. U.S.A.* **72**, 2284–2288.
Iglewski, B. H., Liu, P. V. and Kabat, D. (1977). *Infect. Immun.* **15**, 138–144.
Inatomi, K., Suzuki, M., Kudo, H., Takahashi, Y., Chizimatsu, Y., Washizaki, M. and Homma, H. (1980). Proc. 14th Meeting of Japan *Pseudomonas aeruginosa* Society, p. 15.
Kamimura, T., Mine, Y., Nonoyama, S., Nishida, M., Goto, S. and Kuwahara, S. (1980). *Infect. Immun.* **29**, 13–16.
Karlsson, K. A., Kull, K. E. and Svanholm, R. (1971). *Nord. Veterinabrmed.* **23**, 345–351.
Kawaharajo, K., Abe, C., Homma, J. Y., Kawano, M., Gotoh, E., Tanaka, N. and Morihara, K. (1974). *Jpn J. Exp. Med.* **44**, 435–442.

Kawaharajo, K., Homma, J. Y., Aoyama, Y., Okada, K. and Morihara, K. (1975a). *Jpn J. Exp. Med.* **45**, 79–88.
Kawaharajo, K., Homma, J. Y., Abe, C., Aoyama, Y. and Morihara, K. (1975b). *Jpn J. Exp. Med.* **45**, 89–100.
Kawaharajo, K. and Homma, J. Y. (1975c). *Jpn J. Exp. Med.* **45**, 515–524.
Kawaharajo, K. and Homma, J. Y. (1976). *Jpn J. Exp. Med.* **46**, 155–165.
Kawaharajo, K. and Homma, J. Y. (1977). *Jpn J. Exp. Med.* **47**, 495–500.
Klinger, J. D., Straus, D. C., Hilton, C. B. and Bass, J. A. (1978). *J. Inf. Dis.* **138**, 49–58.
Knox, B. (1953). *Nord. Veterinabrmed.* **5**, 731–760.
Kodama, H. and Ishimoto, M. (1976). *Jpn J. Exp. Med.* **46**, 383–397.
Kojima, Y., Homma, J. Y. and Abe, C. (1971). *Jpn J. Exp. Med.* **41**, 493–496.
Kono, M. and Sei, S. (1977). *Jpn J. Exp. Med.* **47**, 1–7.
Komiyama, T., Aoyagi, T., Takeuchi, T. and Umezawa, H. (1975). *Biochem. Biophys. Res. Commun.* **65**, 352–357.
Kreger, A. S. and Griffin, O. (1974). *Infect. Immun.* **9**, 828–834.
Lieberman, M. M. (1978). *Infect. Immun.* **21**, 76.
Liu, P. V. (1966). *J. Infect. Dis.* **116**, 112–116.
Lutz, F. (1979). *Toxicon* **17**, 467–475.
Maejima, K. (1977). *Jpn J. Bacteriol.* **32**, 48.
Mansi, W., Schofieid, P. B. and Bellard, A. R. M. (1965). *Vet. Rec.* **77**, 1415.
Mashimo, K., Ishiyama, S., Fujii, R., Homma, J. Y., Yoshioka, H. and Nishimura, T. (1980). Proc. 14th Meeting of Japan *Pseudomonas aeruginosa* Society. pp. 2–6.
Mates, A. and Zand, P. (1973). *J. Hyg., Comb.* **73**, 75–83.
McManus, A. T., Moody, E. E. and Mason, A. D. (1980). *Burns* **6**, 235–239.
Meinke, G., Barum, J., Rosenberg, B. and Berk, R. S. (1970). *Infect. Immun.* **2**, 583–589.
Montie, T. C., Craven, R., Wheeler, R. and Holder, I. A. Personal communication.
Morihara, K. (1963). *Biochim. Biophys. Acta* **73**, 113–124.
Morihara, K. (1964). *J. Bacteriol.* **88**, 745–757.
Morihara, K., Tsuzuki, H., Oka, T., Inoue, H. and Ebata, M. (1965). *J. Biol. Chem.* **240**, 3295–3304.
Morihara, K. and Tsuzuki, H. (1977). *Infect. Immun.* **15**, 679–685.
Morihara, K. and Tsuzuki, H. (1978). *Jpn J. Exp. Med.* **48**, 81–84.
Morihara, K., Tsuzuki, H. and Oda, K. (1979). *Infect. Immun.* **24**, 188–193.
Moulton, R. C., Young, L. and Montie, T. C. (1980). *In* "Asstr. Annu. Meet. Am. Soc. Microbiol., 1980", B 102, p. 34.
Nishida, M., Mine, Y., Nonoyama, S. and Goto, S. (1975). 1st ISC-IAMS Proceedings Vol. 4, pp. 277–281.
Nomoto, K. (1977). *Jpn J. Bacteriol.* **32**, 50.
Nonoyama, S., Kojo, H., Mine, Y., Nishida, M., Goto, S. and Kuwahara, S. (1979a). *Infect. Immun.* **24**, 394–398.
Nonoyama, S., Kojo, H., Mine, Y., Nishida, M., Goto, S. and Kuwahara, S. (1979b). *Infect. Immun.* **24**, 399–403.
Nordstoga, K. (1968). *Acta Vet. Scand.* **9**, 33–40.
Ohman, D. E., Burns, R. P. and Iglewski, B. H. (1980). *J. Inf. Dis.* **142**, 547–555.
Oishi, M., Nishizuka, K., Motoyama, M. and Ogawa, T. (1977). Proc. 11th Meeting of The Japan *Pseudomonas* Soc. p. 20.
Okada, K., Kawaharajo, K., Homma, J. Y., Aoyama, Y. and Kubota, Y. (1976). *Jpn J. Exp. Med.* **46**, 245–256.
Okada, K., Kawaharajo, K., Kasai, T. and Homma, J. Y. (1980). *Jpn J. Exp. Med.* **50**, 61–69.

Pavlovskis, O. R., Voelker, F. A. and Shackelford, A. H. (1976). *J. Inf. Dis.* **133**, 253–259.
Pavlovskis, O. R., Pollack, M., Callahan, L. T., III and Iglewski, B. H. (1977). *Infect. Immun.* **18**, 596–602.
Pavlovskis, O. R., Iglewski, B. H. and Pollack, M. (1978). *Infect. Immun.* **19**, 29–33.
Pavlovskis, O. R. and Wretlind, B. (1979). *Infect. Immun.* **24**, 181–187.
Pavlovskis, O. R., Edman, D. C., Leppla, S. H., Wretlind, B., Lewis, L. R. and Martin, K. E. (1981). *Infect. Immun.* **32**, 681–689.
Pennington, J. E. (1979). *In* "*Pseudomonas aeruginosa*" (R. G. Doggett, ed.) pp. 192–215 Academic Press, New York and London.
Pier, G. B., Sidberry, H. F., Zolyomi, S. and Sadoff, J. C. (1978a). *Infect. Immun.* **22**, 908–918.
Pier, G. B., Sidberry, H. F. and Sadoff, J. C. (1978b). *Infect. Immun.* **22**, 919–925.
Pier, G. B., Sidberry, H. F. and Sadoff, J. C. (1981). *J. Inf. Dis.* **34**, 461–468.
Pollack, M., Callahan, L. T., III and Taylor, N. S. (1976). *Infect. Immun.* **14**, 942–947.
Pollack, M., Taylor, N. S. and Callahan, L. T., III (1977). *Infect. Immun.* **15**, 776–780.
Pollack, M. and Young, L. S. (1979). *J. Clin. Invest.* **63**, 276–286.
Reynolds, H. Y., Levine, A. S., Wood, R. E., Zierdt, C. H., Dale, D. C. and Pennington, J. E. (1975). *Ann. Intern. Med.* **82**, 819–831.
Reynolds, H. Y., DiSant'Agnese, P. A. and Zierdt, C. H. (1976). *J.A.M.A.* **236**, 2190–2192.
Sadoff, J. C. (1974). *J. Inf. Dis.* **130** (suppl.), 561–564.
Saelinger, C. B., Snell, K. and Holder, I. A. (1977). *J. Infect. Dis.* **136**, 555–561.
Sakaguchi, G. and Oishi, I. (1976). *In* "Proteins, Nucleic Acids and Enzymes" Suppl., 76–11, pp. 45–54.
Sanai, Y., Takeshi, K., Homma, J. Y. and Kamata, H. (1978). *Jpn J. Exp. Med.* **48**, 553–556.
Sasaki, M., Ito, M. and Homma, J. Y. (1975). *Jpn J. Exp. Med.* **45**, 335–343.
Sasaki, J., Henmi, H., Otsuka, T. and Nishimura, N. (1980). Proc. 14th Meeting of Japan *Pseudomonas aeruginosa* Society, p. 14.
Scharmann, W. (1976a). *J. Gen. Microbiol.* **93**, 283–291.
Scharmann, W. (1976b). *J. Gen. Microbiol.* **93**, 292–302.
Scharmann, W., Jacob, F. and Porstendorfeer, J. (1976). *J. Gen. Microbiol.* **93**, 303–308.
Schultz, D. R. and Miller, K. D. (1974). *Infect. Immun.* **10**, 128–135.
Schultz, W. W., Phipps, T. J. and Pollack, M. (1979). *J. Clin. Microbiol.* **9**, 705–708.
Schwartzmann, S. and Boring, J. R., III (1971). *Infect. Immun.* **3**, 762–767.
Sensakovic, W. and Bartell, P. F. (1974). *J. Inf. Dis.* **129**, 101–109.
Shimizu, T., Homma, J. Y., Abe, C., Aoyama, Y., Onodera, T. and Noda, H. (1974). *Infect. Immun.* **10**, 16–20.
Shimizu, T., Homma, J. Y., Abe, C., Tanamoto, K., Aoyama, Y., Okada, K., Yanagawa, R., Fujimoto, Y., Noda, H., Takashima, I., Honda, E. and Minamide, S. (1976). *Amer. J. Vet. Res.* **37**, 1441–1444.
Shionoya, H., Arai, H. and Ohtake, S. (1977). *Jpn J. Exp. Med.* **47**, 185–194.
Sinozaki, T., Fiujii, R., Sanai, Y. and Homma, J. Y. (1981). *Jpn J. Exp. Med.* **51**, 165–170.
Sompolinsky, D., Hertz, J. B., Høiby, N., Jensen, K., Mansa, B., Pedersen, V. B. and Samra, Z. (1980a). *Acta Path. Microbiol. Scand. Sect. B.* **88**, 143–149.
Sompolinsky, D., Hertz, J. B., Høiby, N., Jensen, K., Mansa, B., Pedersen, V. B. and Samra, Z. (1980b). *Acta Path. Microb. Scand. Sect. B.* **88**, 253–260.
Stieritz, D. D. and Holder, I. A. (1975). *J. Infect. Dis.* **131**, 688–691.

Stieritz, D. D. and Holder, I. A. (1978). *J. Med. Microbiol.* **11**, 101–109.
Suda, H., Aoyagi, T., Takeuchi, T. and Umezawa, H. (1973). *J. Antibiol.* **26**, 621–623.
Tachibana, A., Suzuki, K., Nakata, K., Okano, H. and Tanimoto, H. (1980). Proc. 14th Meeting of Japan *Pseudomonas aeruginosa* Society. pp. 14–15.
Takashima, K., Homma, J. Y., Shimizu, T., Noda, H. and Yanagawa, K. (1975). *J. Japan Vet. Med. Assoc.* **28**, 524–528.
Takeshi, K., Homma, J. Y., Kato, I. and Saito, H. (1977). *Jpn J. Exp. Med.* **47**, 323–325.
Takeshi, K. and Homma, J. Y. (1978). *Jpn J. Exp. Med.* **48**, 497–501.
Takeuchi, S., Ghoda, A., Homma, J. Y. and Abe, C. (1979). Unpublished.
Tanaka, N., Sanai, T., Ohzeki, T., Miyaji, S. and Kawano, M. (1972). *Acta Soc. Ophthalmol. Japan* **76**, 408–415.
Tanaka, N., Sasaki, T., Tanaka, I., Kinoshita, N. and Homma, J. Y. (1978). *Documen. Ophthal. Proc. Series* **20**, 19–22.
Tanamoto, K., Abe, C., Homma, J. Y., Kuretani, K., Hoshi, A. and Kojima, Y. (1978). *J. Biochem.* **83**, 711–718.
Tanamoto, K., Abe, C., Homma, J. Y. and Kojima, Y. (1979). *Eur. J. Bioch.* **97**, 623–629.
Teplits, C. (1965). *Arch. Pathol.* **80**, 297–307.
Terada, Y., Sugiyama, J. and Orikasa, M. (1977). *Jpn J. Exp. Med.* **47**, 203–208.
Tomiyama, T., Homma, J. Y., Abe, C. and Yoichi, M. (1973). *Jpn J. Exp. Med.* **43**, 185–189.
Trautwein, G., Helmboldt, C. F. and Nielsen, S. M. (1962). *J. Amer. Vet. Med. Assoc.* **140**, 701–704.
Ueda, Y., Homma, J. Y. and Abe, C. (1982). *Amer. J. Vet. Res.* **43**, 55–60.
Woods, D. E., Straus, D. C., Johanson, W. G., Jr, Berry, V. K. and Bass, J. A. (1980). *Infect. Immun.* **29**, 1146–1151.
Yabuuchi, E., Miyajima, N. and Furu, Y. (1976). *Jpn J. Exp. Med.* **46**, 393–397.
Yamamoto, A. and Homma, J. Y. (1978). *Jpn J. Exp. Med.* **48**, 545–551.
Yamamoto, A., Homma, J. Y., Ghoda, A., Ishihara, T. and Takeuchi, S. (1979). *Jpn J. Exp. Med.* **49**, 383–390.
Young, L. S. and Armstrong, D. (1972). *J. Inf. Dis.* **126**, 257–276.
Young, L. S. and Pollack, M. (1979). *In* "*Pseudomonas aeruginosa*" (L. D. Sabath, ed.) pp. 119–132. Hans Huber, Bern.
Zierdt, C. H. and Williams, R. L. (1975). *J. Clin. Microbiol.* **1**, 521–526.

11 Immunostimulatory and antineoplastic activities of propionibacteria

W. ROSZKOWSKI, K. ROSZKOWSKI, S. SZMIGIELSKI, G. PULVERER and J. JELJASZEWICZ

Halpern *et al.* (1964) have shown that the introduction of heat-killed cells of *Corynebacterium parvum* results in considerable stimulation of the reticulo-endothelial system in mice. These authors, together with Woodruff and Boak (1966) have demonstrated that this stimulation is accompanied by inhibition of growth of transplantable tumours. Since that time, *Corynebacterium parvum* and other related strains of anaerobic coryneform bacteria, classified by Johnson and Cummins (1972) as *Propionibacterium* species, have become widely applied as a useful tool for investigation of immunostimulatory and antineoplastic activities of these microorganisms. A summary of their known effects is presented in Table 1.

Results of studies with experimental animals have encouraged the investigation of the usefulness of propionibacteria in treatment of cancer in man in a number of clinical centres.

I. IMMUNOSTIMULATORY PROPERTIES

A. Stimulation of reticulo-endothelial system

A single intravenous injection of propionibacteria into mice results in marked enlargement of spleen, liver, and sometimes also of lymph nodes (Adlam and Scott, 1973; Castro, 1974a; Halpern *et al.*, 1964; McBride *et al.*, 1974; Milas *et al.*, 1975a). An increase in the mass of these organs is demonstrable after a few

Table 1   Some biological effects of propionibacteria after systemic and local application

	Route of administration	
Property	Systemic	Local
Antineoplastic activity	Increase or no change	Increase
Antibacterial activity	Increase	No change
Antiviral activity	Increase	No change
Cell-mediated immunity	Decrease	Increase
Humoral immunity (adjuvant reaction)	Increase	Increase
Liver, spleen, and lung mass	Increase	No change
Lymph node mass	No change	Increase
Macrophage activation	Increase	No change
Interferon induction	Increase	No change
Natural killer activity	Increase or decrease	Increase
Stimulation of haemopoiesis	Increase	Increase or no change

days, reaching a maximum about two weeks after the injection of propionibacteria. The return to original mass is slow taking several weeks. The dynamics of these changes are independent of the dose of injected propionibacteria. It has also been demonstrated that the lung mass may considerably increase (Adlam and Scott, 1972). At the time of enlargement of spleen, liver and lymph nodes, thymus mass and the number of Thy 1 positive cells decreases (Castro and Sadler, 1975).

The subcutaneous injection of propionibacteria causes at most only slight enlargement of spleen and liver, though lymph nodes draining the injection site do increase in size (Scott, 1974a; Tuttle and North, 1975).

Histological examination has shown enlarged proliferation of macrophages, histiocytes and haemopoietic cells in the enlarged spleen (Brozovic et al., 1975; Milas et al., 1975a) and of the lymphocytes and histiocytes in lymph nodes and lungs (O'Neil et al., 1973; Scott, 1974; Tuttle and North, 1975). Liver enlargement seems to be associated with the infiltration of monocytes and macrophages, while the number and distribution of Kupfer cells undergoes no change (Brozovic et al., 1975; Milas et al., 1974; Warr and Sljivic, 1974a).

The increase in mass and the histological changes in these organs are preceded by the marked stimulation of bone marrow with proliferation of monocyte precursors being followed by their increased release to peripheral blood (Baum and Breese, 1976; Chare and Baum, 1978; Eliopoulos et al.,

1978; Wolmark and Fisher, 1974). After a short period of increase in bone marrow, the number of nondifferentiated stem cells in the peripheral blood rapidly rises (Roszkowski et al., 1980a). The appearance of bone marrow stimulation suggests that enlargement of spleen and liver may result not only from proliferation of resident macrophages within these organs but also through an increased influx of monocytes originating from bone marrow.

Following activation by propionibacteria, macrophages exhibit increased and more rapid adherence to glass, enlarged vacuolization, and a changed distribution of lysosomes (Olivotto and Bomford, 1974; Puvion et al., 1976). The activity of lysosomal enzyme is also increased (McBride et al., 1974; Wilkinson et al., 1973a,b). Changes in the structure of the cell membrane of stimulated macrophages are also noted (Puvion et al., 1976). Such macrophages exert in vitro and in vivo, as demonstrated with colloidal carbon (Raynaud et al., 1972; Warr and Sljivic, 1974b), [^{51}Cr]-labelled sheep erythrocytes (Warr and Sljivic, 1974b), bovine albumin (McBride et al., 1974) and bacteria (Adlam et al., 1972; Collins and Scott, 1974; Halpern et al., 1973). Increased clearance of foreign particles from blood after the application of propionibacteria seems to be directly related to the degree of enlargement of the liver and spleen, where phagocytosed substances accumulate (O'Neil et al., 1973; Warr and Sljivic, 1974b). In these organs, macrophage-related bactericidal activity is also observed (Collins and Scott, 1974; Fauve and Hevin, 1974). This activity may be the basis of the increased resistance of mice injected with propionibacteria to infection with bacteria such as Staphylococcus aureus (Adlam et al., 1972), Bordetella pertussis (Fauve and Hevin, 1974), Brucella abortus (Halpern et al., 1973), Salmonella enteritidis (Collins and Scott, 1974), or Listeria monocytogenes (Fauve and Hevin, 1971; Ruitenberg and Van Noorle Jansen, 1975). The protective effect has also been achieved by application of a phospholipid fraction extracted from these micro-organisms instead of the whole cell suspension (Fauve, 1975).

Propionibacteria injected intravenously also protect mice against infection with herpes simplex virus (Kirchner et al., 1977a, 1978; Szmigielski et al., 1981), even when the mice are immunosuppressed before infection (Kirchner et al., 1977b; Hirt et al., 1978). Increased levels of interferon have been found in the serum of mice within 5 to 12 days after the intravenous or intraperitoneal injection of propionibacteria (Fig. 1). Propionibacteria-stimulated lymphocytes are able to induce increased interferon production in cultures of human lymphocytes (Hirt et al., 1978b) and murine lymphocytes (Hirt et al., 1978a). The effect exerted by propionibacteria is much more pronounced than that observed after application of some nonspecific mitogens (Table 2). Kirchner et al., 1977a, 1977b, 1969) suggest that in cultures of spleen cells stimulated with propionibacteria, a biphasic reaction occurs. The primary phase, expressed by interferon induction in B lymphocytes, is

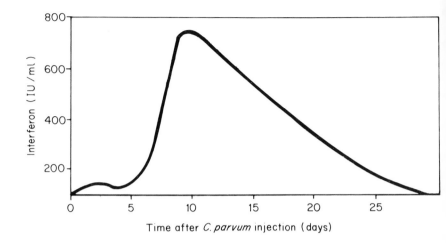

Fig. 1 Interferon production by human lymphocytes after stimulation by *Corynebacterium parvum* (according to Kirchner *et al.*, 1978).

followed by a secondary phase of macrophage activation by interferon (Table 2).

According to Cerutti (1975), propionibacteria-stimulated macrophages may release antiviral substances distinct from interferon as suggested in his experiments on the protective effect of propionibacteria against infection with Newcastle diseases, encephalomyocarditis, and vesicular stomatitis viruses.

Table 2   Proliferation and interferon production by human lymphocytes cultured *in vitro*[a]

Stimulator	DNA synthesis ³H-TdR index	Interferon titre index
None	1	1
Phytohaemagglutinin	400	9
Concanavalin A	350	10
Lipopolysaccharide	3	3
Corynebacterium parvum	130	650

[a] Based on data published in papers of Kirchner *et al.* (1977a, 1977b, 1978, 1979).

B. Humoral immunity

The propionibacteria, being immunogenic, also act as adjuvants, enhancing the humoral response to several antigens. Following intravenous or intra-

peritoneal injection, propionibacteria increase the production of antibodies against thymus-dependent antigens, such as sheep erythrocytes (Biozzi
et al., 1968; Howard *et al.*, 1973a; James *et al.*, 1974) or bovine albumin (James
et al., 1974). This enhancement affects both primary and secondary antibody
responses (IgG and IgM) (Parlebas and Halpern, 1978).

The response to thymus-independent antigens, such as the capsular
polysaccharide of *Streptococcus pneumoniae* S-III (Howard *et al.*, 1973) or
dinitrophenol conjugated with a carrier (Del Guercio, 1972), is also increased.
Pincard *et al.* (1967, 1968) have demonstrated that the primary and secondary
humoral response of rabbits to bovine albumin, may be enhanced by the
injection of strains of propionibacteria that do not possess the ability to
stimulate the reticulo-endothelial system. These authors were also able to
block the induction of immunological tolerance induction to this antigen by
the injection of such strains of propionibacteria. This effect cannot be
reproduced in mice given large doses of pneumococcal polysaccharide
together with "active" strains of propionibacteria (Howard *et al.*, 1973b).

Enhancement of the humoral response is dependent both on the dose of
antigen and on the interval between the injection of propionibacteria and
antigen. Mice immunized with high doses of antigen show the greatest
enhancement of immune response, as measured by number of plaque-forming
cells, when propionibacteria are given 4–7 days before antigen. Propionibacteria given seven days before smaller doses of antigen only produced
slight immunostimulation. When given less than 4 days before antigen
propionibacteria even caused immunodepression.

A similar relationship between dose of antigen and time of injection of
propionibacteria has been demonstrated for type III pneumococcal polysaccharide (Warr and Sljivic, 1974b). It seems that the route of administration of
propionibacteria is also important. Their adjuvant properties are most
strongly expressed after intravenous or intraperitoneal injection, whereas the
subcutaneous route results in only a slight increase in the number of antibody-
producing cells demonstrable in local lymph nodes draining the site of
injection. This last route can enhance the immune response in guinea pigs but
only when the propionibacteria are given together with incomplete Freund
adjuvant (Neveu *et al.*, 1964).

The stimulation of antibody production is most probably associated with
macrophage activation. Increased lability of cell membranes, increased
phagocytic activity, and the prolonged presence of an antigen on the cell
membrane, all enhance the helper function of macrophages as both antigen
carriers and as cells co-operating with T and B lymphocytes in the induction of
the immune response (Winere and Bandieri, 1975). Wiener (1975) has
demonstrated that macrophages derived from mice injected with propionibacteria are much more active in stimulating the immune response to
sheep erythrocytes *in vitro* than macrophages isolated from untreated

animals. In addition to better processing of antigen and its increased presentation to lymphocytes, the possibility cannot be excluded that increased lymphocyte trapping by organs containing stimulated macrophages, thus increasing the chances of co-operation between these cells, may also play an essential part in this process (Frost and Lance, 1973). The possibility of mutual changes in T and B lymphocyte relationships in induction of the immune response, has also to be considered. It has been shown that athymic mice, which are therefore unable to react immunologically to thymus-dependent antigens requiring the helper function of T lymphocytes, acquire this property after application of propionibacteria. In this way, using sheep erythrocytes as the antigen, an IgG response has been obtained in T-lymphocyte-deprived mice (Halpern et al., 1973). This experiment indicates that propionibacteria may activate a mechanism which allows direct stimulation of B lymphocytes without requiring the co-operation of T lymphocytes. Direct mitogenic effects on B lymphocytes have been described (Zola, 1975), but it seems unlikely that this phenomenon can be the mechanism which substitutes for the helper function of T lymphocytes. Other, often more powerful, B cell mitogens than propionibacteria, exhibit neither adjuvant properties nor an ability to substitute for helper T lymphocytes. It is possible that direct stimulation of B lymphocytes occurs through factors released from macrophages activated either by propionibacteria, or antigen bound with the macrophage cell membrane. While activation of the immune response to the thymus-dependent antigens may be related to these mechanisms, in a similar way to several other immunological adjuvants, the explanation of the enhancement by propionibacteria of the response to thymus-independent antigens is not clear. Such enhancement (not requiring the helper function of T lymphocytes and participation of macrophages) is seen only when the propionibacteria are given before immunization. It is possible that in the period between the application of propionibacteria and immunization, proliferation of lymphocytes in lymph nodes and the spleen occurs. This may lead to an increase of the total pool of lymphocytes, including B lymphocytes, thus giving a greater number which can participate in evoking the immune response. In patient receiving propionibacteria for local anticancer treatment, an increased number of T and B lymphocytes is frequently observed in the peripheral blood 2–3 weeks after treatment (Pincard et al., 1967). This cannot, however, be considered as a definite proof of the total increase of lymphocyte pool in the host.

C. Cell-mediated immunity

Together with the enhancement of humoral response, which appears after the administration of propionibacteria, a depression of cell-mediated immunity and of delayed hypersensitivity is frequently observed. Delayed type hypersensitivity to oxazolone, picryl chloride (Alwood and Asherson, 1972; Asherson and Alwood, 1971) or sheep erythrocytes (Scott, 1974b) is clearly reduced in experimental animals given propionibacteria intravenously or intraperitoneally prior to immunization. The rejection of C3H mice skin grafts by DBA mice is significantly delayed (Castro, 1974a). Prolongation of survival time of the first graft has also been noted with other strains of mice, while the survival time of the second graft remained unchanged (Milas et al., 1975a). In graft versus host reactions during which F_1 heterozygotic mice received propionibacteria, a protective effect of these micro-organisms against the lethal activity of lymphocytes originating from one of the parent strains has been described (Biozzi et al., 1965). Immunological attack by donor lymphocytes starts by their extensive proliferation, especially in the spleen of the recipient. It has been demonstrated that after the application of propionibacteria, proliferation of lymphocytes is inhibited by macrophages (Howard et al., 1973a). Splenic lymphocytes from mice receiving pro-pionibacteria are less reactive to mitogens and in the mixed lymphocyte culture (Scott, 1972). Inhibition of proliferation of T lymphocytes in vitro seems to be associated with presence of stimulated adherent cells, as their removal from the culture results in complete recovery of response to phytohaemagglutinin and in mixed cultures (Kirchner et al., 1975; Scott, 1972).

Scott (1974b), investigating the mechanism of depression of delayed type hypersensitivity to sheep erythrocytes evoked by propionibacteria, has demonstrated that this phenomenon does not occur in splenectomized animals. Because stimulated macrophages may cause increased trapping of sensitized lymphocytes by the spleen, he has suggested that this immunosup-pression is related to changed distribution of lymphocytes in the host, with their relative deficiency in peripheral tissues and accumulation in the spleen. This view has not been confirmed by results of studies by Castro (1974a,b), who has found lowered number of T lymphocytes in lymph nodes and spleen. This author suggested that steroid hormones excreted during stress resulting from application of propionibacteria may be responsible for the pheno-menon, but this hypothesis has no experimental support. Our own observations (Roszkowski et al., 1980b) indicate that the application of propionibacteria causes significant changes in the distribution of syngeneic lymphocytes labelled with ^{51}Cr, followed by their accumulation mostly in the liver. This can be prevented by blockade of macrophages and this suggests the participation of these cells in lymphocyte trapping.

The examples of decreased cell-mediated reactivity discussed above are observed only after the intravenous or intraperitoneal injection of pro-pionibacteria. Injection of these bacteria together with the antigen by the subcutaneous route leads to enhancement of the immune response (Bomford, 1975; Scott, 1975a,b). The use of neoplastic cells as antigen in such circumstances, results in the increased induction of cytotoxic activity directed against these cells.

II. ANTINEOPLASTIC ACTIVITY

The antineoplastic activity of propionibacteria is composed of three major effects: immunoprophylaxis, i.e. the prevention of development and/or growth of transplantable and virally or chemically induced tumours, inhibition of tumour growth, and partial or total regression. These latter two properties are defined as the immunotherapeutic effect.

Woodruff and Boak (1966) obtained a definite delay in solid tumour growth and a prolongation of survival time in experimental animals after intravenous application of propionibacteria introduced before subcutaneous implantation of syngeneic tumour cells. Using various experimental models, numerous investigators have since demonstrated the ability of propionibacteria to delay or even totally inhibit tumour growth.

Sisher et al. (1970) described antineoplastic effects of propionibacteria in chemically induced fibrosarcoma. Similar observations were made by Milas et al. (1974b), Castro (1974b) and Bomford (1975).

Antineoplastic activity of the immunoprophylactic type has been observed in several variants of transplantable or spontaneously growing tumours, such as mastocytoma (Scott, 1974a), mammary carcinoma (Woodruff and Inchley, 1971), osteosarcoma (Van Putten et al., 1975), plasmocytoma (Smith and Scott, 1972) or lymphoma (Halpern et al., 1975a,b).

In most of these studies, similar doses of propionibacteria were used, but sometimes quite different antineoplastic effects were observed. These differences, according to most of the investigators, resulted not only from differing susceptibility of the neoplasms to immunotherapy, but also from the choice of route of application of propionibacteria. The strongest effect is obtained after systemic application, and intravenous and intraperitoneal routes seem to be equally successful (Bomford and Olivotto, 1974; Milas et al., 1974a). In some experimental systems, however, a pronounced immunoprophylactic effect is obtained after systemic or local application of propionibacteria. For instance, Milas et al. (1975b) have demonstrated successfully the protective effect evoked by subcutaneous injection of propionibacteria against intravenously introduced fibrosarcoma cells. Besides differences in the efficacy of the immunoprophylactic activity of propionibacteria, variations in lasting of antineoplastic effect have also been noted. According to Smith and Scott (1972), the duration of protection induced by propionibacteria depends on the immunogenecity of neoplastic cells. For weakly immunogenic neoplasms, such as line I lung cancer, this amounts to 10 days; for more immunogenic tumours like fibrosarcoma, pronounced antineoplastic effect has been seen for 25 days (Yuhas and Ullrich, 1976; Castro, 1974a,b).

The immunotherapeutic activity of propionibacteria was demonstrated for the first time by Woodruff and Boak (1966), who described a delay in the growth of syngeneic transplantable mammary carcinoma in mice. As in the case of the prophylactic effect, therapeutic activity has been shown in several types of transplantable carcinomas in animals, such as mastocytoma (Scott, 1974a,b), fibrosarcoma (Milas *et al.*, 1975b), Lewis lung carcinoma (Sadler and Castro, 1976a), melanoma (Houchens and Gaston, 1976), and spontaneous tumours (Kreider *et al.*, 1978). The observed therapeutic effects of treatment with propionibacteria are quite varied, probably as a result of the differing susceptibility of individual types of tumours to this therapy, their immunogenicity, and the route of application of the propionibacteria. The stage of disease and the duration of therapy also seem to be important. Our investigations indicate that initiation of immunotherapy during advanced growth of the tumour exerts no visible effect (Roszkowski *et al.*, 1981). This, however, does not apply to local therapy based on the intratumoural injection of propionibacteria which can inhibit growth or even cause the regression of advanced tumours (Milas *et al.*, 1975b; Woodruff and Dunbar, 1975; Likhite and Halpern, 1973; Roszkowski *et al.*, 1981). Using local immunotherapy, these authors have succeeded in inducing complete regression of neoplasms in some animals. Such animals were later found to be highly resistant to any secondary challenge with neoplastic cells of the same type. These observations suggest that propionibacteria may have different mechanisms of antineoplastic activity, depending on whether introduced systemically or locally. The combination of nonspecific immunostimulation, induced with propionibacteria, with specific immunotherapy using irradiated autologous neoplastic cells was also highly effective. Propionibacteria given subcutaneously with neoplastic cells inhibited the growth of mouse fibrosarcoma (Bomford, 1975), mastocytoma (Scott, 1975a) or carcinoma (Yuhas *et al.*, 1975).

Clinically, propionibacteria are of greatest value combined with conventional methods of cancer treatment, because they are only effective in limiting tumour mass when given early in the course of the disease, a consideration which prevents the application of immunotherapy with propionibacteria as the sole method of treatment.

Experimental studies have shown that the combination of propionibacteria and radiotherapy may be additive or even synergistic. The antineoplastic effect of a combination of these two methods is dependent on several factors such as the sequence of application, the dose of radiation and the route of injection of the propionibacteria. Most reports suggest that the best antineoplastic effect is obtained when propionibacteria are given few days before irradiation of the tumour (Milas *et al.*, 1975c; Suit *et al.*, 1976). It seems that irradiation produces local damage to cells of the reticulo-endothelial system (RES) which markedly decreases the effectiveness of any subsequent immunostimulation. The stimulation of this system before irradiation, however, may significantly help the survival of local RES cells.

Propionibacteria injected locally into tumours are more effective in inducing regression than when followed by irradiation. Given systemically, however, propionibacteria significantly sensitize the tumour for irradiation (Milas *et al.*, 1976).

Another conventional method of treatment, used in combination with immunostimulation by propionibacteria, is chemotherapy; with this, too, an additive antineoplastic effect is noticed. It is known that the simultaneous application of propionibacteria and cyclophosphamide causes regression in 70% of mice with fibrosarcoma (Currie and Bagshawe, 1970). Similar results have been obtained in murine leukaemia (Pearson *et al.*, 1975) and murine mammary carcinoma (Fisher *et al.*, 1976). Most investigators agree that the additive effect of the combined action of propionibacteria and cyclophosphamide occurs when bacteria are given a few days after the initiation of chemotherapy. However, with prolonged asynchronous combinations of these two drugs, the sequence of their application is not essential for effective treatment (Fisher *et al.*, 1976). Propionibacteria have also been combined with other chemotherapeutic drugs. Given with adriamycin propionibacteria produced a prolongation of the mean survival time in mice with leukaemia, when compared with animals given either agent alone (Houhens and Gaston, 1976). Similar results were obtained with propionibacteria and procarbazine (Amiel and Bernardet, 1970), bromcyclonitrosourea (Pearson *et al.*, 1974), mitomycin and 5-fluorouracil (Hattori and Yamagota, 1977).

1. Mechanism of antineoplastic activity

The mechanisms of antineoplastic activity of propionibacteria are as poorly understood as their influence on individual elements of the immune response. Inhibition or regression of tumour growth induced by propionibacteria may result from the stimulation of both specific and nonspecific antineoplastic defence mechanisms. It has been established that systemic application of these bacteria may depress cell-mediated immunity (see above). However, it has also been shown that normal functioning of the cell-mediated immune system is not essential for the antineoplastic effects of propionibacteria as these can be elicited in animals immunodepressed by X-irradiation (Bomford and Olivotto, 1974). Similar results have been obtained with animals deprived of T lymphocytes by thymectomy, lethal X-irradiation, and reconstitution with bone marrow cells (Woodruff et al., 1973; Scott, 1974a), and after application of the antilymphocyte serum (Hattori and Mori, 1973).

Others, however, have reported that the antineoplastic action of propionibacteria is related to cell-mediated immunity. Sadler and Castro (1976b) have demonstrated that the immunotherapeutic effect of propionibacteria in Lewis lung carcinoma may be completely abolished by antilymphocyte serum. Halpern et al. (1973) have shown increased cytotoxic activity in lymph node cells from leukaemic mice given propionibacteria intraperitoneally. Most investigators conclude that whereas the systemic application of this immuno-modulator does have a decisive influence on specific antineoplastic cellular immunity, this mechanism is important in local immunotherapy. This view is supported by the demonstration of specific immunity to secondary implantations of neoplastic cells in animals exhibiting complete regression of tumours after local immunotherapy. Woodruff and Dunbar (1975) have shown in fibrosarcoma that, although local injections of propionibacteria into animals deprived of T lymphocytes have no antineoplastic effect, systemic applications of this immunostimulator in absence of T cells are fully effective. The demonstration of increased cytotoxic activity in vitro in animals with mammary carcinoma after intratumoural therapy, provides further evidence (Fisher et al., 1974). Similar effects have also been observed in mastocytoma (Scott, 1975a).

Serious attention is now being paid to the importance of natural killer cells (NK) in antineoplastic immunity. The cytolytic activity of NK cells has been demonstrated in various types of experimental and spontaneous tumours (Lotzova and McCredie, 1978). The work of Ojo (1979) and Ojo et al. (1978) has shown that NK-cell activity can be correlated with the resistance of animals to the implantation of syngeneic tumour cells. This activity depends on the route of an application of the immunostimulator. Increased NK-cell activity occurs only after the local or intraperitoneal application of propionibacteria, whereas the intravenous injection of these micro-organisms may even diminish the spontaneous cytotoxic reaction.

The specific humoral response is important in resistance to tumours. It seems, however, that humoral immunity plays little part in the mechanisms of tumour destruction effected by propionibacteria. Splenectomy has no effect on their antitumour activity (Castro, 1974b), and this is not diminished in animals with a genetically conditioned low level antibody response (Biozzi et al., 1972). Attempts to transfer antineoplastic resistance to normal mice with serum obtained from animals immunized with killed cancer cells, have failed (Scott, 1975a). It is still a matter of debate whether the paradoxical effect of immunotherapy based on enhanced tumour growth is associated with the generation of blocking antibodies. It is generally accepted, however, that this effect depends on the activation of cells with suppressive properties.

According to many authors, the antineoplastic effect of propionibacteria is associated with non-specific stimulation of macrophages. Activation of these cells by propionibacteria is shown by an increase of macrophage numbers and intensification of their proliferation. Gold salts, which inhibit macrophage lysosomal enzymes, also block the antineoplastic activity of immunostimulators for fibrosarcoma (Scott, 1975b). Peters et al. (1977) have provided convincing evidence for the importance of macrophages, activated by propionibacteria, in inhibiting tumour growth. Fibrosarcoma cells injected subcutaneously with macrophages taken from animals treated with propionibacteria, failed to proliferate.

In vitro studies have shown that propionibacteria-activated macrophages exert both cytostatic and cytolytic effects on neoplastic cells. Peritoneal macrophages, isolated from propionibacteria-treated mice, inhibit the incorporation of [^{3}H]-thymidine by isogenic YC8 tumour cells. Prior X-ray irradiation did not decrease the cytostatic action of macrophages in this system (Halpern et al., 1975a,b). Similar activity has also been shown against fibrosarcoma (Scott, 1974a).

As discussed earlier, propionibacteria not only inhibit tumour growth but can also cause partial and sometimes complete regression. What, then, are the mechanisms by which propionibacteria effect the destruction of malignant cells? Peritoneal macrophages obtained from animals treated with propionibacteria, are cytostatic for murine YC8 tumour cells (Puvion et al., 1975). Basic et al. (1975, 1975) have demonstrated in vitro destruction of fibrosarcoma cells, transformed ovary carcinoma hamster cells and human melanoma cells, by macrophages activated by this immunostimulator. Morphological proof for the destruction of tumour cells by activated macrophages has been obtained by electron microscopy. Direct contact of both these cells was well documented, and the presence of "holes" on the surface of the tumour cell seems to be a consequence of this contact and may result from the cytolytic action of macrophages (Puvion et al., 1975). Stimulated macrophages appear to inhibit or destroy tumour cells without having any effect on normal cells in the culture (Basic et al., 1975). The reasons for this selective destruction of cancer cells are unclear. Perhaps this phenomenon is associated with changes in the surface of the tumour cell surface. Electron microscopy evidence supports such a hypothesis. Tumour cells have a smooth surface folded or covered with digitate axons. The destructive action of stimulated macrophages was most frequently directed against cells with a smooth surface. Tumour cells were destroyed only by macrophages derived from propionibacteria-treated animals. Observations in vivo have demonstrated that cytostatic or cytolytic effects also occur during immunotherapy of transplantable solid tumours (Ando et al., 1978; Janik et al., 1980). This was established by a precise analysis of the life cycle of the malignant cell by calculations of tumour growth parameters during therapy with propionibacteria which showed that during treatment with propionibacteria the proportion of proliferating cells fell. The presence of increased numbers of macrophages in tumour during immunotherapy, also supports these ideas about the role of macrophages in destruction of cancer cells (Roszkowski et al., 1981).

2. Clinical application of propionibacteria in the therapy of cancer in man

The establishment of the immunostimulatory and antineoplastic properties of propionibacteria in animals led to the use of these bacteria in the treatment of human cancer. Trials were started in 1967 (Israel and Halpern, 1972). Propionibacteria are increasingly often used in oncological practice although, despite 13 years of careful observation period, it has still not been possible to prove that they exert any direct anticancer effect in man. It is difficult to arrive at any definite conclusion about their therapeutic efficacy because of differences in the strains and methods of administration encountered in different clinical trials. Immunostimulatory treatment has usually been initiated only at very advanced stages of cancer and in combination with other, conventional methods of therapy. This makes proper evaluation even more difficult.

Israel and Halpern (1972) injected propionibacteria subcutaneously in patients being treated with chemotherapy because of disseminated cancer with various primary localizations of the disease. They noted that patients treated with this combination survived twice as long as those who only received cytostatic drugs. Significant prolongation of life in patients given chemo- and immunotherapy has been observed in breast cancer (Mayr et al., 1978), various histological types of lung cancer (Bjornsson et al., 1978; Israel, 1973), sarcoma, melanoma, ovary carcinoma, stomach and colon carcinoma, seminoma and teratoma (Israel, 1975; Bottino et al., 1978). Similar effects were obtained in patients with malignant head and neck cancer previously subjected to radiotherapy (Mahe et al., 1975).

There are, however, reports which do not confirm the effectiveness of treatment with propionibacteria. Issel et al. (1978) did not find any difference either in survival time or decrease of the tumour mass after therapy with combination of cytostatics and propionibacteria in patients with lung cancer. Immunostimulation by propionibacteria often follows intravenous injection. However, the antineoplastic effect obtained by this route of treatment is also disputed. Kokoschka et al. (1978) compared the efficacy of combined chemo- and immunotherapy with that of chemotherapy alone in patients with melanoma, using a 1 mg dose of propionibacteria. Patients subjected to immunotherapy survived much longer, and partial remissions were more frequent. In lung carcinoma, treatment with cytostatic drugs and intravenous infusions of propionibacteria resulted in a decrease of tumour mass by half (Sarna et al., 1978). These observations have been confirmed by Bjornsson et al. (1978), who noted significant prolongation of survival time in patients with lung cancer receiving cytostatics and intravenous propionibacteria, when compared with those treated with cytostatics only. Other authors, however, have found that the intravenous application of propionibacteria does not significantly influence the course of neoplastic disease. Such reports have been published on breast cancer (McIntosh et al., 1978; Mitcheson and Castro, 1978), osteosarcoma and fibrosarcoma (Bottino et al., 1978) or acute myelobastic leukaemia (Gordon, 1978).

Although views concerning the efficacy of propionibacteria given subcutaneously or intravenously are partly contradictory, this is not generally felt to be so with local application of this immunostimulator. Intratumoural introduction of propionibacteria in a dose of 4–8 mg for five consecutive days caused complete regression of malignant melanoma in all 11 patients treated by this method; one total regression out of 2 cases of skin metastases in oat cell carcinoma; and partial regression of cancer of the stomach infiltrating the peritoneal cavity (Israel, 1975). Further studies by other authors have demonstrated the effectiveness of this method of treatment of other types of cancer, such as breast cancer, oral plano-epithelial carcinoma, and soft-tissue sarcoma (Cheng et al., 1978).

The side-effects of such treatment were very slight and limited to the site of injection. They consisted of local pain lasting from 30 min to 12 hours, accompanied by occasional but transient infiltration and/or thickening of the subcutaneous tissue; this disappeared spontaneously. The suspension of propionibacteria in lignocaine or hyaluronidase completely eliminated these symptoms. In few cases, small sterile abscesses appeared at the site of injection. Generalized symptoms were never reported after intratumoural application of propionibacteria.

The risk of development of generalized side-effects must be considered, when propionibacteria are applied parenterally. Symptoms seen after intravenous injection include chills and increases in body temperature lasting 3–24 hours (Gill and Morris, 1977; Palmer et al., 1978). In some cases, other symptoms such as gastric irritation, vomiting, hypertension and head and bone pain, have also been reported, but it is difficult to ascribe them solely to injection of propionibacteria (Palmer et al., 1978).

Israel (1976) has observed over 100 patients treated with intravenous infusions of propionibacteria over a number of years and has never noted any serious immediate or delayed complications. However, reports have been published describing serious side-effects linked to such immunotherapy. Perhaps the most dramatic were described by Dosik et al. (1978): in 3 out of 87 patients treated intravenously with propionibacteria, symptoms of oliguria, haematuria, azotaemia, and bilateral disseminated infiltrations in lungs were noted. Histopathological investigation of kidney biopsies showed proliferative glomerulonephritis, with deposits of immune complexes in the glomerular basal membrane epithelium. Renal insufficiency in these patients disappeared spontaneously after discontinuation of immunotherapy.

A marked antineoplastic effect was seen after the application of propionibacteria directly into lungs or peritoneal cavity in cases of pleural effusion or ascites in patients with advanced ovarian carcinoma (Cheng et al., 1978), adenocarcinoma and melanoma (Webb et al., 1978). In these patients, a prolongation of survival time and inhibition or marked slowing down of ascites formation was found.

Summarizing the results of clinical investigations, it must be stated that the antineoplastic action of propionibacteria in the therapy of human tumours has not been as impressive as in experimental animal studies. It is frequently postulated that human tumours are biologically totally different and that no suitable experimental models exist which are close enough to human disease. Without rejecting this view totally, it seems likely that one of the causes of the reported discrepancies in the assessment of therapeutic efficacy may be the very low doses of propionibacteria used in human treatment as compared with animal experimental models. The highest doses used in the therapy of human tumours amount to 0.1–0.2 mg kg^{-1} body weight, whereas in experimental conditions the anticancer therapeutic effect is obtained with doses of 20–50 mg kg^{-1} body weight.

The dose of propionibacteria used for treatment is of course closely associated with the problem of toxicity. The subcutaneous injection of these micro-organisms is well tolerated, and no serious side-effects have ever been reported. Introduction of propionibacteria into body cavities may be associated with symptoms similar to those observed after intravenous injection (Cheng et al., 1978). Such symptoms have not as yet been described, but experience with the application of propionibacteria into body cavities is limited.

III. SUMMARY

A schematic presentation of the possible mechanisms of immunomodulation by propionibacteria is presented in Fig. 2. It must remain largely hypothetical, as there in insufficient information available on many details of this complex and fascinating phenomenon. Clinical investigations on the treatment of various types of cancer with cell suspensions of propionibacteria suggest that this form of treatment offers an adjunct to other forms of anticancer therapy. The isolation from propionibacteria of an identifiable active component which is capable of exerting anticancer effect, may help in understanding the mode of action of these micro-organisms.

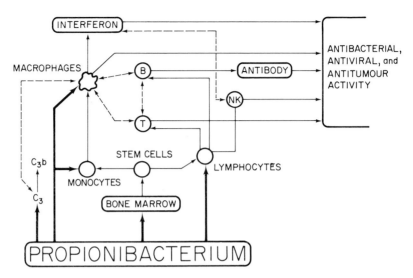

Fig. 2 Possible mechanisms of antimicrobial and antitumour activities of propionibacteria.

REFERENCES

Adlam, C., Broughton, E. S. and Scott, M. (1972). *Nature* **235**, 219–220.

Adlam, C. and Scott, M. T. (1973). *J. Med. Microbiol.* **6**, 261–274.

Allwood, G. G. and Asherson, G. L. (1972). *Clin. Exp. Immunol.* **11**, 579–584.

Amiel, J. L. and Berardet, M. (1970). *Eur. J. Cancer* **6**, 557–559.

Ando, K., Urano, M. and Koike, S. (1978). *Cancer Res.* **38**, 1769–1773.

Asherson, G. L. and Allwood, G. G. (1971). *Clin. Exp. Immunol.* **9**, 249–258.

Basic, I., Milas, L., Grdina, D. J. and Withers, H. R. (1974). *J. Natl Cancer Inst.* **52**, 1839–1842.

Basic, I., Milas, L., Grdina, D. J. and Withers, H. R. (1975). *J. Natl Cancer Inst.* **55**, 589–596.

Baum, M. and Breese, M. (1976). *Brit. J. Cancer* **33**, 468–473.

Biozzi, G., Howard, J. G., Mouton, D. and Stiffel, C. (1965). *Transplantation* **3**, 170–177.

Biozzi, G., Stiffel, C., Mouton, D., Bouthillier, Y. and Decreusefond, C. (1968). *Immunology* **14**, 7–20.

Biozzi, G., Stiffel, C., Mouton, D., Bouthillier, Y. and Decreusefond, C. (1972). *Ann. Inst. Pasteur* **122**, 685–694.

Bjornsson, S., Takita, H., Kuberka, N., Preisler, H., Catane, H., Highby, D. and Henderson, E. (1978). *Cancer Treat. Rep.* **62**, 505–510.

Bomford, R. (1975). *Brit. J. Cancer* **32**, 551–557.

Bomford, R. and Christie, G. H. (1975). *Cell. Immunol.* **17**, 150–155.

Bomford, R. and Olivotto, M. (1974). *Int. J. Cancer* **14**, 226–235.

Bottino, J. C., Rossen, R. D., Hersh, F. M., Rios, A., Hester, J. P. and McBride, C. M. (1978). *J. Artif. Organs* **1**, 53–60.
Brosovic, B., Sljivic, V. S. and Warr, G. W. (1975). *Brit. J. Exp. Path.* **56**, 183–192.
Castro, J. E. (1974a). *Eur. J. Cancer* **10**, 115–120.
Castro, J. E. (1974b). *Eur. J. Cancer* **10**, 121–127.
Castro, J. E. and Sadler, T. E. (1975). In "*Corynebacterium parvum*: Application in Experimental and Clinical Oncology" (B. Halpern, ed.) pp. 252–267. Plenum Press, New York.
Cerutti, I. (1975). In "*Corynabacterium parvum*: Application in Experimental and Clinical Oncology" (B. Halpern, ed.) pp. 84–90. Plenum Press, New York.
Cahre, M. J. B. and Baum, M. (1978). *Develop. Biol. Standard.* **38**, 195–200.
Cheng, V. S., Suit, H. O., Wang, C. C., Raker, J., Weymuller, E. and Kaufman, S. (1978). *Cancer* **42**, 1912–1915.
Collins, F. M. and Scott, M. T. (1974). *Infect. Immun.* **9**, 863–869.
Currie, G. A. and Bagshawe, K. D. (1970). *Brit. Med. J.* **1**, 541–544.
Del Guercio, P. (1972). *Nature* **238**, 213–215.
Dosik, G. M., Gutterman, J. U., Hersh, F. M., Akhtar, M., Sonoda, M. and Horn, R. G. (1978). *Ann. Intern. Med.* **89**, 41–46.
Eliopoulos, G., Andres, S. and Halpern, B. (1978). *Develop. Biol. Standard.* **38**, 183–188.
Fauve, R. M. and Hevin, H. B. (1971). *Ann. Inst. Pasteur* **120**, 399–411.
Fauve, R. M. and Hevin, H. B. (1974). *Proc. Natl Acad. Sci. USA* **71**, 573–577.
Fauve, R. M. (1975). In "*Corynebacterium parvin*: Application in Experimental and Clinical Oncology" (B. Halpern, ed.), pp. 77–83. Plenum Press, New York.
Fisher, J. C., Grace, W. R. and Mannick, J. A. (1970). *Cancer* **26**, 1379–1382.
Fisher, B., Wolmark, N. and Coyle, J. (1974). *J. Natl Cancer Inst.* **53**, 1793–1801.
Fisher, B., Wolmark, N., Rubin, H. and Saffer, E. (1976). *J. Natl Cancer Inst.* **55**, 1147–1153.
Frost, P. and Lance, E. M. (1973). In "Immunopotentiation", Vol. 18, pp. 29–45. Ciba Foundation Symposia, London.
Gill, P. G., Morris, P. J. and Kettlewell, M. (1977). *Clin. Exp. Immunol.* **30**, 229–232.
Gordon, D. S. (1978). *Develop. Biol. Standard.* **38**, 567–572.
Halpern, B., Crepin, Y. and Rabourdin, A. (1975a). In "*Corynebacterium parvum*: Application in Experimental and Clinical Oncology" (B. Halpern, ed.), pp. 191–199. Plenum Press, New York.
Halpern, B., Fray, A., Crepin, Y., Platica, O., Lorinet, A. M., Rabourdin, A., Sparros, L. and Isac, R. (1973). In "Immunopotentiation", Vol. 18, pp. 217–236. Ciba Foundation Symposia, London.
Halpern, B., Lorinet, A. M., Sparros, L. and Fray, A. (1975b). In "*Corynebacterium parvum*: Application in Clinical and Experimental Oncology" (B. Halpern, ed.) pp. 181–186. Plenum Press, New York.
Halpern, B., Prevot, A. R., Biozzi, G., Stiffel, C., Mouton, D., Morard, J. C., Bouthillier, Y. and Decreusefond, C. (1964). *J. Reticuloendothel. Soc.* **1**, 77–96.
Hattori, T. and Yamagota, S. (1977). *Gann* **68**, 115–120.
Hattori, T. and Mori, A. (1973). *Gann* **64**, 15–27.
Hirt, H. H., Becker, H. and Kirchner, H. (1978a). *Cell. Immunol.* **38**, 168–175.
Hirt, H. H., Schwenteck, M., Becker, H. and Kirchner, H. (1978b). *Clin. Exp. Immunol.* **32**, 471–476.
Houchens, D. P. and Gaston, M. R. (1976). *Proc. Amer. Ass. Cancer Res.* **17**, 53.
Howard, J. G., Christie, G. H. and Scott, M. T. (1973a). *Cell. Immunol.* **7**, 290–301.

Howard, J. G., Scott, M. T. and Christie, G. H. (1973b). *In* "Immunopotentiation", pp. 101–120. Ciba Foundation Symposia, London.

Israel, L. (1973). *Cancer Chemother. Rep.* **4**, 283–285.

Israel, L. (1975). *In "Corynebacterium parvum*: Application in Clinical and Experimental Oncology" (B. Halpern, ed.) pp. 389–410. Plenum Press, New York.

Israel, L. (1976). *In* "International Conference on Immunotherapy of Cancer" (C. M. Southam, ed.) pp. 241–251. The New York Academy of Sciences, New York.

Israel, L. and Halpern, B. (1972). *Nouv. Presse Méd.* **1**, 19–23.

Issel, B. F., Valdiveso, M., Hersh, F. M., Richman, S., Gutterman, J. U. and Bodey, G. P. (1978). *Cancer Treat. Rep.* **62**, 1059–1063.

James, K., Ghaffar, A. and Milne, L. (1974). *Brit. J. Cancer* **29**, 11–20.

Janik, P., Roszkowski, W., Ko, H. L., Szmigielski, S., Pulverer, G. and Jeljaszewicz, J. (1980). *Cancer Res. Clin. Oncol.* **98**, 51–58.

Johnson, J. M. and Cummins, C. S. (1972). *J. Bacteriol.* **109**, 1047–1066.

Kirchner, H., Hirt, H. H., Becker, H. and Munk, K. (1977a). *Cell. Immunol.* **31**, 172–176.

Kirchner, H., Hirt, H. H. and Munk, K. (1977b). *Infect. Immun.* **16**, 9–11.

Kirchner, H., Holdern, H. T. and Herberman, R. B. (1975). *J. Immunol.* **115**, 1212–1216.

Kirchner, H., Hirt, H. H. and Munk, K. (1979). *In* "Natural and Induced Cell Mediated Cytotoxicity" (H. Kirchner, ed.) pp. 227–232. Academic Press, New York and London.

Kirchner, H., Scott, M. T., Hirt, H. H. and Munk, K. (1978). *J. Gen. Virol.* **41**, 97–106.

Kokoschka, E. M., Luger, T. and Micksche, M. (1978). *Onkologie* **1**, 98–103.

Kreider, J., Bartlett, T. G. L., Purnell, D. M. and Webb, S. (1978). *Cancer Res.* **38**, 4522–4526.

Likhite, V. V. and Halpern, B. (1973). *Int. J. Cancer* **12**, 699–704.

Lotzova, E. and McCredie, K. B. (1978). *Cancer Immunol. Immunother.* **4**, 215–221.

Mahe, E., Bourdin, J. S., Gest, J., Saracino, R., Burnet, M., Halpern, B., Debaud, B. and Roth, F. (1975). *In "Corynebacterium parvum*: Application in Experimental and Clinical Oncology" (B. Halpern, ed.) pp. 376–382. Plenum Press, New York.

Mayr, A. C., Westerhausen, M. and Senn, H. J. (1978). *Develop. Biol. Standard.* **38**, 523–527.

McBride, W. H., Jones, J. T. and Weir, D. M. (1974). *Brit. J. Exp. Path.* **55**, 38–46.

McIntosh, I. H., Thynne, G. S., Bejrajati, P., Walsh, G. and Greening, W. P. (1978). *Develop. Biol. Standard.* **38**, 477–482.

Milas, L., Basic, I., Kogelnik, H. D. and Withers, H. R. (1975a). *Cancer Res.* **35**, 2365–2374.

Milas, L., Gutterman, J. U., Basic, I., Hunter, N., Mavligit, G. M., Hersh, E. M. and Withers, H. R. (1974a). *Int. J. Cancer* **14**, 493–503.

Milas, L., Hunter, N., Basic, I., Mason, K., Grdina, D. J. and Withers, H. R. (1975b). *J. Natl Cancer Inst.* **54**, 895–902.

Milas, L., Hunter, N. and Withers, H. R. (1974b). *Cancer Res.* **34**, 613–620.

Milas, L., Mason, K. and Withers, H. R. (1976). *Cancer Immunol. Immunother.* **1**, 233–237.

Milas, L., Withers, H. R. and Hunter, N. (1975c). *Proc. Amer. Assoc. Cancer Res.* **16**, 154–160.

Mitcheson, H. D. and Castro, J. E. (1978). *Develop. Biol. Standard.* **38**, 509–514.

Neveu, T., Branellec, A. and Biozzi, G. (1964). *Ann. Inst. Pasteur* **106**, 771–777.

Ojo, M. (1979). *Cell. Immunol.* **45**, 182–187.

Ojo, M., Haller, O., Kimura, A. and Wigzel, H. (1978). *Int. J. Cancer* **21**, 444–452.
Olivotto, M. and Bomford, R. (1974). *Int. J. Cancer* **13**, 478–488.
O'Neil, G. J., Henderson, D. C. and White, R. G. (1973). *Immunology* **24**, 977–995.
Palmer, B. V., Walsh, G., Smedley, P., McIntosh, I. H. and Greening, W. P. (1978). *Develop. Biol. Standard.* **38**, 529–533.
Parlebas, J. and Halpern, B. (1978). *Develop. Biol. Standard.* **38**, 201–204.
Pearson, J. W., Chirigos, M. A., Charapas, S. D. and Sher, N. A. (1974). *J. Natl Cancer Inst.* **52**, 463–468.
Pearson, J. W., Perk, K., Chirigos, M. A., Pryam, J. W. and Fuhrman, F. S. (1975). *Int. J. Cancer* **16**, 142–152.
Peters, L. J., McBride, W. H., Mason, K. A., Hunter, N., Basic, I. and Milas, L. (1977). *J. Natl Cancer Inst.* **59**, 881–887.
Pinkcard, R. N., Weir, D. M. and McBride, W. H. (1967). *Clin. Exp. Immunol.* **2**, 343–350.
Pinkcard, R. N., Weir, D. M. and McBride, W. H. (1968). *Clin. Exp. Immunol.* **3**, 413–421.
Puvion, F., Fray, A. and Halpern, B. (1975). In *"Corynebacterium parvum*: Application in Experimental and Clinical Oncology" (B. Halpern, ed.) pp. 137–144. Plenum Press, New York.
Puvion, F., Fray, A. and Halpern, B. (1976). *J. Ultrastruct. Res.* **54**, 95–108.
Raynaud, M., Kouznetzova, B., Bizzini, B. and Cherman, J. C. (1972). *Ann. Inst. Pasteur* **122**, 685–695.
Roszkowski, K., Roszkowski, W., Ko, H. L., Pulverer, G. and Jeljaszewicz, J. (1981). *Oncology* (in press).
Roszkowski, W., Lipski, S., Ko, H. L., Szmigielski, S., Jeljaszewicz, J. and Pulverer, G. (1980a). *Strahlentherapie* **156**, 729–733.
Roszkowski, K., Roszkowski, W., Ko, H. L., Szmigielski, S., Pulverer, G. and Jeljaszewicz, J. (1980b). *Cancer Immunol. Immunother.* **10**, 33–37.
Ruitenberg, E. J. and Van Noorle Jansen, L. M. (1975). *Zbl. Bakt, Parasit. Infektionskr. Hyg. Abt. I; Reihe A* **231**, 197–201.
Sadler, T. E. and Castro, J. E. (1976a). *Brit. J. Cancer* **34**, 291–295.
Sadler, T. E. and Castro, J. E. (1976b). *Brit. J. Surg.* **63**, 292–296.
Sarna, G. P., Lowitz, B. B., Haskell, C. M. and Dorey, F. J. (1978). *Cancer Treat. Rep.* **62**, 681–687.
Scott, M. T. (1972). *Cell. Immunol.* **5**, 459–468.
Scott, M. T. (1974a). *J. Natl Cancer Inst.* **53**, 855–860.
Scott, M. T. (1974b). *Cell. Immunol.* **13**, 251–263.
Scott, M. T. (1975a). *J. Natl Cancer Inst.* **55**, 65–72.
Scott, M. T. (1975b). *J. Natl Cancer Inst.* **54**, 789–792.
Smith, S. E. and Scott, M. T. (1972). *Brit. J. Cancer* **26**, 361–367.
Suit, H. D., Sadlacek, R., Wagner, M., Orsi, L., Silbrcic, V. and Rothman, J. (1976). *Cancer Res.* **35**, 1305–1314.
Szmigielski, S., Kobus, M., Gil, J., Jeljaszewicz, J. and Pulverer, G. (1980). *Zbl. Bakt. Parasit. Infektionskr. Hyg. Abt. I; Reihe A* **248**, 286–295.
Tuttle, R. L. and North, R. J. (1975). *J. Natl Cancer Inst.* **55**, 1403–1411.
Warr, G. W. and Sljivic, V. S. (1974a). *Tissue Cell Kinet.* **7**, 559–565.
Warr, G. W. and Sljivic, V. S. (1974b). *J. Reticuloendoth. Soc.* **16**, 193–197.
Webb, H. F., Oaten, S. W. and Pike, C. P. (1978). *Brit. Med. J.* **1**, 338–340.
Wiener, E. (1975). *Cell. Immunol.* **19**, 1–7.
Wiener, E. and Bandieri, A. (1975). *Immunology* **29**, 265–274.

Wilkinson, P. C., O'Neil, G. J., and Wapshaw, K. G. (1973a). *Immunology* **24**, 997–1006.
Wilkinson, P. C., O'Neil, G. J., McInroy, R. J., Cater, J. C. and Roberts, J. A. (1973b). *In* "Immunopotentiation", pp. 121–140. Ciba Foundation Symposia, London.
Wolmark, N. and Fisher, B. (1974). *Cancer Res.* **34**, 2869–2872.
Woodruff, M. F. A. and Boak, J. L. (1966). *Brit. J. Cancer* **30**, 345–355.
Woodruff, M. F. A. and Dunbar, N. (1975). *Brit. J. Cancer* **32**, 34–41.
Woodruff, M. F. A., Dunbar, N. and Ghaffar, A. (1973). *Proc. Roy. Soc. London, Ser. B* **184**, 97–102.
Woodruff, M. F. A. and Inchley, M. P. (1971). *Brit. J. Cancer* **25**, 584–593.
Van Putten, L. M., Kram, L. K. J., Van Dierendonck, H. H. C., Smink, T. and Fuzy, M. (1975). *Int. J. Cancer* **15**, 588–595.
Yuhas, J. M., Toya, R. E. and Wagner, E. (1975). *Cancer Res.* **35**, 242–244.
Yuhas, J. M. and Ulrich, R. L. (1976). *Cancer Res.* **36**, 161–166.
Zola, J. (1975). *Clin. Exp. Immunol.* **22**, 514–521.

Index